Diagnostic Procedure Handbook

with

Key Word Index

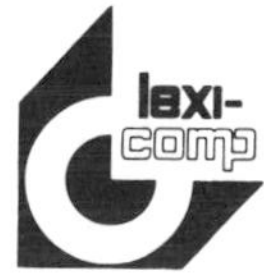

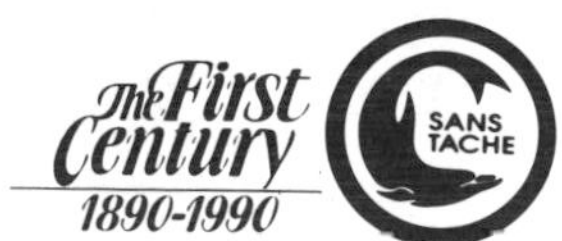

Diagnostic Procedure Handbook

with

Key Word Index

Joseph A. Golish, MD, FACP, FCCP
Editor
Department of Pulmonary Disease
Cleveland Clinic Foundation
Cleveland, Ohio

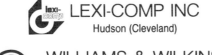

LEXI-COMP INC
Hudson (Cleveland)

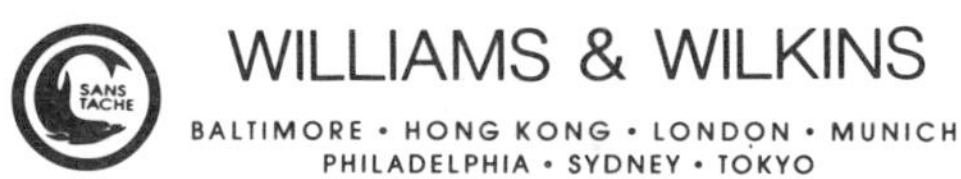

WILLIAMS & WILKINS
BALTIMORE • HONG KONG • LONDON • MUNICH
PHILADELPHIA • SYDNEY • TOKYO

1992

This manual was produced using the Pathfinder™ Program — a complete publishing service of Lexi-Comp Inc.

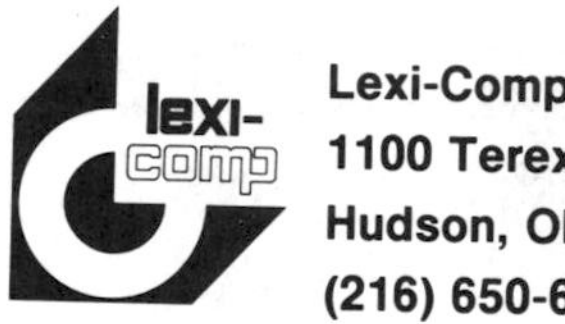

Lexi-Comp Inc
1100 Terex Road
Hudson, Ohio 44236
(216) 650-6506

ISBN 0-683-03619-X

TABLE OF CONTENTS

AUTHORS

Robert K. Desai, MD
Staff Radiologist
St. John and West Shore Hospital
Cleveland, Ohio
Ultrasound

Michael A. Geisinger, MD
Residency Training Program Director
Hospital Radiology
Diagnostic Radiology Department
Cleveland Clinic Foundation
Cleveland, Ohio
Invasive Radiology

Carlos M. Isada MD
Fellow
Department of Infectious Disease
Cleveland Clinic Foundation
Cleveland, Ohio
Allergy, Immunology/Rheumatology and Infectious Disease
Critical Care
Gastroenterology
Nephrology, Urology, and Hematology
Neurology
Pulmonary Medicine

Lawrence E. Lohman, MD, FACS
Northeast Ohio Eye Surgeons
Kent, Ohio
Ophthalmology

Kevin McCarthy, RCPT
Assistant Technical Director
Pulmonary Function Lab
Cleveland Clinic Foundation
Cleveland, Ohio
Pulmonary Function

James K. O'Donnell, MD
Director
Department of Nuclear Medicine
Marymount Hospital
Cleveland, Ohio
Nuclear Medicine

Peter B. O'Donovan, MD, BCh, BAO
Head, Section of Chest Imaging
Diagnostic Radiology Department
Cleveland Clinic Foundation
Cleveland, Ohio
Computed Tomography
Diagnostic Radiology

Jeffrey S. Ross, MD
Administrative Director
Magnetic Resonance Imaging Department
Cleveland Clinic Foundation
Cleveland, Ohio
Magnetic Resonance Imaging

Ernesto E. Salcedo, MD
Head, Section of Cardiac Function Laboratory
Department of Cardiology
Cleveland Clinic Foundation
Cleveland, Ohio
Cardiology

FOREWORD

Supporting the difficult to achieve national goal of providing the best and most cost-effective medical care dictates that today's medical practitioners take into account a significant array of factors when selecting the appropriate diagnostic procedure for their patients. The dynamics of medical technology, everchanging and expanding regulatory or reimbursement requirements, and the increasing medical awareness on the part of patients are just a few of the important considerations that are likely to affect a practitioner's ultimate approach to use of a diagnostic procedure.

This *Diagnostic Procedure Handbook with Key Word Index (DPH),* which details 294 common and less common procedures, is offered as a handy comprehensive yet concise quick reference for practitioners and other healthcare professionals at all levels of experience or training. The authors, as practicing physicians, have attempted to provide up-to-date information with emphasis on consensus interpretations and practical considerations concerning the diagnostic procedures described in their specialty section.

All procedures covered in this reference are logically structured, with specifications of the procedure presented in a functional and consistent format that allows rapid review of an area of specific interest. Salient points of information pertinent to each major aspect of the procedure are provided: procedure name, abstract, patient care/scheduling, method, specimen (when appropriate), interpretation, footnotes, and references. To be useful, the information contained within a book must be quickly accessible to the user. Therefore, heavy emphasis also has been placed on providing comprehensive indexing and extensive cross-referencing within procedure sections as well as in the Key Word Index, CPT-4 Coding Index, and the Alphabetical Index. The arrangement of sections by major diagnostic specialties facilitates access to related procedures or ready review of a specific diagnostic discipline.

The concept for this handbook evolved from the widely used *Laboratory Test Handbook*, *Quick Look Drug Book*, and the *Pediatric Dosage Handbook* publications produced by Lexi-Comp Inc. All of these handbooks are targeted for use by clinicians, practicing physicians, residents, nurses, medical students, technologists, quality assurance, medical record and medical review personnel, and other allied health professionals. The availability of state-of-the-art computer driven typesetting, data base management, and indexing systems (which are Lexi-Comp's specialty) contribute substantially to the ease with which this handbook can be used by the reader.

We hope that this handbook will prove to be not only a valued quick reference but that it will also serve as a useful base to help broaden the user's general knowledge of the many diagnostic tools available today.

ACKNOWLEDGMENTS

This handbook exists in its present form as a result of the concerted efforts of many individuals. The publisher and president of Lexi-Comp Inc, Robert D. Kerscher deserves much of the credit for bringing the concept of such a book to fruition.

Strong support for this project and for the concept of delivering a series of concise reference publications to the healthcare marketplace has been received from Joan D. Caldwell, vice-president and publisher, Reference Division, Williams & Wilkins Medical Publishing and Cordelia W. Slaughter, production manager, Williams & Wilkins.

Other members of the Lexi-Comp staff whose contributions were invaluable and whose patience with the editors' enumerable drafts, revisions, deletions, additions, and enhancements was inexhaustible include: Leonard L. Lance, RPh, pharmacy editor, Diane Harbart, MT (ASCP), medical editor, Lynn Coppinger and Barbara F. Kerscher, production managers, Alexandra Hart, Jil Neuman, Jeanne Eads, and Deborah Burns, production assistants, Jeff J. Zaccagnini and Brian B. Vossler, sales managers, Edmund A. Harbart, vice-president, custom publishing division, and Jack L. Stones, vice-president, reference publishing division. The complex computer programming required for the typesetting of the book was provided by Dennis P. Smithers, Jay L. Katzen, and David C. Marcus, system analysts, under the direction of Thury L. O'Connor, vice-president, and David K. Ream, vice-president, development.

In addition, sincere appreciation to Vaughn W. Floutz, PhD and Priscilla Jane Frank, MT (ASCP) who served as editorial consultants and contributors.

In addition, the authors wish to thank their families, friends, and colleagues who supported them in their efforts to complete this handbook.

HOW TO USE THIS HANDBOOK

The *Diagnostic Procedure Handbook with Key Word Index (DPH)* is divided into two primary sections: (1) Clinical Procedures and (2) Imaging Procedures. Major diagnostic disciplines in each section and the related procedures within the specified discipline are listed alphabetically. Listed under **Clinical Procedures** are: Allergy/Rheumatology and Infectious Disease, Cardiology, Critical Care, Gastroenterology, Nephrology/Urology and Hematology, Neurology, Ophthalmology, Pulmonary Function, and Pulmonary Medicine. Listed under **Imaging Procedures** are: Radiology, Computed Tomography, Invasive Radiology, Ultrasound, and Nuclear Medicine.

A general introduction and overview, covering the purpose and intended utility of the handbook, precedes the individual sections. Author credentials and an introduction to each discipline section are presented at the beginning of a section. Sections and the procedures within are arranged alphabetically and are cross-referenced with synonyms referring the user to the preferred (appropriate) procedure name.

Each procedure is presented in a consistent format. Information relevant to the given procedure is provided under seven major headings: Name, Abstract, Patient Care/Scheduling, Method, Specimen (when appropriate), Interpretation, and References.

Procedure Name

The specific procedure **name** is indicated along with Current Procedural Terminology (CPT-4) coding appropriate to than procedure. Other procedures that contain **related information** to the named procedure are listed and cross-referenced by page number. **Synonyms** are noted and procedures which are not exact synonyms but have similar instructions or require similar consideration are also referred to under the **applies to** heading. In cases where a procedure is **replaced by** another (updated) procedure, a replaces statement is provided.

Abstract

An abstract of what the **procedure commonly includes** as well as **indications** (current use) and **contraindications** of the procedure are provided for each named procedure.

Patient Care/Scheduling

The patient care/scheduling section contains **patient preparation, aftercare,** and **special instructions.** Patient preparation information includes patient care considerations prior to performance of the diagnostic procedure or collection of a specimen. Aftercare information includes patient care considerations following performance of the procedure or specimen collection. Special instructions cover the logistical (scheduling, timing, etc) aspects necessary to appropriately accomplish the procedure or obtain a specimen.

Method

The method section depicts **equipment** and **technique** involved in performing the named procedure. **Data acquired** from the procedure is also discussed.

Specimen

The specimen section of each procedure description includes, when appropriate, the specific **specimen** to be acquired, the **container, sampling time,** detailed **collection** instructions, and **causes for rejection** of the specimen by a laboratory.

Interpretation

The interpretation section contains a discussion of basic information relevant to the clinical application of the named procedure, including **normal findings, critical values,** and **limitations** of the diagnostic method. **Additional information** which may contribute to interpretation or utilization of the procedure is also included.

Footnotes and References

Bibliographic information provided with listed procedures may include **footnotes** referring to specific literature quotations, specific points of information, or opinions. Selected general **references** are presented as sources of research.

Acronyms and Abbreviation Glossary

This glossary is a useful listing of acronyms and abbreviations commonly associated with diagnostic procedures. The glossary is not offered as an exhaustive authoritative list, but more as a guide to assist in interpreting frequently used terminology.

Key Word Index

The Key Word Index provides a reference to the procedure name based on diagnostic property, disease entity, organ system, or syndrome in which the diagnostic procedure is useful or medically significant. This reference helps to focus the user's attention on specific diagnostic procedures available to support a clinical diagnosis or rule out other diagnostic possibilities.

Current Procedural Terminology (CPT-4) Index

CPT-4 codes are given for most named procedures as a basis for documenting the diagnostic procedure and to facilitate financial and patient record keeping. The codes shown are current as of the date of publication. Application of the codes may vary by region of the country and, in some instances, the application of a specific code to a given procedure is a matter of individual interpretation of terms.[1]

Alphabetical Index

The most expedient method for locating a certain procedure is the alphabetical index in the last section of the handbook. Procedure names and synonyms are listed alphabetically and the page number on which the procedure description may be found is given.

[1] Kirschner CG, Edwards NK, May DM, et al, eds, *Physicians' Current Procedural Terminology (CPT 1991),* 4th ed, Chicago, IL: American Medical Association, 1990.

CLINICAL PROCEDURES

ALLERGY, IMMUNOLOGY/RHEUMATOLOGY, AND INFECTIOUS DISEASES

Carlos M. Isada, MD

The subspecialty fields of allergy, immunology/rheumatology, and infectious diseases cover a wide spectrum of human disease. Yet, these three disciplines are related clinically; there are common derangements of the immune system, similarities in patient presentation, and some overlap in diagnostic testing. This relationship is exemplified by the adult immunodeficiency syndrome (AIDS). It is well established that AIDS is primarily an infectious disease caused by the human immunodeficiency virus (HIV). One of the main targets of the retrovirus is the CD4 cell, a key component of the host immune system. As infection progresses and the CD4 count falls, the ability of the host to modulate the immune system is impaired. Patients may exhibit immune system deficiency (recurrent and unusual infections), immune system overactivity or allergy (psoriasis), and rheumatologic manifestations (Sjögren's syndrome, vasculitis, and polymyositis).

The appropriate use of diagnostic procedures in the patient with suspected allergic disease remains controversial. Practitioners vary considerably in their threshold for ordering these tests; some authorities have wondered whether certain allergic conditions warrant testing at all (eg, food allergy). In the following section, emphasis has been placed on the more common diagnostic tests for allergic disease. Whenever possible, general recommendations are in accord with position statements from the American College of Physicians.

Diagnostic procedures within the field of immunology/rheumatology are somewhat fewer in number. Much of the clinical diagnostic testing is serologic in nature and clearly the discovery and refinement of serologic markers for connective tissue diseases have revolutionized the field. Standard procedures such as arthrocentesis and the Schirmer test are covered in some detail. Also included are newer diagnostic techniques (used routinely in some centers) such as nailfold capillaroscopy and labial salivary gland biopsy. Serologic tests such as the antinuclear antibody, Sjögren's antibody, and rheumatoid factor are discussed in the companion *Laboratory Test Handbook*.

Similarly, there is a limited number of diagnostic procedures unique to the field of infectious diseases. The majority of procedures utilized in this subspecialty are often invasive, but are simply part of general internal medicine. Procedures such as bronchoscopy, colonoscopy, CT scan biopsies, and thoracentesis are frequently used to establish the presence of infection. These procedures are covered elsewhere in this book. In recent years, the use of nuclear medicine techniques to localize infection has gained some popularity (and controversy). These include the gallium scan, bone scan, and indium-labeled WBC scan; these are also included in other sections. The tuberculin skin test, commonly ordered by general physicians and infectious disease specialists alike, is discussed in some detail due to its popularity and the known difficulties in interpretation.

The entries which follow should be used as general guidelines only. Current references are cited, but the use and interpretation of many procedures are still evolving.

Allergy Testing, Intracutaneous (Intradermal)

CPT 95014 (antibiotics, biological, stinging insects, local anesthetics, 1-5 tests); 95020 (allergenic extracts up to 10 tests)

Related Information

Allergy Testing, Percutaneous *on page 7*
Penicillin Allergy Skin Testing *on page 29*

Synonyms Immediate Hypersensitivity Skin Test; Intracutaneous (Intradermal) Allergy Testing

Abstract **PROCEDURE COMMONLY INCLUDES:** Injection of one or more allergenic substances into the skin, including certain inhalants (grasses, molds, trees, weeds), epidermals (animal dander and house dust), ingestants (foods and food additives), and insect venoms. Intradermal testing is an objective, *in vivo* means of evaluating IgE-mediated hypersensitivity. **INDICATIONS:**

- objectively demonstrate the presence of immediate-type hypersensitivity to foreign substances (allergens) suspected from the clinical history; potential test substances include common allergens to which the atopic individual is often sensitive: pollens, grasses, animal dander, as well as individual substances such as antibiotics (prototype penicillin), stinging insect venom, and certain foods
- determine if allergic disease underlies difficult to manage cases of asthma, rhinitis, dermatitis, angioedema-urticaria, or anaphylaxis
- further evaluate "indeterminate" test results obtained on prior skin prick testing (percutaneous allergy testing)
- follow up on negative skin prick tests when the clinical suspicion for a particular allergen remains high
- document immediate hypersensitivity prior to provocative allergy testing or prior to allergy desensitization therapy (immunotherapy)

CONTRAINDICATIONS:

- recent use of medications known to inhibit the wheal and flare skin response; this includes antihistamines, hydroxyzine, tricyclic antidepressants, and phenothiazines. Newer antihistamines with longer half-lives may interfere with testing for more than 1 week.
- documented anaphylactic reaction on prior skin testing; any foreign substance causing a serious systemic reaction under controlled test conditions should never be retested in the same individual. Unrelated substances are not necessarily contraindicated but should be approved by the physician.
- known hypersensitivity to a stabilizer or diluent found in some commercial allergen preparations; 0.03% human serum albumin is often used as a stabilizer in solutions used for intradermal testing. The patient should be routinely questioned prior to testing regarding egg allergy.

Patient Care/Scheduling **PATIENT PREPARATION:** Requisition should include current medications, including last dose of antihistamines or other drugs which may interfere with testing; contact physician if these medications have been recently used (see Contraindications). Procedure and risks are explained. Once in testing center, the nurse or physician should perform a brief dermatologic exam to ensure adequate areas of normal appearing skin and to identify the rare patient with dermographism. **AFTERCARE:** If no procedural complications have occurred, patient may be discharged from testing center. Skin sites should be kept clean until well healed. Patient should contact physician immediately if 6-8 hours later symptoms of wheezing, lightheadedness, or shortness of breath develop (the unusual case of a "late phase response"). **SPECIAL INSTRUCTIONS:** A physician must be immediately available if skin testing is performed by a nurse or other trained personnel. Emergency equipment should be close by in the rare case of anaphylaxis. Materials such as tourniquets, aqueous epinephrine for injection, needles and syringes should be conveniently available. **COMPLICATIONS:** Intradermal testing is generally safe, but the possibility of a systemic reaction does exist as with any mode of allergy skin testing. During intradermal testing, inadvertent overpenetration of the needle beyond the dermis may lead to injection of the allergen into the subepidermal capillary bed (and from there, into the systemic circulation). In contrast, with skin prick testing, the allergen is introduced only into the epidermis and penetration into deeper layers is unlikely. In theory, this may lead to less profound adverse reactions. The incidence of systemic reaction with intradermal testing has been estimated between 0.03% and 0.49%, with at least 14 documented fatalities.[1,2] Systemic reactions include generalized urticaria, hypotension, and anaphylaxis. Local complications are generally minor and resolve quickly; these include subcutaneous hemorrhage (clinically negligible), localized pruritus, and nonspecific irritant reactions. The risk of bacterial infection or hepatitis B is diminishingly small if proper technique is followed and needles are not reused between patients. A "late phase response" has been described and is an unusual and unpredictable occurrence. This occurs 6-18 hours after a positive wheal and flare response; test site(s) develop inflammatory edema or induration which resolves in 24 hours without specific treatment.

Method **EQUIPMENT:** Allergens used for intradermal testing are commercially prepared extracts of foreign substances, buffered in saline solution and stabilized with human serum albumin. Commonly tested substances include:

- inhalants such as trees and shrubs (ash, birch, cottonwood poplar, maple, and others), weeds (ragweed, English plantain, cocklebur, sheep sorrel, and others), grasses (Bermuda, bluegrass, fescue), molds and fungi (*Alternaria*, *Aspergillus*, *Fusarium*, *Mucor*)
- epidermals such as house dust, house mites, feathers, cat and dog dander
- ingestants such as foods, food additives, drugs (penicillin)
- injectants such as drugs or stinging insect venom (*Hymenoptera*)

Hundreds of standardized extracts are available, but not all foreign substances are suitable for intradermal testing. Some have not undergone proper biologic standardization in terms of potency, purity, and efficacy, while others cause immediate irritant skin reactions (not IgE-mediated). Also required are 0.5 mL or 1 mL tuberculin syringes, alcohol swabs, sterile gauze, and 26- to 30-gauge needles. A separate needle and syringe is needed for each allergen.

TECHNIQUE: Physician reviews and confirms selection of allergens. The volar aspect of the arm or forearm is the preferred site for testing. Each allergen is individually drawn up into the tuberculin syringe and bubbles are eliminated to avoid nonspecific "splash reactions". The allergen is then injected into the dermis using a 27-gauge needle angled at approximately 45°. The volume of solution injected should be enough to raise a small bleb 2 mm in diameter, usually 0.01-0.02 mL. Larger volumes (>0.05 mL) may result in nonimmunologic irritant skin reactions (false-positives). Needle and syringe are discarded. Serial intradermal injections may be made in this fashion but must be adequately spaced (>2 cm apart) to avoid errors in interpretation. A negative and positive skin test control is often included, consisting of saline and histamine, respectively. **DATA ACQUIRED:** Test sites are examined at 15-20 minutes for a wheal and flare reaction. Late phase reactions occurring more than 6 hours later are not recorded because their significance is not known. The largest diameter of the wheal and/or erythema is measured and recorded in millimeters.

Interpretation **NORMAL FINDINGS:** No wheal or erythema found at allergen test sites. The histamine control site should be positive and saline control site (if used) should be negative. **CRITICAL VALUES:** A wheal >5 mm with accompanying erythema is considered a positive test. This was defined in a position paper from the American College of Physicians.[3] (A number of alternative grading schemes are also commonly used in clinical practice. However, the specific criteria applied in these grading schemes vary considerably, and this lack of consistency is a potential source of confusion and error.[4] One such system is as follows:

- 0: wheal and erythema <5 mm
- 1+: wheal 5-10 mm; erythema 11-20 mm
- 2+: wheal; erythema 21-30 mm
- 3+: pseudopods; erythema 31-40 mm
- 4+: wheal >15 mm or pseudopods; erythema >40 mm)

Intradermal allergy testing plays an integral role in the evaluation of the patient with suspected allergic disease. Following the history and physical examination, it is considered by some as the initial diagnostic test of choice to objectively confirm the presence of allergic disease. Some individuals have symptomatic IgE-mediated hypersensitivity to multiple common environmental substances (pollens, grass, animal dander, etc), and are termed

(Continued)

Allergy Testing, Intracutaneous (Intradermal) *(Continued)*

"atopic". These allergic reactions in atopic individuals represent a type I Gell and Coombs' reaction. That is, an individual exposed to a relevant allergen (one to which he has been previously sensitized) manifests a characteristic series of immunologic events. Mast cells are activated, leading to release of inflammatory mediators such as histamines, leukotrienes, and eosinophil chemotactic factors. This process is mediated by IgE antibodies. Clinical manifestations of this immediate hypersensitivity are variable and include bronchospasm, urticaria, rhinitis, food allergy, and even anaphylaxis. Nonatopic individuals may also develop IgE-mediated hypersensitivity. Often, there is sensitivity to only one substance, such as stinging insect venom. Intradermal testing is useful in documenting IgE-mediated allergy in both atopic and nonatopic individuals. Intradermal testing induces a characteristic inflammatory response in the skin when the proper antigen is reintroduced into a sensitive patient. Mast cells in the skin release histamine, causing increased vascular permeability and dilation of blood vessels. This "wheal and flare" dermal response is seen with IgE-mediated allergy, regardless of whether the patient's main symptoms are located in the airways, skin, nasal mucosa, gastrointestinal tract, etc. Proper interpretation of skin test results requires consideration of the history and physical in each case. Even if technical errors are minimized (see Limitations), test results cannot be interpreted in isolation. A positive test result by itself does not necessarily denote clinical allergy. Strictly speaking, a positive skin response indicates only a state of potential hypersensitivity, a heightened immunologic reactivity towards a particular allergen. Instances of positive skin tests in asymptomatic, nonallergic individuals have been well documented. Symptoms characteristic of allergic disease (rhinorrhea, sneezing, wheezing, etc) may result from:

- true allergic disease with a positively reacting intradermal test
- allergic disease with a negatively reacting skin test (false-negative from technical error)
- allergic disease caused by a substance not tested
- nonimmunologic, non-IgE mediated disease

By itself, the intradermal test does not definitively discriminate between these possibilities and does not prove causality. If a positive skin test occurs in response to an allergen strongly suspected from the history, most clinicians would consider that allergen the likely etiology of symptoms. A negative skin test occurring with a substance not suspected from the history strongly rules out that substance as the cause of allergic symptoms. The relevance of a positive test occurring with an allergen not suspected from the history and physical is problematic and may require repeat testing or further serologic or provocative allergy testing. A negative skin test occurring with an allergen strongly suspected from the history should be repeated carefully with attention to technical factors; a repeatedly negative result casts doubt on the substance as the cause of symptoms.

LIMITATIONS: False-positives may result from the following:

- nonspecific irritant skin reactions interpreted as positive. This is a significant problem with intradermal testing. The volume of test substance introduced with intradermal injection is considerably greater than that used with skin prick testing, making the intradermal test potentially "too sensitive".
- hemorrhage at injection site interpreted as erythema
- dermographism interpreted as a wheal
- allergen contaminating neighboring sites
- test sites too close together
- impurities or contaminants in allergen preparations or the use of nonstandardized test materials
- small wheals (eg, 2 mm) interpreted as positive

False-negatives may result from the following:

- subcutaneous (not intradermal) injection of allergen
- waning allergen potency or improper volume or concentration
- drugs such as H_1 antagonists, hydroxyzine, tricyclic antidepressants, phenothiazines, dopamine
- active skin disease such as atopic dermatitis
- possibly extremes of age

ADDITIONAL INFORMATION: Intradermal testing is more expensive and time-consuming than the skin prick test. Both procedures evaluate the presence of IgE-mediated hypersensitivity. Although some physicians screen patients with suspected allergic disease by using intradermal testing exclusively, others begin with the more convenient prick test and follow up on negative or equivocal results with the more sensitive intradermal test. Positive results obtained on the skin prick test generally do not mandate further intradermal testing with the same antigen. Technically, intradermal allergy tests and the tuberculin skin test are performed in a nearly identical manner. However, the latter evaluates type IV cell-mediated immunity (delayed hypersensitivity) rather than type I antibody-mediated immunity (immediate hypersensitivity). This is due to the nature of the host immune response. Individuals exposed to *Mycobacterium tuberculosis* (MTB), for example, characteristically develop type IV cell-mediated immunity rather than IgE-mediated hypersensitivity. The skin response to intradermal injection of MTB antigen usually consists of erythema and induration at 24-48 hours, not an immediate wheal and flare reaction.

Footnotes

1. Bousquet J, "*In Vivo* Methods for Study of Allergy: Skin Tests, Techniques, and Interpretation," *Allergy, Principles and Practice*, 3rd ed, Chapter 19, Middleton E Jr, Reed CE, Ellis EF, et al, eds, St Louis, MO: CV Mosby Co, 1988, 419-36.
2. Nelson HS, "Diagnostic Procedures in Allergy. I. Allergy Skin Testing," *Ann Allergy*, 1983, 51:411-8.
3. Terr AI, "Allergic Diseases," *Basic and Clinical Immunology*, 6th ed, Stites DP, Stabo JD, and Wells JV, eds, Norwalk, CT: Appleton and Lange, 1987, 435-56.
4. Van Arsdel PP Jr and Larson EB, "Diagnostic Tests for Patients With Suspected Allergic Disease: Utility and Limitations," *Ann Intern Med*, 1989, 110(4):304-12.

Allergy Testing, Percutaneous

CPT 95000 (allergenic extracts, up to 30 tests); 95005 (antibiotics, biologicals, stinging insects, local anesthetics, 1-5 tests)

Related Information

Allergy Testing, Intracutaneous (Intradermal) *on page 4*
Fungal Skin Testing *on page 18*
Penicillin Allergy Skin Testing *on page 29*

Synonyms Immediate Hypersensitivity Skin Test; Percutaneous Allergy Testing; Prick Test; Puncture Test; Scratch Test; Skin Prick Test

Abstract PROCEDURE COMMONLY INCLUDES: Skin testing patients with suspected immediate-type hypersensitivity to one or more environmental substances. The test is performed by placing a drop of allergen(s) on the skin and making a needleprick through the drop(s) and into the underlying epidermis. Puncture sites are examined over the next 20 minutes for a wheal and flare skin response which, if present, indicates antibody-mediated (IgE) hypersensitivity to the test allergen. INDICATIONS:

- confirm the presence of immediate-type hypersensitivity to foreign substances (allergens) suspected from the patient's clinical history; in addition to commonly encountered allergens (eg, pollens, animal dander, grasses, molds, house dust) other potential test substances include antibiotics, stinging insect venom, and a variety of foods
- determine whether environmental allergens are playing a role in difficult to manage cases of asthma, urticaria, eczema, or anaphylaxis
- document immediate hypersensitivity prior to more elaborate allergy testing, such as provocation testing (bronchial provocation, oral food provocation) or prior to allergy desensitization therapy (immunotherapy)

CONTRAINDICATIONS:

- use of antihistamine medications (HI antagonists) within 48 hours of skin testing; antihistamines may inhibit the wheal and flare response, potentially causing false-negative results. Newer antihistamines with longer half-lives may interfere with testing for more than 1 week.
- use of hydroxyzine (Atarax®) within 1 week of testing
- documented anaphylactic reaction on prior percutaneous testing; allergens causing systemic reaction under test conditions should never be retested in the same patient. Unrelated substances, however, are not necessarily contraindicated but require physician approval.

(Continued)

Allergy Testing, Percutaneous *(Continued)*

- known systemic reaction to stabilizers or diluents contained in some allergen preparations; albumin is sometimes used as a stabilizer in commercial preparations; some testing centers routinely question patients regarding egg allergy.

Patient Care/Scheduling **PATIENT PREPARATION:** Requisition should include current medications, including last dose of antihistamines if applicable. Contact physician if there has been recent use of antihistamines or hydroxyzine (see Contraindications). Procedures and risks are explained to the patient beforehand. Once in the testing center, a brief dermatologic exam should be performed to ensure adequate areas of normal appearing skin for test purposes (and to identify the rare case of dermographism). **AFTERCARE:** If no adverse reaction has occurred postprocedure, patient is free to leave testing area. Instruct patient to keep the skin puncture sites clean until well healed. Patient should contact physician immediately if symptoms of dyspnea, wheezing, lightheadedness, severe pruritus, etc develop later that day (the rare case of "late phase response"). **SPECIAL INSTRUCTIONS:** Prior to testing, patient ideally should undergo a complete medical history and physical, with attention to allergy-related signs and symptoms. This allows a more directed and rational selection of antigens to be tested. Although skin testing may be performed by nurses or other trained personnel, a physician must be immediately available at all times to treat the rare case of anaphylaxis. Emergency equipment should be conveniently located and should include tourniquets, aqueous epinephrine, syringes, etc. **COMPLICATIONS:** The most common complication is a mild pruritus localized to positive test sites, usually resolving overnight. The incidence of significant bleeding or superficial skin infection is diminishingly low. However, as with other types of allergy skin testing, the possibility of systemic reaction exists. The exact incidence is unclear, but is felt to be rare and only at a case report level. It is generally regarded as safer than the closely related intradermal allergy test (estimated incidence of systemic reaction in the latter is >0.03%). Reported complications include generalized urticaria and anaphylaxis.

Method **EQUIPMENT:** Allergens used for prick testing are commercially prepared liquid extracts of a wide variety of foreign substances, numbering in the hundreds. It should be noted that some commercial allergens have not undergone biologic standardization for potency and purity. In addition, other allergen extracts are known to cause nonimmunologic irritant skin reactions which cannot be interpreted (codeine, radiographic contrast dye). Thus, not all foreign substances are suitable for skin testing. Commonly used allergen extracts include:

- trees (cottonwood, poplar, ash, birch, maple, oak, elm, hickory, pecan, and others)
- weeds (including ragweed, English plantain, sorrel-dock, pigweed)
- grasses (Timothy, Johnson, Bermuda, fescue, bluegrass)
- molds or fungi (*Alternaria*, *Fusarium*, *Hormodendrum*, *Aspergillus*, *Mucor*); hypersensitivity to *Aspergillus fumigatus* is often tested in patients with suspected allergic bronchopulmonary aspergillosis (ABPA)
- epidermals (house dust, house mites, feathers, cat and dog dander)

Standardized extracts are also available for foods, antibiotics, and insect venoms. Most prick test allergens are stabilized in 50% glycerol to prevent spontaneous degradation (human serum albumin is more often used as a stabilizer with intradermal testing). A supply of 27-gauge disposable hypodermic needles is also required, one needle for each allergen. Various automatic lancet devices and reusable solid needles are being promoted as alternatives to the hollow needle (possibly with some cost savings), but these devices remain optional.

TECHNIQUE: The physician reviews and confirms selection of allergens to be tested. Preferred test areas are the back or volar aspect of the forearm. A drop of each allergen is individually placed in a predetermined location on the skin. Usually less than 30 allergens are tested in one session and drops are placed in parallel rows approximately 2 cm apart. A 27-gauge needle is then passed through the drop at a 20° angle and the epidermis is penetrated with a stabbing motion. The needle tip is lifted slightly to tent the skin upwards, with care taken not to induce bleeding, and the needle is then removed. This constitutes the "prick" or "puncture". Over 30 separate pricks may be made in this fashion in several minutes using a new needle for each allergen. The drop of solution is wiped off 1 minute after needle puncture (some physicians prefer to wait up to 20 minutes). Frequently a negative and positive skin test control is included in the test battery consisting of glycerol and histamine, respectively. Minor variations in the overall techniques may be necessary if optional devices (such as the Morrow Brown needle) are used. Important differences exist between the prick test (described previously) and the technically similar "scratch test". In the scratch test a superficial linear abrasion is made in the epidermis (instead of a "prick") and a drop of allergen is placed on the scratch. Multiple scratches are often required. This technique has fallen out of favor due to a high incidence of nonimmunologic irritant reactions, patient discomfort, scar formation, and poor reproducibility.

DATA ACQUIRED: Test sites are examined for a wheal and erythema reaction, maximal at 15-20 minutes. Late phase reactions (6-8 hours) are not recorded routinely since their significance is unclear. Largest diameter of the wheal and/or erythema is measured and recorded in millimeters. Alternatively, the shape of wheal and flare may be permanently recorded by placing transparent paper directly onto the patient's back and outlining the skin reaction with a pen. Advanced techniques using ultrasound or Doppler flowmetry of the skin reaction are still primarily research tools.

Interpretation **NORMAL FINDINGS:** No wheal or erythema at test sites except for histamine control **CRITICAL VALUES:** A wheal <5 mm in transverse diameter is of questionable significance. A wheal >5 mm with accompanying erythema constitutes a positive test, as defined in a position paper issued by the American College of Physicians.[1] In clinical practice, grading systems are often employed, but grading criteria lack uniformity. One example is as follows:

- negative – no reaction
- 1+ – no wheal, erythema <20 mm
- 2+ – no wheal, erythema >20 mm
- 3+ – definite wheal and erythema
- 4+ – pseudopods, wheal and erythema

In this system, grades 2+ through 4+ are considered positive. The evaluation of the patient with suspected allergic disease is based on the history, physical examination, and allergy skin tests. Some individuals suffer from antibody (IgE) – mediated sensitivity to multiple commonly encountered substances, such as pollens, grass, and animal dander. These symptomatic individuals are termed "atopic" and represent approximately 10% of the population in the United States. Nonatopic individuals may also develop IgE-mediated allergy, as in the case of acquired hypersensitivity to insect venom. Percutaneous allergy testing is an *in vivo* method of identifying afflicted individuals in both these groups and identifying the most likely causative agents. Allergic reactions of the immediate hypersensitivity variety represent type I Gell and Coombs' reactions. Exposure to a relevant allergen (true antigen) leads to mast cell activation with release of mediators of inflammation such as histamine, leukotrienes, and eosinophil chemotactic factors. This process is mediated by IgE antibodies. A wide spectrum of symptoms may be seen in association with allergic disease and ranges from rhinitis, dermatitis, and asthma to urticaria-angioedema and anaphylaxis. It should be noted that each of these conditions may also be caused by nonallergic mechanisms without direct involvement of the host immune system. Percutaneous allergy testing may be useful in this setting, as in differentiating allergic from nonallergic asthma. When a sensitized individual is re-exposed to antigen by means of the prick test, the skin undergoes characteristic inflammatory changes. Mast cells in the skin release histamine causing increased vascular permeability and vasodilatation. This dermal response, the wheal and flare, is uniformly seen in patients with IgE-mediated disease regardless of the location of the patient's presenting symptoms: nasal mucosa, skin, airways, or gastrointestinal tract. Prick testing has been critically evaluated in the medical literature and found to have acceptable sensitivity, specificity, and reliability for clinical practice. The challenge in prick testing lies not in its technical aspects but in the interpretation of a positive or negative result. A number of potential false-positive and false-negative results may complicate interpretation (see Limitations). Yet, even if these usually procedural errors are eliminated, correct interpretation requires consideration of the clinical history and physical along with skin test results. A positive test by itself indicates only a state of potential hypersensitivity, a heightened immunologic reactivity towards a particular allergen. In a study involving scratch testing of college students, 17% of asymptomatic subjects had one or more positive skin tests, indicating that immunologic sensitivity may exist in the absence of symptoms.[2] There is no guarantee that a positive reacting allergen is the cause of a patient's

(Continued)

Allergy Testing, Percutaneous *(Continued)*

symptoms (rhinorrhea, bronchospasm, etc). Symptoms of allergic disease may be caused by:

- a positive reacting test material (true positive)
- a negative reacting test material (false-negative)
- a foreign substance not tested
- nonimmunologic, non-IgE-mediated disease

By itself, the prick test does not prove causality. If a positive skin test occurs with an allergen strongly suspected from the history, most clinicians consider this presumptive evidence of causality. Similarly, a negative test occurring with a test substance of low suspicion effectively rules out that substance as the cause of a patient's symptoms. The clinical relevance of a positive test occurring with an allergen not suspected from clinical presentation is very problematic and may require repeat testing or further serologic or provocative testing. A negative skin test occurring with an allergen strongly suspected from the history may require follow-up with the somewhat more sensitive intradermal allergy test.

LIMITATIONS: False-positives: nonspecific irritant reactions; dermographism interpreted as a wheal; hemorrhage at prick site interpreted as erythema; allergen spread from one site to another when the same needle is reused; small wheals (eg, 2 mm) interpreted as significant; impurities or contaminants in allergen preparations; test sites improperly spaced; inappropriate allergen concentrations

False-negatives: waning potency of allergens; inadequate concentration of allergen; technical errors in epidermal puncture; drugs such as HI antagonists, hydroxyzine, tricyclic antidepressants, phenothiazines, dopamine; skin diseases such as atopic dermatitis; possibly extremes of age

ADDITIONAL INFORMATION: Some allergists test for immediate hypersensitivity exclusively with the prick test, while others use intradermal testing instead. The prick test is simpler, faster, safer, and possibly less painful to the patient than intradermal testing. However, there is a higher rate of false-negatives and sensitivity is somewhat less. A common compromise is to begin evaluation of the allergic individual with the prick test and follow up indeterminate reactions or negative reactions of strongly suspected allergens with the intradermal test.

Footnotes

1. American College of Physicians, "Allergy Testing," *Ann Intern Med*, 1989, 110(4):317-20.
2. Hagy GW and Settipane GA, "Prognosis of Positive Allergy Skin Tests in an Asymptomatic Population: A Three-Year Follow-up of College Students," *J Allergy*, 1971, 48:200-11.

References

Bousquet J, "*In Vivo* Methods for Study of Allergy: Skin Tests, Techniques, and Interpretation," *Allergy, Principles and Practice*, 3rd ed, Middleton E Jr, Reed CE, Ellis E, et al, eds, St Louis, MO: CV Mosby Co, 1988, 419-36.

Council on Scientific Affairs, "*In Vivo* Diagnostic Testing and Immunotherapy for Allergy: Report 1 of the Allergy Panel," *JAMA*, 1987, 258:1363-7, 1505-8.

Lessof MH, Buisseret PD, Merrett J, et al, "Assessing the Value of Skin Prick Tests," *Clin Allergy*, 1980, 10:115-20.

Nelson HS, "Diagnostic Procedures in Allergy. I. Allergy Skin Testing," *Ann Allergy*, 1983, 51:411-8.

Terr AI, "Allergic Diseases," *Basic and Clinical Immunology*, 6th ed, Stites DP, Stabo JB, and Wells JV, eds, Norwalk, CO: Appleton and Lange, 1987, 435-56.

Van Arsdel PP and Larson EB, "Diagnostic Tests for Patients With Suspected Allergic Disease. Utility and Limitations," *Ann Intern Med*, 1989, 110(4):304-12.

Anergy Control Panel *see* Anergy Skin Test Battery *on next page*

Anergy Skin Test Battery

CPT 95030 (intracutaneous tests with allergenic extracts, delayed reaction, 24-72 hours, 2 tests); 95031 (3-4 tests)

Related Information

Fungal Skin Testing *on page 18*
Tuberculin Skin Testing, Intracutaneous *on page 33*

Synonyms Anergy Control Panel; Anergy Skin Testing; Delayed Reaction Intracutaneous Tests; Skin Test Battery

Abstract PROCEDURE COMMONLY INCLUDES: Injection of several common antigenic substances into the skin, such as *Candida*, *Trichophyton*, and mumps antigens. Anergy skin testing is an *in vivo* means of evaluating the cell-mediated immune system. Skin injection sites are examined at 24, 48, and 72 hours. The development of local erythema and induration indicates an adequate delayed hypersensitivity response and implies competent T-cell function. Failure to respond to any skin test antigen is termed cutaneous anergy and is seen in a variety of systemic disorders. INDICATIONS:

- objectively demonstrate cutaneous anergy in cases of suspected cellular immune system deficiency (T-cell dysfunction); often this procedure is performed as part of an initial immune system assessment, but may also be repeated in a serial fashion in cases of protracted or chronic illness
- serve as a "control" skin test accompanying the tuberculin skin test (or other specific antigen tests); this allows more accurate interpretation of a negative tuberculin test; patients with generalized cutaneous anergy predictably fail to react to injected tuberculin despite prior exposure to *M. tuberculosis*
- establish the presence of cutaneous anergy prior to more extensive *in vitro* evaluation of lymphocyte and monocyte function
- less commonly, to help predict postoperative morbidity and mortality, especially in patients with sepsis[1]
- occasionally, to provide general prognostic information in patients with cancer[2]

CONTRAINDICATIONS:

- prior systemic reaction to any antigen included in the skin test battery; alternate antigens may be substituted in most cases
- known hypersensitivity to a stabilizer or diluent used in commercial antigen preparations; for example, mumps skin test antigen is derived from virus incubated in chicken embryo and preserved in thimerosal. Patients should therefore be questioned regarding feather and egg allergy as well as sensitivity to thimerosal prior to administering mumps antigen. Depending on the particular antigens selected, published manufacturer's warnings should be reviewed and potential hypersensitivity reactions avoided.

Patient Care/Scheduling PATIENT PREPARATION: Procedure and risks are explained to the patient. No specific skin preparation is necessary. However, those patients with generalized skin disease, such as psoriasis, should be examined beforehand to ensure that there are suitable areas of normal appearing skin. Although testing need not be performed by a physician, one should be immediately available in the event of a systemic reaction. AFTERCARE: If no adverse reaction has occurred within 30 minutes, patient may be discharged from the testing center. Test sites should be kept reasonably clean for 72 hours. No restrictions on bathing are necessary. Patient should contact physician if severe local reactions develop, extensive erythema beyond the test site occurs, or if fever, dyspnea, or lightheadedness develops. SPECIAL INSTRUCTIONS: Requisition should include a list of all current medications, with attention to corticosteroids or other immunosuppressive agents. COMPLICATIONS: Anergy skin testing is generally quite safe. However, as with other forms of skin testing, immediate local reactions to antigens are distinctly unusual but possible. These reactions are usually IgE-mediated and lead to an immediate wheal and flare reaction. Rarely, serious local reactions have been reported to various antigens commonly included in the test battery. These include vesiculation, skin necrosis, and extensive erythema. Systemic reactions have been reported only on an individual case basis.

Method EQUIPMENT: Antigens used for anergy testing are commercially prepared liquid extracts of a variety of foreign substances. These antigens are chosen because ubiquitous exposure to these substances is expected in the general population. Thus, in any randomly selected subgroup, a high rate of delayed hypersensitivity skin reactions would be antic-

(Continued)

Anergy Skin Test Battery *(Continued)*

ipated. Commonly used bacterial antigens include streptococcal antigen (derived from *Streptococcus* group CH 46A), *Proteus* antigen (often from *Proteus mirabilis* IM 2104 strain), and in some centers, tuberculin is also included. Fungal antigens frequently employed include *Candida* antigen (derived from *Candida albicans* strain 2111), *Trichophyton* antigen (from *Trichophyton mentagrophytes*), and frequently histoplasmin is used (from *Histoplasma capsulatum* – see Fungal Skin Testing). Toxoids are also included in the test battery, usually tetanus toxoid (from *Clostridium tetani*, Harvard strain 401) and diphtheria toxoid (from *Corynebacterium diphtheriae*). Mumps skin test antigen is a viral antigen derived from inactivated mumps virus cultured in chick embryo. The choice of antigens and total number employed has yet to be standardized. Most test centers use less than five antigens in their routine battery, but considerable variation exists, with the total number ranging from 1-11. Palmer et al discovered that 90% of 750 hospitalized patients reacted to one or more of the following: mumps, *Candida*, *Trichophyton*, and tuberculin.[3] Increasing the total number of antigens improved the rate of skin reactions by only 1%. With respect to the individual selection of antigens, a representative battery might therefore include mumps, *Candida*, and *Trichophyton*; this combination is commonly seen in practice. However, in one literature review, more than 30 different antigens were found to be in routine use at major centers.[4] Disposable plastic or glass tuberculin syringes, 0.5-1 mL are also required, along with 26- or 27-gauge short (1/4" – 1/2") beveled needles, some alcohol pads, and gauze. An alternative anergy testing technique has been developed in recent years to address the aforementioned lack of standardization in antigen selection and number. Termed the Multitest® CMI system, seven standardized antigens and one control are simultaneously injected by means of a multiple puncture device. Antigens used here are tetanus toxoid, diphtheria toxoid, streptococcal antigen, *Proteus*, tuberculin, *Candida*, and *Trichophyton*. This device obviates the need for separate syringes, needles, and antigens.

TECHNIQUE: Traditional method: Antigens are injected separately. Antigens are individually drawn up into tuberculin syringes immediately prior to testing. The volar aspects of the arms or forearms are the preferred test sites. Only normal appearing skin should be used. Sites are prepared with alcohol swabs. Using a 26- or 27-gauge needle, each antigen is injected intradermally at a 45° angle, bevel down. A small bleb approximately 2-3 mm in diameter should be raised; usually an injected volume of 0.05 mL is sufficient. Care should be taken to avoid deeper subcutaneous injections. Each antigen is separately planted in this fashion with adequate spacing between injection sites (>2 cm).

Multipuncture method: Antigens are placed simultaneous by means of the Multitest® CMI device. Seven antigens and one glycerol control are standardized with respect to selection and concentration and are preloaded onto this disposable plastic device. A different antigen coats each of seven multiple puncture heads, which are spaced approximately 2 cm apart, in two parallel rows of four. The skin over the forearm is held taut. The device is then oriented per manufacturer's instructions ("T" bar towards the head) and applied to the skin with a rocking motion. Each head must sufficiently puncture the skin. Regardless of technique, all test sites should be examined immediately and at 24, 48, and 72 hours. Date and time of injection must be recorded. The precise location, identity, and concentration of each antigen should be recorded, most often in a pictorial format or standardized table. It may be helpful to circle and label each antigen with a waterproof pen directly onto the skin, but this must not replace formal notations in the medical chart.

DATA ACQUIRED: The transverse diameter of induration at each test site should be carefully measured by both inspection and palpation. Results are recorded in millimeters at the appropriate 24-hour intervals. Areas of erythema are also measured but play a minor role in most grading schemes.

Interpretation **NORMAL FINDINGS:** Normal individuals should demonstrate a positive skin reaction to one or more test antigens. **CRITICAL VALUES:** A positive skin test is usually defined as the presence of induration and accompanying erythema ≥5 mm in transverse diameter at an injection site at 24, 48, or 72 hours. Immediate skin reactions (ie, within minutes) are due to mechanisms other than cellular immunity and do not define a positive test. When the Multitest® CMI system is used, induration ≥2 mm in transverse diameter is considered significant. This disparity in definition between the intradermal and multiple puncture technique results from a variety of technical factors including volume of antigen introduced, depth of skin penetration, etc. A state of anergy is defined as an inability to mount an appropriate delayed hypersensitivity response. In clinical practice this is manifested as a complete absence of reactivity to a skin test battery of at least four to five antigens. Some authorities require repetition of the test battery at least once before labeling a patient "anergic". Normal individuals are expected to develop a positive skin test in response to at least one antigen, barring technical error. Anergy may be present as a generalized defect in T-cell function, as in sarcoidosis, AIDS, or tuberculosis, or as a specific defect in cellular immunity, as in mucocutaneous candidiasis where T-cell response to *Candida* is selectively deficient. There are numerous causes of anergy and may be categorized as follows:

- infections: bacterial, tuberculosis, disseminated fungal infections, viral (influenza, mumps, mononucleosis, hepatitis, and others), parasitic
- congenital: cell-mediated deficiency (DiGeorge syndrome), combined cellular and humoral deficiency (Nezelof's, Wiskott-Aldrich syndrome, etc)
- acquired/iatrogenic: neoplasms (solid tumors, lymphomas, leukemias), medications (corticosteroids, antineoplastic agents, methotrexate, and others), AIDS
- rheumatic diseases: rheumatoid arthritis, lupus, Behçet's disease
- miscellaneous: uremia, diabetes mellitus, inflammatory bowel disease, sarcoidosis, extremes of age, malnutrition

However, anergy skin testing by itself does not distinguish amongst these conditions from a diagnostic viewpoint. Clinically, anergy testing is most useful in evaluating the patient who presents with chronic or recurrent infections, or infection with unusual organisms. In such cases, formal evaluation of the immune system may be warranted. This may include assessment of all four major components of the immune system: cell-mediated (T-cell) immunity, antibody-mediated (B-cell) immunity, phagocytic system (polymorphonuclear leukocytes, macrophages), and complement. Often a careful history and physical, with attention to infectious diseases, will identify the particular component deficiency. Anergy testing is an appropriate and recommended screening procedure for suspected deficiencies in cell-mediated immunity, often characterized by fungal, mycobacterial, or disseminated viral infections (eg, varicella-zoster, cytomegalovirus, herpes simplex virus). Among the many laboratory tests available to evaluate host defense, anergy testing is rightfully obtained soon after the history and physical (along with a complete blood count with differential) but prior to more elaborate *in vitro* investigation of T-cell function. These latter tests include T-cell surface marker studies, T-cell subsets, and response to mitogens (such as pokeweed mitogen, phytohemagglutinin, concanavalin A). Some individuals demonstrate partial or inconclusive responses to skin testing. This is seen as a "borderline" skin induration diameter (ie, 1-4 mm) or as a poor reactivity rate when a large antigen battery is employed (ie, 1 positive reaction out of 10 tested). In the literature, these patients have sometimes been called "hypoergic," which implies a partially impaired delayed hypersensitivity response. The clinical significance of this phenomenon is unclear at present.

LIMITATIONS: "Traditional" skin test battery limitations, mentioned previously, include variation in selection and total number of antigens used as well as a lack of standardization of antigen potency. However, some practitioners consider the inability to select and interchange antigens in the Multitest® CMI system a major drawback.

False-positive reactions may occur:

- when an immediate wheal and flare is interpreted as delayed hypersensitivity
- when intradermal bleeding is interpreted as erythema
- when dermographism is present

False-negative reactions may be caused by:

- lack of antigen potency
- subcutaneous injection
- inadequate dose or concentration
- incomplete skin puncture by the Multitest® device
- attenuated skin response, as in atopic dermatitis

ADDITIONAL INFORMATION: For details regarding the cellular mechanisms of the delayed hypersensitivity skin response, see the review by Ahmed (1983).

Footnotes

1. Johnson WC, Ulrich F, Mequid MM, et al, "Role of Delayed Hypersensitivity in Predicting Postoperative Morbidity and Mortality," *Am J Surg*, 1979, 137:536-42.

(Continued)

Anergy Skin Test Battery *(Continued)*

2. Ahmed AR and Blose DA, "Delayed-Type Hypersensitivity Skin Testing," *Arch Dermatol*, 1983, 119:934-45.
3. Palmer D and Reed W, "Delayed Hypersensitivity Skin Testing: I. Response in a Hospitalized Population," *J Infect Dis*, 1973, 130:132-7.
4. Kniker WT, Anderson CT, and Roumiantzeff M, "The Multitest® System: A Standardized Approach to Evaluation of Delayed Hypersensitivity and Cell-Mediated Immunity," *Ann Allergy*, 1979, 43:73-9.

References

Bates SE, Suen JY, and Tranum BL, "Immunological Skin Testing and Interpretation. A Plea for Uniformity," *Cancer*, 1979, 43:2306-14.

Cooper MD and Lawton AR, "Primary Immune Deficiency Diseases," *Harrison's Principles of Internal Medicine*, 12th ed, Chapter 263, Wilson JD, Braunwald E, Isselbacher KJ, et al, eds, New York, NY: McGraw-Hill Book Co, 1991, 1395-402.

Kniker WT, Anderson CT, McBryde JL, et al, "Multitest® CMI for Standardized Measurement of Delayed Cutaneous Hypersensitivity and Cell-Mediated Immunity: Normal Values and Proposed Scoring System for Healthy Adults in the USA," *Ann Allergy*, 1984, 52:75-82.

Arthrocentesis

CPT 20600 (small joint); 20605 (intermediate joint); 20610 (major joint)

Related Information

Ingestion Challenge Test *on page 20*

Synonyms Closed Joint Aspiration; Joint Tap

Abstract **PROCEDURE COMMONLY INCLUDES:** Passing a needle into a joint space and aspirating synovial fluid for diagnostic analysis **INDICATIONS:**

Diagnostic indications include:

- joint effusions of unknown etiology
- arthritis of unclear etiology
- all cases of suspected infectious arthritis (bacterial, fungal, tuberculous)
- confirmation of a diagnosis strongly suspected on clinical grounds, such as suspected gout in patients with podagra
- monitoring synovial fluid response to antibiotic therapy in established cases of septic arthritis

Therapeutic indications include:

- decompression of a tense, painful joint effusion
- evacuation of pus in bacterial arthritis (repeated closed drainage)
- removal of inflammatory cells and crystals in selected cases of gout or pseudogout
- intra-articular injection of corticosteroids

CONTRAINDICATIONS:

- local infection along the proposed needle entrance tract (eg, overlying cellulitis, periarticular infection)
- uncooperative patient, especially if unable to keep the joint immobile throughout procedure
- difficult to identify boney landmarks
- a poorly accessible joint space, as in hip aspiration in the obese patient
- inability to demonstrate a joint effusion on physical examination, except when septic arthritis is strongly suspected (and effusions may be barely detectable)

In addition, some authors consider bacteremia (documented or suspected) a contraindication to arthrocentesis based on the theoretical concern of seeding a sterile joint when the entering needle ruptures surrounding capillaries. No data is available to support or refute this. We feel that clinical judgment must be individualized in each case. If infectious arthritis is suspected, arthrocentesis should be promptly performed even with documented bacteremia. However, more elective indications for the procedure, such as corticosteroid injection, should be deferred, at physician's discretion.

Patient Care/Scheduling **PATIENT PREPARATION:** Procedure and risks are explained and consent is obtained. No intravenous pain medications or sedatives are required. **AFTERCARE:** Determined by results of procedure, as outlined by physician. May range from joint immobilization with passive range of motion, as in septic arthritis, to full weight bearing, as in effusions secondary to osteoarthritis. No specific joint positioning postprocedure has been demonstrated to reduce complications. **COMPLICATIONS:** Arthrocentesis is a generally safe procedure, especially when performed on a large, easily accessible joint such as the knee. Potential complications include:

- iatrogenic joint space infection (if properly performed, incidence has been estimated at 1 in 15,000 cases)
- hemorrhage or hematoma formation (usually when alternative approaches are used and blood vessels are ruptured on the flexor surface of the joint)
- local pain caused by needle trauma to the periosteum
- injury to cartilage, particularly problematic due to slow repair rate
- tendon rupture
- nerve palsies

Method **EQUIPMENT:** Alcohol swabs, povidone-iodine prep solution, sterile gloves and towels, gauze, and forceps. Local anesthesia with ethyl chloride vinyl spray and/or lidocaine 1% with appropriate syringes and subcutaneous needles. If the joint to be aspirated is large, use 18- or 20-gauge 1.5" needle on a 20 mL syringe (additional syringes should be available). If joint is small or effusion minimal, use 20- or 22-gauge 1.5" needle on 3 mL syringe. In this latter case, additional tubes for fluid collection will not be needed. Otherwise, use three sterile tubes for collection, the first one with either EDTA additive or a small amount of heparin. If gonococcal arthritis is suspected, obtain chocolate (Thayer-Martin) media. Glass slides and polarized microscope are necessary if crystalline arthropathy is suspected. **TECHNIQUE:** Procedure should be performed by experienced physician only. The following description details the technique of knee arthrocentesis, a joint commonly aspirated by the generalist. Presence of effusion is confirmed on physical examination. If the effusion appears small, an elastic wrap (or manual pressure) may be placed around the knee to compress mobile fluid into the joint space. Patient is instructed to lie supine and remain relaxed. Ideally, the operator should be seated and the height of patient's bed adjusted accordingly. Physician selects the type of approach: suprapatellar, parapatellar, or infrapatellar. The parapatellar approach is popular and effective with tense effusions. Here, the knee is placed in 20° flexion to relax the quadriceps. The preferred entry site is the midportion of the patella (approximately 2 cm superior to the inferior portion of the patella), preferably the medial aspect. This site is marked by indenting the skin with the retracted end of a ballpoint pen. The skin is prepped with alcohol first then povidone iodine. Some clinicians prefer strict aseptic technique (5-minute scrub, masks, gowns, and drapes) whereas others do not use even sterile gloves or drapes. We prefer a middle-ground approach, using sterile gloves and towels but foregoing masks and gowns. The use of local anesthesia also varies amongst practitioners. If the joint is tense, and anatomical landmarks easily palpable, we prefer cutaneous anesthesia with only a spray of ethyl chloride solution. Alternatively, a subcutaneous wheal of lidocaine may be raised in the usual fashion. Injection of lidocaine into deeper structures is not usually required (where it may potentially interfere with culture results because of bacteriostatic properties). Following this, the needle-on-syringe is passed through the marked skin site and advanced slowly while aspirating. A "pop" may be felt as the needle penetrates the capsule. The needle should be directed parallel to the plane of the synovial capsule if the parapatellar approach is used. Once fluid is returned, the needle should not be advanced further in order to avoid cartilage damage. Only mild suction should be used to aspirate so that trauma and hemorrhage do not occur. In general, joint effusions should be drained completely. A blind "search" with the needle (often with vigorous aspiration) is hazardous and should not be attempted. Forceps may be used to stabilize the needle if several syringe changes are required. Once completed, withdraw the needle, apply pressure, and place adhesive tape over puncture site. If persistent pain is encountered during the procedure, trauma to cartilage or periosteum is likely. Do not reflexly anesthetize these deeper tissues with lidocaine; instead, withdraw the needle and redirect it along a new plane. Correct placement of the needle in the joint space is normally painless. In the case of a "dry tap," folds of synovium may be acting as a valve obstructing the needle lumen. Reposition the needle

(Continued)

Arthrocentesis *(Continued)*

slightly, or if there is fluid in the syringe, inject a small amount to clear the needle bevel. This problem can be avoided by using the infrapatellar approach. The technique for suprapatellar and infrapatellar aspiration has been detailed elsewhere. The suprapatellar approach is most useful in tense effusions where the suprapatellar bursa (usually in communication with the joint space) is visibly distended. While easily performed, there is a potential for sinus tract formation especially if the entry site is directly over the bursa, rather than several centimeters away. The infrapatellar approach has a low risk of cartilage damage compared with the parapatellar approach and is useful for patients with marked flexion contractures of the knee. However, clinicians may not be familiar with the technical details of this approach. Similar principles apply to aspiration of joints other than the knee and are referenced. **DATA ACQUIRED:** A wide array of tests on synovial fluid is available. Routine tests on effusions of unknown etiology include: cell count, glucose, Gram stain and routine culture, and microscopic examination for crystals (urate, calcium, pyrophosphate dihydrate). Optional tests include: viscosity, mucin clot test, uric acid level, and culture for *Neisseria gonorrhoeae*, tuberculosis, etc. Occasionally, ordered tests include: synovial fluid protein, LDH, cytology, rheumatoid factor, complement.

Specimen Synovial fluid **CONTAINER:** For small fluid volumes, send capped syringe without needle to laboratory; otherwise, fluid may be carefully transferred to sterile tubes. **COLLECTION:** Tube 1: Gram stain and culture; tube 2: mucin clot, if ordered (no heparin); tube 3: (add heparin or EDTA) cell count, chemistries, crystals, additional studies. If gonococcal arthritis is suspected, chocolate (Thayer-Martin) agar should be inoculated, either at the bedside or during initial specimen processing. **STORAGE INSTRUCTIONS:** Specimen should be hand carried to the laboratory, preferably by the physician. Delay in processing may spuriously lower synovial fluid glucose levels.

Interpretation **NORMAL FINDINGS:** In the absence of disease, synovial fluid usually cannot be aspirated. Normal synovial fluid is clear and viscous. A drop placed between the thumb and forefinger (or two microscope slides) can form a string >2 cm long as the fingers are separated, indicating high viscosity. Similarly, the mucin clot test is performed by adding 1 mL synovial fluid to a 5% solution of acetic acid. Normally, a firm clot forms. Both tests reflect high viscosity of synovial fluid caused by leukocyte hyaluronic acid. Cell count and differential normally reveal <200 WBCs/mm^3 with <25% neutrophils. Chemistries show protein <2 g/dL, uric acid <8 mg/dL, synovial glucose nearly equal to serum glucose, and synovial LDH less than serum LDH. Gram stain and cultures are negative (acellular). **CRITICAL VALUES:** Abnormal synovial fluid can be divided into four diagnostic categories. Considerable overlap exists among these categories and correlation with the clinical presentation is required.

Group I synovial fluids are seen commonly in degenerative joint disease (osteoarthritis) and trauma. Fluid is clear or yellow tinged, viscous and mucin clot firm. WBC count is <200/mm^3 with <25% neutrophils (often mononuclears >50%). Chemistries including glucose are normal and microbiologic cultures are negative. This is considered a "noninflammatory" effusion. Some inflammatory conditions may at times cause a group I fluid, such as acute rheumatic fever and systemic lupus erythematosus.

Group II fluids are "inflammatory" in nature. Diseases leading to this category include: crystal-induced arthropathies (gout, CPPD or "pseudogout"), rheumatoid arthritis, connective tissue diseases (SLE, polymyositis, etc), ankylosing spondylitis and other seronegative spondyloarthropathies (Reiter's syndrome, psoriatic arthritis), and acute rheumatic fever. Synovial fluid appears opaque and turbid from cellular fragmentation. Viscosity is similar to water and the "string test" yields only short strings. Mucin clot testing results in a friable gel rather than a tight, rope-like clot. WBC counts are elevated, 5000 to 75,000/mm^3 with >50% neutrophils. Synovial glucose tends to be lower than serum glucose, especially if synovial WBCs are elevated (neutrophils consume glucose). Gram stain and cultures are negative.

Group III effusions are characteristic of septic arthritis. Fluid appears grossly turbid and may be frankly purulent. WBC count as a rule is >50,000/mm^3 and may be >1,000,000/mm^3. Differential shows preponderance of neutrophils (>90%), with the exception of tuberculous arthritis where lymphocytes may comprise 50% of leukocytes. Synovial glucose is characteristically <50% of simultaneous serum glucose and this finding strongly suggests septic arthritis. Glucose values <10 mg/dL have been reported and support classification into group III (rather than group II) in cases where WBC count is moderately elevated. However, sensitivity of low glucose levels in the septic joint is approximately 50%. Gram stain yield in group III effusions varies with the bacteria isolated. In patients with staphylococcal septic arthritis, the Gram stain is diagnostic in 75% of cases, with gram-negative arthritis, 50% of Gram stains are diagnostic, but with gonococcal arthritis, only 25% of Gram stains are positive. In nongonococcal septic arthritis, the bacterial culture is more helpful than the Gram stain, the former being positive in 85% to 95% of cases (provided no recent antibiotic use). However, with gonococcal arthritis, the culture is less sensitive, with only a 25% positive yield.[1]

Group IV synovial effusions are grossly hemorrhagic. Etiologies include: systemic abnormalities (eg, excessive heparin anticoagulation, severe thrombocytopenia) and local joint pathology (eg, femur fracture, neuropathic joint).

As mentioned earlier, diagnostic groups are not mutually exclusive. Certain disease entities may fall into more than one diagnostic category. For example, synovial fluid in acute rheumatic fever may appear as either a group I or a group II effusion; neuropathic arthropathy may appear as group I or IV, and lupus-associated effusions as group I or II. In addition, an individual patient may befall more than one pathologic process over the course of time. It has been demonstrated that rheumatoid arthritis (group II effusion) is a predisposing factor for the later development of bacterial arthritis (group III) and both may be present in the same patient. Finally, some diseases may change from one diagnostic category to another over a short time period. For example, septic arthritis in an early stage may present with a low synovial WBC count and normal glucose (group I) and only later on progress to a typical septic arthritis (group III) picture on subsequent arthrocentesis.

ADDITIONAL INFORMATION: Arthrocentesis is indispensable for the accurate diagnosis (or exclusion) of septic arthritis and crystal-induced arthropathy and therein lies its greatest utility. Despite the difficulties with the classification scheme described above, synovial fluid findings in both these treatable conditions is often pathognomonic. Practically, the procedure carries a low risk of complications and can be performed in minutes when an accessible joint is involved. The general physician often handles aspirations of the knee, elbow, and first metatarsal phalangeal joint. When septic arthritis is suspected in a less accessible area, such as the sacroiliac joint, aspiration should not be delayed due to a lack of familiarity. Rheumatologic consultation should be obtained promptly.

Footnotes

1. Goldenberg DL and Reed JI, "Bacterial Arthritis," *N Engl J Med*, 1985, 312(12):764-71.

References

Gatter RA, "Arthrocentesis Technique and Intrasynovial Therapy," *Arthritis and Allied Conditions: A Textbook of Rheumatology*, 11th ed, Chapter 39, McCarty DJ, ed, Philadelphia, PA: Lea & Febiger, 1989.

Rodnan GP and Schumacher HR, "Examination of Synovial Fluid," *Primer on the Rheumatic Diseases*, 8th ed, Chapter 90, Atlanta, GA: Arthritis Foundation, 1983.

Simon RR and Brenner BE, "Orthopedic Procedures," *Procedures and Techniques in Emergency Medicine*, Chapter 7, Baltimore, MD: Williams & Wilkins, 1982.

Closed Joint Aspiration *see* Arthrocentesis *on page 14*

Contact Dermatitis Skin Test *see* Patch Test *on page 27*

Delayed Hypersensitivity Fungal Skin Tests *see* Fungal Skin Testing *on next page*

Delayed Reaction Intracutaneous Tests *see* Anergy Skin Test Battery *on page 11*

Epicutaneous Patch Test *see* Patch Test *on page 27*

Food Allergy Test *see* Ingestion Challenge Test *on page 20*

Fungal Skin Testing

CPT 86455 (anergy testing, 1 or more antigens); 86490 (coccidioidomycosis); 86510 (histoplasmosis)

Related Information

Allergy Testing, Percutaneous *on page 7*
Anergy Skin Test Battery *on page 11*
Tuberculin Skin Testing, Intracutaneous *on page 33*

Synonyms Delayed Hypersensitivity Fungal Skin Tests; Skin Tests for Histoplasmosis, Blastomycosis, Coccidioidomycosis

Abstract **PROCEDURE COMMONLY INCLUDES:** Intradermal injection of fungal antigen(s) to determine if a delayed hypersensitivity reaction is present to a given fungus. Skin test sites are examined at 24, 48, and 72 hours for induration which, if present, implies prior infection with the tested fungus. **INDICATIONS:** Fungal skin testing has been applied for the following reasons:

- as an epidemiologic tool for defining geographic regions of endemic fungal infection
- as a diagnostic aid in individual cases of suspected primary fungal infection (limited usefulness)
- as a prognostic indicator in culture-proven cases of fungal infection (particularly coccidioidomycosis)
- as a component of a comprehensive cutaneous anergy panel, used to assess the integrity of a patient's cell-mediated immune system (T-cell function); this standardized panel is usually comprised of *Candida*, mumps, and *Trichophyton* antigens

CONTRAINDICATIONS: Prior systemic reaction to fungal skin testing; known immediate hypersensitivity (IgE-mediated) to the specific fungus to be tested; known immediate hypersensitivity to mercury, which is contained in some commercial preparations of *Coccidioides* antigen; the presence of erythema nodosum (high risk for adverse reaction – see following information).

Patient Care/Scheduling **PATIENT PREPARATION:** Procedure and risks are explained to the patient. No specific skin preparation is necessary. However, those patients with generalized skin disorders such as extensive psoriasis should be examined beforehand for suitable areas of normal appearing skin. If immediate hypersensitivity to the fungal antigen is even remotely suspected, physician should be in attendance. **AFTERCARE:** Fifteen to 30 minutes after injections, sites should be examined for adverse reactions ranging from the IgE wheal and flare response to systemic reactions; otherwise, close observation postprocedure is generally not necessary and patients should be instructed to keep test sites clean for 72 hours. No restrictions on bathing or cleaning injection sites are necessary.

SPECIAL INSTRUCTIONS: Requisition should state the specific fungal antigens to be planted, as well as whether a simultaneous skin anergy panel is desired. Current medications should also be included in the requisition, with attention to corticosteroids or other immunosuppressive agents. **COMPLICATIONS:** As with other forms of skin testing, immediate IgE-mediated local reactions are possible, although unusual. Erythema, vesiculation, and skin necrosis may be seen, at times involving large areas. Systemic reactions, including anaphylaxis, have rarely been reported. Patients with infection with *Coccidioides immitis* who manifest erythema nodosum may be at an increased risk of a major systemic reaction after skin testing. However, in the vast majority of cases, fungal skin testing is safe.

Method **EQUIPMENT:** Skin test materials are derived from cultures of the appropriate fungi and most are available commercially in standardized concentrations. Common fungal antigens tested include *Histoplasma capsulatum*, *Coccidioides immitis*, *Blastomyces dermatitidis* (not available commercially), *Candida*, and *Trichophyton*. Disposable plastic or glass tuberculin syringes are required along with 26- or 27-gauge short (1/4" to 1/2") beveled needles. **TECHNIQUE:** The volar aspect of the forearm is prepped with alcohol swabs. Skin test material(s) are injected intradermally so that discrete wheals are raised. Generally, 0.1 mL skin test antigen is injected, but more dilute solutions may be used if a severe reaction is anticipated. Subcutaneous injections should be avoided. Multiple fungal antigens may be injected at separate sites using this method. Test sites should be examined at 24, 48, and 72 hours. Date and time of injection should be recorded along with the location of each fungal antigen. **DATA ACQUIRED:** The transverse diameter of induration should be carefully measured by inspection and palpation and results recorded (in millimeters) at 24-hour intervals. Areas of erythema, however, are not as important as induration and are excluded in most grading schemes unless extensive (>10 mm).

Interpretation **NORMAL FINDINGS:** No induration or erythema **CRITICAL VALUES:** A positive skin test is defined by many authorities as a diameter of induration ≥5 mm.[1] Induration of 0-4 mm is considered negative. Alternatively, a standardized grading scale, which is popular with general delayed-type hypersensitivity skin testing, may be used:[2]

- 0: no reaction
- 1+: erythema >10 mm and/or induration 1-5 mm
- 2+: induration 6-10 mm
- 3+: induration 11-20 mm
- 4+: induration >20 mm

The interpretation of a positive (or negative) skin test is so problematic that the clinical utility of fungal skin testing is significantly limited. A positive reaction indicates only that exposure to the relevant fungus has occurred at some time in the past, whether recent or remote. In addition, fungal infections are endemic in many areas of the United States, where >90% of the local population may be skin test positive following asymptomatic or subclinical infections (eg, histoplasmosis in the Ohio River Valley). Thus, in the individual patient with suspected active fungal infection, a positive skin test adds little new diagnostic information and fails to establish the fungus as the infecting agent.[1] This becomes especially relevant if the patient has ever lived in a known endemic area. In the patient with pulmonary nodules, the importance of a positive test is also unclear. Some authorities consider a positive histoplasmin test in an area of low prevalence as strong evidence for histoplasmosis.[3] Others argue that lung nodules may still be due to bronchogenic carcinoma despite a positive histoplasmin test, and skin testing adds little to clinical decision making. Similarly, a negative skin test presents major problems in interpretation. Lack of reactivity may be seen in the following situations:

- no previous fungal infection
- previous fungal infection in an immunocompromised patient
- acute systemic fungal infection, where skin test positivity is often delayed for 2-4 weeks
- waning skin test reactivity to a given fungus, as occurs in the elderly
- technical errors in antigen placement

Even the documentation of skin test conversion (ie, negative test converting to positive or serial testing) is regarded as only indirect evidence of fungal exposure In the interim and does not necessarily imply active infection. Regarding the specific fungal antigens, the derivative of *Histoplasma capsulatum* is termed histoplasmin. An older preparation of histoplasmin cross reacted frequently with *Blastomyces* and *Coccidioides* and caused a rise in complement fixation titers to *Histoplasma*. A newer histoplasmin preparation ameliorates, but does not entirely eliminate, these problems. The histoplasmin skin test may cause a spurious increase in *Histoplasma* complement fixation titers. Since the CF serologic test is clinically more useful than the histoplasmin skin test, serologies should be drawn first in suspected cases. Coccidioidomycosis skin testing shares many of the same interpretive difficulties as histoplasmosis testing, such as waning reactivity over time, delay in test positivity during acute fungal infection, and areas of high prevalence. Two preparations of *Coccidioides* antigen are available, the older coccidioidin (derived from the mycelia phase) and Spherulin® (derived from lysed spherules). Spherulin® may have superior sensitivity and has been found to be positive in 30% more cases than coccidioidin. Although testing is not useful in the individual with suspected *Coccidioides* pneumonia, it may provide prognostic information in culture proven cases. In a classic study, patients with disseminated coccidioidomycosis had a higher survival rate if their skin test was positive (75%) compared with those who tested negative (15%).[4] Patients with limited coccidioidomycosis almost always develop a positive test; failure to do so may predict impending disseminated disease.[5] Use of the coccidioidin preparation may cause false-positive histoplasmosis serologic tests, but neither Spherulin® nor coccidioidin interferes with serologic tests for coccidioidomycosis. Coccidioidal skin tests are generally positive before coccidioidal serologic tests; some clinicians use this fact to justify skin testing in acute cases (despite its limited diagnostic utility). Skin tests for blastomycosis are presently of questionable

(Continued)

Fungal Skin Testing *(Continued)*

value due to poor sensitivity and specificity, even in the study of epidemics. Fungal antigens derived from *Candida albicans* and *Trichophyton* are primarily used only for anergy testing because of high prevalence of positive skin tests in the general population.

ADDITIONAL INFORMATION: Fungal skin testing is a form of delayed hypersensitivity skin testing and as such is an assessment of cell-mediated immunity. Delayed hypersensitivity is a clinical phenomenon based on the reaction of the skin to intradermal injection of an antigen. It is a common form of immune protection against a wide range of infectious agents, including fungi. Following initial exposure to a fungus, a population of transformed T-lymphocytes is created, the so-called memory cells. When fungal antigen is introduced intradermally at a later date, these sensitized T cells are activated and initiate a cascade involving lymphokines, neutrophils, and macrophages. Clinically this is manifested by the delayed formation of significant skin induration. Delayed hypersensitivity fungal skin testing should be differentiated from immediate hypersensitivity skin testing. The former is primarily T-cell mediated and the latter is mediated by IgE mechanisms. Skin testing for common allergies to molds or fungi is carried out using the percutaneous allergy testing method (see Allergy Testing, Percutaneous) and is IgE-mediated. Similarly, skin tests for immediate hypersensitivity to *Aspergillus fumigatus* also use this method. This is commonly obtained in the evaluation of patients with suspected allergic bronchopulmonary aspergillosis.

Footnotes

1. Davies SF and Sarosi GA, "Role of Serodiagnostic Tests and Skin Tests in the Diagnosis of Fungal Disease," *Clin Chest Med*, 1987, 8:135-46.
2. Bates SE, Suen JY, and Tranum BL, "Immunological Skin Testing and Interpretation. A Plea for Uniformity," *Cancer*, 1979, 43:2306-14.
3. Ahmed AR and Blose DA, "Delayed-Type Hypersensitivity Skin Testing," *Arch Dermatol*, 1983, 119:934-45.
4. Smith CE, Whiting EG, Baker ES, et al, "The Use of Coccidioidin," *Am Rev Respir Dis*, 1948, 57:330-60.
5. Drutz D and Catanzaro A, "Coccidioidomycosis," *Am Rev Respir Dis*, 1978, 17:559-85.

Immediate Hypersensitivity Skin Test *see* Allergy Testing, Intracutaneous (Intradermal) *on page 4*

Immediate Hypersensitivity Skin Test *see* Allergy Testing, Percutaneous *on page 7*

Ingestion Challenge Test

CPT 95075

Related Information

Arthrocentesis *on page 14*

Bronchial Challenge Test *on page 215*

Synonyms Food Allergy Test; Oral Provocation Test

Abstract **PROCEDURE COMMONLY INCLUDES:** *In vivo* testing of patients with suspected food allergy. This procedure is useful in evaluating patients with a clinical history consistent with IgE-mediated hypersensitivity to specific foods. Other substances may also be tested, such as food additives (metabisulfites) and certain medications (nonsteroidal anti-inflammatory agents). The patient is asked to ingest capsules containing fixed amounts of a specific food (or food additive) and is then observed for the development of allergic symptoms. **INDICATIONS:** Ingestion challenge testing is useful in the following situations:

- clinical history typical for IgE-mediated food allergy but relevant skin prick tests are negative or nondiagnostic
- clinical history of nonspecific "food intolerances" of uncertain significance but skin tests are positive
- prior diagnosis of "food allergy" established by unknown or unproven methods

Formal testing is not required in every case of suspected food allergy; this procedure yields useful clinical information in only a limited number of situations. When the patient's clinical history is compatible with IgE-mediated food allergy and subsequent skin prick tests confirm the diagnosis, formal oral testing is probably unnecessary. Under these circumstances many clinicians would simply instruct the patient to avoid the food (or food additive) in question. If the results of this are equivocal, then ingestion challenge testing may be indicated.

CONTRAINDICATIONS:

- documented anaphylactic reaction in the past to food substance in question (eg, anaphylaxis from prior skin testing)
- inadequate medical supervision or resuscitation equipment

Patient Care/Scheduling **PATIENT PREPARATION:** In general, a patient with suspected food allergy should undergo a careful history and physical examination before any laboratory testing. Following this, if a formal oral challenge test appears indicated, the purpose, risks, and technique of this procedure should be reviewed with the patient. All foods suspected of causing allergy should be avoided prior to testing in order to simplify test interpretation. Antihistamines should also be discontinued before testing, since H_1 antagonists depress the IgE response. All such medication changes must be reviewed and approved by the physician. **AFTERCARE:** Per protocol of the individual testing center. In general, the patient is carefully observed for varying lengths of time after completion of the study, depending on the nature and severity of the allergic reaction. Rarely, complications may develop some hours after discharge from the testing center; patient should be instructed to contact a physician immediately. **COMPLICATIONS:** A number of physiologic reactions may occur as a result of a positive test. These "complications" include potentially life-threatening events such as anaphylactic shock, acute asthma, and angioedema. Other complications are less severe and include nausea, diarrhea, rhinitis, and urticaria. These complications are not unique to oral provocation testing, and are shared by other allergy tests which evaluate immediate hypersensitivity.

Method **EQUIPMENT:** Several food preparations are available for oral provocation testing. One such preparation is a gelatin capsule containing 500 mg of a single food substance. These are popular and well tolerated. Placebo capsules may also be necessary if a blinded challenge is planned. **TECHNIQUE:** Specific protocols for testing vary. Usually, the patient ingests food capsules at specific time intervals and is carefully observed by a physician for signs of allergy. Placebo capsules are included in single-blinded or double-blinded trials. If no reaction has occurred after 12 capsules, the test is terminated. If a severe allergic reaction is expected based on the clinical history, smaller doses are given at 1 hour intervals.

Interpretation **NORMAL FINDINGS:** No adverse reactions after ingestion of multiple food capsules **CRITICAL VALUES:** Test is considered positive when typical symptoms of food allergy develop shortly after administration of a specific food capsule, but not after placebo. The validity of such allergic reactions relies on the clinical judgment of the testing physician. Typical symptoms are urticaria, wheezing, angioedema, and rhinitis. Other possible symptoms include nausea, vomiting, diarrhea, and abdominal pain, which may be difficult to interpret. **ADDITIONAL INFORMATION:** The ingestion challenge test has also been used to evaluate allergy to certain drugs, particularly nonsteroidal anti-inflammatory agents. Often, bronchial provocation is used in conjunction with the oral ingestion of the medication (see Bronchial Challenge Test). In this way, bronchospasm may be objectively documented in response to the oral challenge. Much controversy surrounds the subject of food allergy in general. The medical literature is filled with various testing techniques for food intolerance, but they are often uncontrolled and anecdotal. A position paper, issued by the American College of Physicians[1], addressed the many controversies in allergy testing, including the ingestion challenge test. The information presented in this entry is in keeping with the recommendations of the American College of Physicians.

Footnotes

1. American College of Physicians, "Allergy Testing," *Ann Intern Med*, 1989, 110(4):317-20.

References

Lessof MH, Wraith DG, Merrett TG, et al, "Food Allergy and Intolerance in 100 Patients – Local and Systemic Effects," *Q J Med*, 1980, 195:259-71.

Metcalfe DD, "Diagnostic Procedures for Immunologically-Mediated Food Sensitivity," *Nutr Rev*, 1984, 42:92-7.

(Continued)

Ingestion Challenge Test *(Continued)*

Van Arsdel PP and Larson EB, "Diagnostic Tests for Patients With Suspected Allergic Disease. Utility and Limitations," *Ann Intern Med*, 1989, 110(4):304-12.

Intracutaneous (Intradermal) Allergy Testing *see* Allergy Testing, Intracutaneous (Intradermal) *on page 4*

Joint Tap *see* Arthrocentesis *on page 14*

Labial Salivary Gland Biopsy

CPT 42405

Synonyms Lower Lip Biopsy for Sjögren's Syndrome; LSG Biopsy; Minor Salivary Gland Biopsy

Abstract **PROCEDURE COMMONLY INCLUDES:** Incisional biopsy of the minor salivary glands in the lower lip. This procedure is carried out by a surgeon in an ambulatory care setting, using local anesthesia only. It is a safe but invasive means of confirming the diagnosis of Sjögren's syndrome. **INDICATIONS:** Labial salivary gland (LSG) biopsy is useful in selected cases of Sjögren's syndrome (keratoconjunctivitis sicca), especially when the diagnosis remains in doubt. Biopsy is indicated when histologic confirmation of salivary gland involvement is necessary for clinical management. **CONTRAINDICATIONS:**

- patient refusal
- severe coagulopathy (thrombocytopenia, elevated PT/PTT)
- systemic anticoagulation (eg, heparin, warfarin)
- hypersensitivity to lidocaine or epinephrine
- local infection, mouth ulcers (relative contraindications)

Patient Care/Scheduling **PATIENT PREPARATION:** Procedure and possible complications are discussed in detail with patient and informed consent is obtained. The details of scheduling (date of procedure, time, location, etc) are handled by the surgical team following a formal evaluation. All aspirin and aspirin-containing products should be discontinued 5-7 days prior to procedure; nonsteroidal anti-inflammatory agents should also be held at least 2-3 days beforehand. Routine patient medications may be taken on the morning of surgery. If a bleeding disorder is suspected, obtain a complete blood count, PT, and PTT. **AFTERCARE:** As per surgical team recommendations. In general, solid foods are avoided for several hours postprocedure. The patient should be instructed to contact surgeon or primary physician promptly if complications arise. A follow-up visit is usually arranged by the surgical team. **COMPLICATIONS:** LSG biopsy is considered a very safe procedure. Reported complications include:

- persistent numbness in the lower lip, at the incision site; this may occur if small sensory branches are severed during incision or, less commonly, dissection. This complication has been associated with the use of older surgical techniques, which include the blind "punch biopsy" (skin trephine technique), where a core of labial tissue was removed; elliptical incisions with removal of nearly all tissue above the orbicularis oris; and labial midline biopsies. With newer surgical approaches, the incidence of lip numbness is estimated at <1%.
- excessive bleeding at the biopsy site. This is an unusual complication and associated more with earlier surgical techniques, such as palatal biopsy.
- local discomfort, seen in the majority of patients, usually resolving in 24-48 hours.

Method **TECHNIQUE:** As previously mentioned, a variety of surgical techniques may be employed; only recent techniques will be described. The procedure is carried out on an alert patient, seated comfortably in a dental chair. The lower lip is anesthetized using lidocaine with epinephrine, then everted. Only areas of normal mucosa are suitable for biopsy. Daniels (1984) advocates making a single horizontal incision approximately 2 cm long between the midline and commissure. Following this, blunt dissection is carried out to free the salivary glands from the surrounding fascia. This technique allows direct visualization of sensory nerves, which are then easily avoided. At least five glands should be removed; due to their small size, histologic findings (eg, lymphocytic infiltration) may not be present in all glands.

Specimen At least five salivary glands. Tissue processing is supervised by the surgical staff. Routine histologic processing is sufficient in most cases; electron microscopy, microbiological culture, and cytology may be obtained at physician discretion.

Interpretation **NORMAL FINDINGS:** General histopathology and degree of glandular inflammation is determined by a pathologist. There is some disagreement in the rheumatologic literature concerning the precise pathologic criteria for Sjögren's syndrome. The "focus scoring method" is the most widely accepted method of interpretation and involves semiquantitative grading of salivary gland inflammation. Based on the early work of Chisholm and Mason (1968), more than one focus of lymphocytes/4 mm^2 of minor salivary gland tissue accurately distinguishes Sjögren's syndrome from normal controls. A focus of lymphocytes has been defined as an aggregate of 50 or more round cells. Focus score of 0 or 1 is normal. Scattered foci of lymphocytes may still yield a focus score of 0-1 if the number of lymphocytes in a given focus is small (<50 cells), or foci are widely spaced (>4 mm^2 of gland). Background glandular tissue must be normal as well. **CRITICAL VALUES:** A focus score >1 is consistent with Sjögren's syndrome. In other words, two or more focal aggregates of lymphocytes (>50 cells each) are seen consistently in most glands of the specimen. It is important that normal-appearing acini are found adjacent to lymphocyte aggregates. Salivary glands which show evidence of duct obstruction or nonspecific injury must be excluded from analysis. **LIMITATIONS:** Authorities disagree over the optimal histologic criteria for diagnosing Sjögren's syndrome. The focus scoring method is only one of several interpretive schemes. False-positive results have been reported if the biopsy is taken in an area of chronic mucosal inflammation, such as lichen planus, repeated trauma, mucocele, etc. Potential sampling bias may occur if small number of glands are obtained. The procedure establishes the presence of the salivary component of Sjögren's syndrome only, not the ocular component. **ADDITIONAL INFORMATION:** The diagnosis of xerostomia is difficult, if not impossible, to make on the basis of clinical grounds alone. The sensation of dry mouth is highly subjective and variable; physical examination of the parotid region and oral mucosa is often normal in Sjögren's syndrome. The diagnosis of primary Sjögren's syndrome is particularly problematic, since by definition no other connective tissue disease is present, and the clinician must rely on symptoms of dry mouth and dry eyes. Xerostomia has been criticized as a poor diagnostic criterion due to subjectivity and lack of specificity (xerostomia is commonly seen as a medication side effect). LSG biopsy is a well accepted, low-risk procedure for objectively confirming oral involvement. However, other diagnostic procedures have been introduced to assess salivary Sjögren's involvement. These less invasive techniques include:

- parotid salivary flow rate, measured with Carlson-Crittenden cups positioned over the parotid ducts (specificity is low and correlation of flow rate with subjective symptoms is poor)
- secretory sialography; contrast dye is injected into the orifice of the parotid duct
- salivary scintigraphy with ^{99m}Tc pertechnetate scanning
- sialochemical studies

To date, no clinical trials comparing these various techniques directly have been performed. Before performing a LSG biopsy, the appropriateness of alternative techniques should be considered on a case-to-case basis.

References

Daniels TE, "Labial Salivary Gland Biopsy in Sjögren's Syndrome," *Arthritis Rheum*, 1984, 27:147-56.

Daniels TE, "Salivary Histopathology in Diagnosis of Sjögren's Syndrome," *Scand J Rheumatol Suppl*, 1986, 61:36-43.

Segerberg-Konttinen M, "Focus Score in Sialolithiasis," *Scand J Rheumatol*, 1988, 17:87-9.

Talal N, "Sjögren's Syndrome and Connective Tissue Diseases Associated With Other Immunologic Disorders," *Arthritis and Allied Conditions: A Textbook of Rheumatology.*, 11th ed, Chapter 76, McCarty DJ, ed, Philadelphia, PA: Lea & Febiger, 1197-213.

Lower Lip Biopsy for Sjögren's Syndrome *see* Labial Salivary Gland Biopsy *on previous page*

LSG Biopsy *see* Labial Salivary Gland Biopsy *on previous page*

Mantoux Test *see* Tuberculin Skin Testing, Intracutaneous *on page 33*

Minor Salivary Gland Biopsy *see* Labial Salivary Gland Biopsy *on previous page*

Nailfold Capillaroscopy *see* Widefield Capillary Microscopy *on page 36*

Nailfold Capillary Microscopy *see* Widefield Capillary Microscopy *on page 36*

Nasal Endoscopy

CPT 31250

Synonyms Rhinolaryngoscopy; Rhinopharyngoscopy

Abstract **PROCEDURE COMMONLY INCLUDES:** Direct examination of the nasal passages, nasopharynx, oropharynx, and larynx by means of a flexible fiberoptic endoscope. This procedure permits visualization of upper airway structures inaccessible to the conventional otoscope or nasal speculum. Nasal endoscopy is carried out by an allergist or otolaryngologist in an outpatient setting. It is a safe and rapid (10-15 minutes) means of evaluating complicated upper airway and sinus disorders, particularly those refractory to standard medical therapy. **INDICATIONS:** The precise role of nasal endoscopy in clinical practice is still evolving. Although it has been applied to a wide variety of clinical situations, some experts warn against its indiscriminate use. Clearly, not every patient who presents with symptoms referable to the nasopharynx need undergo endoscopy.

General indications for this procedure are:

- upper airway disease of unclear etiology
- chronic or recurrent upper airway disease, despite appropriate therapy

Specific indications for nasal endoscopy include:

- suspected nasal polyposis (or when polyps are seen on speculum exam); to confirm the diagnosis, assess extent of disease, check response to treatment, and screen for recurrence after polypectomy
- chronic or recurrent sinusitis; purulent material may be visualized directly and the source located (sphenoid, maxillary, ethmoid ostia)
- persistent nasal obstruction, not due to septal deviation and not responding to decongestants
- chronic nasal discharge of unknown etiology, especially if unilateral (ie, undiagnosed nonallergic rhinitis)
- anosmia
- recurrent epistaxis or serosanguineous nasal discharge
- persistent hoarseness
- chronic use of steroid nasal sprays for perennial rhinitis, especially after several years of therapy
- suspected cases of adenoidal hypertrophy (eg, young child with sleep apnea)
- suspected cases of eustachian tube obstruction (eg, child with recurrent otitis after tympanic tubes placed)
- evaluation of "pseudoasthma," where stridor and wheezing are due to vocal cord apposition and not bronchospasm (possibly psychiatric in origin)
- suspected nasopharyngeal carcinoma (persistent pain, history of cigarette use, Oriental ancestry, etc)
- suspected nasopharyngeal candidiasis in an immunocompromised patient even if conventional examination reveals a normal oropharynx
- postoperative evaluation of upper airway surgical sites
- evaluation of patients with known or suspected granulomatous disease (sarcoidosis, Wegener's disease), to rule out upper airway granulomas or ulcerations in selected cases

Emergency indications include:

- suspected epiglottitis
- laryngeal trauma
- difficult endotracheal intubations, to provide direct visualization for tube placement
- stridor, to rule out foreign body (diagnosis only)

Nasal endoscopy is less useful in:

- uncomplicated allergic rhinitis; procedure is generally not required to establish this diagnosis
- random screening for nasal polyps in asymptomatic patients or patients with simple allergic rhinitis

CONTRAINDICATIONS: The procedure is contraindicated when a severe, uncontrolled coagulopathy is present. Mucosal trauma is always a possibility (although unusual) and local tamponade of bleeding sites is difficult. In addition, the sphenopalatine artery lies in the posterior nares, and trauma to this vessel may cause serious arterial hemorrhage. Since nasal endoscopy may theoretically induce cardiac arrhythmias or vasovagal syncope, it is contraindicated in the patient with a tenuous cardiopulmonary status. However, serious morbidity or mortality of this nature has yet to be reported.

Patient Care/Scheduling **PATIENT PREPARATION:** Technique and risks of the procedure are discussed with the patient and verbal consent is obtained. (Some experts consider this procedure an extension of the clinical examination and do not obtain formal written consent.) Nasal endoscopy is generally performed as an elective, outpatient procedure with scheduling issues handled by the allergist or otolaryngologist. Often, endoscopy is carried out during the initial visit to the allergist's office, at physician's discretion. The patient need not be fasting prior to procedure. Routine medications may be taken the morning of endoscopy. Some endoscopists will require the patient to discontinue aspirin products and nonsteroidal anti-inflammatory agents several days beforehand, especially if significant epistaxis is anticipated. Premedication with sedatives is not usually required. **AFTERCARE:** Food and water should be avoided until gag reflex returns (gag may be depressed by Xylocaine® solution or spray), otherwise; no specific postprocedure restrictions are necessary. **COMPLICATIONS:** Nasal endoscopy appears to be a very safe procedure. Rohr (1983) reported no complications out of 230 rhinopharyngoscopies. A similar safety profile was documented by Selner (1985) with a single nosebleed (mild) out of 400 examinations. Transient complications include coughing, sneezing, and nasal comfort, resolving soon after termination of the procedure. Potential complications include:

- epistaxis
- nasal discomfort (<5%)
- bronchospasm
- laryngospasm (avoided by keeping the instrument above the vocal cords)
- syncope/arrhythmias

Method **EQUIPMENT:** A number of fiberoptic nasal endoscopes are available, either rigid or flexible. Currently, the flexible endoscope is the preferred instrument due to its superior safety profile, patient acceptance, and technical convenience. The flexible endoscope is usually 300 mm in length, with a diameter of 3.7-4 mm; deflection angle of the tip is 90° down and 130° up. The rhinolaryngoscope is connected with a cold light source. In some centers, the instrument is part of a camera-mount-cine system, with video camera, monitor, and recorder suspended from the ceiling. The physician views the images on a standard video monitor, which also provides a permanent audiovisual record of the examination. **TECHNIQUE:** At the beginning of the procedure, the patient is comfortably seated in a standard examination chair equipped with head supports. A standard nasal speculum exam is performed. Following this a 4:1 mixture of 4% lidocaine and 1:1000 epinephrine is aerosolized into the nasopharynx. Alternatively, a 4% cocaine aerosol may be used as a topical anesthetic agent and vasoconstrictor. If a detailed examination of the hypopharynx is planned, some physicians will have the patient gargle with a Xylocaine® solution. Others, however, feel this is unnecessary and avoid this step due to frequent patient discomfort. Additional anesthetic effect may be obtained using 2% viscous lidocaine applied directly to the turbinates with a cotton swab. After 3-5 minutes, the examiner guides the endoscope into the nostril, where the septum and turbinates may be clearly seen. The sinus orifices may also be examined for signs of inflammation or discharge. After the nasal fossa examination is completed, the tip of the endoscope is advanced through the choana and into the nasopharyngeal cavity. A number of important structures are visualized, such as the eustachian tube orifice, Rosenmueller's fossa, and adenoids. The patient may be asked to swallow several times to confirm the location of the eustachian tube orifice. Following inspection of the inferior portion of the oropharynx, the instrument is advanced into the hypopharynx. Here, structures such as the lingular tonsil, posterior tongue, piriform sinuses, and epiglottis are visualized. The vocal cords are easily seen and vocal cord function is assessed with the patient phonating. In general, the endoscope is not passed through the vocal cords, thus avoiding bronchospasm. Anatomy can be reviewed as the instrument is withdrawn. The procedure is then repeated through the other nostril.

Interpretation **NORMAL FINDINGS:** No abnormalities seen. A preliminary written report is completed immediately after procedure. **CRITICAL VALUES:** Numerous findings of clinical

(Continued)

Nasal Endoscopy *(Continued)*

Clinical Findings on 400 Consecutive Nasal Endoscopies

Nose		
Concha (turbinates)	28	Clefting conchal sinus, polypoidal changes, bullosa, papillary hyperplasia, fibromatous hypertrophy, telangiectasia, atrophy
Septum	42	Deviation, perforation, spurs
Polyps	51	
Inflammatory mucosa	23	Mucous pus, hypertrophy, cystic changes, mucocele, vessel injection, inflammation of ostea of sphenoethmoidal recess, edema
Nasopharynx and Superior Pharynx		
Adenoids	63	
Eustachian orifice	5	Torus cyst, lymphoid inclusion, adenoid enchroachment
Inflammation — edema	7	Vessel injection, ulceration
Pharyngeal wall	17	Osteophyte, aneurysm, lymphoid hypertrophy
Other	4	Rathke pouch cyst, cystic lymphoid involution
Inferior Pharynx–Hypopharynx–Larynx		
Lingular tonsils	28	Significant enlargement
Post tongue	2	Circumvallate papillary cyst
Vallecula	6	Cystic changes, papillomata
Epiglottis	15	Mucocele, inflammation, displacement, petiole prominence
Glottis	24	Erythema, displacement
Vocal cord	23	Polyp papillomata, contact ulceration, paralysis, granuloma, web
Arytenoids	6	Contact ulcer, asymmetry, edema
Other	10	Laryngocele (2), cord trauma (3), inflammatory granuloma (2), paralysis (3)

Reproduced with permission from Selner JC and Koepke JW, "Rhinolaryngoscopy in the Allergy Office," *Ann Allergy*, 1985, 54:480.

significance may be encountered, including anatomic abnormalities (polyps, hyperplasia, ulcers, carcinoma, cysts), inflammation, edema, and infections. Selner (1985) outlined his findings in 400 consecutive rhinolaryngoscopies in the previous table. **LIMITATIONS:** Rhinopharyngoscopes do not permit biopsy of suspicious lesions or therapeutic interventions (eg, electrocautery) **ADDITIONAL INFORMATION:** Conventional examination of the upper airways consists of otoscopic evaluation with a nasal speculum. This visualizes only 2.5 cm of the nasal passage due to a short focal length, which leaves significant areas (>11 cm) of the nasopharynx unexamined. Nasal endoscopy allows rapid examination of these areas. The figure on the following page depicts the areas of the upper respiratory tract which are difficult to examine using conventional techniques (eg, otoscope, nasal speculum).

References

Rohr A, Hassner A, and Saxon A, "Rhinopharyngoscopy for the Evaluation of Allergic-Immunologic Disorders," *Ann Allergy*, 1983, 50:380-4.

Schumacher MJ, "Fiberoptic Nasopharyngolaryngoscopy: A Procedure for Allergists?" *J Allergy Clin Immunol*, 1988, 81(5 Pt 2):960-2.

Selner JC and Koepke JW, "Rhinolaryngoscopy in the Allergy Office," *Ann Allergy*, 1985, 54:479-82.

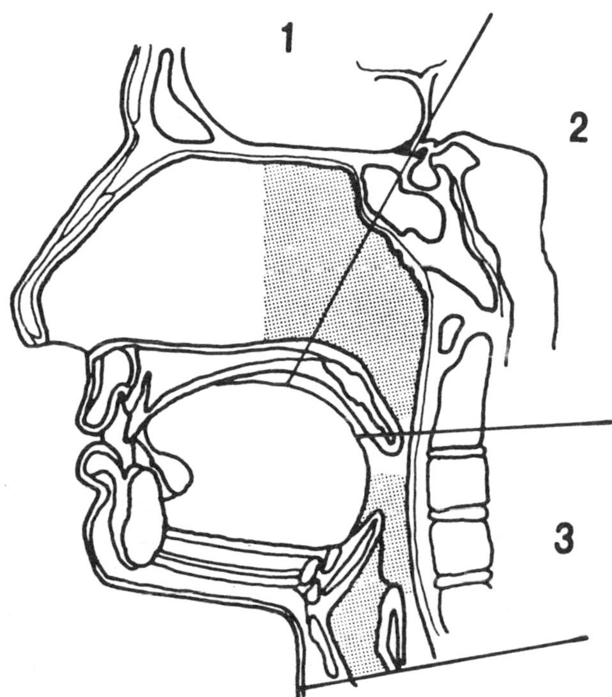

Reproduced with permission from Selner JC and Koepke JW, "Rhinolaryngoscopy in the Allergy Office," *Ann Allergy,* 1985, 54:480.

Patch Test

CPT 95040 (patch or application tests (up to 10 tests)); 95041 (11-20 tests); 95042 (21-30 tests); 95043 (more than 30 tests)

Synonyms Contact Dermatitis Skin Test; Epicutaneous Patch Test

Abstract PROCEDURE COMMONLY INCLUDES: Application of multiple test materials to the skin surface in order to demonstrate allergic contact dermatitis (ACD). Suspected allergens are taped in rows onto the patient's back and the underlying skin is examined 48 hours later for erythema, signifying delayed-type hypersensitivity. INDICATIONS: In general, this procedure is used diagnostically to identify causes of ACD.

The patch test is most useful in the following situations:

- confirming the diagnosis of ACD already suspected from history and physical exam
- determining the individual allergen causing ACD when many are suspected
- exploring causes of chronic dermatitis unresponsive to usual therapies
- excluding the presence of ACD in complicated dermatological cases (by means of negative patch testing)

CONTRAINDICATIONS: Patch testing with a substance previously implicated in an anaphylactic reaction in a particular patient represents a relative contraindication; physician supervision is necessary.

Patient Care/Scheduling PATIENT PREPARATION: No special skin preparation is required. Whenever possible, patient should bring additional suspected allergens (eg, personal cosmetics) to the testing area for physician review. AFTERCARE: The following instructions should be given to the patient. Patch test sites must be kept dry initially. Heavy exercise is not permitted in order to avoid excess perspiration. Any test material causing severe pruritus or pain must be removed promptly and the physician notified. On the evening

(Continued)

Patch Test *(Continued)*

prior to follow-up appointment, patch tests should be entirely removed by the patient and discarded. Following this, bathing is permissible but vigorous rubbing of test sites should be avoided. **SPECIAL INSTRUCTIONS:** Patch testing requires large areas of normal appearing skin. Thus, patients with known pre-existing dermatitis must undergo careful skin examination prior to patch testing. **COMPLICATIONS:** Adverse reactions may be broadly divided into two categories, nonimmunologic and immunologic (allergic) reactions. The "irritant skin reaction" is considered nonimmunologic; certain materials may be intrinsically damaging to the skin, causing an early onset, painful, macular dermatitis. Another nonimmunologic complication is bacterial or viral infection involving strongly reacting test sites. Adverse reactions which are immunologic are mediated by either immediate or delayed hypersensitivity mechanisms. Contact urticaria is possible within minutes of applying the standard test battery, but is unusual. Rarely, immediate life-threatening anaphylaxis has been reported but this appears most often associated with patch testing drugs and not with commercial test materials. Examples of delayed hypersensitivity complications include the following:

- severe skin reactions (pustules, necrosis) when an allergen causes a flare of underlying contact dermatitis
- persistent positive reactions
- active sensitization to a test material, ie, ACD may actually be induced by a test substance (incidence unclear)

Overall, however, the incidence of all complications is low and serious complications are reportable.

Method **EQUIPMENT:** Patch test materials are standardized and available commercially. Test allergens are available as a standardized battery consisting of approximately 30 items (benzocaine, neomycin, fragrance mix, wood alcohols, etc). Additional allergen batteries are available for specific occupations such as printers, hairdressers, or medical practitioners. Delivery systems are also standardized and several are available. Commonly, an aluminum cup or round cellulose disk is used to affix each test allergen to the surface of the skin. An ultraviolet marking pen or gentian violet is required to label test sites. **TECHNIQUE:** Testing is performed on normal appearing skin. The patient's back is premarked in vertical rows using a fluorescent pen. A small amount of test allergen is applied to the disk (or aluminum cup) and affixed to the skin with nonallergenic tape. Patches remain in place 48 hours and are then removed by the patient. Tape irritation is allowed to resolve for 12-24 hours. Skin response is recorded by the physician by means of a graded scoring system at 24 and 48 hours after patch removal. Certain substances require additional readings at 72 hours (eg, neomycin). The previous steps are only guidelines and subject to physician modification.

Interpretation **NORMAL FINDINGS:** The skin underlying each test substance is examined and graded. Normal skin is graded "–". **CRITICAL VALUES:** Several grading schemes for evaluating positive skin reactions have been proposed. One popular scheme is as follows:[1]

+ = weak positive (faint erythema, no vesicles)
++ = strong positive (vesicles, edema, papules)
+++ = extreme positive (spreading, bullous)
? = doubtful reaction
IR = irritant reaction

The physician must distinguish primary irritant skin reactions (ie, chemical burns) from true allergic reactions. The former tend to occur early and diminish over days and are more painful, demarcated, and erosive.

LIMITATIONS: Spurious results from patch testing are well acknowledged in the literature and represent a major clinical challenge. False-positive rates are significant, the most common cause being the use of excessively high concentrations of test material. Other false-positives include misinterpretation of irritant reactions, misinterpretation of contact urticaria, and the so-called "angry back" syndrome (generalized erythema of the entire back). False-negative results are often related to technical errors in allergen placement, concentration, or timing of readings. In some instances, false-negative results stem from the failure to mimic real-life conditions at the workplace; factors such as perspiration and friction are not considered routinely. **ADDITIONAL INFORMATION:** The economic and social consequences of contact dermatitis are significant. Forty percent to 60% of occupational absenteeism is attributed to some form of contact dermatitis.[2] Patch testing evaluates delayed-type hypersensitivity to various allergens by means of classic type IV immunologic reaction (helper T-lymphocyte mediated). Given this, patch testing does not evaluate either immediate hypersensitivity reactions (contact urticaria) or irritant dermatitis. At present, patch testing is the only objective means of establishing ACD. In practicality, frequency of patch testing varies considerably among physicians; some rarely patch test while others routinely test any patient with eczema. It should be noted that the physician's history and physical exam alone is often inadequate in pinpointing even the more common etiologies of ACD.[3] Thus, despite its limitations, patch testing remains an indispensable tool.

Footnotes

1. Fregert S, *Manual of Contact Dermatitis*, 2nd ed, Copenhagen: Munksgaard, 1981.
2. Johnson MLT, Burdick AE, Johnson KG, et al, "Prevalence, Morbidity, and Cost of Dermatological Diseases," *J Invest Dermatol*, 1979, 73:395-401.
3. Kieffer M, "Nickel Sensitivity: Relationship Between History and Patch Test Reaction," *Contact Dermatitis*, 1979, 5:398.

References

Adams RM, "Patch Testing – A Recapitulation," *J Am Acad Dermatol*, 1981, 5:629-43.

Fischer T and Maibach HI, "Patch Testing in Allergic Contact Dermatitis: An Update," *Semin Dermatol*, 1986, 5:214-24.

Fransway AF, "Epicutaneous Patch Testing: Current Trends and Controversial Topics," *Mayo Clin Proc*, 1989, 64(4):415-23.

Maibach HI, Epstein E, and Lahti A, "Contact Skin Allergy," *Allergy Principles & Practice*, 3rd ed, Middleton E Jr, Reed CE, Ellis E, et al, eds, St Louis, MO: CV Mosby Co, 1988, 1429-63.

Young E and Houwing RH, "Patch Test Results With Standard Allergens Over a Decade," *Contact Dermatitis*, 1987, 17:104-7.

Penicillin Allergy Skin Testing

CPT 95005 (percutaneous tests with antibiotics); 95014 (intracutaneous tests with antibiotics)

Related Information

Allergy Testing, Intracutaneous (Intradermal) *on page 4*

Allergy Testing, Percutaneous *on page 7*

Synonyms Penicillin Skin Tests; Skin Tests for Penicillin Allergy

Abstract **PROCEDURE COMMONLY INCLUDES:** Skin testing patients with suspected IgE-mediated penicillin allergy. The reagents used in this procedure are derivatives of the basic benzylpenicillin molecule. They are introduced into the epidermis by a skin prick or into the dermis by an intracutaneous (intradermal) injection. An immediate wheal-and-flare reaction confirms immediate hypersensitivity (Gell and Coombs' type I reaction). This is an important procedure in clinical practice and accurately identifies those individuals at high risk for a severe allergic reaction to penicillin. **INDICATIONS:** Theoretically, all patients about to receive a beta-lactam antibiotic should be skin tested. However, Adkinson[1] demonstrated that such a comprehensive testing policy has a low yield and is not cost-effective. Most authorities recommend skin testing in the following situations:

- patients with a history of penicillin allergy who require penicillin as the drug of choice (eg, treatment of central nervous system syphilis)
- patients with a history of penicillin allergy who require a beta-lactam antibiotic (eg, semisynthetic penicillin, cephalosporin)
- patients with a history of multiple "antibiotic allergies;" skin testing can determine if a beta-lactam drug is a safe treatment option

CONTRAINDICATIONS:

- documented history of penicillin-induced anaphylaxis, Stevens-Johnson syndrome, exfoliative dermatitis, or status asthmaticus. These conditions are life-threatening and contraindicate the use of penicillins in general; thus, there is little need to skin test.
- recent use of medications known to inhibit the IgE-mediated skin response (wheal and flare); this includes antihistamines, hydroxyzine, tricyclic antidepressants, and phenothiazines.

(Continued)

Penicillin Allergy Skin Testing *(Continued)*

Patient Care/Scheduling **PATIENT PREPARATION:** In some medical centers, penicillin skin testing is permitted only after formal consultation with the allergist performing the procedure. If the procedure appears necessary, the technique, risks, and benefits should be explained to the patient. As a preliminary screening measure, the physician should perform a brief dermatologic exam to ensure adequate areas of normal-appearing skin and to identify the rare patient with dermographism. Patient should be instructed to discontinue the following medications several days prior to testing: antihistamines, tricyclic antidepressants, hydroxyzine, phenothiazines. Newer antihistamines with extended half-lives may interfere with testing for over 1 week. All medication changes should be approved by the primary physician. **AFTERCARE:** If no complications have occurred, the patient may be discharged from the testing center following completion of the test. Skin sites should be kept clean but remain uncovered. Physician should be contacted immediately if symptoms of wheezing, lightheadedness, or shortness of breath develop several hours later (the unusual case of the "late phase response"). **SPECIAL INSTRUCTIONS:** If skin testing is performed by a nurse or physician-assistant, a physician should be immediately available for the rare case of anaphylactic shock. Emergency equipment must be in the testing area, including defibrillation equipment, intubation blades, lidocaine (and other cardiac medications), aqueous epinephrine for injection needles, syringes, and tourniquets. **COMPLICATIONS:** When properly performed, serious adverse reactions are unusual. The incidence of systemic reactions has been estimated at <1%, with the majority of these being mild or self-limited. Local complications are more common, but generally resolve within hours. These include subcutaneous hemorrhage, localized pruritus, and nonspecific irritant reactions. The risk of hepatitis B, local infection, or human immunodeficiency virus (HIV) transmission is diminishingly small since needles are not reused between patients. The "late response" is a rare but reported complication of allergy skin testing (see Allergy Testing, Intracutaneous (Intradermal)).

Method **EQUIPMENT:** The reagents used for skin testing include:

- The "major determinant," a derivative of the benzylpenicillin molecule called benzylpenicillin-polylysine. It is standardized, commercially available, and routinely used.
- The "minor determinant mixture (MDM)," either benzylpenicillin itself or another derivative (such as penicilloate or penicilloyl-amine). The MDM has not yet been standardized and is not commercially available. Nonetheless, the MDM is widely employed by many allergists and is clinically relevant.

Both the major and minor determinants are administered in most cases. If the major determinant is used alone, 10% to 25% of allergic individuals could be missed. If the minor determinant is used alone, perhaps 5% to 10% of cases could remain undetected, including potential cases of anaphylaxis. In addition to these two reagents, positive (histamine) and negative (diluent) controls are often given. Standard tuberculin syringes, 27-gauge needles, and prick test equipment are also needed.

TECHNIQUE: Ideally, skin test reagents are applied first by the prick test, followed by an intradermal test if the prick test is negative. The prick test is carried out by placing a drop of the reagent in a predetermined location on the skin, usually the forearm. A small needle is passed through the drop and into the epidermis, then removed. (For details, see Allergy Testing, Percutaneous.) For intracutaneous testing, each reagent is individually drawn up into a tuberculin syringe. Again, the volar aspect of the forearm is the preferred site for testing. The reagent (or control) is injected into the dermis, using a 27-gauge needle. A small bleb is raised, usually 0.01-0.02 mL. (For details, see Allergy Testing, Intracutaneous (Intradermal.)) **DATA ACQUIRED:** Test sites are examined at 15-20 minutes for a local wheal-and-flare reaction. The largest diameter of the wheal and/or erythema is measured and recorded in millimeters.

Interpretation **NORMAL FINDINGS:** No wheal or erythema after the major determinant, minor determinant, and diluent control. Administration of histamine control should result in a positive skin reaction, with induration >5 mm diameter. **CRITICAL VALUES:** For both the prick test and the intracutaneous test, a wheal >5 mm in diameter (with erythema) is considered a positive test. For proper interpretation, the patient should be questioned regarding a history of penicillin allergy. If a reasonable history of penicillin allergy is obtained, a negative skin test essentially rules out a life-threatening allergic response to therapeutic doses of penicillin. No cases of anaphylaxis have been reported in patients who are skin test negative. However, ≤3% of patients who are skin test negative may develop minor reactions while on therapy, such as rash and pruritus. In the patient who has a positive skin test and a positive history of penicillin allergy, the odds of a serious allergic reaction to penicillin therapy are quite high, perhaps 50% to 70%. If skin tests are administered to patients who provide no history of penicillin allergy, the chances of a positive test are low (about 2%). Unfortunately, anaphylaxis during penicillin therapy has been reported in this patient population, although rare. Skin testing all patients prior to beta-lactam therapy, with or without a history of penicillin allergy, is not practical or cost-effective. **LIMITATIONS:**

- This procedure detects only IgE-mediated allergic reactions. Thus, a variety of adverse drug reactions may still occur in skin test negative patients, including serum sickness, drug fever, antibiotic associated colitis, interstitial nephritis, contact dermatitis, bone marrow suppression, and others.
- A number of factors can cause false-positive and false-negative results, as seen in other forms of skin testing (see Allergy Testing, Intracutaneous, (Intradermal)).
- Test results apply to penicillin-type antibiotics (natural penicillins, semisynthetic penicillins), but not to cephalosporins, aztreonam, or imipenem.

Footnotes

1. Adkinson NF, Spence M, and Wheeler B, "Randomized Clinical Trial of Routine Penicillin Skin Testing (Abstract)," *J Allergy Clin Immunol*, 1984, 73:163.

References

Sarti W, "Routine Use of Skin Testing for Immediate Penicillin Allergy to 6764 Patients in an Outpatient Clinic," *Ann Allergy*, 1985, 55:157-61.

Van Arsdel PP, Martonick GJ, Johnson LE, et al, "The Value of Skin Testing for Penicillin Allergy Diagnosis," *West J Med*, 1986, 144:311-4.

Weiss ME and Adkinson NF, "Beta-lactam Allergy," *Principles and Practice of Infectious Diseases*, 3rd ed, Chapter 21, Mandell GL, Douglas RG, and Bennett JE, eds, New York, NY: Church Livingstone, 1990, 264-9.

Weiss ME and Adkinson NF, "Immediate Hypersensitivity Reactions to Penicillin and Related Antibiotics," *Clin Allergy*, 1988, 18(6):515-40.

Penicillin Skin Tests *see* Penicillin Allergy Skin Testing *on page 29*

Percutaneous Allergy Testing *see* Allergy Testing, Percutaneous *on page 7*

PPD Test *see* Tuberculin Skin Testing, Intracutaneous *on page 33*

Prick Test *see* Allergy Testing, Percutaneous *on page 7*

Prong Test *see* Tuberculin Skin Testing, Multiple Puncture *on page 35*

Puncture Test *see* Allergy Testing, Percutaneous *on page 7*

Purified Protein Derivative (PPD) Test *see* Tuberculin Skin Testing, Intracutaneous *on page 33*

Rhinolaryngoscopy *see* Nasal Endoscopy *on page 24*

Rhinopharyngoscopy *see* Nasal Endoscopy *on page 24*

Schirmer 1 Test *see* Schirmer Test *on this page*

Schirmer 2 Test *see* Schirmer Test *on this page*

Schirmer Test

CPT 92499 (unlisted ophthalmological procedure)

Synonyms Schirmer 1 Test; Schirmer 2 Test

Abstract **PROCEDURE COMMONLY INCLUDES:** *In vivo* measurement of total tear production, both basal and reflex tear output. A strip of filter paper is placed in the lower conjunctival sac. After 5 minutes, the amount of moisture on the paper is determined and compared against normal values. Although the technique is somewhat crude, this is a simple and well-established means of assessing the patient with "dry eyes". **INDICATIONS:**

- evaluation of the patient with suspected Sjögren's syndrome in order to confirm decreased tear secretion objectively

(Continued)

Schirmer Test *(Continued)*

- evaluation of the "dry eye" syndrome, which encompasses a wide variety of conditions (medications, autoimmune diseases, chronic blepharoconjunctivitis, allergies, etc)

CONTRAINDICATIONS: None reported.

Patient Care/Scheduling **PATIENT PREPARATION:** Patient may take routine oral medications on the day of examination but the specific drugs should be recorded in the chart. "Artificial tears" eye drops (or similar ophthalmics) should be discontinued prior to procedure. **AFTERCARE:** Patient may resume previous activity level.

Method **EQUIPMENT:** Standardized filter paper strips are available for Schirmer testing (eg, Whatman No 41, Berens and Halberg filter strips, and others). **TECHNIQUE:** As noted by Mackie and Seal (1980), the Schirmer test has been performed in a variety of ways, leading to some confusion. In the Schirmer 1 test, the patient is seated in a well-lit room. The 5 mm top end of the filter paper is folded back and placed in the lower palpebral conjunctival sac. Most experts prefer an open-end technique. After 5 minutes, the paper is removed and the length of filter paper moistened (in millimeters) is recorded. In the basal secretion test, topical anesthetic eye drops are placed in the conjunctival sac. After the anesthetic has taken effect, the Schirmer 1 test is repeated with the room somewhat darkened. (Note that some authorities call this the "Schirmer 2" test, adding to the confusion.) In the Schirmer 2 test, anesthetic eye drops are again instilled in the conjunctival sac. Filter paper strips are positioned as before, then a cotton swab is inserted high into the nasal passage. By irritating the nasal mucosa, reflex tear secretion is theoretically stimulated.

Interpretation **NORMAL FINDINGS:**

- Schirmer 1 test: 10-30 mm of filter paper moistened
- basal secretion test: >8 mm of filter paper moistened
- Schirmer 2 test: >15 mm of filter paper moistened

CRITICAL VALUES:

- Schirmer 1 test: <10 mm of filter paper moistened is considered abnormal; <5 mm is consistent with Sjögren's syndrome; this test measures abnormalities in both reflex and/or basal secretions
- basal secretion test: <8 mm; suggests impaired basic tear secretion
- Schirmer 2 test: <15 mm; suggests impaired reflex tear secretion

LIMITATIONS: Although test results are quantitative, technique is relatively crude. It offers only a rough approximation of total tear production. Other more sensitive and specific tests are available, such as fluorescein dye staining, Rose Bengal staining, and biomicroscopy. Variations in test technique may complicate interpretation. Test is unreliable in evaluating the moderately dry eye. Its greatest utility lies in distinguishing the normal from the severely dry eye. The ability of this test to separate basal from reflex tear secretion has been disputed. **ADDITIONAL INFORMATION:** The patient who presents with "dry eyes" often poses a challenge to the general practitioner. The differential diagnosis of this condition is broad, and if mild to moderate in severity, the etiology may be difficult to determine on clinical grounds. Even the patient with Sjögren's syndrome may present with a normal ocular examination and absent (or confusing) ocular symptomatology. In these situations, the Schirmer test becomes useful as a rapid screen for Sjögren's syndrome, particularly when markedly decreased tear production is found (<5 mm wetting).

References

Mackie IA and Seal DV, "Confirmatory Tests for the Dry Eye of Sjögren's Syndrome," *Scand J Rheumatol Suppl*, 1986, 61:220-3.

Mackie IA and Seal DV, "The Questionably Dry Eye," *Br J Ophthalmol*, 1981, 65:2-9.

West C, "Corneal Disease," *Principles and Practice of Ophthalmology*, Peyman GA, Sanders DR, and Goldberg MG, eds, Philadelphia, PA: WB Saunders Co, 1980, 446-9.

Scratch Test *see* Allergy Testing, Percutaneous *on page 7*

Skin Prick Test *see* Allergy Testing, Percutaneous *on page 7*

Skin Test Battery *see* Anergy Skin Test Battery *on page 11*

Skin Tests for Histoplasmosis, Blastomycosis, Coccidioidomycosis *see* Fungal Skin Testing *on page 18*

Skin Tests for Penicillin Allergy *see* Penicillin Allergy Skin Testing *on page 29*

Tine Test *see* Tuberculin Skin Testing, Multiple Puncture *on page 35*

Tuberculin Skin Testing *see* Tuberculin Skin Testing, Intracutaneous *on this page*

Tuberculin Skin Testing, Intracutaneous

CPT 86580

Related Information

Anergy Skin Test Battery *on page 11*
Fungal Skin Testing *on page 18*
Tuberculin Skin Testing, Multiple Puncture *on page 35*

Synonyms Mantoux Test; PPD Test; Purified Protein Derivative (PPD) Test; Tuberculin Skin Testing

Abstract PROCEDURE COMMONLY INCLUDES: Intradermal injection of culture extracts of *Mycobacterium tuberculosis* (MTB). This is an *in vivo* means of evaluating delayed hypersensitivity to MTB. Skin test sites are examined at 24, 48, and 72 hours for signs of induration and erythema. A positive skin test indicates prior exposure to MTB (either recent or remote), with an adequate cell-mediated immune response. INDICATIONS: In general, the tuberculin skin test is used to evaluate individuals with suspected MTB infection. Testing is routinely indicated in the following situations:

- patient with clinical signs and symptoms of active tuberculosis, either pulmonary or extrapulmonary
- patient with a chest radiograph compatible with past tuberculosis
- individuals who have been recently exposed to a proven (index) case of active tuberculosis; this includes close household contacts and healthcare workers with significant exposure
- individuals who have a history of tuberculosis in the remote past, never treated
- selected patients who are to start a prolonged course of steroids (or other immunosuppressives), particularly if there has been past exposure to MTB; this includes most solid organ transplantation candidates
- patients at increased risk for developing tuberculosis on the basis of their underlying disease (eg, silicosis, gastrectomy)
- routine surveillance of persons with ongoing exposure to MTB, such as nursing personnel, respiratory therapists, etc
- immigrants from areas where MTB is endemic
- epidemiologic and public health surveys (eg, nursing homes, innercity residents, etc)

Some clinicians will skin test any patient with a serious underlying illness, such as hepatitis, cirrhosis, AIDS, peptic ulcer disease, cardiomyopathy, severe pulmonary disease, end-stage renal failure, carcinoma, leukemia, and others. A positive tuberculin skin test in patients with these conditions is usually an indication for prolonged isoniazid prophylaxis.

CONTRAINDICATIONS: Testing is contraindicated in the rare patient with known sensitivity to tuberculin. This includes severe local reactions (extensive erythema, vesiculations, ulcers) and anaphylaxis. Note that the development of local skin erythema (only) on a prior tuberculin skin test does not usually constitute a true hypersensitivity reaction. Some clinicians feel that the Mantoux test is contraindicated in the patient who has had a clearly documented positive PPD test in the past. The incidence and significance of this complication has not been studied formally; some physicians fear a hyperimmune local response when the patient is rechallenged with tuberculin.

Patient Care/Scheduling PATIENT PREPARATION: The procedure is explained to the patient. Inquiries should be made regarding past PPD reactions. No specific skin preparation is necessary; however, patients with severe skin disease, such as psoriasis, should be examined beforehand to ensure that there are suitable areas of normal appearing skin. Although testing need not be performed by a physician, one should be immediately avail-

(Continued)

Tuberculin Skin Testing, Intracutaneous *(Continued)*

able for systemic reactions. **AFTERCARE:** If no adverse reaction has occurred within several minutes, the patient may be discharged from the testing center. In some centers, patients are given written instructions on measurement and recording of a positive skin reaction at home. Other centers prefer patients to return to the test center at 48 and 72 hours for formal skin test reading by a nurse or physician. Test sites should be kept clean for 72 hours. No bathing restrictions are necessary. Patient should contact physician if a severe local reaction develops or if fever and dyspnea occurs. **SPECIAL INSTRUCTIONS:** If skin testing is performed in a separate department, requisition should state:

- the strength of tuberculin test (1 TU, 5 TU, 250 TU)
- whether an anergy skin battery is also desired

COMPLICATIONS: In general, adverse reactions are uncommon. Rare complications include fever, lymphangitis, adenopathy, and local ulcers or vesicles. If local lesions develop, these should be treated with dry sterile dressings. The use of topical ointments is optional.

Method **EQUIPMENT:** Culture extracts of MTB (tuberculins) are available for injection in preparations termed "purified protein derivatives" or PPD. Commercial preparations of PPD are available in different doses, standard test dose being 5 tuberculin unit dose (5 TU). Also required are a disposable glass or plastic tuberculin syringe, a short 1/4" to 1/2" 26- or 27-gauge needle. **TECHNIQUE:** The standard 5 TU tuberculin test is performed as follows. A skin site on the volar surface of the forearm is cleaned. 0.1 mL 5 TU PPD is drawn up into a tuberculin syringe and the needle is inserted bevel upwards intradermally and a discrete wheel (5-10 mL) is produced. If the test is improperly performed, a second dose can be given at an alternate location. Test sites are examined at 24, 48, and 72 hours for the presence of induration, by palpation and inspection. The largest transverse diameter of induration is measured along the long axis of the forearm. Areas of erythema are disregarded. The following should be **carefully** recorded in the chart: Strength of PPD used, date of testing, date of reading, and size of induration. The applied method described also applies to testing with nonstandard tuberculin doses (1 TU or 250 TU).

Interpretation **NORMAL FINDINGS:** In general, the 5 TU PPD test is considered "insignificant" when induration is <10 mm; however, this cutting point is controversial. **CRITICAL VALUES:** Reactions >10 mm for 5 TU of PPD are classified as "significant" in most areas of the United States. The larger the reaction, the more likely it represents specific MTB. In some instances, higher or lower values are used. In areas where nontuberculous mycobacterium are common (Southeast U.S.) the likelihood of false-positive skin test increases; higher cutting points of 15 mm are more appropriate. Lower cutting points (5 mm) are used in persons who:

- have had recent close contact with a known TB case
- have chest x-ray findings suspicious for TB
- reside in areas devoid of nontuberculous mycobacterium (Alaska)
- have the acquired immunodeficiency syndrome (AIDS)

The foregoing discussion applies only to the 5 TU PPD test. No standardization has yet been devised for the 1 TU or 250 TU PPD test. However, the 1 TU test is commonly used in patients with a history of a significant local reaction to a 5 TU PPD test. The 250 TU test is used to rule out exposure to any mycobacterial organisms (tuberculous or nontuberculous). Some experts feel that a negative 250 TU PPD essentially excludes tuberculosis exposure, providing the patient has a fully reactive anergy panel.

LIMITATIONS: For best results, trained personnel are necessary for administering and reading the test. **ADDITIONAL INFORMATION:** The tuberculin test is a measure of delayed (cellular) immunity to MTB. As such, a positive test indicates only exposure to MTB and does not distinguish current from past infections. False-positive tests may be seen with exposure to nontuberculous (atypical) mycobacterium or previous inoculation with BCG vaccine. False-negative tests are common and can be difficult to interrupt. Causes for false-negative tests relate not only to the technique of administration, but also the age and immune status of the person being tested. Insignificant reactions are commonly seen secondary to anergy from immunosuppressive therapy, neoplastic disease, various bacterial or viral infections, and vaccinations. Thus, the tuberculin test is often performed along with skin tests for common antigens, such as *Candida* and mumps, to assess possible anergic states. In addition, hypersensitivity to tuberculin may diminish gradually with age. A "booster phenomenon" has been described in the elderly whereby waning tuberculin sensitivity is augmented by repeating 5 TU skin testing at 1 week intervals. Although controversy exists concerning the interpretation of both the booster phenomenon and of the standard tuberculin test itself, this test remains an invaluable aid in diagnosing tuberculous infection.

References

Reichman LB, "Tuberculin Skin Testing, The State of the Art," *Chest*, 1979, 76(6);764-70.

The American Thoracic Society, "The Tuberculin Skin Test," *Am Rev Respir Dis*, 1981, 124:356-63.

Thompson NJ, "The Booster Phenomenon in Serial Tuberculin Testing," *Am Rev Respir Dis*, 1979, 119:587-97.

Tuberculin Skin Testing, Multiple Puncture

CPT 86585

Related Information

Tuberculin Skin Testing, Intracutaneous *on page 33*

Synonyms Prong Test; Tine Test

Abstract **PROCEDURE COMMONLY INCLUDES:** Extracts of *Mycobacterium tuberculosis* (MTB) are introduced into the skin by means of a multiple point applicator coated with tuberculin. At 48 and 72 hours, the skin site is examined for papular reaction. **INDICATIONS:** The multiple puncture test is used to identify individuals who have been previously exposed to MTB. Unlike the intracutaneous (Mantoux) tuberculin test, the multiple puncture test is most commonly used to screen large numbers of asymptomatic individuals with a low suspicion of MTB infection. **CONTRAINDICATIONS:** Previously known sensitivity to tuberculin, from a prior Mantoux test or Tine test.

Patient Care/Scheduling **PATIENT PREPARATION:** No special preparation required **AFTERCARE:** Patient should be instructed to keep the test site clean. **SPECIAL INSTRUCTIONS:** Requisition must state medications patient is currently receiving, especially any steroid preparations or other immunosuppressives. **COMPLICATIONS:** Adverse reactions are uncommon. Rarely fever, adenopathy, and local ulcers may be seen. Local lesions should be treated only with dry sterile dressings; the use of topical steroids is optional.

Method **EQUIPMENT:** Several types of applicators are available commercially. Concentrated tuberculin is used in all applicators in either one of two forms: old tuberculin (OT) or purified protein derivative (PPD). The device consists of an applicator with points coated with dried tuberculin. **TECHNIQUE:** Tuberculin is introduced into the skin by pressing an applicator firmly onto a clean skin surface, preferably the volar aspect of the forearm. Test site is examined at 48 and 72 hours for evidence of papules or vesicles. In the first case, if a papular reaction occurs, the largest single papule is examined and the diameter of induration recorded. If several papules are found coalesced, the largest diameter of induration is recorded. In the second case, if a vesicular reaction occurs, it is not necessary to record the diameter of induration; documentation of a significant vesicular reaction is sufficient.

Interpretation **NORMAL FINDINGS:** No papular or vesicular skin reaction **CRITICAL VALUES:** A multiple puncture test is considered potentially positive if a papular skin reaction evolves. In all such cases, further tests using formal intracutaneous (Mantoux) tuberculin testing is warranted. Vesicular reactions are considered strongly positive tests and no further confirmatory testing is necessary. **LIMITATIONS:** The tine test shares many of the same limitations as the intracutaneous tuberculin test, including false-negative reactions in patients with impaired immune systems. In addition, the tine test delivers a variable dose of highly concentrated tuberculin and thus, false-positive reactions are relatively common. It is not intended for strict diagnostic use and thus, few management decisions can be made using isolated tine test results. **ADDITIONAL INFORMATION:** Tuberculin skin testing remains an invaluable tool in the diagnosis of tuberculosis. Infection with MTB results in skin sensitivity to culture extracts of MTB (tuberculins), an example of delayed or cellular hypersensitivity. The tine test has several advantages over the intracutaneous test. These include the following:

- little equipment necessary
- less expensive
- no training required for administration

(Continued)

Tuberculin Skin Testing, Multiple Puncture *(Continued)*

The tine test is most useful when screening large numbers of asymptomatic individuals in whom the suspicion for tuberculous infection is low. In general, completely negative tine tests are felt to correlate highly with negative Mantoux tests; tine tests with vesicular reactions are felt to correlate strongly with significant (>15 mm) Mantoux tests. Interpretation of a papular reaction with a tine test is more problematic. Since doses of delivered tuberculin are uncontrolled with a multiple point applicator, false-positive cross reactions with nontuberculous mycobacterium are common. Further testing using the Mantoux test with its attendant cost and time is necessary to interpret the papular reaction. In spite of these caveats, the tine test is a convenient and inexpensive screen for MTB exposure for the practicing physician.

References

Reichman LB, "Tuberculin Skin Testing, the State of the Art," *Chest*, 1979, 76(6):764-70.

Reichman LB and O'Day R, "Tuberculous Infection in the Large Urban Population," *Am Rev Respir Dis*, 1978, 117:705-12.

The American Thoracic Society, "Screening for Pulmonary Tuberculosis in Institutions," *Am Rev Respir Dis*, 1977, 115:901.

The American Thoracic Society, "The Tuberculin Skin Test," *Am Rev Respir Dis*, 1981, 124:356-63.

Widefield Capillary Microscopy

Synonyms Nailfold Capillaroscopy; Nailfold Capillary Microscopy

Abstract PROCEDURE COMMONLY INCLUDES: *In vivo* examination of finger nailfold capillaries with a wide-angle microscope or ophthalmoscope. Abnormalities in the magnified appearance of nailfold capillaries have been well-described in several connective tissue diseases such as scleroderma, dermatomyositis, systemic lupus erythematosus (SLE), and mixed connective tissue disease (MCTD). A distinctive capillary pattern of capillary enlargement accompanied by avascular areas has been reported in >80% of patients with systemic sclerosis. This procedure has found its greatest use in the early detection of systemic sclerosis. INDICATIONS: Nailfold capillaroscopy is a relatively new procedure and clinical applications are still evolving. Common indications include:

- evaluation of the patient with isolated Raynaud's phenomenon (ie, not associated with other connective tissue diseases), particularly if the duration of symptoms is less than 2 years. Normal nailfold capillaroscopy suggests a benign course. Abnormal microscopy may identify those patients with Raynaud's phenomenon who will develop systemic sclerosis (scleroderma) months or years later; thus, this procedure is useful in the early recognition of scleroderma.
- evaluation of the patient with mixed connective tissue disease (MCTD), where there are combined features of scleroderma, systemic lupus erythematosus, and polymyositis; nailfold capillaroscopy may predict the subset of patients with MCTD who will go on to manifest diffuse systemic sclerosis.
- evaluation of the patient with known scleroderma, in order to estimate the severity of visceral involvement; severity of capillary lesions correlates reasonably well with the degree of multisystem organ disease and survival rate

CONTRAINDICATIONS: None reported. However, extensive nail disease (eg, onychomycosis) may preclude a thorough examination and represents a relative contraindication.

Patient Care/Scheduling PATIENT PREPARATION: Technique is explained to the patient and verbal consent is obtained. Female patients should remove fingernail polish beforehand. AFTERCARE: No specific activity restrictions afterwards COMPLICATIONS: None reported; this procedure is risk-free.

Method EQUIPMENT: A variety of instruments have been advocated for microscopy, including a handheld magnifying glass, ophthalmoscope, an inverted 10x microscope eyepiece, and a stereomicroscope. Some authorities advocate the conventional ophthalmoscope due to its effectiveness and easy availability but the viewing field is quite narrow. Maricq (1981) argues for the stereomicroscope with magnification of 12-14x which allows depth perception and wide-angle viewing. TECHNIQUE: In some centers all 10 nailfolds are routinely examined; others advocate testing of the fourth nailfolds only. A drop of oil is placed on the nailfold, usually grade B immersion oil (fairly viscous). Nailfold capillaries are examined with the magnifying instrument of choice; incident lighting usually is provided by a fiberoptic cool light source. Photographs of abnormal capillary anatomy may be obtained using specialized techniques.

Interpretation **NORMAL FINDINGS:** No abnormalities in nailfold capillary pattern seen. Results interpreted by rheumatologist familiar with this procedure. **CRITICAL VALUES:** The pattern of capillary abnormalities seen in scleroderma is characterized by:

- enlarged capillary loops, "giant loops" 4-10x normal size
- loss of capillaries (reduction in number)
- increased tortuosness and disorganization of remaining capillaries, or "budding"
- regions of avascularity
- capillary hemorrhages

Some of these features may be absent in a given patient and nail-to-nail variability is not uncommon. Rating scales have been developed (semiquantitative) to classify the degree of capillary involvement. Capillary abnormalities may be seen in a wide variety of connective tissue diseases in addition to scleroderma. Enlarged capillary loops have been reported in patients with SLE and rheumatoid arthritis. However, the complete "scleroderma pattern" (described previously) is found in 80% to 90% of patients with scleroderma, but only rarely in SLE, RA, or normal controls. The presence of avascular regions in the nailfold appears specific for scleroderma. Some authors feel that capillaroscopy findings are sufficiently specific to diagnose scleroderma and rule out other connective tissue diseases, but further studies are needed to confirm this.

ADDITIONAL INFORMATION: Although the technique of capillary microscopy has gained clinical acceptance in the past decade, it was first described as far back as 1912. The pathologic basis of this procedure – anatomic derangements of cutaneous microvessels in systemic sclerosis – was originally documented in the 1920s; this included the existence of "giant" nailfold capillaries. The introduction of Widefield technique helped popularize this noninvasive procedure in recent years. A high degree of correlation has been demonstrated between findings on capillary microscopy and histologic features on nailfold biopsy.

References

Lee P, Leung F, Alderdice C, et al, "Nailfold Capillary Microscopy in the Connective Tissue Diseases: A Semiquantitative Assessment," *J Rheumatol*, 1983, 10:930-8.

Lee P, Sarkozi J, Bookman AA, et al, "Digital Blood Flow and Nailfold Capillary Microscopy in Raynaud's Phenomenon," *J Rheumatol*, 1986, 13:564-9.

Lovy M, MacCarter D, and Steigerwald JC, "Relationship Between Nailfold Capillary Abnormalities and Organ Involvement in Systemic Sclerosis," *Arthritis Rheum*, 1985, 28:496-501.

Maricq HR, "Widefield Capillary Microscopy: Technique and Rating Scale for Abnormalities Seen in Scleroderma and Related Disorders," *Arthritis Rheum*, 1981, 24:1159-65.

McGill NW and Gow PJ, "Nailfold Capillaroscopy: A Blinded Study of its Discriminatory Value in Scleroderma, Systemic Lupus Erythematosus, and Rheumatoid Arthritis," *Aust N Z J Med*, 1986, 16:457-60.

CARDIOLOGY

Ernesto E. Salcedo, MD

In the past three years there has been an explosion of technology for the diagnosis and management of patients with cardiovascular disorders. A sound understanding of the methodology, clinical applications, and limitations for the use of these techniques will enhance their proper application.

As in the rest of the handbook, this section has been organized in alphabetical order and descriptions of the most common cardiologic procedures are described in detail.

Although traditionally cardiovascular procedures have been classified as invasive versus noninvasive, this differentiation is somewhat arbitrary and their borders are becoming blurred. This review covers information regarding cardiac catheterization, stress testing, cardiac ultrasound, electrocardiography, Holter and pacemaker testing, and phonocardiography and systolic time intervals. Although the list of cardiovascular testing is probably much larger than this, this review is not intended to be a comprehensive review of all cardiovascular testing, but an easily accessible source of information regarding the most common procedures performed in cardiology today.

Adult Cardiac Catheterization *see* Cardiac Catheterization, Adult *on next page*

Ambulatory Electrocardiography *see* Holter Monitorization *on page 47*

Ambulatory Holter Electrocardiography *see* Holter Monitorization *on page 47*

Arm Ergometer Stress

Abstract INDICATIONS: Musculoskeletal, neurologic or vascular disease of lower extremities are conditions in which arm ergometer stress testing is used in place of stress testing on the treadmill or bicycle. Used to evaluate the potential for rhythm disturbances, to screen for coronary artery disease, to write an exercise prescription, and to determine exercise capacity. CONTRAINDICATIONS: Acute myocardial infarction.

Patient Care/Scheduling PATIENT PREPARATION: The skin is prepared and electrodes are applied to the chest. Patient is instructed how to use an arm wheel. SPECIAL INSTRUCTIONS: Patients are instructed not to eat, drink, or smoke for 2 hours prior to test and to wear clothes suitable for exercise. Physician in charge of stress testing should be present to witness the test unless the patient's own physician requests to do so. Patients on cardiac medication will be instructed accordingly. Consent form informs patients of the benefits and risks of test.

Method TECHNIQUE: The arm ergometer stress is a means of testing patients with significant musculoskeletal, neurologic, or vascular disease of the lower extremities. The patient is prepared in the same manner as in the treadmill stress test. The exercising is done on an arm wheel. The patient turns the arm wheel which is set at different workloads, becoming more difficult at each higher workload. The patient exercises for 3 minutes, then rests for 1 minute while the physician records the blood pressure. The workload is then increased and the patient continues every 4 minutes at higher workloads until chest pain, fatigue, or the physician discontinues the test. Resting tracings are then taken every minute for 5-10 minutes.

Specimen TURNAROUND TIME: 24-48 hours.

References

Acker J Jr and Martin D, "Angina and ST Segment Depression During Treadmill and Arm Ergometer Testing in Patients With Coronary Artery Disease," *Phys Ther*, 1988, 68(2):195-8.

Hollingsworth V, Bendick P, Franklin B, et al, "Validity of Arm Ergometer Blood Pressures Immediately After Exercise," *Am J Cardiol*, 1990, 65(20):1358-60.

Bicycle Stress Testing

CPT 93015

Abstract INDICATIONS: Determine presence of coronary artery disease or exercise related rhythm disturbances and blood pressure response to exercise.

Patient Care/Scheduling PATIENT PREPARATION: The skin is prepared and electrodes are attached to the patient's chest. Patient is instructed how to exercise on a bicycle to the rhythm of a metronome. Patient is also asked to hyperventilate (short, fast, deep breathing for 30 seconds) to give the physician witnessing the test a preview of how the heart will react to exercise. AFTERCARE: Patient is advised not to shower or bathe for 1 hour following the test. SPECIAL INSTRUCTIONS: The patient is instructed to eat 2 hours prior to the test and not to eat, smoke, or drink anything thereafter until the test is completed. Patients are also instructed to wear clothing suitable for exercise, preferably tennis shoes and shorts. The physician in charge of stress testing or a qualified representative should be present to witness the test unless the patient's own physician requests to do so. Patients on cardiac medication will be instructed accordingly. A consent form may be used to explain the benefits and risks of the test.

Method TECHNIQUE: The procedure followed for a bicycle stress test is the same as described under treadmill stress testing. The patient will exercise on a bicycle to determine the presence of coronary artery disease or exercise related rhythm disturbances. The patient will be instructed to bicycle to the rhythm of a metronome. The workload is increased every 4 minutes by tightening the tension on the bicycle wheel. The workload ranges from

(Continued)

Bicycle Stress Testing *(Continued)*

300-1200 kpm. A preliminary report will be given verbally to the patient by the physician after completion of the exam. A final typed report will be sent to the referring physician within 24 hours.

Specimen TURNAROUND TIME: 24-48 hours.

Cardiac Catheterization, Adult

CPT 93501 (right heart); 93510 (left heart); 93526 (combined right and retrograde left heart)

Related Information

Pericardiocentesis *on page 63*

Stress Test *on page 52*

Swan-Ganz Catheterization *on page 71*

Synonyms Adult Cardiac Catheterization; Cineangiocardiography; Coronary Arteriography; Left Heart Catheterization; Right and Left Heart Catheterization; Right Heart Catheterization

Applies to HIS Bundle Electrograms

Abstract INDICATIONS:

- evaluate patients being considered for coronary bypass surgery
- evaluate patients to determine whether angina is the result of aortic stenosis or coronary artery disease
- determine if bypass grafts are patent
- evaluate patients in whom surgical repair of suspected left ventricular aneurysm, perforated interventricular septum, or mitral insufficiency is being considered
- definitive determination of the presence of coronary artery disease as a cause of angina
- evaluate structural, valvular, and vascular abnormalities

Patient Care/Scheduling PATIENT PREPARATION: Patients scheduled for cardiac catheterization must have a written and properly identified consultation from a cardiologist recorded in the chart prior to procedure. The consultant's note should state indications for procedure and evaluation of risk to patient.

Left heart catheterization: CBC, BUN, and EKG should be recorded in chart the day before the test; a serum potassium should also be ordered the day before the test on all patients receiving diuretics; if the Judkin's technique will be used, shave patient's groins on the day before the procedure; two units of blood must be "on call" in the Blood Bank. Requesting physician may need to obtain signed procedure permit for invasive diagnostic cardiac test or specific procedure ordered. Patients younger than 18 years of age must have parent or legal guardian sign permit. Patients receiving digitalis should be given usual dose on the morning of catheterization. A sedative such as Valium® 10 μg I.M. should be given "on call" from the Adult Cardiac Catheterization Laboratory. For AM patients, omit breakfast on day of test. For PM patients, juice and coffee may be given at breakfast time. Water may be consumed ad lib. Weigh patient on day of procedure and record on chart. All patients should be sent to laboratory on a stretcher wearing a hospital gown and regular slippers. Send with patients: all charts, angiograms, and x-rays. An I.V. is not necessary. If the patient is edentulous, he/she should wear all dentures.

AFTERCARE: Right heart catheterization (including HIS bundle electrograms): Remove dressing in 4 hours. Check for hematoma or bleeding at catheter insertion site twice in 1 hour. If a cutdown was performed, remove sutures in 5-7 days.

Left heart catheterization (including coronary arteriograms): Check the following: heart rate, blood pressure, arterial puncture site, and distal pulses four times at 15-minute intervals, then four times at 30-minute intervals, then four times at 1-hour intervals. If the femoral approach has been used, enforce absolute bedrest for 8 hours. Keep a 5 lb sandbag on puncture site for 4 hours unless otherwise instructed.

Pericardiocentesis: Check the following: heart rate, blood pressure, and neck vein distention four times at 15-minute intervals, then four times at 30-minute intervals, then four times at 1-hour intervals. Call physician in charge (Director or Assistant Director) for any suspected complications of the procedure.

SPECIAL INSTRUCTIONS: These studies are arranged by the requesting physician.

Specimen TURNAROUND TIME: Preliminary reports will be recorded in the chart on the day of the procedure. Final reports will be sent to the chart approximately 72 hours after the procedure.

References

Ross J, Branderburg RD, Dinsmore RE, et al, "Guidelines for Coronary Angiography. A Report of The American College of Cardiology/American Heart Association Taskforce on Assessment of Diagnostic and Therapeutic Procedures," Subcommittee on Coronary Angiography, *Circulation*, 1987, 76:963A, 977A.

Cardiogram, Electro *see* Electrocardiography *on page 44*

Cineangiocardiography *see* Cardiac Catheterization, Adult *on previous page*

Color Doppler

CPT 93325

Synonyms Color Flow Doppler; Color Flow Mapping

Abstract PROCEDURE COMMONLY INCLUDES: Color Doppler echocardiography integrates the structural information provided by 2-D echocardiography with pulsed Doppler color coded flow maps that depict the direction, velocity, and turbulence of blood flow through the cardiac chambers and great vessels. Thus, a true noninvasive angiogram is now part of the cardiac ultrasound technologies. INDICATIONS: Color Doppler complements two-dimensional echocardiography and conventional Doppler techniques by providing color flow maps that improve the spatial characterization of flow disturbances. It has proven to be of most value in the detection and specifically the quantitation of regurgitant lesions. The gradation of aortic, mitral, tricuspid, and pulmonic insufficiency can now be made with certainty with the help of color Doppler. The localization and direction of the regurgitant jets, through color Doppler, has provided useful insight in the etiology of the regurgitant lesions. Color Doppler can also assist in the evaluation of stenotic lesions by providing a clear visual display of the jet directions from which continuous wave Doppler velocities can be measured. It also aids in determining the exact size of the valve orifices. Additionally, the diagnosis of intracardiac shunts in congenital heart disease has been greatly enhanced by color Doppler echocardiography. CONTRAINDICATIONS: There are no contraindications for color Doppler but like all other forms of cardiac ultrasound, technically poor studies may be obtained in patients with chronic lung disease or obesity. Additionally, the registration of color Doppler decreases in the far field and flow abnormalities may not be obvious in areas distant to the transducer.

Patient Care/Scheduling PATIENT PREPARATION: See Two-Dimensional Echocardiography listing for patient care/scheduling information. Similar principles apply to color flow Doppler.

Method TECHNIQUE: The color Doppler study is performed simultaneously with the 2-D echocardiogram. After obtaining the initial echocardiographic views and optimizing the settings, the color Doppler is switched on to survey the flow pattern through the cardiac chambers and great vessels, then the operator focuses on the specific flow abnormalities of interest. The long axis left parasternal view is most useful to evaluate flow through the mitral valve into the left ventricle and out of the left ventricle through the outflow tract and aortic valve. Mitral insufficiency and aortic insufficiency can be evaluated from this view. The left parasternal short axis view at the base of the heart best depicts flow through the tricuspid valve into the right ventricle and through the pulmonic valve out to the pulmonary artery. The apical 4-chamber view allows for study of the flows through the tricuspid and mitral valves into the right ventricle and left ventricle. This view also permits the evaluation and quantification of mitral and tricuspid regurgitation. The apical 5-chamber view permits the study of flow through the outflow tract of the left ventricle. It also allows for the evaluation and quantification of aortic insufficiency when present. The subcostal view permits study of the right ventricle and left ventricle inflow tract through the tricuspid and mitral valves. It also allows determination of the presence and severity of mitral and tricuspid insufficiency. The suprasternal view provides for the study of flow in the ascending aorta, aortic arch and descending aorta. Conditions such as aortic stenosis and coarctation of the aorta can be best studied from this region.

Interpretation NORMAL FINDINGS: Good understanding of normal and abnormal cardiac physiology is needed to adequately interpret color Doppler echocardiography. It is also very important to recognize that mild degrees of valvular incompetence, especially tricuspid and mitral, is frequently seen in normal subjects. When significant insufficiency is pres-

(Continued)

Color Doppler *(Continued)*

ent, this must be evaluated from different orthogonal planes so that the best volumetric estimation of the regurgitant jet is made. A detailed description of the size, direction, and number of the jets helps in assessing the severity and etiology of the regurgitant lesion. Similar detailed analysis should be made in intracardiac shunt lesions so that the precise anatomic site and size can be determined. Additionally, the direction, right to left, left to right, or bidirectional, of the flow should be described. In patients with stenotic lesions, color flow can further the definition of the site of obstruction and aid in the precise determination of orifice areas. The degree of flow disturbance is also related to the severity of the stenosis.

References

Omoto R, *Color and Atlas of Real-Time Two-Dimensional Doppler Echocardiography*, 2nd ed, Philadelphia, PA: Lea & Febiger, 1987.

Color Flow Doppler *see* Color Doppler *on previous page*

Color Flow Mapping *see* Color Doppler *on previous page*

Coronary Arteriography *see* Cardiac Catheterization, Adult *on page 40*

Cross-Sectional Echocardiography *see* Two-Dimensional Echocardiography *on page 57*

2-D Echo *see* Two-Dimensional Echocardiography *on page 57*

Doppler Echo *see* Doppler Echocardiography *on this page*

Doppler Echocardiography

CPT 93320

Related Information

Pericardiocentesis *on page 63*

Synonyms Doppler Echo; Doppler Ultrasound

Abstract **PROCEDURE COMMONLY INCLUDES:** The clinical application of Doppler echocardiography is based on the Doppler shift principle by which sound waves increase or decrease their frequency as the object that produces or reflects them approximates or moves away from a given point. A transducer that acts as a transmitter and receiver is placed so that ultrasound waves are sent parallel to cardiac flow, the red cells reflect these waves and alter the frequency of the ultrasound wave proportionally to the velocity in which they are moving. By knowing the velocity of ultrasound through cardiac tissue, the frequency of the transmitted and received sound waves and the angle of incidence, it is possible to calculate the velocity of the blood flow. Volume measurements can be calculated by measuring, with echocardiography, the diameter or area of a given vessel or chamber and multiplying this by the Doppler derived velocity through them. Pressure gradients can be measured by Doppler using the simplified Bernoulli's equation: $P=4V^2$ where P is the pressure gradient and V is the Doppler derived velocity. Doppler echocardiography can be used as a stand alone technique with a Piddof transducer or it can be image guided by 2-D echocardiography. Doppler can be pulsed or continuous wave depending on the transducer sending and receiving ultrasound waves intermittently or continuously. The pulsed wave Doppler has the advantage that allows for precise location of the Doppler flow (range resolution) but is limited to the velocity of the flow it can detect, usually 1-1.5 m/second. Continuous wave Doppler does not have range resolution but it can detect high velocities of flow as seen in stenotic or regurgitant lesions. In most situations both forms of Doppler are required, the pulsed wave form to determine the origin and extent of the flow disturbance and the continuous wave Doppler to detect the maximal velocities present in a given condition. **INDICATIONS:** Doppler echocardiography has complemented 2-D echocardiography by providing hemodynamic information not available through conventional echocardiography. The most common applications of Doppler include evaluation of stenotic and regurgitant valve lesions and the study of intracardiac shunts. Continuous wave Doppler echocardiography permits precise measurement of gradients in aortic stenosis and, when combined with 2-D echo, allows through the continuity equation to calculate aortic valve area. In mitral stenosis, it permits the measurement of transmitral gradient and through the use of pressure half-time calculations it allows for estimation of mitral valve area. Pulsed wave Doppler permits not only the diagnosis but the quantification of aortic and mitral insufficiency. Other applications of Doppler echocardiography include cardiac output calculations and intracardiac pressure measurements such as right ventricular and pulmonary artery systolic pressure. **CONTRAINDICATIONS:** There are no contraindications to Doppler echocardiography. Similar to 2-D echocardiography, technical difficulties may exist in patients with chronic lung disease or obesity. The utmost care must be used to obtain the best spectral display in every patient. This frequently requires the use of multiple transducer locations to best evaluate the flow disturbance.

Patient Care/Scheduling **PATIENT PREPARATION:** No special patient preparation is required. Fasting is not necessary. No special time of the day is preferred. **SPECIAL INSTRUCTIONS:** A complete Doppler study takes approximately 45 minutes. If a patient is going to have a Doppler and an echocardiogram 60-90 minutes of schedule time will be necessary. A note in the chart or a requisition form detailing the reason for requesting the Doppler study will help the Echo Laboratory personnel in providing the best possible study. Other useful information includes age, weight, and height.

Method **TECHNIQUE:** Most patients will have a Doppler study in conjunction with a 2-D echocardiogram. The initial patient interaction is similar in both cases. After the 2-D echocardiogram is completed, a Doppler study can then be performed and can be tailor-made to address specific unanswered questions. Routinely, a Doppler study will include flow interrogations of the aortic valve from the apex, right parasternal window, and suprasternal window. The mitral and tricuspid valves can be best interrogated from the left parasternal window and from the apex. The pulmonic valve is best interrogated from the left parasternal window and the epigastric region. Recordings at all these levels are made on a strip chart recorder and/or on a video cassette recorder. All necessary measurements are made either from the strip chart recordings or from the video recordings through the computer measurement packages which most instruments now have.

Peak Doppler Velocities (m/sec)

	Children		Adults	
Mitral flow	1.0	(0.8–1.2)	0.9	(0.4–1.3)
Tricuspid flow	0.6	(0.5–0.8)	0.5	(0.3–0.7)
Pulmonary artery	0.9	(0.7–1.1)	0.75	(0.6–0.9)
Left ventricle	1.0	(0.7–1.2)	0.9	(0.7–1.1)
Aorta	1.5	(1.2–1.8)	1.35	(1.0–1.7)

Reproduced with permission from Hatle L and Angelson B, *Doppler Ultrasound in Cardiology: Physical Principles and Clinical Applications,* 2nd ed, Lee & Febiger, Philadelphia, PA: 1985.

Interpretation **NORMAL FINDINGS:** Adequate interpretation of Doppler echocardiograms requires good understanding of cardiovascular physiology and hemodynamics, and knowledge of the normal flow patterns plus range of velocities through the different values and cardiac chambers (see table). Distinct abnormalities have been characterized by Doppler echocardiography in most cardiovascular disorders.

References

Hatle L and Angelsen B, *Doppler Ultrasound in Cardiology: Physical Principles and Clinical Applications*, 2nd ed, Philadelphia, PA: Lea & Febiger, 1985.

Doppler Ultrasound *see* Doppler Echocardiography *on previous page*

Dynamic Electrocardiography *see* Holter Monitorization *on page 47*

ECG *see* Electrocardiography *on next page*

EKG *see* Electrocardiography *on next page*

EKG, 2-Step Test *replaced by* Electrocardiogram, Adult, Exercise ECG Test *on next page*

Electrocardiogram, Adult, Exercise ECG Test

CPT 93015

Synonyms Multistage Exercise Electrocardiographics Test; MEET

Replaces EKG, 2-Step Test

Abstract PROCEDURE COMMONLY INCLUDES: The skin is prepared and electrodes are attached. A set of three control electrocardiograms is taken (resting, standing, and post-1-minute hyperventilation). The patient is instructed and shown by a nurse how to walk on the treadmill. The test is performed with a qualified professional present. A 12-lead EKG is taken each minute of exercise. Every 2-3 minutes the speed and incline of the treadmill are increased until such time as a near maximum heart rate is achieved, ischemia changes are present, or the supervisor of the test decides to terminate the exercise. Once the exercise is terminated the patient lies down and an EKG is recorded every minute for 5 minutes or until ischemic changes have returned to normal and/or heart rate has returned to normal. INDICATIONS:

- determine the presence of exercise induced myocardial ischemia
- evaluate patient's exercise tolerance
- evaluate blood pressure response to exercise
- evaluate the presence of exercise induced arrhythmia
- evaluate the results of medical and surgical therapy

CONTRAINDICATIONS: Inability to walk on treadmill, unstable angina, severe hypertension, fever, low serum potassium, presence of left bundle branch block precludes diagnosis of cardiac ischemia and use of thallium treadmill might need to be considered.

Patient Care/Scheduling PATIENT PREPARATION: Instruct patient not to eat or drink anything except water after midnight if appointment is in the morning. Patients to be tested in the afternoon should have nothing to eat or drink after a light breakfast, coffee or juice and toast at least 4 hours before test. When clinically feasible it is preferred that the patient be off digitalis at the time of testing; 3 days for digoxin and 10-14 days for long-acting preparation. Patients need tennis shoes, shorts, or pants; women also need to wear a bra. No jumpsuits, loose clothing is suggested. AFTERCARE: Patient may need wheelchair to return to room. Patient should rest following test.

Method TECHNIQUE: Treadmill.

Specimen TURNAROUND TIME: Final report is given within 2 work days after the test.

Interpretation LIMITATIONS: Patients must be able to walk to perform test ADDITIONAL INFORMATION: The test is supervised by a physician who may cancel the test at his discretion.

References

Lachterman B, Lehmann KG, Detrano R, et al, "Comparison of ST Segment/Heart Rate Index to Standard ST Criteria for Analysis of Exercise Electrocardiogram," *Circulation*, 1990, 82(1):44-50.

Electrocardiography

CPT 93000

Synonyms Cardiogram, Electro; ECG; EKG

Abstract PROCEDURE COMMONLY INCLUDES: The electrocardiogram (ECG) remains the basic cardiologic test and is widely applied in patients with suspected or known heart disease and as a basic reference for most other cardiologic tests. Although 1-lead ECG is used as reference for most other cardiologic diagnostic procedures, the electrocardiogram, in the present context, will be the full 12-lead ECG recording. INDICATIONS: In patients without known heart disease, the ECG is used as a screening test for occult coronary artery disease, cardiomyopathies, or left ventricular hypertrophy. ECG is used as a baseline for future reference and comparison and preoperatively, to rule out silent coronary artery disease. The ECG may also provide useful insight in the presence of metabolic alterations, such as hypercalcemia and hypocalcemia and hyperkalemia and hypokalemia. In patients with known heart disease, the ECG serves as a useful marker for the severity and progression of the disease process. The ECG is invaluable in the evaluation of patients with chest pain and in the management of patients with suspected or known to have acute myocardial infarction or coronary insufficiency. Most patients with myocardial, valvular, and congenital heart disease will eventually demonstrate ECG abnormalities and an ECG is warranted in these cases for diagnostic as well as management purposes. Rhythm disorders can be evaluated through ECG rhythm strips. CONTRAINDICATIONS: There are no contraindications for ECG recordings.

Patient Care/Scheduling PATIENT PREPARATION: No special patient preparation is needed, patients do not need to fast before the ECG is taken and no special time of the day is preferable. SPECIAL INSTRUCTIONS: Inpatients will have a bedside ECG and outpatients will go to the ECG Laboratory. Patients can be scheduled to have a routine ECG (to be done within 24 hours of request) or stat ECG to be done immediately. The reason for the request should be noted in the chart or in the requisition form. Additional information of interest includes patient's age, sex, and race, as well as any cardiac medications they may be taking. Situations that require special lead placement should be noted. These include use of back leads if a posterior myocardial infarction is suspected and use of right precordial leads if a right ventricular infarction is suspected. If the patient has a rhythm disturbance a rhythm strip may be requested.

Method TECHNIQUE: After checking the appropriateness and type of ECG to be taken, a brief description of the procedure is provided to the patient. With the patient in a supine and relaxed position, the wrists and ankles are prepared for the extremity leads. The precordium is prepared and marked for the precordial leads and the electrodes are put in place with contact gel and supported by elastic straps in the extremities and suction cups in the precordium. After making sure the calibration settings are adequate, registration of the 12 leads is accomplished. This can be done by selecting lead by lead or, with the newer ECG recorders, by simultaneous recordings of 3-6 leads. The recordings are usually made at a paper speed of 25 mm/second. Usually one copy is left in the chart or is given to the patient and one copy goes to the ECG Laboratory for interpretation and findings.

Interpretation NORMAL FINDINGS: Proper interpretation of electrocardiograms is essential for all physicians and especially for those who take care of patients with potential heart problems. The interpretation of the normal electrocardiogram and its variants needs to be emphasized at all levels of medical training and continued interpretation and education is required if a person is to maintain proficiency in ECG interpretation. Distinct abnormalities exist in the ECG in the presence of chamber dilatation or hypertrophy, in the presence of acute or remote myocardial infarction, pericarditis, ventricular aneurysms, and conduction abnormalities.

References

Grauer K and Curry RW, *Clinical Electrocardiography: A Primary Care Approach*, Oradell, NJ: Medical Economics Books, 1986.

Wilson RF, Marcus ML, Christensen BV, et al, "Accuracy of Exercise Electrocardiography in Detecting Physiologically Significant Coronary Arterial Lesions," *Circulation*, 1991, 83(2):412-21.

Electrophysiologic Studies

CPT 93600

Synonyms EPS; HIS Bundle Recordings; Invasive Cardiac Electrophysiologic Studies; Programmed Electrical Stimulation

Abstract PROCEDURE COMMONLY INCLUDES: Invasive cardiac electrophysiologic studies have been developed to evaluate patients with complex arrhythmias and conduction abnormalities. Electrode catheters are introduced percutaneously via peripheral veins and are directed to cardiac chambers with the aid of fluoroscopy for the recording of the electric phenomena within the heart. INDICATIONS: Electrophysiologic studies are performed for diagnostic and therapeutic purposes. The most common diagnostic indications for EPS include:

- evaluating patients with sinus node dysfunction through the measurement of sinus node recovery time
- evaluation of atrioventricular conduction to identify the site of conduction malfunction early and to determine by those means who are better candidates for permanent pacing
- differential diagnosis of wide complex QRS tachycardia
- to define the mechanism and differential diagnosis of supraventricular tachycardia
- diagnosis and management of patients with ventricular tachycardia
- evaluation and management of survivors of sudden cardiac death

The most common therapeutic uses of EPS include:

- pharmacologic control of tachycardia where tachycardia is induced, an intravenous therapeutic agent is administered, reinduction is tried and the response is evaluated

(Continued)

Electrophysiologic Studies *(Continued)*

- selecting patients for nonpharmacologic control of tachycardias such as ablation therapy antitachycardia pacemakers and the implantable defibrillators

CONTRAINDICATIONS: There are no absolute contraindications for EPS but, as with all invasive procedures, a careful risk to benefit analysis should be obtained before proceeding with it.

Patient Care/Scheduling **PATIENT PREPARATION:** The procedure takes from 2-4 hours. Electrophysiologic studies are performed in the postabsortive state and are usually carried out without sedation, although in apprehensive patients mild sedation is advisable. Sufficient time is allowed for the elimination of drugs that alter the electric system of the heart, roughly the duration of five half-lives of a given drug. There is no need to discontinue other cardiac medications that patient may be taking for other cardiac problems. For the introduction of the catheters the groin is scrubbed and shaved prior to the patient coming to the EP Laboratory. On arrival to the laboratory the patient is greeted and given a detailed explanation of the procedure and is then placed in the electrophysiologic table where he/she is draped and prepared for the EPS. At the completion of the EPS, gentle pressure is applied in the area of catheter insertion and patients are allowed to ambulate after 4-6 hours of bedrest.

Method **TECHNIQUE:** Routinely, at least three surface electrocardiographic leads are recorded as reference. A temporary pacemaker is generally placed under local anesthesia and with fluoroscopic guidance at least three catheters are advanced to the appropriate area. Usually these will include one in the right atrium or coronary sinus, one across the tricuspid valve near the bundle of HIS, and one in the right ventricle. A multichannel oscilloscope and a multichannel recorder is used to register the electrophysiologic data and for later analysis and study. Well placed catheters with appropriate amplification and filtering should provide diagnostic recordings in most patients. Depending on the clinical need, the site and type of a specific protocol will be applied.

Interpretation **ADDITIONAL INFORMATION:** Appropriate interpretation of electrophysiologic studies requires knowledge of the site and specific EPS protocol used as well as precise understanding of the electrophysiologic properties of the heart in health and disease. Measurement of electrophysiologic intervals obtained from intracardiac recordings at the level of the coronary sinus, atrioventricular (A-V) node, HIS bundle, and right ventricle are usually obtained. These include the A-V, atrial-HIS (A-H), and HIS-ventricular (H-V) intervals. Abnormalities in these intervals will suggest the presence of different types of A-V conduction problems. By these means it is possible to diagnose malfunction of the sinus node, to characterize intra-atrial, A-V node, HIS bundle system, and intramyocardial conduction, and to determine the presence, location, and electrophysiologic properties of accessory pathways when present. Additionally, the site and form of initiation and termination of supraventricular and ventricular tachycardias can be characterized by EPS.

Endomyocardial Biopsy

CPT 93505

Synonyms Heart Biopsy; Right Ventricular Endomyocardial Biopsy

Abstract **PROCEDURE COMMONLY INCLUDES:** The skin is prepared with a surgical scrub of hexachlorophene soap followed by lodophor. A #8 French arterial introducer is placed percutaneously in the superior vena cava. A sterile biopsy forceps is then advanced into the right ventricle of the heart and samples are taken from the right ventricular wall. **INDICATIONS:** The test is used to evaluate the histology of the heart in cases of cardiac transplantation and to screen for patients with myocardiopathies or myocarditis. Since right sided intracardiac pressures are measured during the procedure, an evaluation of hemodynamics is also available. The test is used in the diagnosis of treatable cardiac lesions and in the follow-up evaluation of therapy of these lesions.

Specimen **CAUSES FOR REJECTION:** If the patient is found to have significantly elevated right ventricular and pulmonary artery blood pressure, the test may be cancelled. **TURNAROUND TIME:** A report of the immediate procedure is written on the chart at the time of the biopsy. Results are usually available from the Pathology Department within 48 hours of the arrival of the specimen.

References

Billingham ME, "Endomyocardial Biopsy Diagnosis of Acute Rejection in Cardiac Allografts," *Prog Cardiovasc Dis*, 1990, 33(1):11-8.

EPS *see* Electrophysiologic Studies *on page 45*

Esophageal Echo *see* Transesophageal Echocardiography *on page 56*

ETT *see* Stress Test *on page 52*

Exercise Tolerance Test *see* Stress Test *on page 52*

Graded Exercise Test *see* Stress Test *on page 52*

GXT *see* Stress Test *on page 52*

Heart Biopsy *see* Endomyocardial Biopsy *on previous page*

HIS Bundle Electrograms *see* Cardiac Catheterization, Adult *on page 40*

HIS Bundle Recordings *see* Electrophysiologic Studies *on page 45*

Holter ECG *see* Holter Monitorization *on this page*

Holter Monitorization

CPT 93224

Synonyms Ambulatory Electrocardiography; Ambulatory Holter Electrocardiography; Dynamic Electrocardiography; Holter ECG

Abstract PROCEDURE COMMONLY INCLUDES: Holter monitorization is a method for recording the electrocardiogram (ECG) from an ambulatory subject over extended periods of time. Holter monitoring has emerged as the most sensitive and specific means of detecting and evaluating supraventricular and ventricular arrhythmias. The conventional Holter recording obtains ECG data comparable to leads V_1 through V_5 positions of the standard 12-lead ECG. The electrical signal is recorded onto a reel-to-reel recorder or cassette magnetic tape. The usual recording time on Holter monitorization is 24 hours, but newer recorders allow for up to 5 days of continued monitorization. Using a light portable tape recorder, prolonged recordings can be made while the patient engages in usual daily activities and records these activities as well as any symptoms in a diary. INDICATIONS: The clinical indications for ambulatory electrocardiography include:

- assessment of symptoms that may be related to arrhythmias
- assessment of RR interval characteristics
- assessment of risk in patients with or without symptoms of arrhythmia
- assessment of efficacy of antiarrhythmic therapy
- assessment of pacemaker function
- detection of myocardial ischemia

Patient Care/Scheduling PATIENT PREPARATION: To maximize the usefulness of ambulatory electrocardiography, the following information should be provided: general patient information (age, sex, phone number, etc), reason for performing test, medications, presence and type of pacemaker. On scheduling Holter monitorization, the request should specify if the monitorization should be continuous, intermittent, or patient activated or event recording. The routine Holter monitorization is continuous, but some laboratories offer any of these three choices, and if that is the case the specific type of request should be noted. No specified patient preparation is required. Patients are instructed to perform their normal daily activities and to record these activities as well as any symptoms in a diary.

Method TECHNIQUE: When the patient arrives at the Holter Laboratory he/she is greeted by the Holter Laboratory personnel and a detailed explanation of the procedure is given. Previous history of allergic reaction to tape or electrode gel is obtained. The chest is prepared and the electrodes are firmly put in place. The electrodes are looped and securely taped to minimize movement and artifact. The operation of the recorder and event marker is explained to the patient and information on how to complete the diary is provided. The patient is given instructions on continuing their normal daily activities, except they should avoid taking a bath while carrying the Holter monitor. Instructions on how to turn off the instrument, how to change batteries, and how to disconnect the monitor are provided.

Interpretation ADDITIONAL INFORMATION: The interpretation of Holter monitorization is done with the aid of an analysis system which includes a playback deck for either reel-to-reel or

(Continued)

Holter Monitorization *(Continued)*

cassette tapes and a screen for operator interaction with the system. Modern scanners have analog-to-digital converter and electronic memories, allowing for the ECG to be memorized and played back to provide real-time ECG strip documentation. The scanner will provide information regarding duration of taping, amount of time deleted from analysis because of artifact, maximal and minimal heart rate, number of ventricular and supraventricular complexes, and number of runs if present. The Holter technician will select strips of areas of interest for further analysis and interpretation. Most recorders have dual channel ECG monitorization to facilitate arrhythmic and ST displacement interpretation. Some systems provide "full disclosure" capability in which every complex occurring during the recording is plotted on compressed time and voltage scale. This is particularly helpful to detect sequence of premature ventricular complex and runs of ventricular tachycardia. Since the patient keeps a diary of activities, symptoms and time of medication, and the scanner can determine the time of occurrence of any given arrhythmia, it is possible to associate symptoms with the presence or absence of rhythm abnormalities.

References

DiMarco JP and Philbrick JT, "Use of Ambulatory Electrocardiographic (Holter) Monitoring," *Ann Intern Med*, 1990, 113(1):53-68.

Knoebel SB, Crawford MH, Dunn MI, et al, "Guidelines for Ambulatory Electrocardiography," *Circulation*, 1989, 79(1):206-15.

Sheffield LT, Berson A, Bragg-Rehmschel D, et al, "Recommendations for Standards of Instrumentation and Practice in the Use of Ambulatory Electrocardiography," *Circulation*, 1985, 71:626A-636A.

Invasive Cardiac Electrophysiologic Studies *see* Electrophysiologic Studies *on page 45*

Left Heart Catheterization *see* Cardiac Catheterization, Adult *on page 40*

MEET *see* Electrocardiogram, Adult, Exercise ECG Test *on page 44*

M-Mode Echo *see* M-Mode Echocardiography *on this page*

M-Mode Echocardiography

CPT 93307

Synonyms M-Mode Echo; Unidimensional Echo

Abstract **PROCEDURE COMMONLY INCLUDES:** M-mode echocardiography, the first form of cardiac ultrasound used in clinical practice, takes its name from the motion of the cardiac structures that was possible to visualize when this diagnostic method was introduced. M-mode echocardiography provides an "ice pick" view of the heart with a very high temporal and unidimensional space resolution, so that it provides an excellent method to measure chamber dimensions and to time cardiac events. **INDICATIONS:** The most common indications for this test include:

- wall thickness measurement of interventricular septum, posterior left ventricular wall and right ventricular free wall
- measurement of end-diastolic and end-systolic left ventricular internal dimensions
- percent of fractional shortening (difference between end-diastolic and end-systolic dimensions divided by end-diastolic dimension)
- measurement of right ventricular dimension; measurement of the anteroposterior diameter of the ascending aorta and left atrium

M-mode echocardiography is **most useful** in:

- diagnosis of pericardial effusion
- left ventricular hypertrophy
- generalized left ventricular dysfunction
- hypertrophic obstructive cardiomyopathy
- mitral valve prolapse
- mitral stenosis
- left atrial myxoma

CONTRAINDICATIONS: There are no contraindications for M-mode echocardiography but patients with chronic obstructive lung disease or marked obesity will usually have tests of poor diagnostic quality.

Patient Care/Scheduling PATIENT PREPARATION: No special patient preparation is required. Fasting is not necessary. The procedure can be done at any time. In scheduling patients that will have multiple cardiac diagnostic procedures it will be best to order the echocardiogram before Holter monitoring since the multiple electrodes placed on the chest for this procedure may interfere with the performance of the echocardiogram. Also, if a patient is to have a stress test on the same day, enough time (2-3 hours) should be allowed after the exercise test to perform the echocardiogram under basal conditions. SPECIAL INSTRUCTIONS: In most cases the M-mode echocardiogram is performed as part of a more complete cardiac ultrasound study that includes either 2-D echocardiography and/or Doppler echocardiography. The test that provides the most information should be requested, although sometimes this decision is left to the personnel in the Echo Laboratory. A complete cardiac ultrasound study takes anywhere from 60-90 minutes, the "M-mode" part of it takes approximately 30 minutes. To optimize the diagnostic yield of the echocardiogram a note relating the reason for the request should be made in the patient's chart or in a requisition form. Other useful information to be presented includes patient's age, weight, and height.

Method TECHNIQUE: A patient arriving at the Echo Laboratory is greeted by the laboratory personnel. He/she is asked about any previous experience with the procedure and is given a brief description of the test. Patient is asked to undress from the waist up and is given a gown with the opening in the front. Three electrodes for EKG monitorization are placed on the chest and the patient is asked to lie in a left lateral decubitus position. Currently, most M-mode echocardiograms are obtained by using a 2-D echocardiographic probe and selecting M-mode information from it. Briefly, the transducer is placed at the left parasternal border, the long axis view is selected, and the M-mode line is moved from the left ventricle to the mitral valve and finally to the aorta and left atrium. Recordings at these levels are registered in a strip chart recorder, a video recorder, or a page printer. These recordings become part of the report and of the Echo Laboratory file.

Interpretation NORMAL FINDINGS: Adequate interpretation of M-mode echocardiography requires knowledge of the normal values of the dimension of the cardiac chambers and great arteries (see table), and an understanding of the normal motion of the valves and different walls of the cardiac system. Distinct abnormalities can be characterized by M-mode echocardiography for many cardiovascular disorders.

Normal M-Mode Echocardiographic Values

	Mean (cm)	Range (cm)
RVD	1.7	0.9–2.6
LVIDD	4.7	3.5–5.7
PLVWT	0.9	0.6–1.1
IVSWT	0.9	0.6–1.1
LA	2.9	1.9–4.0
AO	2.7	2.0–3.7
FS	36%	34%–44%

RVD = Right ventricular dimension
LVIDD = Left ventricular internal dimension in diastole
PLVWT = Posterior left ventricular wall thickness
IVSWT = Interventricular wall thickness
LA = Left atrium
AO = Aorta
FS = Fractional shortening

Reproduced with permission from Feigenbaum H, *Echocardiography,* 4th ed, Philadelphia, PA: Lea & Febiger, 1986.

References

Sahn DJ, DeMaria A, Kisslo J, et al, "Recommendations Regarding Quantitation in M-Mode Echocardiography: Results of a Survey of Echocardiographic Measurements," *Circulation*, 1978, 58:1072.

Multistage Exercise Electrocardiographics Test *see* Electrocardiogram, Adult, Exercise ECG Test *on page 44*

Pacemaker Check

CPT 93731 (electronic analysis of dual chamber pacemaker, without programming); 93732 (with programming); 93733 (telephonic analysis)

Synonyms Pacemaker Follow-up; Pacer Check

Abstract **PROCEDURE COMMONLY INCLUDES:** Pacemaker checks are part of the routine follow-up of all patients with permanent pacemakers and are designed to anticipate failure and define its cause so that appropriate and timely preventive measures can be undertaken. As pacemakers have become more sophisticated so has the follow-up required for them. Although some routine check-ups can be made in the physician's office with the aid of an ECG alone, most medical centers that implant a large volume and variety of pacemakers have an electronic surveillance center with transtelephonic transmission and devices to underscore and analyze the pacemaker wave form and to carry a full programming routine in the programmable pacemakers. **INDICATIONS:** All patients with permanent pacemakers qualify as candidates for routine pacemaker follow-up. The frequency and depth of the check-up depends on the type of pacemaker, the time elapsed since implantation, and the underlying rhythm disorder. **CONTRAINDICATIONS:** No contraindications exist for pacer check.

Patient Care/Scheduling **PATIENT PREPARATION:** No special patient care or preparation is required for the routine pacemaker check. It is essential to instruct the patient to bring to the pacer check visit all pertinent information regarding the pacemaker. This is usually provided by the pacemaker manufacturing company in the form of a personalized card with the type and serial number of the device, as well as the date of implantation when appropriate instruction for transtelephonic transmission is given to the patient.

Method **TECHNIQUE:** A routine pacemaker check should include an initial clinical evaluation including history, physical exam, chest x-ray, fluoroscopy, and a 12-lead ECG with a long rhythm strip. Additionally, and at intervals mandated by the type and length of implantation of the device, a detailed oscilloscopic analysis of the pacemaker wave form should be performed, including analysis of precise pace rate (accurate to at least 1/10 of a beat/minute), amplitude, duration and contour of the impulse, and proof of appropriate pacing by analyzing a rhythm strip with the pacer turned into the asynchronous mode by a magnet placed on the surface of the device. In programmable pacemakers a full programming routine should be carried at appropriate intervals. A highly successful extension of the pacemaker check center has been developed through the use of transtelephonic monitoring. This has permitted many of the pacemaker check functions routinely carried out in the hospital or physician's office to be performed through the telephone from the patient's home. Transtelephonic monitoring has facilitated the follow-up of distant patients and increased the frequency of evaluation without the logistic problems of patient transport.

Pacemaker Evaluation

Abstract **PROCEDURE COMMONLY INCLUDES:** History, blood pressure check, monitoring, reprogramming, patient education, and electronic surveillance **INDICATIONS:** To determine the function of a pacemaker, evaluate battery reserve and lead function, and reprogram parameters as needed by each patient.

Patient Care/Scheduling **PATIENT PREPARATION:** The skin is prepared. Electrodes are then placed on patient's arms and legs. The procedure will take from 15-30 minutes. **SPECIAL INSTRUCTIONS:** Outpatients are by appointment only. Inpatients are performed as ordered. The patient should know the type of pacemaker and the date it was implanted.

Method **TECHNIQUE:** A magnet is placed over the pacemaker implantation site and a recording is obtained to determine configuration and rate of paced rhythm. A small computer is placed on the patient's chest to determine rate, pulse width, and pacing intervals.

Specimen **TURNAROUND TIME:** 24-48 hours except in emergencies.

Pacemaker Follow-up *see* Pacemaker Check *on this page*

Pacer Check *see* Pacemaker Check *on this page*

Phonocardiography and Pulse Tracings

CPT 93201 (phonocardiogram with ECG lead); 93205 (with ECG lead, indirect carotid artery and/or jugular vein tracing, and/or apex cardiogram); 93210 (intracardiac)

Synonyms Pulse Tracings: Phono, Carotid, Apex, and Venous

Abstract **PROCEDURE COMMONLY INCLUDES:** Phonocardiography refers to the technique of recording heart sounds and murmurs. As commonly used, the term phonocardiography also embraces carotid, apex, and venous pulse tracings. Low frequency vibrations in the order of 1-30 cycles/second are produced by myocardial contractility and distention of veins or arteries reach the neck and surface of the chest and can be graphically recorded as an apex cardiogram, carotid pulse, or venous jugular pulse. Higher frequency vibrations in the order of 30-1000 cycles/second are provided by the opening and closure of valves and flow through different valves or chambers. These vibrations are registered as sound by the human ear and with selective filtering can be registered by phonocardiography as heart sounds, clicks, and murmurs. An ECG is commonly used as reference. **INDICATIONS:** Phonocardiography and pulse tracings are used to graphically document normal and abnormal heart sounds and pulsations. Phono is most commonly used to clarify the origin of normal and abnormal heart sounds or murmurs, to help timing of cardiac events, to determine systolic time intervals (see listing), and as a teaching tool for bedside diagnostic skills. By analyzing the timing, duration, and intensity of the recorded vibrations it is possible to differentiate physiologic from pathologic heart murmurs. Phonocardiography and pulse tracings afford clues to many specific cardiovascular diagnoses including aortic stenosis, mitral stenosis, hypertrophic obstructive cardiomyopathy, mitral valve prolapse, atrial septal defect, constrictive cardiomyopathy, and many others. **CONTRAINDICATIONS:** No contraindications exist for phonocardiography and pulse tracings.

Patient Care/Scheduling **PATIENT PREPARATION:** No special patient preparation is required. Fasting is not necessary. **SPECIAL INSTRUCTIONS:** A phonocardiogram usually is performed in association with M-mode echocardiography or Doppler echocardiography. The phonocardiogram and pulse tracing recordings will require an additional 20-30 minutes. To optimize the diagnostic yield of the phonocardiogram and pulse tracings a note relating the reason for the request should be made in the patient's chart or on a requisition form.

Method **TECHNIQUE:** For best results of phonocardiographic and pulse recordings, the room where this is to be done should be free of noise and the patient must be lying comfortably in the supine position. The placement of transducers should be supervised by a physician with knowledge of the clinical problem and the most informative location on the chest wall in a given patient. For the phonocardiogram, the microphones are usually applied in the second right intercostal space, the left lower sternal border, and the cardiac apex. A choice of filters can be used in order to accentuate low frequency diastolic sound or murmurs or, alternatively, the higher frequency heart sound or murmurs. For the apex cardiogram, the patient is usually placed in a left lateral position and the transducer is applied at the point of maximal apical displacement. The transducer is either held by hand or by a strap around the chest. Simultaneous recordings of an ECG and phonocardiogram are usually obtained. For the carotid pulse tracing, the patient is placed in a supine position with a pillow between the shoulders to hyperextend the neck and make the carotid pulse easier to register. A handheld transducer is usually placed over the carotid pulsation and registered simultaneously with an ECG and a phono recording from the aortic area. For the jugular venous pulse recording, the patient is placed in the supine position with the head of the bed elevated to 45° or to the point where venous pulsations are more apparent. The transducer is held by hand over the internal jugular vein in the supraclavicular fossa between the attachment of the sternocleidomastoid muscle.

Interpretation **NORMAL FINDINGS:** For best interpretation of the phonocardiogram and pulse tracings good knowledge of cardiac physical diagnosis is required. Clear understanding of the characteristics and wave forms of the normal phonocardiogram and normal pulse tracings is essential before attempting to interpret abnormal findings. The phonocardiogram is used to evaluate normal versus abnormal splitting of the first and second heart sounds. It can also differentiate normal versus single, wide, and paradoxic or fixed splitting of the second sound. It is also used in the evaluation of ejection sounds, opening snaps, clicks, third and fourth heart sounds, friction rubs, and prosthetic valve sound. The carotid pulse tracing is applied to time acoustic events, to calculate systolic time intervals, and to evaluate through its contour pattern the velocity and force of left ventricular ejection. The apex

(Continued)

Phonocardiography and Pulse Tracings *(Continued)*

cardiogram has characteristic abnormalities in the presence of left ventricular hypertrophy, left ventricular aneurysm, constrictive pericarditis, congestive cardiomyopathy, and mitral insufficiency. Characteristic abnormalities in the jugular venous pulse are seen in patients with tricuspid stenosis and insufficiency, constrictive pericarditis, and atrioventricular dissociation.

References

Mills P and Crage E, "Echophonocardiography," *Prog Cardiovasc Dis*, 1978, 20:337.

Tavel ME, *Clinical Phonocardiography and External Pulse Recording*, 3rd ed, Chicago, IL: Year Book Medical Publishers Inc, 1978.

Programmed Electrical Stimulation *see* Electrophysiologic Studies *on page 45*

Pulse Tracings: Phono, Carotid, Apex, and Venous *see* Phonocardiography and Pulse Tracings *on previous page*

Right and Left Heart Catheterization *see* Cardiac Catheterization, Adult *on page 40*

Right Heart Catheterization *see* Cardiac Catheterization, Adult *on page 40*

Right Ventricular Endomyocardial Biopsy *see* Endomyocardial Biopsy *on page 46*

STI *see* Systolic Time Intervals *on page 54*

Stress Test

CPT 93015

Related Information

Cardiac Catheterization, Adult *on page 40*

Synonyms ETT; Exercise Tolerance Test; Graded Exercise Test; GXT

Abstract **PROCEDURE COMMONLY INCLUDES:** The skin at the electrode sites is vigorously prepared with alcohol and mild abrasion to remove superficial layers of skin. Electrodes are attached using the Mason-Likar lead system. Baseline, pretest 12-lead electrocardiograms are recorded in the supine and standing positions and compared to previous standard 12-lead EKGs for new changes. (Post 30-second hyperventricular electrocardiograms are often performed to identify ventilatory induced stress test changes.) The test procedure is explained to the patient and informed consent is obtained. The technician verbally instructs and demonstrates for the patient how to walk on the treadmill. The test is performed with a technician and at least one other qualified professional present. The physician is available in the testing area. An appropriate exercise protocol is selected based on the clinical questions asked, the patient's medical status, and the predicted ability of the patient. Every 2-3 minutes the speed and/or grade of the treadmill are increased to yield an increment of 1/2-2 METS increase per stage. At least one channel (V_5) and preferably three channels of the electrocardiogram are continuously monitored on a real-time visual display. Twelve-lead electrocardiograms and blood pressures are recorded at least once at every stage (usually the last 30 seconds of each stage). Heart rate, ST segments, arrhythmias, symptoms, and subjective patient responses regarding the activity are also continuously monitored. The test is terminated when the patient achieves a subjective maximal effort, significant ischemic changes are observed, significant rhythm disturbances are observed, hemodynamic status is compromised, the patient requests to stop the test, the equipment fails or a predetermined endpoint is achieved. At the conclusion of the exercise test, the treadmill speed and grade are lowered to a base level and the patient is encouraged to ambulate as tolerated to avoid venous pooling and a vasovagal response. Patients ambulate for 3-5 minutes or until heart rate and blood pressure plateau. Patients are then observed in the sitting or supine position. If patients cannot ambulate after the test or if ambulation is contraindicated, patients should be placed in the prone position immediately and monitored. During recovery, the EKG is continuously monitored and recorded along with blood pressure and symptoms every minute until the patient is hemodynamically stable and has returned to a near pretest level. **INDICATIONS:**

- determine the presence and severity of exercise induced myocardial ischemia

- evaluate potential for rhythm disturbances
- evaluate hemodynamic responses to activity
- evaluate the effect of medical or interventional therapy
- prescribe appropriate activity guidelines
- evaluate patient's exercise/work tolerance
- evaluate the impact of cardiac rehabilitation intervention

CONTRAINDICATIONS:

- acute MI
- severe valvular heart disease
- uncontrolled ventricular arrhythmias
- uncontrolled supraventricular arrhythmias compromising cardiac function
- unstable or at-rest angina
- uncontrolled congestive heart failure
- suspected or known dissecting aneurysm
- thrombophlebitis
- recent embolism
- left ventricular outflow tract (LVOT) obstruction
- clinically significant acute pericarditis or myocarditis
- complete heart block
- intracardiac thrombus
- acute infection
- significant psychiatric disturbance
- neuromuscular complications that prevent or severely limit ambulation

Patient Care/Scheduling **PATIENT PREPARATION:** The patient is examined and cleared for exercise by a physician. Test procedure, risks, and benefits are explained to the patient and informed consent is obtained. The patient is weighed prior to the test. All clothes above the waist are removed. Female patients may wear a loose fitting hospital gown that offers easy access to electrodes and lead wires. Large breasted women may require binding to minimize EKG artifact. The skin at electrode sites is vigorously prepared with abrasion to remove superficial skin layer and alcohol to remove dirt and oils. Electrodes are attached using the Mason-Likar lead system. Electrodes and lead wires are secured to minimize motion artifact. Resting, supine, and standing 12-lead EKGs are recorded and compared to previous EKGs to identify changes. (A 30-second posthyperventilation EKG is often recorded prior to exercise to identify ventilatory induced changes in the ST segments.) Patient receives instruction and demonstration regarding walking on the treadmill. Patient is encouraged to walk upright, take long steps, and rely on the treadmill bar only for balance and not for support. After a brief trial period when the patient is adapted to treadmill ambulation, the protocol is initiated. **AFTERCARE:** The patient is monitored until hemodynamically stable and values return to a near-baseline level. A neutral temperature shower may be taken following the test but extremes of water temperature should be avoided. Vigorous activity is not recommended for 12-24 hours following the test. Patients should check-out with laboratory personnel when leaving the area. **SPECIAL INSTRUCTIONS:** Outpatients are by appointment only. Inpatients are scheduled as soon as possible (usually within 24 hours of request). Patients are instructed not to eat or drink for 3-4 hours before test, and are also instructed to bring or wear clothes suitable for exercise; preferably tennis, jogging, or rubber soled walking shoes and shorts. Patients are requested to discontinue long-acting nitrates. Other medications should be taken as prescribed unless instructed differently. Insulin dependent diabetics should not take premeal dose of insulin if they skip that meal. The procedure, risks and benefits, should be explained by the physician and receipt of patient consent should be documented prior to beginning the test.

Method **EQUIPMENT:** Motor driven treadmill, multichannel electrocardiograph with real-time monitor display and printer; sphygmomanometer; cardiac emergency equipment (defibrillator, oxygen, suction, I.V. kits and fluid, emergency drugs, airway management equipment). **DATA ACQUIRED:** 12-lead EKG, heart rate, arrhythmias, ST segment values, blood pressure, symptoms, patient subjective responses (eg, rating of perceived exertion, angina scale, dyspnea scale).

Interpretation **NORMAL FINDINGS:** Shortening of the PR and QT intervals and a J point depression may occur. Less than 1 mm ST depression 60-80 msec after the J point as compared to resting measures. A linear increase in heart rate with activity ≥85% predicted (Continued)

Stress Test *(Continued)*

maximal heart rate (if not on a chronotropic medication – most commonly beta blocker). A continuous increase of 7-12 mm Hg in SBP/MET to a peak ≤220 mm Hg. A fall, no change, ≤20 mm increase in DBP to a peak ≤120 mm Hg. Occasional ventricular or supraventricular ectopy that does not significantly increase with activity. Test termination because of leg or general fatigue and appropriate SOB. Nausea and dizziness early in recovery are not uncommon. **CRITICAL VALUES:** 1 mm or more upright, horizontal or down sloping ST segment depression, 60-80 msec beyond J point as compared to rest (without any compounding medication, metabolic or EKG abnormalities). Horizontal or down sloping ST segment depression carries a greater probability of significant CAD than rapid up sloping depression. ≥1 mm ST segment elevation of the J point in leads without significant Q waves. >10 mm Hg fall in SBP with increasing workloads recorded on two separate readings at least 30 seconds apart (especially if associated with symptoms of exercise intolerance). PB >10 mm Hg above rest during activity. Increase SBP >250 mm Hg. Increasing ventricular ectopy to >30% of all complexes. Onset of bundle branch blocks. Onset of second degree or third degree heart block. Lightheadedness, cyanosis, ataxia, confusion, or nausea during activity. **LIMITATIONS:**

- ST segments cannot be accurately interpreted if patient has LBBB, LVH, WPW, digitalis, ventricular pacing, cardiomyopathy, hypokalemia, MVP, pectus excavation or baseline ST-T wave abnormalities.
- Sudden intense activity can cause false-positive ST segment depression.
- Medications (beta blockers, calcium channel blockers, vasodilators and after load reducing agents) may reduce myocardial oxygen demand and prevent expression of ischemia during activity.
- Early termination of test by patient or investigator limits predictive ability.
- Exercise stress testing has an average sensitivity of 60% to 70% and specificity of 80% to 90%.
- The less severe the disease the lower the sensitivity.
- Orthopedic complications or lack of patient motivation or compliance limit predictive ability of test if peak myocardial oxygen demand is not achieved.
- Women yield a higher false-positive rate than men.

References

American College of Sports Medicine, *Guidelines for Exercise Testing and Prescription*, 3rd ed, Philadelphia, PA: Lea & Febiger, 1986.

American Heart Association, Committee on Exercise, *Exercise Testing and Training of Individuals With Heart Disease or at High Risk for Its Development: A Handbook for Physicians*, Dallas, TX: American Heart Association, 1975.

American Heart Association, *The Exercise Standards Book*, Dallas, TX: American Heart Association, 1979.

Ellestad MH, *Stress Testing, Principles and Practice*, Philadelphia, PA: FA Davis Co, 1980.

Froelicher VF, *Exercise Testing and Training*, New York, NY: LeJacq Publishing Inc, 1983.

Systolic Time Intervals

CPT 93201

Synonyms STI

Abstract **PROCEDURE COMMONLY INCLUDES:** Systolic time intervals are measurements obtained through phonocardiography carotid pulse tracing and electrocardiography in an attempt to give insight into systolic ventricular function. Although they can be measured in relation to right ventricular function, they usually imply left ventricular systolic times unless specified otherwise. **INDICATIONS:** Systolic time intervals are used as a simple noninvasive quantitative method to assess left ventricular performance. However, it should be remembered that systolic time intervals are nonspecific and their simplicity may be misleading. As with other noninvasive techniques, their proper application requires they be used in conjunction with careful appraisal. **CONTRAINDICATIONS:** No contraindications exist for the measurement of systolic time intervals, but it should be remembered that often conflicting effects may coexist in the same patient and if the effects of digitalis or other inotropic agents are added to this, the resulting data may indeed be confusing.

Patient Care/Scheduling PATIENT PREPARATION: Since systolic time intervals are usually obtained by recording a phonocardiogram, ECG, and carotid pulse, the patient preparation and scheduling is similar to that discussed in the section on phonocardiography.

Method TECHNIQUE: The most widely used method to calculate systolic time intervals utilizes a configuration of an ECG lead recording with clear delineation of the beginning of the QRS complex, a carotid pulse tracing with clear definition of the beginning of the upstroke and the dicrotic notch, and a phonocardiogram with clear recording of the beginning of the A_2 component of the second heart sound. From the simultaneous registration of these three signals at fast paper speed (usually 100 mm/second) the following measurements are made: total electromechanical systole (QS_2) measured from the beginning of the QRS to the beginning of the second heart sound, left ventricular ejection time (LVET) measured from the beginning of the carotid upstroke to the dicrotic notch, and pre-ejection period (PEP) calculated by substantiating LVET from QS_2.

Interpretation NORMAL FINDINGS: Good understanding of the factors that alter the duration of each of the components of the systolic time interval is needed before attempting to apply them in clinical practice (see table). The most widely used measurement of systolic

Factors That Alter Systolic Time Intervals

	Chronotropism		Inotropism		Afterload		Preload	
	Increased	Decreased	Increased	Decreased	Increased	Decreased	Increased	Decreased
PEP	↓	↑	↓	↑	±	↓	↓	↑
LVET	↓	↑	↑	↓	↑	±	↑	↓
QS_2	↓	↑	±	±	↑	±	±	±

↑ = lengthen; ↓ = shorten; ± = variable or no change

time interval, that is applied clinically, is the PEP over LVET ratio. This has been found to be the most sensitive and specific marker for evaluating left ventricle function with systolic time intervals. In chronic myocardial disease on the basis of cardiomyopathy, coronary artery disease, hypertensive cardiovascular disease, or valvular heart disease, the PEP/LVET ratio increases as a consequence of prolongation of the PEP and shortening of the LVET. In acute myocardial infarction there is obstruction of the QS_2 interval. In aortic stenosis there is prolongation of the LVET and shortening of the PEP. In aortic insufficiency there is also prolongation of the LVET with shortening of the PEP with a corresponding low PEP/LVET.

References

Salcedo EE and Siegel W, "Systolic Time Intervals," *Noninvasive Cardiac Diagnosis*, Chang E, ed, Chapter 11, Philadelphia, PA: Lea & Febiger, 1976.

TEE *see* Transesophageal Echocardiography *on next page*

Thallium Stress Testing

CPT 78461

Abstract INDICATIONS: Thallium imaging.

Patient Care/Scheduling PATIENT PREPARATION: The skin is prepared. Electrodes are attached to the chest. The patient is instructed on how to walk on the treadmill. The patient is also hyperventilated (deep fast breathing for 30 seconds) to give the physician a preview of how the heart will react to exercise. SPECIAL INSTRUCTIONS: By appointment only. Must be scheduled 24 hours in advance. Patient is instructed to eat 2 hours prior to the test and not to eat, smoke, or drink anything after that until the test is completed. Patient is also instructed to wear clothes suitable for exercise, preferably tennis shoes and shorts. Physician in charge of stress testing should be present to witness the test unless patient's own physician requests to do so. Patients on cardiac medication will be instructed accordingly. Consent form informs patient of benefits and risks.

(Continued)

Thallium Stress Testing *(Continued)*

Method TECHNIQUE: A thallium stress test is the same as a treadmill stress test except that the patient is given a radioactive material, thallium-201, approximately 45 seconds before the cessation of exercise. To administer the thallium, an I.V. is started. Inpatients' I.V.s are started in the patient's room. Outpatients' I.V.s are started in the Heart Station by a technician. Once the thallium is administered and exercise has stopped, the patient is placed under a gamma camera for the thallium imaging. See Nuclear Medicine.

Specimen TURNAROUND TIME: 24-48 hours.

Transesophageal Echocardiography

CPT 93312

Synonyms Esophageal Echo; TEE

Abstract PROCEDURE COMMONLY INCLUDES: Transesophageal echocardiography (TEE) has been developed to solve one of the limitations of echocardiography, that is, the poor imaging quality seen in some patients in whom the bony structures as well as increased lung interface degrade the quality of the images obtained with conventional echocardiography. By placing an echo transducer at the tip of a gastroscope and advancing it into the esophagus, the heart can be imaged from behind without any lung or chest cage interference. Additionally, the closer proximity to the heart allows for utilization of higher frequency transducers which provide higher resolution images. Transesophageal echocardiography has provided a new window through which the heart can be examined with far greater detail than was once thought possible. The mild inconvenience of having to pass a transesophageal probe has been by far outweighed by the enhanced images obtained with it. Presently, transesophageal echocardiography includes 2-D echocardiography, pulsed Doppler, and color flow imagings. Continuous wave Doppler should be incorporated in the near future. INDICATIONS: Transesophageal echocardiography currently is being used intraoperatively to follow cardiac function during cardiac and noncardiac surgery, in the intensive care units to follow and evaluate critically ill patients, and in the study of ambulatory patients to better evaluate a variety of cardiovascular disorders. Transesophageal echocardiography has been found most useful in the evaluation of prosthetic valve dysfunction, particularly mitral valve prosthesis, in the quantitation and diagnostic characterization of native mitral valve insufficiency, in the evaluation of left atrial thrombosis and masses, in the evaluation of bacterial endocarditis and its complications, and in the evaluation of intracardiac shunts. CONTRAINDICATIONS: TEE is contraindicated in patients with esophageal obstructions or with respiratory failure if not intubated.

Patient Care/Scheduling SPECIAL INSTRUCTIONS: To minimize the risk of aspiration, a period of 6-8 hours fasting is recommended. An intravenous line to keep a vein open for administration of I.V. antibiotics is needed, and sedation as required is advised. Patients with prosthetic valves, native valve stenosis or insufficiency, and congenital heart disease should receive I.V. antibiotic prophylaxis as recommended by the American Heart Association. After the antibiotics have been given the patient should be expected to be in the laboratory for approximately 1 hour to allow for the performance of the procedure and recovery from sedation and analgesic when used. There is no need for repeated antibiotic prophylaxis after initial dose is completed. Most patients will be able to resume full activity after the procedure, but outpatients are advised to have a companion drive them back home to minimize risks from sedation and analgesics when used.

Method TECHNIQUE: A patient arriving at the Echo Laboratory is greeted by the laboratory personnel, a fasting period of 6-8 hours is confirmed, the reasons indicated for the test are reviewed, vital signs are obtained, symptomatic status is determined, history of allergies is determined, and a detailed explanation of the procedure is made. SBE antibiotic prophylaxis is completed as recommended by the AHA. The patient is asked to undress from the waist up and is gowned with the opening in the front. Electrocardiographic and blood pressure monitorization will be made throughout the procedure. The laboratory should be prepared for cardiopulmonary resuscitation. A local anesthetic is given to the back of the throat through a spray, and a fast-acting hypnotic and analgesic is given I.V. (currently we use Versed® 0.5-2 mg I.V. and Demend® 25-100 mg I.V.). The patient is then placed on left lateral decubitus and the esophageal probe is passed. A dental suction set minimizes flow of saliva out of the mouth. Patient stays awake and comfortable throughout the procedure in most cases. A systematic and complete study should be performed on each patient. Additionally, the area of specific concern should be evaluated with further detail. A complete study will include 2-D imaging and color flow Doppler study of all cardiac chambers, valves, and great vessels. The study is initiated with the probe placed most distally, which provides a short axis view of the left ventricle as the probe is removed a view equivalent to an apical 4-chamber is obtained. This allows for the best view of the mitral and tricuspid valves. Further removal of the probe allows for visualization of the outflow tract of the left ventricle and aortic valve, after this the left atrium atrial appendage, interatrial septum, and pulmonary veins can be studied. Finally, with further removal of the probe, the aortic arch is visualized. The color Doppler is turned on during the study to evaluate normal and abnormal flow patterns. A continuous video recording is obtained throughout the study for later study and analysis. After completion of the study, the transesophageal probe is removed and the patient is kept under observation until regaining a prestudy status.

Interpretation NORMAL FINDINGS: Transesophageal echocardiography has provided a new window to the heart, but the operator must recognize and become familiar with the different orientation of the cardiac structures and tomographic planes as seen from a different perspective. Also, there is a limitation in the number of tomographic planes than can be obtained through TEE since the motion of the probe is somewhat limited in the esophagus. With these limitations in mind, the interpretation of images through TEE is similar to that described in the section of color Doppler echocardiography.

References

Seward JB, Khandheria BK, Oh JK, et al, "Transesophageal Echocardiography: Technique, Anatomic Correlations, Implementation, and Clinical Applications," *Mayo Clin Proc*, 1988, 63(7):649-80.

Two-Dimensional Echocardiography

Synonyms Cross-Sectional Echocardiography; 2-D Echo

Abstract PROCEDURE COMMONLY INCLUDES: Two-dimensional echocardiography is the most common cardiac ultrasound technique in use today. It provides real time, high resolution tomographic images of the heart and great vessels. It is the preferred noninvasive imaging technique for a variety of cardiovascular disorders. INDICATIONS: Two-dimensional echocardiography provides information for the diagnosis and management of patients with congenital, pericardial, myocardial, and valvular heart disease. It provides accurate information regarding chamber size and ventricular function. The high resolution and clear anatomic detail provided by 2-D echo makes this technique ideally suited for the analysis of common and complex congenital heart disease. It permits not only the diagnosis but the classification of interatrial and interventricular septal defects as well as atrioventricular canal defects. The diagnosis of pulmonic stenosis, bicuspid aortic valve, tetralogy of Fallot, transposition of the great arteries and Ebstein anomaly is greatly enhanced by the use of 2-D echocardiography. Two-dimensional echocardiography allows for the diagnosis and sizing of pericardial effusions and can be used as a guide to perform pericardiocentesis. The diagnosis and characterization of left ventricular dilatation and dysfunction has been greatly aided by 2-D echo; it permits differentiation between congestive, restrictive, and obstructive cardiomyopathies. Ejection fraction obtained by 2-D echo correlates well with that obtained by angiography and nuclear ventriculography. Two-dimensional echocardiography is firmly established as an ideal imaging technique to evaluate patients with valvular heart disease. In mitral stenosis it not only provides an accurate diagnosis but it allows for gradation of severity, pliability, presence of calcification, and aids in determining timing for surgery plus feasibility of commissurotomy or need for valve replacement. In patients with mitral insufficiency it provides accurate assessment of the physiopathologic process responsible for the cause of the regurgitation and its effects in ventricular function. In patients with aortic valve disease, 2-D permits one not only to establish the diagnosis but to ascertain the etiology and severity. Two-dimensional echocardiography has also been most useful in the evaluation of intracardiac tumor, clots, and vegetations. CONTRAINDICATIONS: There are no contraindications for 2-D echocardiography, but as with M-mode echocardiography, patients with COPD or obesity may have tests of poor diagnostic quality. An advantage of 2-D over M-mode echo in this respect is the possibility of performing studies with the 2-D echo technique from the apical and subcostal windows which may be the only

(Continued)

Two-Dimensional Echocardiography *(Continued)*

areas from where the heart can be visualized with echo in patients with chronic lung disease.

Patient Care/Scheduling **PATIENT PREPARATION:** No special patient preparation is required. Fasting is not necessary. The procedure can be done at any time. When scheduling patients that will have multiple cardiac diagnostic procedures, it would be best to order the echocardiogram before Holter monitoring since the multiple electrodes from this procedure may interfere with the performance of the echocardiogram. Also, if a patient is to have a stress test on the same day as the 2-D echo, enough time (2-3 hours) should be allowed after the exercise test to perform the echocardiogram under basal conditions. **SPECIAL INSTRUCTIONS:** A 2-D echocardiogram takes approximately 45 minutes to perform. Most laboratories allot 1 hour per test to allow for patient preparation and chart handling. To optimize the diagnostic yield of the echocardiogram a note relating the reason for the request should be made in the patient's chart or in a requisition form. Other useful information to be presented include patient's age, weight, and height.

Method **TECHNIQUE:** A patients arriving at the Echo Laboratory is greeted by the laboratory personnel. He/she is asked about previous experience with the procedure and is given a brief description of the test. The patient is asked to undress from the waist up and is given a gown with the opening in the front. Three electrodes for EKG monitorization are placed on the chest and the patient is asked to lie in a left lateral decubitus position. A complete 2-D echocardiogram includes multiple tomographic views from the left parasternal area, the apex, subcostal region, and suprasternal fossa. Recordings at all these levels are made on a video cassette recorder and selected frames are registered for the final report. All necessary measurements are made from either freeze frames during the study or afterwards from the video tape.

Interpretation **NORMAL FINDINGS:** Adequate interpretation of 2-D echocardiography requires knowledge of the normal values of the dimensions of the cardiac chambers and great arteries (see following table) and understanding of the normal motion of the valves and different walls of the cardiac system. Distinct abnormalities can be characterized by 2-D echocardiography for most cardiovascular disorders (see References).

Two-Dimensional Echocardiography

	Males	Females
Left ventrical end diastolic volume	130 ± 27 (73–201) mL	92 ± 19 (53–146) mL
Left atrial volume	50 mL	36 mL
Left ventricular mass	135 g	99 g

Reproduced with permission from Schiller NB, "Cardiology," *Echocardiography and Doppler in Clinical Cardiology,* Chapter 41, Parmley WW and Chartarjee K, eds, Philadelphia, PA: Lippincott Co, 1987.

References

Henry WL, DeMaria A, Gramiak R, et al, "Report of the American Society of Echocardiography Committee on Nomenclature and Standards in Two-Dimensional Echocardiography," *Circulation*, 1980, 62:212.

Salcedo EE, *Atlas of Echocardiography*, 2nd ed, Philadelphia, PA: WB Saunders Co, 1985.

Tajik AJ, Seward JB, Hagler DJ, et al, "Two-Dimensional Real-Time Ultrasonic Imaging of the Heart and Great Vessels, Technique, Image Orientation, Structure Identification, and Validation," *Mayo Clin Proc*, 1978, 53:271.

Unidimensional Echo *see* M-Mode Echocardiography *on page 48*

CRITICAL CARE

Carlos M. Isada, MD

The field of critical care has been revolutionized by the introduction of the flow-directed pulmonary artery (PA) catheter (the Swan-Ganz catheter). In many large institutions, invasive hemodynamic monitoring at the bedside has become routine, both in critical care units and in "step-down" units. Terms such as the "wedge" and "SVR" are now part of the daily conversations of resident house staff. In some coronary intensive care units, invasive monitoring is considered mandatory in the post-MI patient. It is considered bold (or negligent) to manage a complicated infarct without a PA catheter.

Although several million PA catheters have been used since 1970, the therapeutic impact of this invasive procedure remains controversial. Some experts believe that this device fails to influence the ultimate outcome of the critically ill patient. In a large retrospective series by Gore at al[1] (1987), the use of the PA catheter displayed no benefit in patient with acute MI. Critically ill patients who were managed without this catheter had the same average length of hospitalization and long-term prognosis. In an editorial in the journal *Chest*, Robin[2] reviewed the literature regarding harmful effects of the Swan-Ganz catheter and advocated a nationwide "moratorium" on the use of such devices. Certainly, the controversy regarding the utility of invasive monitoring (and the entire field of critical care) is likely to continue for years to come. The growing trend in U.S. hospitals is to accept only the more acutely ill patients; thus, the role of the critical care unit appears secure despite this scrutiny.

The following section outlines the procedures most commonly carried out in the critical care unit. Many procedures are included in the Pulmonary Medicine section and are also applicable, such as thoracentesis, oximetry, arterial blood gases, and others. In all such procedures, there is considerable variation in technique, even amongst physicians in the same institution.

---

[1] Gore JM, Goldberg RJ, Spodick DH, et al, "A Community-Wide Aassessment of the Use of Pulmonary Artery Catheter in Patients With Acute Myocardial Infarction," *Chest*, 1987, 92(4):727-31.

[2] Robin ED, "Death by Pulmonary Artery Flow-Directed Catheter (editorial)," *Chest*, 1987, 92(4):727-31.

Arterial Cannulation

CPT 36620 (arterial catheterization or cannulation for sampling, monitoring, or transfusion); 36625 (cutdown)

Related Information

Arterial Blood Gases *on page 206*
Pulse Oximetry *on page 241*
Swan-Ganz Catheterization *on page 71*

Synonyms Arterial Catheterization; Arterial Line Placement; Direct Arterial Pressure Monitoring

Abstract **PROCEDURE COMMONLY INCLUDES:** Insertion of an indwelling catheter directly into the arterial circulation for continuous blood pressure (BP) monitoring. **INDICATIONS:** May be divided into three categories:

- hemodynamic monitoring of the unstable patient (acutely hypotensive or hypertensive) including those on vasopressor or vasodilator agents
- multiple sampling of arterial blood, particularly in the mechanically ventilated patient
- determination of cardiac output (less common)

CONTRAINDICATIONS: Poor collateral circulation around the artery to be cannulated constitutes a relative contraindication. Thrombus formation at the catheter site is common and can result in distal extremity ischemia if collaterals are inadequate. Also, coagulopathies, systemic anticoagulation (eg, heparin), and interventional thrombolysis are considered contraindications and reversal may be required.

Patient Care/Scheduling **PATIENT PREPARATION:** The risks and benefits of the procedure are explained. After the site of cannulation is selected by the physician, the area is prepared using povidone-iodine scrub for a minimum of 30 seconds. A sterile technique should be maintained. **AFTERCARE:** Meticulous care is required to avoid line-related infections. Recommendations by the Centers for Disease Control include:[1]

- handwashing prior to any manipulation of the system
- applying topical antiseptics to the insertion site immediately after catheter is placed
- covering the site with sterile dressing
- recording date of catheter insertion and each dressing change
- daily inspection of catheter site
- replacing sterile dressing every 48-72 hours with new antibiotic ointment
- flushing of line using normal saline in a closed flush system
- changing flush solution every 24 hours
- changing arterial line site every 4 days or less
- removing catheter promptly at the first sign of infection

COMPLICATIONS: Estimates of significant complications range from 15% to 40%. Thrombosis is the most frequent complication. Incidence of thrombosis increases if:

- the catheter is left in place more that 3-4 days
- a large diameter catheter is used
- multiple puncture attempts are required
- hypotension, decreased cardiac output, atherosclerosis, or hypothermia are present
- prolonged pressure is required to control bleeding after catheter removal; thrombosis rate under optimal conditions is approximately 5% to 8%; symptomatic occlusion requiring surgery is much less (<1%).

Infectious complications are also frequent, with the catheter serving as either a primary or secondary site of bacteremia. Factors predisposing to infection include prolonged (more than 4 days) catheter insertion, the use of cutdown for insertion, local inflammation, and infection from a secondary source. Other complications include hemorrhage or hematoma formation, pseudoaneurysms, vasovagal reactions, and local skin necrosis. Distal embolization of small clots or air may occur if improper line-flush technique is used.

Method **EQUIPMENT:** Varies somewhat depending on artery selected. A 19- or 20-gauge teflon catheter-over-needle is used in most instances. 16 cm catheters are used for femoral and axillary sites, shorter (1 1/4" to 2") catheters are used for radial, brachial, and dorsalis pedis sites. If the Seldinger technique is used, a flexible guidewire is also needed. Other equipment includes sterile gloves, hair covers, povidone-iodine, 1% lidocaine without epinephrine, and 3-0 or 4-0 silk suture and suture equipment. **TECHNIQUE:** The radial artery is generally considered the site of choice; alternate sites include femoral, axillary, brachial and dorsalis pedis arteries. For radial artery cannulation, the presence of collateral flow must first be established using the modified Allen test. Following this, the wrist is dorsiflexed 60° and using a sterile technique 1% lidocaine is used to infiltrate overlying skin. Catheter-over-needle is inserted at a 30° angle to skin and advanced until arterial blood is seen in the needle hub. The needle is held fixed while the surrounding catheter is advanced into the artery. The needle is removed and the catheter hub is attached to the connecting tubing. After suturing the catheter in place, a wrist board may be used to stabilize the neutral wrist position. The Seldinger technique may be used for larger arteries. Here, the artery is located with a simple 20-gauge needle. Once arterial blood is returned, a flexible guidewire is passed through the needle; the needle is removed and the teflon catheter is threaded over the guidewire into the artery. **DATA ACQUIRED:** Graphic waveform of arterial pressure, with pressure on the vertical axis (mm Hg) and time on the horizontal axis.

Interpretation **NORMAL FINDINGS:** A typical arterial pressure tracing for a normal individual is depicted in Figure A. The peak of each waveform represents the systolic blood pressure

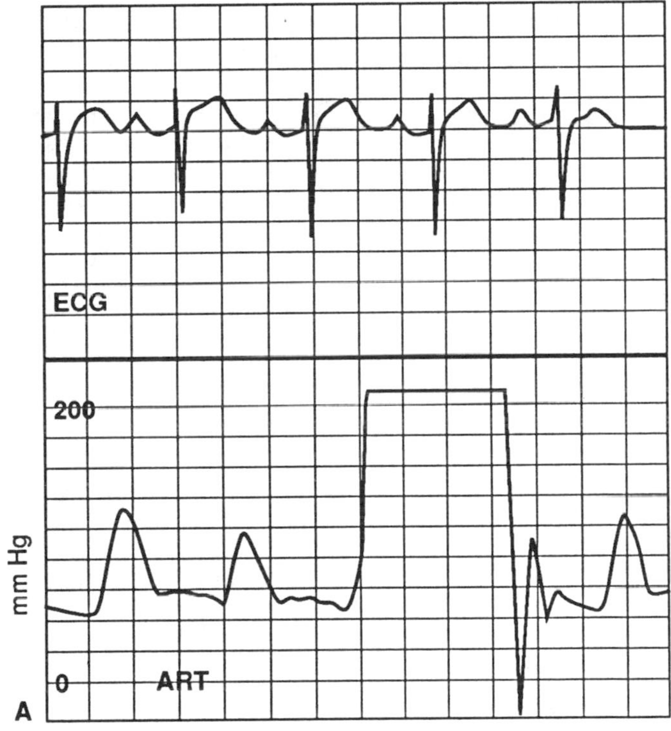

Normal arterial pressure tracing (lower panel) with simultaneous electrocardiogram (upper). Marker indicates start of square wave. Reproduced with permission from *Textbook of Advanced Cardiac Life Support*, American Heart Association, 1987.

and the trough represents the diastolic blood pressure (in mm Hg). Normal values for blood pressure obtained by arterial cannulation are slightly higher than those obtained by routine sphygmomanometry, ranging from 5-20 mm Hg higher. This is due to a combination of physiologic and technical factors, reviewed elsewhere.[2] If indirect pressure readings (ie, cuff pressures) are greater than arterial line readings, instrument error is likely. The entire system (tubing, calibration, seals, catheter, etc) should be carefully inspected; the transmitted arterial waveforms may also appear "damped," further suggesting technical error. A normal "square wave" response is also shown in Figure A. This waveform is

(Continued)

Arterial Cannulation *(Continued)*

seen whenever the tubing system is flushed. Most monitoring systems are equipped with a "flush valve" which can be opened and closed rapidly (routinely performed by nursing staff). A rapid-velocity stream flows through the tubing, removing bubbles and debris. The resulting waveform is by nature artifactual, but abnormalities in its configuration suggest underlying technical problems. See Figure B. In normal individuals peak systolic blood

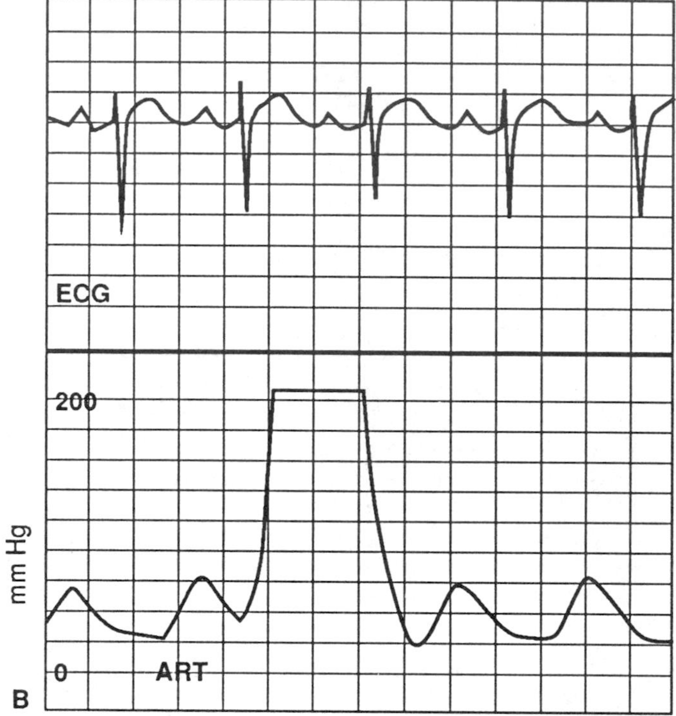

Damped arterial pressure tracing (lower panel) with simultaneous normal electrocardiogram (upper). Configuration of square wave is also damped, suggesting technical error. Reproduced with permission from *Textbook of Advanced Cardiac Life Support*, American Heart Association, 1987.

pressures vary somewhat with respiration, a finding difficult to appreciate with bedside sphygmomanometry, but easily observed with direct arterial blood pressure monitoring. When a healthy person inspires, there is a transient fall in blood pressure. On the blood pressure monitoring screen, this appears as a "dip" in the pressure tracings, which returns to baseline during expiration. The maximum drop in systolic blood pressure (pulsus paradoxus) should not exceed 8-10 mm Hg. Values less than this are physiologic and should not be confused with cardiac tamponade. **CRITICAL VALUES:** Cutoff values for hypertension, as defined in textbooks, are the same for blood pressure obtained by arterial cannulation and routine sphygmomanometry. A "hypertensive urgency" is characterized by marked elevations in diastolic (and sometimes systolic) blood pressure, accompanied by retinal hemorrhages, exudates, and papilledema. End-organ damage is likely within several days if blood pressure is not adequately controlled. In a "hypertensive emergency" (malignant hypertension), the retinal findings described are present along with such alarming features as acute renal failure, seizures, blurred vision, mental status deterioration, stroke, and congestive heart failure. End-organ damage is already apparent. Although both hypertensive urgencies and emergencies show marked blood pressure elevations (eg, diastolic blood pressure >120-140 mm Hg), there are no precise cutoff values. These syndromes should not be arbitrarily diagnosed or excluded on the basis of arterial line blood pressure readings alone; they are complex clinical diagnoses. Similarly, no black-and-white cutoff values exist for defining hypotension. Most physicians would consider a systolic blood pressure in the 70-80 mm Hg range abnormal if the individual was previously healthy. However, systolic blood pressures in the 80-90 mm Hg range are not unheard of in the patient with end stage cardiac disease or on multiple vasodilatory agents. Conversely, a "normal" systolic blood pressure of 110 mm Hg may indicate significant hypotension in the dialysis patient whose baseline is 200 mm Hg. A drop in systolic blood pressure during inspiration >10 mm Hg is significant. This increased paradoxical pulse may be seen in cardiac tamponade, severe asthma, pulmonary embolism, and other conditions. Arterial cannulation is useful in monitoring the patient with cardiac tamponade, but is seldom used to make the diagnosis. Disparity in blood pressure readings between direct and indirect measurements >20 mm Hg may occur in shock states. This is due to reflex peripheral vasoconstriction (increased systemic vascular resistance). Korotkoff sounds may be barely audible when direct measurement of central arterial pressures are low-normal. Large discrepancies may also be seen in patients with severe peripheral atherosclerosis (arteriosclerosis obliterans), where systolic pressure drops off dramatically distal to a luminal occlusion. It should be emphasized that inaccuracies may occur in **both** direct and indirect systems. Clinical importance should be placed on the trends in blood pressure values, regardless of the system used. **LIMITATIONS:** Accuracy is limited by errors introduced by the equipment, which transforms mechanical energy (pulse) into electrical energy (tracing). Factors such as the natural frequency of the transducer, clamping, and compliance may cause artifact. Other sources of error include improper leveling of equipment, improper assembly, and air in the tubing. **ADDITIONAL INFORMATION:** Arterial cannulation is generally considered a procedure of low technical difficulty. The true difficulty lies in avoidance of thrombosis and infection and careful patient selection.

Footnotes

1. Center for Disease Control Working Group Guidelines for Prevention of Intravascular Infections, "Guidelines for the Prevention and Control of Nosocomial Infection," U.S. Department of Health and Human Services, Public Health Service, 1981.
2. American Heart Association, *Textbook of Advanced Cardiac Life Support*, 1987.

References

Baud JD and Maki DG, "Infections Caused by Indwelling Arterial Catheters for Hemodynamic Monitoring," *Am J Med*, 1979, 67:735-41.

Downs JB and Rackstein AD, "Hazards of Radial-Artery Catheterization," *Anesthesiology*, 1973, 38:283-6.

Mandel MA and Dauchot PJ, "Radial-Artery Cannulation in 1000 Patients: Precautions and Complications," *J Hand Surg*, 1977, 2:482-5.

Venus B, Mathru M, and Smith RA, "Direct Versus Indirect Blood Pressure Measurements in Critically Ill Patients," *Heart Lung*, 1985, 14:228-31.

Arterial Catheterization *see* Arterial Cannulation *on page 60*

Arterial Line Placement *see* Arterial Cannulation *on page 60*

Arterial Lines *see* Swan-Ganz Catheterization *on page 71*

Aspiration of Pericardial Fluid by Paracentesis *see* Pericardiocentesis *on this page*

Closed Pleural Biopsy *see* Pleural Biopsy *on page 68*

Direct Arterial Pressure Monitoring *see* Arterial Cannulation *on page 60*

Echocardiography *see* Pericardiocentesis *on this page*

Pericardial Effusion Tap *see* Pericardiocentesis *on this page*

Pericardiocentesis

CPT 33010 (initial); 33011 (subsequent)

Related Information

Cardiac Catheterization, Adult *on page 40*
Doppler Echocardiography *on page 42*
Swan-Ganz Catheterization *on page 71*
(Continued)

Pericardiocentesis *(Continued)*

Synonyms Aspiration of Pericardial Fluid by Paracentesis; Pericardial Effusion Tap

Applies to Echocardiography; Pulmonary Artery Catheterization

Abstract **PROCEDURE COMMONLY INCLUDES:** Aspiration of pericardial fluid for microbiologic, biochemical, or cytologic analysis. Pericardiocentesis is also commonly performed to relieve cardiac tamponade on an urgent basis. In either case, this procedure may be carried out in a "blind" fashion or under direct echocardiographic (or fluoroscopic) guidance. **INDICATIONS:** The precise indications for pericardiocentesis are still controversial.[1] Published opinions from cardiologists, intensivists, and thoracic surgeons vary considerably. Some authorities advocate pericardiocentesis as a first-line diagnostic test in selected cases of pericardial effusion of unknown etiology. Due to its convenience and diagnostic yield, pericardiocentesis is important in ruling out the following:

- suspected bacterial (purulent) pericarditis
- tuberculous pericarditis
- malignant pericardial effusion

Other experts maintain that pericardiocentesis should be limited to emergency situations only. The indications for pericardiocentesis (listed previously) also apply to an open surgical drainage procedure, that is, direct drainage of the pericardial sac (ie, pericardiotomy, pericardiectomy). A surgical approach, it is argued, has several potential advantages over needle pericardiocentesis:

- superior safety profile
- easily obtained pericardial biopsy
- rapid and thorough drainage of the pericardial sac

In addition to having equal or superior diagnostic yield, surgical drainage is the therapeutic procedure of choice in certain instances, such as purulent pericarditis. Thus, these experts believe that pericardiocentesis is rarely needed for elective, diagnostic purposes, with the possible exception of the critically ill, poor surgical candidate. The exact role of surgical drainage versus needle pericardiocentesis continues to be debated. Most would agree, however, that the presence of a large pericardial effusion in and of itself is **not** an indication for pericardiocentesis. In clinical practice, many pericardial effusions are not tapped. The nontoxic patient who presents with a pericardial effusion of unknown etiology (and without hemodynamic compromise) poses a difficult clinical problem. Based on limited clinical studies, some authorities believe pericardiocentesis is not routinely indicated in this situation, due to a 6% diagnostic yield.[2] The major therapeutic indication for pericardiocentesis is the emergency relief of cardiac tamponade. On occasion, this procedure is also performed as part of a terminal resuscitation effort, where the presence of an effusion has not been established. Often, pericardiocentesis is performed for both therapeutic and diagnostic reasons. For example, the complex, ICU patient may undergo urgent pericardiocentesis primarily for relief of tamponade, but fluid samples are also sent for diagnostic analysis.

CONTRAINDICATIONS: No demonstrable pericardial effusion, by CT scan, fluoroscopy, chest x-ray, echocardiography, etc; severe thrombocytopenia or noncorrectable coagulopathy; skin or soft tissue infection at proposed needle entry site. Other high risk situations, not necessarily representing contraindications include:

- small pericardial effusion by echocardiography (estimated <200 mL)
- no anterior effusion by echocardiography
- loculated effusion
- acute hemopericardium secondary to trauma, where the reaccumulation rate of blood often exceeds the maximum rate of needle aspiration

Patient Care/Scheduling **PATIENT PREPARATION:** Technique and risks of the procedure are discussed in detail with the patient and consent is obtained. If performed in AM nonemergently, omit breakfast that day. If performed in afternoon or PM, restrict diet to clear liquids. Recent PT, PTT, and platelet count should be on the chart, as well as K^+ level if patient is on diuretics. Have chest x-ray and electrocardiogram available for physician review. If a high risk situation is anticipated, have blood typed and crossmatched before starting. A thoracic surgery team may need to be notified in an anticipatory fashion. An infusion of I.V. 0.9% NaCl solution is often begun prior to the procedure and continued throughout, especially if cardiac tamponade is imminent. In addition, full emergency equipment must be set up at bedside, including defibrillator, intubation blades, atropine, epinephrine, antiarrhythmics, and supplemental oxygen. Vital signs should be carefully documented preprocedure and frequently thereafter at physician discretion. Ideally, continuous intra-arterial blood pressure monitoring should be employed to instantaneously detect changes in hemodynamics. Many cardiologists also routinely combine pericardiocentesis with pulmonary artery catheterization; obtain the requisite Swan-Ganz equipment for these additional invasive procedures. At physician discretion, premedication with atropine may be necessary to avoid the transient vasovagal reactions associated with pericardial puncture. **AFTERCARE:** Following pericardiocentesis, monitor pulse, blood pressure, and neck vein distention four times at 15-minute intervals and then every hour for 4 hours. Most patients require ICU observation for at least 24 hours. If a pulmonary artery catheterization is performed as a joint procedure with pericardiocentesis, record right atrial (RA) pressures, pulmonary artery (PA) pressures, cardiac output, and pulmonary artery occlusive pressure ("wedge") immediately after effusion is aspirated and subsequently per physician's order. The following are suggestive of recurrent tamponade:

- reappearance of paradoxical pulse
- elevation of neck veins
- decreasing cardiac output
- increasing pulmonary artery (PA) diastolic pressure
- increasing right ventricular (RV) diastolic pressure
- hypotension or respiratory distress

Due to the highly invasive nature of this procedure, physician should be contacted immediately if complications arise (see Complications). An intrapericardial catheter is sometimes left in place postprocedure as part of a closed-drainage system. If no drainage is seen accumulating over a several hour period, the lumen of this catheter may be obstructed by cellular debris. Hemorrhagic or fibrin rich pericardial effusions predispose to this. Gentle flushing of the catheter with sterile saline may be requested by the physician. Some centers prefer a dilute heparin solution for flush. This carries a theoretical risk of increased bleeding, the clinical significance of which is unclear.

COMPLICATIONS: The exact incidence of complications is unknown. Published reports in the 1960s estimated the incidence of life-threatening complications near 20% for "blind" bedside pericardiocentesis. Subsequent studies have demonstrated a more favorable safety profile, reflecting the widespread use of echocardiography and/or fluoroscopy in guiding this procedure. Direct comparison from study to study is problematic due to methodological differences, patient variables, and technical variables.

Known complications include:

- malignant ventricular arrhythmias including cardiac arrest
- puncture of ventricles or atria (commonly RA)
- laceration of coronary arteries
- laceration of lung with hemothorax or pneumothorax
- cardiac tamponade from myocardial laceration
- air embolism
- acute pulmonary edema from sudden ventricular dilation following relief of tamponade (rare)

If a percutaneous pericardial catheter is left in place, local catheter infection is possible, especially if not removed after 48 hours. Fredrickson reported 3 cardiac chamber punctures out of 21 pericardiocenteses in 1971.[3] Six years later Silverberg noted 1 cardiac arrest following 21 total attempts.[4] Krikorian (1978) reported that out of 123 procedures, complications included 1 case of ventricular tachycardia, 5 patients with hemopericardium, and 5 deaths.[5] Wong et al (1979) published a retrospective and relatively favorable series. Out of 52 consecutive pericardiocenteses, there were 8 major complications but only 1 expiration.[6] The authors attributed their low complication rate to liberal use of echocardiography and cardiac laboratory facilities. Based on these studies, estimates of the complication rate in the era of echocardiography have ranged from 0% to 5%.

Method **EQUIPMENT:** Some variation in equipment exists. Required are:

- a long, 9 cm 16- to 18-gauge pointed needle
- 50 mL sterile syringe

(Continued)

Pericardiocentesis *(Continued)*

- standard EKG recording machine with the "V" lead attached to a sterile alligator clip
- 3-way stopcock with sterile connecting tubing
- No 11 scalpel blade
- povidone-iodine, sterile gauze, alcohol prep pads
- sterile drapes, gowns, hair caps, masks, etc
- 1% lidocaine without epinephrine along with assorted small needles and syringes for local anesthesia
- sterile tubes for specimen collection, culture media, heparin additive if cytology desired

Optional equipment includes:

- transducer-manometer apparatus for monitoring intrapericardial pressure directly
- intrapericardial catheter with multiple side holes for prolonged pericardial fluid drainage (soft teflon Gensini catheter); also needed is a soft J-tip guidewire
- intra-arterial blood pressure monitoring apparatus
- pulmonary artery catheterization tray

TECHNIQUE: Only an experienced physician should attempt needle pericardiocentesis. In some centers this procedure is limited to cardiologists. Ideally, the procedure should be carried out in a Cardiac Catheterization Laboratory or designated procedure room with hemodynamic monitoring capabilities. EKG should be continuously monitored, at the minimum. Among the various published methods of performing pericardiocentesis, the subxiphoid approach is the one preferred by the American Heart Association.[7] This approach minimizes the chances of coronary artery, internal mammary artery, or pleural surface laceration. Briefly, the patient is placed in the supine position with head of bed raised 20° to 30°. Under sterile conditions the subxiphoid region is shaved and prepped in the usual fashion. The needle entry site is located directly below the xiphoid approximately 1 cm left of midline. The region is infiltrated with 1% lidocaine into the skin and deeper tissues. The 16-gauge needle-on-syringe is advanced through the skin entry site, at a 30° angle, directed towards the right shoulder. The EKG "V" lead may be connected directly to the 16-gauge needle via a sterile alligator clip to help guide needle placement. While the needle is being advanced towards the pericardium, this technique provides continuous intrathoracic EKG monitoring. Periodically, the operator gently aspirates with the syringe. Eventually, some resistance will be felt as the pericardial surface is encountered. A "pop" may be felt as the needle penetrates the pericardium and enters the sac. However, if the needle is advanced too far, and the myocardium is irritated, the EKG V lead will show ST or PR segment elevation; needle should be pulled back slightly. With proper needle placement, fluid may be freely aspirated. The pericardial sac is then drained "dry" unless an intrapericardial catheter is placed (see following information). Intrapericardial pressures may be directly measured as one variation of this described technique. This is most useful with suspected tamponade. Before starting, a pressure transducer is attached to the 16-gauge needle and 50 mL syringe by means of a 3-way stopcock. The procedure is carried out as before. When the needle is correctly placed in the pericardial sac, the stopcock is turned so the needle and transducer form an open circuit and the syringe is "off". Direct pressure waveforms are recorded from within the pericardial sac, both initially and serially, as each aliquot of fluid is aspirated. As another variation, a temporary intrapericardial catheter may be placed for continuous drainage of pericardial fluid. This is done when the needle first enters the pericardial sac. A flexible guidewire with a J-tip is threaded through the lumen of the 16-gauge needle into the pericardial space. The needle is then completely removed over the wire and a sterile (teflon) catheter with multiple side holes is threaded back over the guidewire. This helps ensure proper placement of the catheter tip in the pericardial sac. After guidewire removal, fluid can then be collected continuously. Echocardiography is used in some centers to guide this procedure. This technique should not be confused with surgical procedures such as the pericardial window (limited pericardiectomy) or the subxiphoid limited pericardiotomy. **DATA ACQUIRED:** Analytic tests on pericardial fluid should be chosen based upon clinical impression. Commonly obtained tests include pericardial fluid cell count, hematocrit (if grossly hemorrhagic), glucose, LDH, and protein. If infectious pericarditis is suspected, Gram stain and AFB smear may be obtained, along with cultures for bacteria, *M. tuberculosis* (MTB), and fungi. Culture of pericardial fluid for viral agents is associated with a disappointingly low yield and is infrequently ordered. Cytologic examination is warranted if lymphoma or metastatic solid tumor is suspected. Optional tests include cholesterol, amylase, CEA, complement, rheumatoid factor, and others. Data concerning intrapericardial pressures may be obtained along with preprocedure and post-procedure hemodynamic profiles.

Specimen **CONTAINER:** Sterile tubes for pericardial fluid. Add heparin to tubes sent for cell count and cytology. Alternatively, use lavender top tube for cell count (EDTA-containing), and red top for chemistries. Inoculate appropriate culture media without delay. **COLLECTION:** Samples should be hand carried to respective laboratories immediately, preferably by physician. **STORAGE INSTRUCTIONS:** Specimens should not be refrigerated or stored overnight. **CAUSES FOR REJECTION:** Specimens stored or refrigerated for prolonged period of time, samples for culture sent in inappropriate containers (eg, sterile swabs for anaerobic culture), cytology specimen submitted without heparin additive **TURNAROUND TIME:** Cell count and chemistries, less than 24 hours. Most aerobic bacterial cultures within 2-3 days, but anaerobic and fungal cultures may be more than 5 days. Gram stain and AFB smear are immediate but MTB culture requires several weeks. Cytology may be run "stat" with results in less than 1 day.

Interpretation **NORMAL FINDINGS:** 15-50 mL fluid is normally contained in the pericardial sac, in the absence of disease. Characteristically, this fluid is clear and colorless, with <500 WBCs/mm^3 (<25% polymorphonuclear cells) and 0 RBCs. However, pericardial fluid sufficient in volume to be safely aspirated by standard pericardiocentesis is never a normal finding. In this sense, no "normal" values exist for pericardial fluid obtained using this technique. Normal values for intrapericardial pressure monitoring have been established using micromanometer measurements and average approximately 0 mm Hg with some slight respiratory variation. In normal individuals, with only 50 mL fluid, intrapericardial monitoring using standard technique is technically impossible (and hazardous). Again, no truly "normal" values can exist, although some cardiologists consider a fall in intrapericardial pressure from a high initial value (eg, 15 mm Hg) to 0 mm Hg as evidence of successful pericardiocentesis for tamponade.[1] **CRITICAL VALUES:** Pericardial effusions may be generally classified as "transudates" or "exudates" based on the underlying mechanism of fluid accumulation. Transudative effusions result from an imbalance in the various Starling forces across the pericardium, but the pericardial surface itself is normal and free of disease. Exudative effusions result from disease processes which cause active inflammation of the pericardium with subsequent breakdown of its permeability. Unlike the analysis of pleural effusions, strict biochemical criteria for differentiating transudative and exudative pericardial effusions have **not** been developed. Only rough guidelines exist; exudates tend to have higher values for protein, LDH, specific gravity, and total WBC counts and lower values for glucose. No accurate "cutoffs" for any of these variables have been established, limiting clinical utility. **ADDITIONAL INFORMATION:** Pericardial effusion often develops following injury to the parietal pericardium. Etiologies are numerous and include all the following causes of pericarditis:

- infections: viral, tuberculosis, fungal, parasitic, bacterial
- neoplastic: especially lung, breast, lymphoma, leukemia
- radiation-induced
- uremia
- autoimmune diseases: lupus, rheumatoid arthritis, Wegener's granulomatosis, scleroderma, and others
- acute MI, postmyocardial infarction syndrome (Dressler's), postpericardiotomy syndrome
- severe hypothyroidism
- nephrotic syndrome
- trauma with hemopericardium
- drugs
- sarcoidosis, inflammatory bowel disease, amyloidosis
- idiopathic

Pericardiocentesis is useful in diagnosing only a few of the listed conditions. A definitive diagnosis of tuberculous pericarditis can be made by isolation of *M. tuberculosis* from pericardial fluid. However, acid-fast bacillus (AFB) stain is relatively insensitive and failure of

(Continued)

Pericardiocentesis *(Continued)*

MTB to grow on appropriate media has been reported. Pericardial biopsy during an open surgical drainage procedure (eg, pericardial window) will improve diagnostic yield over analysis of pericardial fluid alone. Bacterial pericarditis usually presents as an acute, prostrating illness with spiking fevers, rigors, and dyspnea. Pericardial fluid analysis shows many PMNs and sometimes frank pus. Other pericardial fluid abnormalities include a markedly decreased glucose and elevated protein and LDH. Viable bacteria may be isolated in Gram stain and culture, but sterile purulent effusion is sometimes seen in late meningococcal pericarditis. Pericardiocentesis is indispensable in establishing the initial diagnosis of purulent pericarditis but appropriate management usually entails early surgical drainage. In cases of neoplastic pericardial effusion, gross appearance of fluid is usually hemorrhagic, but this may also be seen in radiation pericarditis. Cytology is diagnostic in roughly 85% of all cases of malignant pericarditis. False-negative results are highest in lymphoma and mesothelioma but uncommon with solid tumor metastases. Carcinoembryonic antigen level in pericardial fluid may be useful as an adjunctive test. In viral pericarditis, specific serum viral antibody titers are probably more useful in establishing the etiology of an effusion than analysis of pericardial fluid. Virus is only rarely isolated from pericardial effusions. Pericarditis with effusion may be seen in SLE but analysis of fluid is not specific enough to justify routine pericardiocentesis for diagnostic confirmation alone. Fluid profile in SLE is characterized by a grossly bloody appearance, increased protein, decreased glucose, decreased complement (with respect to serum), WBC $<10,000\ mm^3$ (usually PMNs).

Footnotes

1. Lorell BH and Braunwald E, "Pericardial Disease," *Heart Disease: A Textbook of Cardiovascular Medicine*, 3rd ed, Chapter 44, Braunwald E, ed, Philadelphia, PA: WB Saunders Co, 1988, 1484-534.
2. Permanyer-Miralda G, Sagristá-Savleda J, and Soler-Soler J, "Primary Acute Pericardial Disease: A Prospective Series of 231 Consecutive Cases," *Am J Cardiol*, 1985, 56:623-30.
3. Fredriksen RT, Cohen LS, and Mullins CB, "Pericardial Windows or Pericardiocentesis for Pericardial Effusion," *Am Heart J*, 1971, 82:158-62.
4. Silverberg S, Oreopoulos DG, Wise DJ, et al, "Pericarditis in Patients Undergoing Long-Term Hemodialysis and Peritoneal Dialysis," *Am J Med*, 1977, 63:874-80.
5. Krikorian JG and Hancock EW, "Pericardiocentesis," *Am J Med*, 1978, 65:808-14.
6. Wong B, Murphy J, Chang CJ, et al, "The Risk of Pericardiocentesis," *Am J Cardiol*, 1979, 44:1110-4.
7. American Heart Association, "Invasive Therapeutic Techniques. Part II: Pericardiocentesis," *Textbook of Advanced Cardiac Life Support*, Chapter 13, Dallas, TX: American Heart Association, 1987, 187-205.

References

Hancock EW, "Cardiac Tamponade," *Med Clin North Am*, 1979, 63:223-7.

Hancock EW, "Management of Pericardial Disease," *Med Concepts Cardiovasc Dis*, 1979, 48:1-6.

Wei JY, Taylor GJ, and Achuff SC, "Recurrent Cardiac Tamponade and Large Pericardial Effusions: Management With an Indwelling Pericardial Catheter," *Am J Cardiol*, 1978, 42:281-2.

Pleural Biopsy

CPT 32400

Related Information

Swan-Ganz Catheterization *on page 71*

Thoracentesis *on page 267*

Synonyms Closed Pleural Biopsy

Abstract **PROCEDURE COMMONLY INCLUDES:** Percutaneous needle biopsy of the pleura under local anesthesia, often performed in conjunction with thoracentesis. A blunt-tipped Cope or Abrams needle is advanced through an intercostal space and several specimens of parietal pleura are obtained. Biopsy samples are sent for histologic and microbiologic analysis, along with pleural fluid. Pleural biopsy has its greatest applicability in the diagnosis of malignant neoplasms involving the pleura and tuberculous pleural effusions. **INDICATIONS:**

Pleural biopsy is most useful in the following clinical situations:

- pleural effusion of unclear etiology when a prior thoracentesis has failed to establish a diagnosis
- suspected malignant pleural effusion (eg, bronchogenic carcinoma, breast cancer with pleuropulmonary metastases, mesothelioma, lymphoma, and others)
- Suspected tuberculous pleural effusions; the diagnostic yield from thoracentesis alone is low in pleural infections caused by *Mycobacterium tuberculosis*. This procedure allows direct culture of pleural samples for *M. tuberculosis*, as well as pathologic analysis for caseating granulomas.

CONTRAINDICATIONS:

- severe, uncorrectable coagulopathy
- platelet count <50,000/mm^3 (in many cases may be temporarily corrected with platelet transfusion)
- inadequate volume of pleural effusion, usually determined radiographically. To perform a pleural biopsy safely, pleural fluid should be present in a large enough volume to physically separate the lung parenchyma from the pleura. The risk of pneumothorax and lung laceration increases with smaller volumes of pleural fluid.

Patient Care/Scheduling **PATIENT PREPARATION:** Technique and risks of the procedure are explained to the patient and informed consent is obtained. Pleural biopsy may be safely performed as an outpatient and hospitalization postprocedure is not required in most cases. Patient should be referred to a chest physician. Details regarding procedure scheduling are generally handled by the subspecialist performing the biopsy. In all cases, a recent PA and lateral chest x-ray must be performed and should be readily available for physician review. Decubitus chest radiographs are frequently performed before thoracentesis and pleural biopsy to determine the size of the effusion, degree of fluid loculation, and presence of an underlying lung infiltrate. If coagulopathy is suspected, complete blood count (CBC) and clotting parameters (prothrombin time, partial thromboplastin time) should be drawn and the results placed on the chart without delay. Bleeding time measurement is optional and not usually necessary. Other studies may be necessary prior to the procedure, at physician discretion (arterial blood gas, pulse oximetry, etc). If a thoracentesis is performed simultaneously with pleural biopsy, the same considerations apply as outlined previously (see Thoracentesis entry). **AFTERCARE:** Following pleural biopsy a "stat" chest x-ray is routinely performed to rule out iatrogenic pneumothorax. Often this film is taken with the patient at end-expiration (ie, an expiratory radiograph) to accentuate a small pneumothorax. Vital signs are usually obtained frequently postbiopsy, depending in part on the patient's baseline cardiopulmonary condition. For example, pulse and blood pressure may be obtained four times at 30-minute intervals for the first 2 hours and then every hour for the next 4 hours followed by routine measurement. If a large volume of pleural fluid is also removed, some pulmonologists recommend low flow (1-2 L/minute) supplemental oxygen by nasal cannula, but this is probably optional. **SPECIAL INSTRUCTIONS:** If performed in an outpatient setting, patient should contact a physician immediately if dyspnea or severe chest pain should develop after discharge. **COMPLICATIONS:**

- pneumothorax; probably the single most common adverse outcome. Risk increases with smaller pleural effusions. Pneumothorax is a relatively common complication but is often negligible and only observed with serial chest x-rays. Tension pneumothorax requiring immediate tube thoracostomy has been reported but is unusual.
- hemothorax; secondary to laceration of intercostal vessels. May be potentially life-threatening. Standard biopsy techniques are designed to minimize their risk (ie, no pleural samples taken at the "12 o'clock" position when in the intercostal space).
- lung perforation
- vasovagal reactions
- local infection at the needle entrance site (rare)
- implantation of malignant cells along the needle entrance tract with the lung parenchyma (rare, but reported)
- local pain

Method **EQUIPMENT:** The two most popular biopsy needles are the Cope and Abrams needle although others are available. Both needles are blunt-tipped and wide-bore, with an

(Continued)

Pleural Biopsy *(Continued)*

outer trocar, inner cannula, and central stylet. The Abrams needle has a special hook on the outer trocar to grip and cut the pleura. The Cope needle has a similar sharp biopsy chamber in an inner trocar. Pleural fluid can be withdrawn using either needle. The efficacy and safety of both Abrams and Cope needles are similar. Standard thoracentesis equipment is also required. **TECHNIQUE:** In most hospitals, pleural biopsies are performed exclusively by pulmonologists or thoracic surgeons, despite it being a "bedside" procedure. Unlike conventional thoracentesis, a procedure commonly performed by internists and resident house staff, pleural biopsy has remained a subspecialty technique. The patient is placed in a comfortable sitting position (as with conventional thoracentesis). The margins of the pleural effusion are located by the physician using physical examination techniques. The appropriate intercostal space is located and the area cleaned with povidone-iodine in a standard sterile fashion. One percent lidocaine is used for cutaneous anesthesia following the sterile prep. Superficial skin incision is made using a scalpel to facilitate needle entry. The Cope or Abrams needle is advanced through the skin incision between ribs and into the pleural space. Pleural fluid may be withdrawn at this time to confirm proper needle positioning and for diagnostic purposes. Following this, the needle is withdrawn slightly until the parietal pleura is engaged. Several passes are made into the pleura using the sharp cutting edge (usually at the 3, 6, and 9 o'clock positions). Once adequate pleural samples have been collected, the remainder of the pleural fluid may be evacuated. The needle is then removed. **DATA ACQUIRED:** In most cases, pleural specimens are sent for:

- acid-fast stain (ie, for *M. tuberculosis*)
- culture for acid-fast bacilli (AFB)
- pathologic analysis; routine light microscopy, H & E stain, silver stain, AFB stain, etc

Less commonly:

- routine Gram stain, culture and sensitivity
- fungal culture

Specimen Fresh specimens of parietal pleura and any pleural fluid collected separately. Biopsy specimens are usually sent to both the Microbiology and Pathology Laboratories. As with other fresh biopsy specimens, pleural specimens should be hand-carried immediately to the Microbiology Laboratory in a sterile container, with or without sterile saline. No formalin should be added to samples bound for culture. Samples sent to the Pathology Laboratory may be either fresh or placed in fixative (such as formalin).

Interpretation **NORMAL FINDINGS:** Normal parietal pleura by microscopy and special staining along with negative results of routine and AFB cultures. Microscopy findings are reported by Pathology Department; culture results per Microbiology Laboratory. **CRITICAL VALUES:** Abnormalities as reported. In many cases, the diagnosis of primary bronchogenic or metastatic carcinoma may be established using standard histologic technique. In addition, the finding of caseating granulomas (with or without a positive AFB culture) is suggestive of infection with *M. tuberculosis*. **LIMITATIONS:** Although pleural biopsy is quite specific for both malignancy and tuberculosis, the sensitivity is more limited. The histologic finding of "nonspecific pleural inflammation" is very common, approaching 50% to 70% of biopsies in the published literature.[1] Such a finding may prompt a repeat pleural biopsy since $\leq$25% of patients with nonspecific inflammatory biopsies may develop malignancy.

Footnotes

1. American College of Physicians, "Diagnostic Thoracentesis and Pleural Biopsy in Pleural Effusions," *Ann Intern Med*, 1985, 103:799-802.

References

Escudero BC, Garcia CM, Cuesta CB, et al, "Cytologic and Bacteriologic Analysis of Fluid and Pleural Biopsy Specimens With Cope's Needle," *Arch Intern Med*, 1990, 150(6):1190-4.

Kinasewitz GT and Fishman AP, "Pleural Dynamics and Effusions," *Pulmonary Diseases and Disorders*, 2nd ed, Chapter 135, Fishman AP, ed, New York, NY: McGraw-Hill Book Co, 1988.

Murray JF and Nadel JA, "Bronchoscopy, Lung Biopsy, and Other Procedures," *Textbook of Respiratory Medicine*, Chapter 29, Philadelphia, PA: WB Saunders Co, 1988.

Poe RH, Israel RH, Utell MJ, et al, "Sensitivity, Specificity, and Predictive Values of Closed Pleural Biopsy," *Arch Intern Med*, 1984, 144:325-8.

Prakash UBS and Reiman HM, "Comparison of Needle Biopsy With Cytologic Analysis for the Evaluation of Pleural Effusion: Analysis of 414 Cases," *Mayo Clin Proc*, 1985, 60:158-64.

Scerbo J, Keltz H, and Stone DH, "A Prospective Study of Closed Pleural Biopsies," *JAMA*, 1971, 218:377-80.

Pulmonary Artery Catheterization *see* Swan-Ganz Catheterization *on this page*

Pulmonary Artery Catheterization *see* Pericardiocentesis *on page 63*

Right Heart Catheterization *see* Swan-Ganz Catheterization *on this page*

Swan-Ganz Catheterization

CPT 36010

Related Information

Arterial Cannulation *on page 60*
Cardiac Catheterization, Adult *on page 40*
Pericardiocentesis *on page 63*
Pleural Biopsy *on page 68*

Synonyms Pulmonary Artery Catheterization; Right Heart Catheterization

Applies to Arterial Lines

Abstract **PROCEDURE COMMONLY INCLUDES:** Insertion of a flexible, balloon-tipped catheter into the pulmonary artery for hemodynamic monitoring of the critically ill patient. Although Swan-Ganz catheterization is considered an invasive procedure, it may be safely performed at the bedside in an intensive care unit setting, using continuous EKG and blood pressure monitoring. In brief, this technique involves cannulation of a large vein, such as the subclavian or internal jugular vein. A flow-directed catheter is advanced through the central venous system into the right atrium (RA), right ventricle (RV), and pulmonary artery (PA). If desired, the catheter may be further "wedged" briefly into a small pulmonary artery branch. Direct pressure measurements are obtained in the respective cardiac chambers and pulmonary artery. An indirect measurement of left atrial filling pressure is obtained when the catheter is "wedged". In addition, other hemodynamic parameters may be easily measured, such as the cardiac output, systemic vascular resistance (SVR), mixed venous oxygen saturation, and intrapulmonary shunt fraction. Swan-Ganz catheterization has become an integral (and sometimes routine) procedure in the modern intensive care unit and has revolutionized the practice of critical care medicine. **INDICATIONS:** Pulmonary artery catheterization is indicated in the following situations:

- acute myocardial infarction with hemodynamic instability
- severe hypotension of unknown etiology, especially if the response to initial therapy is inadequate (eg, volume loading)
- selected cases of septic shock
- adult respiratory distress syndrome, to confirm the diagnosis of noncardiogenic pulmonary edema (normal "wedge" pressure) and to aid in subsequent fluid and ventilator management
- suspected cases of cardiac tamponade, to confirm the diagnosis, monitor hemodynamics during pericardiocentesis, and follow response to therapy
- suspected papillary muscle rupture
- possible ventricular septal defect or atrial septal defect following myocardial infarction
- congestive heart failure responding poorly to diuretics, especially when intravascular volume status is uncertain
- intraoperative monitoring of patients undergoing open heart surgery, particularly coronary artery bypass procedures involving multiple vessels; patients undergoing abdominal aortic aneurysm repair may also benefit from PA catheterization perioperatively

Swan-Ganz catheterization may also be useful in the following scenarios:

- drug overdose, especially when the risk of acute lung damage is high (eg, heroin, aspirin)

(Continued)

Swan-Ganz Catheterization *(Continued)*

- exacerbations of chronic obstructive lung disease requiring intubation; hemodynamic monitoring may detect occult or superimposed causes of respiratory failure not suspected clinically (eg, left ventricular dysfunction)
- end-stage liver failure with deteriorating renal function
- suspected cases of pulmonary hypertension

In general, Swan-Ganz catheterization is indicated when measurement of right atrial, pulmonary artery, and pulmonary artery occlusive pressures will significantly alter patient management. The threshold for performing this procedure varies considerably amongst clinicians; some authorities feel this technique is overutilized and is indicated in only rare circumstances.

CONTRAINDICATIONS:

- severe, uncorrectable coagulopathy
- presence of a left bundle branch block (LBBB) on EKG; placement of a right heart catheter may lead to complete heart block (A-V dissociation) if an underlying LBBB is present
- local infection at the skin insertion site
- severe hypothermia; in this situation the myocardium is highly irritable and prone to malignant arrhythmias induced by the catheter
- inadequate monitoring equipment; continuous EKG monitoring with blood pressure measurements is necessary during catheter insertion
- patient refusal

Patient Care/Scheduling

PATIENT PREPARATION: Technique and risks of the procedure are explained to the patient. When patient is comatose or disoriented, the appropriate guardians should be contacted. Catheterization may be safely performed in an intensive care unit, specialized procedure room with telemetry and fluoroscopy, or a formal Cardiac Catheterization Laboratory. A standard emergency room or regular nursing floor is generally not equipped for this procedure. No specific patient preparation is required and often this procedure is performed on an urgent basis. Whenever possible, aspirin and nonsteroidal anti-inflammatory agents should be discontinued in advance, but this is not absolutely necessary. Effects of heparin or warfarin, however, should be reversed prior to catheterization. If an underlying coagulopathy is suspected (eg, disseminated intravascular coagulation, thrombocytopenia), appropriate laboratory studies should be obtained immediately including a platelet count and PT/PTT. In most cases parenteral sedation is unnecessary; however the use of agents such as meperidine (Demerol®) is at the physician's discretion.

COMPLICATIONS:

- balloon rupture
- conduction disturbance (ie, new right bundle branch block 5%)
- arrhythmias (3% ventricular tachycardia, 2% ventricular fibrillation)
- pulmonary infarction/pulmonary hemorrhage
- perforation or rupture of the pulmonary artery
- knotting of the catheter
- thrombosis of a blood vessel (ie, 1% to 2% superior vena cava syndrome)
- pulmonary emboli
- infection (0% to 5%)
- blood loss, including hemothorax, retroperitoneal bleed, etc
- inadvertent arterial puncture (6% femoral)
- pneumothorax and tension pneumothorax (0% to 6%)
- valvular trauma
- disconnection of the introducer apparatus with disappearance into the vein.

Method

EQUIPMENT:

- I.V. pole and pressure monitor manifold, pressure monitor
- normal saline (250-500 mL) with heparin (1000 units) for flush
- pressure bag
- pressure tubing
- stopcocks (3-way)
- cutdown tray (for peripheral approach)
- vein introducer kit

- Swan-Ganz catheter kit
- 1% lidocaine for local anesthesia
- bowl of sterile saline (flush and balloon integrity check)
- suture
- instrument set
- 3 and 5 mL syringes
- 25-gauge needle for anesthesia
- gloves, gowns, masks
- sterile dressing kit (surgical drapes)
- bedside table on which to place instruments
- telemetry monitor for heart rate and rhythm automatic blood pressure cuff, A-line
- Betadine® scrub

TECHNIQUE: Swan-Ganz catheterization can take place via a variety of approaches including internal jugular vein, subclavian vein, femoral vein, or brachial vein. The last of these approaches most commonly entails direct visualization of the brachial vein from a cut-down exposure. The procedure should be performed in a closely monitored setting, enabling constant recording of heart rate, rhythm, and frequent blood pressure readings, usually an intensive care unit. The procedure may be performed at the patient's bedside with or without the assistance of fluoroscopic guidance. Sterile technique is required for catheter insertion. The skin at the site of approach is most commonly prepped with a Betadine® scrub. Often, if the internal jugular or subclavian veins are utilized, the patient is placed in a Trendelenburg position to assist with central venous distension and ease of access. The physician should scrub and wear gown, mask, and gloves. The patient is then draped with sterile sheets (most institutions drape the patient from head to toe, while others require a sterile field only at the site of access). The patient should be cooperative for catheter insertion. If a patient is uncooperative or becomes uncooperative during the procedure, sedation may be given at the discretion of the physician. Upon initiation of the procedure, the skin and subcutaneous tissue is infiltrated with lidocaine (1%) and a small gauge needle. Deeper tissues may then be infiltrated with lidocaine for the comfort of the patient. A thin gauged needle (21-gauge, 1 1/2") is usually attached to a 5 mL syringe and used to localize the vessel of interest for a central venous approach. Once the vessel has been located, a large gauge needle (16- or 18-gauge) is then attached to a syringe and placed into the vessel following the course of the "finder needle." When blood is aspirated easily into the syringe, the syringe is disconnected from the needle and a flexible guidewire is threaded through the needle into the vein. Wire placement can cause a variety of complications, most often ventricular ectopy. If an increase in ectopy is observed, the guidewire should be withdrawn several centimeters. Once the guidewire has been passed into the vessel, the needle is removed from the patient. At no time should the physician lose control of the tip of the guidewire. Failure to control the guidewire can cause serious complications and death if lost in the patient. Once the needle is removed, a dilator is advanced over the guidewire and through the skin, to facilitate passage of a venous introducer. The introducer should be flushed with heparinized saline prior to insertion to avoid air emboli. Once the tract along the guidewire is dilated, the dilator should be slipped off the guidewire (maintaining guidewire position **in** the vein). The introducer and dilator can then be put together as a unit (dilator within introducer) and slid over the guidewire into the vein, again taking care to control the tip of the guidewire outside the patient's body. After the placement of the introducer and guidewire assembly, the guidewire and dilator should be removed from the patient. This leaves only the venous introducer sheath within the patient. At this point, if the introducer has a side port lumen, venous blood should be aspirated and the introducer then flushed. If blood cannot be aspirated via a side-port lumen, the introducer is incorrectly placed and must be reinserted. No blood should come from the center of the introducer since this piece is usually accompanied by a one-way ball valve which does not allow blood leakage. The introducer should then be secured to the patient's skin with sutures. When the venous introducer has been placed, the Swan-Ganz catheter can then be inserted. Prior to catheter insertion, the balloon tip should be checked under sterile water for leaks and the catheter flushed. The catheter should then be connected to the appropriate pressure monitoring lines and flushed again via the pressure tubing to ensure that the catheter is bubble-free and that a column of uninterrupted fluid exists from the tubing through the tip of the catheter. The

(Continued)

Swan-Ganz Catheterization *(Continued)*

catheter can then be guided via the introducer, through the central venous system, through the right atrium, right ventricle, pulmonary artery, and into the wedge position. The catheter usually passes smoothly through the circulation, with the aid of the inflated balloon at its tip. The catheter should never be withdrawn with the balloon inflated. Catheter position can be ascertained by pressure wave forms, although fluoroscopy can be quite helpful in guiding the catheter into the wedge position. A chest radiograph is usually obtained after catheter insertion to verify position, as well as to rule out the possibility of pneumothorax if the subclavian or internal jugular approach was utilized.

Interpretation NORMAL FINDINGS: Normal resting hemodynamic values:

- right atrium → mean: 0-8 mm Hg; A wave: 2-10 mm Hg; V wave: 2-10 mm Hg
- right ventricle → systolic: 15-30 mm Hg; end diastolic: 0-8 mm Hg
- pulmonary artery → systolic: 15-30 mm Hg; end diastolic: 3-12 mm Hg
- wedge → A wave: 3-15 mm Hg; V wave: 3-12 mm Hg; mean: 5-12 mm Hg
- AVO_2 difference (mL/L) → 30-50
- cardiac output (L/minute) → 4.0-6.5 (varies with patient size)
- cardiac index (L/minute/m^2) → 2.6-4.6
- pulmonary vascular resistance (dynes - second - cm^{-2}) → 20-130
- systemic vascular resistance (dynes - second - cm^{-2}) → 700-1600

The right atrial waveform normally has two major positive deflections, the A wave and the V wave. The A wave is due to atrial systole and follows the P wave inscribed on the EKG. The X descent follows this initial positive deflection and is often interrupted by a small positive deflection called the C wave, which occurs with tricuspid valve closure. At the nadir of the X descent, full atrial relaxation has occurred and pressure in the right atrium begins to rise again with atrial refilling. Rise in right atrial pressure during ventricular systole is called the V wave and it reaches its peak prior to tricuspid valve opening. The Y descent then occurs as the tricuspid valve opens and the right atrium empties into the right ventricle. The pulmonary artery wedge pressure normally has a waveform similar to left atrial pressure, but is delayed in transmission through the capillary vessels. A normal wedge should show clear A and V waves; however, C waves are most often not visible. X and Y descents should be fairly clear as long as the pressure tracing is not overdamped.

CRITICAL VALUES: Pressure tracings may be virtually diagnostic of certain conditions. For example, mitral stenosis is associated with a pressure gradient in diastole across the mitral valve (wedge or left atrial pressure vs left ventricular pressure). A large V wave in the pulmonary artery wedge tracing may be seen with mitral regurgitation, since the amplitude of the V wave is affected by left atrial filling from the pulmonary veins as well as the regurgitant volume from the left ventricle. Stenotic and regurgitant lesions of the pulmonic and tricuspid valves can also be documented by right sided heart catheterization using simultaneous recordings or by pull back techniques. With regard to the hemodynamic profile rendered by the Swan-Ganz catheter, certain general parameters can be quite useful. Decreases in right atrial pressure, pulmonary capillary wedge pressure, and cardiac index/output can indicate hypovolemia. In cases of elevated right atrial pressures with concomitant low wedge pressures and low cardiac index/output (especially in the face of an inferior wall myocardial infarction) one may suspect right ventricular involvement and failure. Pulmonary congestion due to left ventricular failure or volume overload will increase the pulmonary artery wedge pressure, ie, congestion usually occurs at a wedge pressure in excess of 18 mm Hg and frank pulmonary edema occurs with a wedge pressure in the upper twenties and above. Cardiogenic shock and pulmonary edema are characterized by signs of hypoperfusion, with hemodynamic data including systemic hypotension, markedly decreased cardiac index (<2.1 L/minute/m^2), and elevated wedge pressures (often well >18 mm Hg). Septic shock is also characterized by clinical signs of hypoperfusion, but may be differentiated from cardiogenic shock by certain hemodynamic data which often include a normal or near normal wedge pressure, an elevated cardiac index/output, and a marked decrease in systemic vascular resistance. Caution should be exercised in that these parameters are only general guidelines, and during the course of a patient's illness, such information may not always be exact. As always, history and physical examination are critical in the diagnostic assessment of each patient. The catheter can aid with diagnostic dilemmas, but is most useful as a management tool. Pulmonary artery catheters can also be useful in the diagnosis of ventricular septal defects by sampling O_2 saturations as the catheter is advanced from the great veins to the right atrium to the right ventricle and out into the pulmonary artery. An oxygen "step-up" from the right atrium to the right ventricle of approximately 10% is indicative of left to right shunting. In the appropriate setting of acute myocardial infarction and sudden deterioration after a stable course, this diagnosis may be a consideration; right heart catheterization is one method to establish the diagnosis. Other causes of an O_2 step-up include coronary fistula draining into the RV, primum atrial septal defects, and pulmonic insufficiency with a patent ductus arteriosus. Cardiac tamponade is another diagnosis which can be documented by pulmonary artery catheter measurements. Rising intrapericardial pressures interfere with diastolic filling of the heart. Marked increases in the end-diastolic pulmonary artery (PA), right ventricular (RV) , and right atrial (RA) pressures to the same value ("equalization of the pressures") strongly suggest tamponade. Somewhat similar findings may be seen with constrictive and restrictive diseases, discussion of which is beyond this outline. Pulmonary hypertension and increased pulmonary vascular resistance can suggest such diagnoses as pulmonary embolism or even mitral stenosis. Care must be taken in the interpretation of all hemodynamic data derived from the catheter.[1]

Footnotes

1. Raper R and Sibbald WJ, "Misled by the Wedge? The Swan-Ganz Catheter and Left Ventricular Preload," *Chest*, 1986, 89(3):427-34.

References

Amin DK and Shah PK, "The Swan-Ganz Catheter," *J Crit Illness*, 1986, 1(4): 24-45, 1(5):40-61.

Forrester JC, Diamond G, Chatterjee K, et al, "Medical Therapy of Acute Myocardial Infarction by Application of Hemodynamic Subsets," *N Engl J Med*, 1976, 295:1356-62, 1404-13.

Matthay MA and Chatterjee K, "Bedside Catheterization of the Pulmonary Artery: Risks Compared With Benefits," *Ann Intern Med*, 1988, 109(10):826-34.

Shoemaker WC, "Use and Abuse of the Balloon Tip Pulmonary Artery (Swan-Ganz) Catheter: Are Patients Getting Their Money's Worth?" *Crit Care Med*, 1990, 18(11):1294-6.

Wiedemann HP, Matthay MA, and Matthay RA, "Cardiovascular-Pulmonary Monitoring in the Intensive Care Unit," *Chest*, 1985, 85(4):537-49, 656-67.

GASTROENTEROLOGY

Carlos M. Isada, MD

The fiberoptic endoscope has clearly revolutionized the practice of both gastroenterology and general medicine. This breakthrough in optical technology has allowed the early diagnosis and treatment of a wide variety of GI disorders, particularly mucosal abnormalities. The safety profile of endoscopy is generally quite good, and with its growing availability in even smaller centers, this technique has become routine in evaluating many GI diseases.

However, GI endoscopy is particularly operator dependent. "Negative" tests performed by inexperienced or hurried endoscopists may have disastrous consequences. The cost of these procedures is considerable, even in comparison with established radiologic tests, such as the barium enema. The medical literature is filled with editorials addressing the inappropriate use of gastroenterologic endoscopy.

General guidelines have been established by several respected physician organizations. These recommendations have been incorporated in many of the entries which follow.

Contributing to this section is the following author:

Agnes Saleski, MD	Biliary Drainage Breath Hydrogen Analysis Esophageal Dilation Hollander Test I.V. Secretin Gastrin Levels

Abdominal Paracentesis *see* Paracentesis *on page 111*

Acid Infusion Test *see* Bernstein Test *on page 81*

Acid Perfusion Test for Esophagitis *see* Bernstein Test *on page 81*

Acid pH Measurement *see* Hollander Test *on page 105*

Anal Rectal Motility *see* Anorectal Manometry *on this page*

Anorectal Manometry

CPT 91122

Synonyms Anal Rectal Motility; ARM; Balloon Manometry for Fecal Incontinence; Rectosphincteric Manometry

Abstract PROCEDURE COMMONLY INCLUDES: Direct measurement of pressures in the anal canal, including the internal and external anal sphincters, along with assessment of rectal sensation and reflexes. This is performed by using either a manometry probe or a 3-balloon apparatus with external pressure transducers. It is most useful in the evaluation of suspected Hirschsprung's disease and difficult cases of fecal incontinence. INDICATIONS: Only carefully selected patients should undergo anorectal manometry (ARM). Certainly, not every patient presenting with fecal incontinence warrants invasive testing. The procedure is indicated in the following situations:

- to evaluate cases of suspected Hirschsprung's disease, in both children and adults; particularly useful in patients with megacolon of unknown etiology or adults with possible "short-segment" Hirschsprung's disease
- to evaluate difficult cases of fecal incontinence especially if one of the following is suspected: surgical trauma to anal sphincters or nerve structures; invasive perianal disease compromising regional nerve or muscle; impaired motor function and/or sensory innervation involving one or both anal sphincters from systemic disease (eg, scleroderma, polymyositis, etc); impaired sensation of rectal distention, as in diabetes mellitus
- to assess fecal continence mechanisms following surgery for defecation disorders (surgery for imperforate anus, Hirschsprung's disease, etc)

In addition to diagnostic indications, ARM has an important therapeutic role in the treatment of fecal incontinence with biofeedback.[1] Retraining the external anal sphincter in patients with weak voluntary contractions has been successful; biofeedback data is based on continuous external sphincter pressure readings.

CONTRAINDICATIONS:

- uncooperative patient
- confused or comatose patient; ARM usually requires the patient to voluntarily squeeze and relax muscles controlling continence
- active lower GI bleeding
- history of allergy to rubber or latex products

Patient Care/Scheduling PATIENT PREPARATION: The details of the procedure are discussed with the patient and consent is obtained. Patient should understand that the procedure involves inflation of a balloon in the rectum. In many centers cleansing of the rectal vault is performed routinely, using saline or Fleet® enemas, sometimes also cathartics. Some specialists do not request any bowel prep unless hard stool is expected. Sedatives should not be automatically given, but instead should be reserved for the very young (and extremely anxious) patient. AFTERCARE: No specific postprocedure restrictions are necessary. Patient may resume previous level of activity. COMPLICATIONS: ARM is a very safe procedure. To date, only one major complication has been reported, that of systemic anaphylaxis.[2] This was presumed to be an IgE-mediated hypersensitivity reaction to the latex manometry balloon, as it came in contact with the rectal mucosa.

Method EQUIPMENT: Two different systems for performing ARM are popular, and equipment for each is different. (The First International Symposium on ARM reported a wide variety of commercial devices in common use, the majority deemed acceptable[3]). In the first system, "perfusion manometry," a small diameter (0.7-2 mm) manometry probe is utilized, resembling an esophageal manometry catheter. In some models there is a large inflatable rectal balloon at the distal tip. This probe is a soft plastic catheter with radially arranged ports

(Continued)

Anorectal Manometry *(Continued)*

(sensing orifices), and uses a standard water perfusion system. Other acceptable devices include stiff, hollow metal catheters and dacron-woven catheters with microtip sensors. Attached to the manometry catheter is a pressure transducer for each sensing orifice. Results are recorded on a multichannel polygraph machine. The second system is a nonperfused or "balloon manometry" system. Here, three balloons are aligned in series on a hollow metal cylinder. The largest balloon (50 mL capacity) is the "rectal balloon," and is attached to the end of the cylinder. After proper placement, it will be located in the upper anal canal. The middle balloon is doughnut-shaped and will be positioned in the anal ampulla, surrounded by the internal (and part of the external) anal sphincter. The external balloon will lie at the anal verge, within the external anal sphincter. Each balloon is connected to its own pressure transducer, which in turn transmits to the multichannel recorder. The large rectal balloon may be inflated or deflated by means of an air-filled syringe. **TECHNIQUE:** The procedure is performed only by an experienced GI specialist in a fully equipped procedure room. Perfusion manometry technique: With patient in supine position (or left lateral), a standard digital examination is carried out and anal wink reflex tested. Manometry probe is advanced per rectum approximately 10 cm (in the adult), then slowly withdrawn using station pull-through technique. Pressures are continuously observed and the area of high pressure corresponding to the anal sphincters is located. (This may require several repetitions to ensure reproducibility of results.) This so-called "basal anal pressure" is recorded with the patient relaxed. The patient is then asked to perform a maximal sphincter squeeze, and again, highest pressures are recorded. This is termed the "maximal squeeze pressure". Following this the manometry catheter is reinserted as before and the 50 mL rectal balloon inflated slowly. Patient reports the first conscious sensation of rectal fullness and the volume of the rectal balloon is recorded at that time. In addition, response of the anal sphincters to rectal distention may be measured with some devices.

Balloon manometry technique: If the three balloon apparatus is used, it is inserted per rectum following a digital rectal exam. This device is advanced approximately 8 cm or until the distal (external) balloon is just inside the anal verge and can barely be visualized. Both the middle and external balloons are then inflated and pressure tracings noted. The large internal rectal balloon is inflated with up to 50 mL air. Patient reports the first sensation of rectal fullness. A "threshold value" of rectal sensation is obtained by deflating the balloon slowly and noting the smallest volume sensed. Following this, the large rectal balloon is reinflated and simultaneous pressures recorded from the middle balloon (reflecting internal and external sphincter in upper anal canal) and external balloon (reflecting external sphincter in anal verge).

Additional pressure tracings reflecting the external sphincter may be obtained during cough, anal pinprick, and other maneuvers.

DATA ACQUIRED: With perfusion manometry:

- basal pressure of sphincter zone (mm Hg)
- maximal squeeze pressure with maximum voluntary sphincter contraction
- squeeze increment (maximal squeeze pressure minus basal pressure)
- rectal sensation and threshold if rectal balloon is used

With balloon manometry:

- rectal sensation and rectal distention sensory threshold
- urge to defecate following rectal distention
- response of internal sphincter to rectal distention
- response of external sphincter to rectal distention
- estimation of rectal compliance

A compliance curve may be generated if the pressure within the large rectal balloon is plotted against its volume over a range of values.

Interpretation **NORMAL FINDINGS:** Testing information is reported by an experienced GI specialist. For basal and squeeze pressures, a wide range of normal values has been reported due to the variety of manometric devices in use. Thus, normal ranges for men and women must be defined by each individual laboratory. Examples are basal pressure roughly 60 mm Hg, squeeze pressure approximately 200 mm Hg in men. The normal response to rectal distention (simulated by the inflated rectal balloon) is reflex relaxation of the internal sphincter. This is the "rectoanal inhibitory reflex" under autonomic nervous system control. This occurs within seconds of rectal distention (often <20 mL in balloon) and a 30-40 mm Hg drop in sphincter pressure is seen. This is measured by the middle balloon of the 3-balloon system. Simultaneously there is contraction of the external anal sphincter, the "rectoanal contraction response". This response to rectal distention is felt to be a learned phenomenon and not a reflex per se. When the large rectal balloon is slowly inflated, most normal individuals can consciously sense distention with approximately 10 mL air. Rectal compliance curves generated from pressure-volume measurements are compared against the norm for an individual laboratory. **CRITICAL VALUES:** Test is considered positive (abnormal) if a measured variable or reflex response consistently falls outside the established normal range. **ADDITIONAL INFORMATION:** In certain disease states, ARM abnormalities may be pathognomonic. In Hirschsprung's disease, for example, rectal distention may lead to paradoxical internal sphincter contraction, rather than relaxation. Aganglionosis invariably involves the internal sphincter, and due to involvement of the intramural plexus, the rectoanal inhibitory reflex is abolished. Accuracy is high enough to obviate the need for deep muscle biopsy in some cases. In the adult with short segment Hirschsprung's disease, ARM may be the only practical means of establishing the diagnosis. Although ARM is rarely diagnostic of a specific disease in patients with fecal incontinence, important information regarding sphincter failure may be obtained. Abnormally low basal pressures (with normal squeeze pressures) indicate isolated internal anal sphincter dysfunction. Abnormally low squeeze pressures (with normal basal pressures) are characteristic of isolated external sphincter dysfunction. Systemic involvement of neuromuscular disease may at times be confirmed by ARM in patients with fecal incontinence. In scleroderma, for instance, incontinence may be due to selective involvement of the smooth muscle in the internal sphincter. Striated muscle characteristically is spared. There is loss of the rectoanal inhibitory reflex, but external sphincter contraction remains intact. In polydermatomyositis only striated muscle is involved. External sphincter contraction is impaired but the rectoanal inhibitory reflex is normal. It should be noted that a number of underlying systemic diseases may also cause fecal incontinence and isolated external sphincter dysfunction, including myotonic dystrophy, hyperthyroidism, myasthenia gravis, and perhaps diabetes mellitus. Abnormal sensory threshold for rectal distention suggests a lesion in sensory neural pathways. This has been demonstrated in some diabetics with fecal incontinence where the required distending volume of the rectal balloon is more than 10 mL greater than normal controls. Decreased rectal compliance is the etiology of fecal incontinence in a limited number of diseases. These include radiation proctitis, inflammatory bowel disease with rectal involvement, rectal ischemia, and (possibly) fecal impaction.

Footnotes

1. Marzuk PM, "Biofeedback for Gastrointestinal Disorders: A Review of the Literature," *Ann Intern Med*, 1985, 103:240-4.
2. Sondheimer JM, Pearlman DS, and Bailey WC, "Systemic Anaphylaxis During Rectal Manometry With a Latex Balloon," *Am J Gastroenterol*, 1989, 84(8):975-7.
3. Mishalany H, Suzuki H, and Yokoyama J, "Report on the First International Symposium of Anorectal Manometry," *J Pediatr Surg*, 1989, 24(4):356-9.

References

Hanauer SB, "Fecal Incontinence in the Elderly," *Hosp Pract [Off]*, 1988, 23(3A):105-12.

Henry MM, "Pathogenesis and Management of Fecal Incontinence in the Adult," *Gastroenterol Clin North Am*, 1987, 16:35-45.

Hirsh EH, Hodges KS, Hersh T, et al, "Anorectal Manometry in the Diagnosis of Hirschsprung's Disease in Adults," *Am J Gastroenterol*, 1980, 74:258-60.

Marshall JB, "Chronic Constipation in Adults. How Far Should Evaluation and Treatment Go?" *Postgrad Med*, 1990, 88(3):49-51, 54, 57-9, 63.

Sandler RS, "Rectal Manometry and Biofeedback Therapy for Fecal Incontinence," *Manual of Gastroenterologic Procedures*, 2nd ed, Drossman DA, ed, New York, NY: Raven Press, 1987, 80-9.

Schiller LR, "Fecal Incontinence," *Gastrointestinal Disease: Pathophysiology, Diagnosis, Management*, 4th ed, Chapter 21, Sleisenger MH and Fordtran JS, eds, Philadelphia, PA: WB Saunders Co, 1989, 317-31.

Schuster MM, "Tests Related to the Colon, Rectum, and Anus," *Bockus Gastroenterology*, 4th ed, Chapter 28, Berk JE, ed, Philadelphia, PA: WB Saunders Co, 1985, 388-401.

(Continued)

Anorectal Manometry *(Continued)*

Wald A, Caruana BJ, Freimanis MG, et al, "Contributions of Evacuation Proctography and Anorectal Manometry to Evaluation of Adults With Constipation and Defecatory Difficulty," *Dig Dis Sci*, 1990, 35(4):481-7.

Anoscopy

CPT 46600 (diagnostic only); 46602 (collection of specimen by brushing or washing); 46606 (biopsy); 46610 (removal of polyp)

Related Information

Colonoscopy *on page 87*
Flexible Fiberoptic Sigmoidoscopy *on page 102*

Synonyms Proctoscopy

Abstract **PROCEDURE COMMONLY INCLUDES:** Direct examination of the lower rectal mucosa and anal canal. The device used, the anoscope, is a rigid metal or plastic instrument 5-8 cm in length. In general, this procedure is useful in the diagnosis of diseases of the distal anal canal. **INDICATIONS:** Common indications include:

- rectal bleeding
- evaluation of the perianal mass discovered on digital rectal examination (eg, hematoma, carcinoma, thrombosed hemorrhoids)
- suspected cases of proctitis; procedure allows visually-directed cultures to be obtained (eg, herpes simplex virus, *Neisseria gonorrhoeae*)
- evaluation of rectal pain, including anal fissures, perianal abscesses, fistulae, hematoma
- diagnosis of internal hemorrhoids

Therapeutic procedures which may be performed along with routine anoscopy include:

- collection of specimens for microbiological staining and culture
- direct dilation
- removal of foreign bodies
- biopsy of suspicious lesions, ulcers, or masses
- removal of polyps, single or multiple
- coagulation of bleeding mucosal lesions
- treatment of hemorrhoids by injection or banding

CONTRAINDICATIONS: There are few absolute contraindications for diagnostic anoscopy. Anoscopy should not be performed if patient refuses to consent, or if severe rectal pain is present. In the latter case, if diagnostic anoscopy is considered crucial (ie, perianal abscess), a formal examination under anesthesia may be warranted. If an uncorrectable coagulopathy is present, biopsy should be avoided.

Patient Care/Scheduling **PATIENT PREPARATION:** An individual patient's candidacy for this procedure is determined by a medical history and physical, including a digital rectal exam. One of the advantages of anoscopy is its convenience. It may be performed in a physician's office on short notice and without bowel preparation. The details of the procedure are explained to the patient and consent is obtained. Often, there is a certain amount of anxiety and embarrassment on the part of the patient. The medical staff can do much to alleviate this problem with some simple reassurance and courtesy. **AFTERCARE:** If no therapeutic procedures have been performed (such as biopsy or fulguration), no specific aftercare is required. The patient may be discharged directly to home in many cases. Since sedatives are not administered routinely, patients are allowed to drive postprocedure. If the procedure is lengthy or complicated, the physician may want to observe the patient for a variable period of time. **COMPLICATIONS:** In skilled hands, anoscopy is a safe procedure. Severe complications are unusual. Potential problems include local pain, hemorrhage, and bowel perforation. If a biopsy is performed, the risk of bleeding will increase, depending on the nature of the lesion.

Method **EQUIPMENT:** The anoscope is a rigid metal or plastic tube. The diameter or the device is about 2 cm and the length is 5-8 cm. A wide variety of models are available. Some models require external illumination but others have a built-in fiberoptic light source. **TECHNIQUE:** In the majority of cases, sedatives or anesthetics are not required. Procedure may be performed in an endoscopy suite or a well-lit physician's office. The patient is appropriately positioned on an examination table according to physician preference (eg, left lateral decubitus). With the instrument's obturator (introducer) in place, the anoscope is lubricated and then advanced gently through the anal canal, angled posteriorly towards the umbilicus. Once fully inserted, the introducer is removed. The lumen of the canal is inspected for abnormalities.

Interpretation NORMAL FINDINGS: The normal rectal mucosa appears pink with visible submucosal vessels. A preliminary report is completed in the patient's chart immediately by endoscopist. CRITICAL VALUES: A variety of local and systemic diseases can cause rectal pathology. The anoscopist usually addresses the following aspects of the examination:

- type of instrument used
- depth of visualization (eg, 10 cm)
- appearance of the mucosa
- presence of blood or pus
- anal fissures, tumors, polyps
- presence of proctitis, vesicles
- hemorrhoids
- foreign bodies
- therapeutic procedures performed
- complications

ADDITIONAL INFORMATION: Proctoscopy is safe and very convenient. It may be performed in a physician's office without a special bowel prep, unlike colonoscopy. In addition, proctoscopy is not limited to the gastroenterologist. Physicians in primary care fields may perform routine cases with safety and accuracy after proper training. Some experts feel that the anoscope provides optimal visualization of the distal rectum, superior to flexible sigmoidoscopy and colonoscopy. As such, it is the procedure of choice for evaluating anal diseases.

References

Jagleman DG, "Anoscopy," *Gastroenterologic Endoscopy*, Chapter 47, Sivak MV, ed, Philadelphia, PA: WB Saunders Co, 1987, 960-5.

Kelly SM, Sanowski RA, Foutch PG, et al, "A Prospective Comparison of Anoscopy and Fiberendoscopy in Detecting Anal Lesions," *J Clin Gastroenterol*, 1986, 8:658.

Schrock TR, "Examination of the Anorectum, Rigid Sigmoidoscopy, Flexible Sigmoidoscopy, and Diseases of the Anorectum," *Gastrointestinal Disease: Pathophysiology, Diagnosis, Management*, 4th ed, Sleisenger MH and Fordtran JS, ed, Philadelphia, PA: WB Saunders Co, 1989, 1570-91.

ARM *see* Anorectal Manometry *on page 77*

Ascites Fluid Tap *see* Paracentesis *on page 111*

Bacterial Overgrowth Testing *see* Breath Hydrogen Analysis *on page 85*

Bag Dilation of Esophagus *see* Esophageal Dilation *on page 96*

Balloon Manometry for Fecal Incontinence *see* Anorectal Manometry *on page 77*

BAO (Basal Acid Output) *see* Hollander Test *on page 105*

Basal Serum Gastrin Determination *see* I.V. Secretin Gastrin Levels *on page 107*

Bernstein Test

CPT 91030

Related Information

Esophageal Motility Study *on page 98*
Standard Acid Reflux Test *on page 124*

Synonyms Acid Infusion Test; Acid Perfusion Test for Esophagitis

Abstract PROCEDURE COMMONLY INCLUDES: Infusion of acid (0.1 N HCl) into the distal esophagus to determine if a patient's complaints of chest pain originate in the esophagus. Both acid and a saline control are alternately infused via a nasogastric (NG) tube, without the

(Continued)

Bernstein Test *(Continued)*

patient being aware of the identity of the solution. Any subjective symptoms of chest or abdominal discomfort are recorded. **INDICATIONS:**

- determine if symptoms in an individual patient are caused by esophageal disease, most commonly gastroesophageal (GE) reflux disease
- help objectively discriminate between angina pectoris and esophageal disease in the patient with atypical chest pain

CONTRAINDICATIONS:

- confused or agitated patient; the Bernstein test requires accurate verbal descriptions of symptoms by the patient during acid infusion
- active upper GI bleeding
- nausea and vomiting at test time
- possibly, severe coronary artery disease (CAD)

Patient Care/Scheduling **PATIENT PREPARATION:** Technique and risks of the procedure are explained and consent is obtained. Requisition from referring physician should specify whether Bernstein test is to be performed alone or in conjunction with formal esophageal manometry testing. Patient should be NPO for at least 8 hours before testing and preferably overnight. Avoid antacids and H_2 blockers prior to procedures (check with GI Laboratory if there are questions regarding medications). **AFTERCARE:** If no complications have occurred, patient may be dismissed from GI procedure room. No particular postprocedure restrictions are required, with activity *ad libitum* as tolerated. Usually, the patient is given 30 mL antacid before leaving. If test is positive, inform the patient that he/she will be contacted by the referring physician for specific antireflux instructions. **COMPLICATIONS:** This procedure is considered quite safe. Minor complications include nausea, vagal reactions, and pyrosis, all usually transient. Mellow et al reported a potential major complication.[1] In patients with documented coronary artery disease (CAD), acid infusion with resultant chest pain was at times associated with significant increase in "double product" (heart rate times systolic blood pressure) and ST segment depression on EKG. These changes were felt to be consistent with transient myocardial ischemia. No evidence of myocardial ischemia during acid infusion was reported in patients without CAD (controls), or in patients with documented CAD who remained asymptomatic during acid perfusion.

Method **EQUIPMENT:** In GI procedure room: nasogastric tube, connecting tubing, 3-way stopcock, solutions of normal saline and 0.1 N HCl, and lubricant. Commonly, this procedure is done in conjunction with esophageal manometry, in which case the manometer replaces the NG tube. **TECHNIQUE:** The procedure is usually performed by a GI specialist. However, if manometry is not desired, the Bernstein test may be safely carried out by a general physician. In the original description of this procedure by Bernstein, patients were positioned in an upright, seated fashion throughout. More recently, however, this has become a matter of preference and many GI specialists opt for the supine position. Following this, the NG tube is lubricated and advanced through the nares 30-35 cm by convention, placing the tip in the distal esophagus. Separate bottles of 0.1 N HCl and saline solution are connected to the NG tube via the 3-way stopcock and clear tubing. Initially, the stopcock is set such that the saline solution is infused first through the NG tube, at a rate of 120 drops/minute for 15 minutes. Patient is instructed to describe any symptoms in detail, whether or not it is typical of the chief complaint. After this 15 minute control period, the stopcock is turned so that the infusing solution is changed from saline to 0.1 N HCl without the patient's knowledge. The acid infusion is continued until symptoms appear or until 30 minutes have elapsed. As a general rule, symptoms of pyrosis or abdominal pain should be persistent as long as acid is infusing and worsening in severity over several minutes. "Twinges" or other transient sensations should be recorded but are probably insignificant. If clearly persistent symptoms of retrosternal burning are described, the infusing solution is changed back to saline (unbeknownst to patient). Saline is continued for at least 5 minutes. Note whether or not symptoms are alleviated; if so, restart acid infusion and record patient reaction. Alternatively, some clinicians give 30 mL antacid after the initial episode of acid-induced chest pain, foregoing the traditional saline "washout". Patient describes degree of pain relief with antacids, if any. Test is then continued with saline or acid as before. **DATA ACQUIRED:** Presence or absence of symptoms with each infusion, along with duration of symptoms. Nature of symptoms is documented carefully, not simply by "positive" or "negative," because this is essential for interpretation.

Interpretation NORMAL FINDINGS: No symptoms during either saline or acid infusion CRITICAL VALUES: A positive test is defined as reproduction of the original chest pain with infusion of acid, but not saline. This should occur consistently with each separate acid infusion. As an aside, some clinicians through the years have asserted that disappearance of symptoms after cessation of acid infusion (or after administration of antacids) is also a requisite for a positive test. This criterion was not a part of the Bernstein test, as originally described. Winnan et al prospectively investigated this issue and found that a significant number of patients with documented GE reflux experienced persistent chest pain following acid infusion, not relieved by antacids or a replacement saline infusion.[2] They concluded that this clinical adage is probably incorrect and need not be used to define a positive test.

An "inconclusive" test is defined as either:

- chest pain with both saline and acid infusions equally or
- development of a new pain, different from the original chief complaint

ADDITIONAL INFORMATION: The Bernstein test has gained clinical acceptance as a rapid and inexpensive means of diagnosing gastroesophageal reflux disease. In some cases of atypical chest pain, a positive result may be quite useful in identifying a sensitive lower esophagus as an origin of symptoms. Richter et al (1982) reviewed the literature relating a positive Bernstein test with gastroesophageal reflux and found a sensitivity of 79% and specificity of 82%. Some authors believe that specificity is increased if the patient experiences symptoms within 7 minutes of acid infusion. However, false-negative tests have been documented in nearly all clinical series. Some experts feel that the Bernstein test may be falsely positive in patients with gastritis, further compromising test specificity.[3] This procedure does not objectively measure acid reflux, nor does it diagnose esophagitis. Despite these limitations, this procedure may still be useful, especially when performed in combination with esophageal manometric studies. This appears to be its most accepted role in recent years, especially with the advent of highly elaborate tests for reflux esophagitis.

Footnotes

1. Mellow MH, Watt L, Haye O, et al, "Cardiovascular Response to Esophageal Acid Perfusion in Coronary Disease," *Gastroenterology*, 1981, 80(5):1230, (abstract).
2. Winnan GR, Meyer CT, and McCallum RW, "Interpretation of the Bernstein Test: A Reappraisal of Criteria," *Ann Intern Med*, 1982, 92:320-2.
3. De Moraes-Filho JPP and Bettarello A, "Lack of Specificity of the Acid Perfusion Test in Duodenal Ulcer Patients," *Dig Dis*, 1974, 19(9):785-90.

References

Behar J, Biancani P, and Sheahan DG, "Evaluation of Esophageal Tests in the Diagnosis of Reflux Esophagitis," *Gastroenterology*, 1976, 71(1):9-15.

Hogan WJ and Dodds WJ, "Gastroesophageal Reflux Disease," *Gastrointestinal Disease: Pathophysiology, Diagnosis, and Management*, 4th ed, Chapter 34, Sleisenger MH and Fordtran JS, eds, Philadelphia, PA: WB Saunders Co, 1989, 594-619.

Richter JE and Castell DO, "Gastroesophageal Reflux," *Ann Intern Med*, 1982, 97:93-103.

Biliary Drainage

Synonyms Biliary Drainage With Cholecystokinin; CCK Test; Duodenal Aspirate; Duodenal Drainage; Gallbladder Stimulation; Transduodenal Drainage With CCK

Applies to Endoscopic Biliary Drainage; Standard Duodenal Intubation Method of Biliary Drainage

Replaces Biliary Drainage With Magnesium Sulfate

Abstract PROCEDURE COMMONLY INCLUDES: Light microscopic and polarized scope examination of "B" bile for cholesterol and calcium bilirubinate crystals INDICATIONS: To evaluate by light and polarized microscopy the "B" bile obtained from patients with persistent symptoms of biliary colic who have had negative or inconclusive oral cholecystograms and biliary ultrasound or who are allergic to radiographic dye. Cholelithiasis or acalculous cholecystitis are suggested by the presence of cholesterol or calcium bilirubinate crystals, by the absence of "B" bile, or by the reproduction of symptoms upon injection of cholecystokinin (CCK). Such supportive evidence of gallbladder disease suggests that symptomatic relief is likely to occur with cholecystectomy. CONTRAINDICATIONS: Blocked common bile duct

(Continued)

Biliary Drainage *(Continued)*

may yield little fluid return during CCK stimulation test and an absence of crystals. Tumor or gallstones may also be the cause of such obstruction.

Patient Care/Scheduling **PATIENT PREPARATION:** Obtain a signed procedure permit for "Biliary Drainage." Patient should have nothing by mouth after the evening meal on the day before the test. Start an I.V. of normal saline. If using the endoscopic method, give 5-10 mg Valium® (no atropine). Anesthetize posterior pharynx with 5% Cetacaine® spray prior to duodenal intubation or endoscopy. **SPECIAL INSTRUCTIONS:** Requisition **must** state name of test. Procedure is approved by consultation with gastroenterology staff.

Method **TECHNIQUE:** Under fluoroscopy a Dreiling-type, radiopaque, double-lumen tube is intubated. The distal lumen is placed just beyond the papilla of vater in the duodenum, thereby placing the proximal lumen in the gastric antrum. Suction is applied to the gastric lumen and continued throughout the procedure. Cholecystokinin (CCK) is administered by I.V. at the dose of 0.1 mL/kg body weight. Suction is then applied to the duodenal lumen. Three types of bile should be recognized and collected separately. Therefore, the specimen trap should be changed upon recognition of each type of bile. The first bile obtained, "A" bile, is clear and comes from the common bile duct. The second or "B" bile is dark green and comes from the gallbladder. The third or "C" bile is yellow and originates from the biliary radicals. It is the "B" bile that is sent for microscopic analysis. If a satisfactory amount of "B" bile has not been obtained within 15 minutes of CCK injection, the dose should be doubled and repeated. If using an endoscope, the method of collection is basically the same except that the duodenal aspirate is obtained through a suction catheter that is inserted through the biopsy channel.[1] **DATA ACQUIRED:** Presence or absence of cholesterol and calcium bilirubinate crystals; presence or absence of "B" bile; total volume of drainage; patient response.

Specimen 20-25 mL dark "B" bile **CONTAINER:** Any clean plastic container with lid. A Daval mucous specimen trap has been suggested. **SAMPLING TIME:** 30 minutes – usually begins 10-15 minutes after CCK injection **CAUSES FOR REJECTION:** Patient not fasting, administration of peristalsis inhibiting medication (if any questions regarding medications, call the department) **TURNAROUND TIME:** 24-48 hours.

Interpretation **NORMAL FINDINGS:** No cholesterol or calcium bilirubinate crystals seen. "B" bile present at least 15-20 mL. Symptoms not reproduced by CCK injection. **CRITICAL VALUES:** Test is considered "suspicious" when 1-10 crystals of either calcium bilirubinate or cholesterol are found per slide. Test is considered "positive" when more than 10 crystals of calcium bilirubinate or cholesterol are spotted per slide. No "B" bile obtained even after repeat CCK injection. Symptoms reproduced by CCK injection. **LIMITATIONS:** Reproduction of symptoms alone is only subjective evidence of gallbladder pathology especially since CCK physiologically produces abdominal discomfort and the urge to defecate. However, the CCK test alone has gained popularity in some of the recent literature.[2,3] Liver or pancreatic diseases may cause failure to produce "B" bile and therefore produce a false-positive. A false-positive may also be obtained due to formation of calcium bilirubinate crystals in the presence of pancreatic and liver diseases as well as hemolytic anemias. There is also evidence that cholesterol crystals may be produced physiologically in the fasting state.[4] A false-positive may also be obtained if "false bilirubin" is interpreted as true crystals. These structures are yellow and somewhat amorphous with a pH <4.5 as opposed to the more alkalotic discrete burgundy to brick-red granules of calcium bilirubinate.[1] **ADDITIONAL INFORMATION:** It is advised to use the cholecystokinin (CCK) stimulation test when other tests to detect gallbladder disease are unsuccessful. This would include an inconclusive finding on a radiology oral cholecystogram test, or when a patient is allergic to the iodine substance contained in most contrast media. Stains and cultures of duodenal aspirates are useful in limited situations. If *Giardia lamblia* or *Strongyloides stercoralis* are suspected but fecal exams remain negative, stains of duodenal aspirates may prove helpful. Cultures have been proven helpful in typhoid or *Salmonella* carriers.

Footnotes

1. Foss DC and Laing RR, "Detection of Gallbladder Disease in Patients With Normal Oral Cholycystograms," *Am J Dig Dis*, 1977, 22:685-9.
2. Sykes D, "Use of Cholecystokinin in Diagnosis of Biliary Pain," *Ann R Coll Surg Engl*, 1982, 64:114-6.

3. Lennard TWJ, Farndon JR, and Taylor RMR, "Acalculous Biliary Pain, Diagnosis and Selection for Cholecystectomy Using Cholecystokinin Test for Pain Reproduction," *Br J Surg*, 1984, 71:368-70.
4. Northfield TC and Hoffman AF, "Biliary Lipid Secretion in Gallstone Patients," *Lancet*, 1973, 1:747-8.

References

Burnstein MJ, Vassal KP, and Strasberg SM, "Results of Combined Biliary Drainage and Cholecystography in 81 Patients With Normal Oral Cholecystograms," *Ann Surg*, 1982, 196(6):627-32.

Biliary Drainage With Cholecystokinin *see* Biliary Drainage *on page 83*

Biliary Drainage With Magnesium Sulfate *replaced by* Biliary Drainage *on page 83*

Blind Liver Biopsy *see* Liver Biopsy *on page 108*

Breath Analysis *see* Breath Hydrogen Analysis *on this page*

Breath Hydrogen Analysis

CPT 91065

Synonyms Breath Analysis; Breath Test; Hydrogen Breath Test; Hydrogen Exhalation Test

Applies to Bacterial Overgrowth Testing; Carbohydrate Malabsorption Tests; Measurement of Intestinal Transit Time

Replaces Carbon-14 Glycine Cholate Test for Bacterial Overgrowth; Carbon-14 Lactose Breath Test; Carbon-14 Stool Excretion; Intestinal Biopsy (for Disaccharidase Deficiency); Intestinal Intubation for Culture; Intestinal Perfusion and Lactose Barium Radiography; Lactose (Sucrose and d-Xylose) Tolerance Test; Stool pH Test; Tests for Fecal Reducing Substances

Abstract PROCEDURE COMMONLY INCLUDES: Carbohydrate intolerance: The patient ingests lactose or other carbohydrate feeding. This is followed by collection of samples of expired air. The H_2 content of the expired air is then determined by gas chromatography. Above average H_2 content is considered a positive test.

Measurement of intestinal transit time: The patient ingests a carbohydrate feeding which is followed by a collection of a series of samples of expired air. The H_2 content of each air sample is determined by gas chromatography. The time period between the ingestion of the carbohydrate meal and the first measured increase in expired H_2 is considered to be the small intestinal transit time.

Bacterial overgrowth: The patient ingests a carbohydrate feeding which is followed by a collection of a series of samples of expired air. The H_2 content of each air sample is determined by gas chromatography. The test is considered positive if two distinct H_2 peaks are detected. The first peak corresponds to carbohydrate fermentation by bacteria in the small bowel, and the second to fermentation in the colon (an abnormal finding). Fasting breath H_2 is also usually elevated in this condition.

INDICATIONS: Diagnosis of carbohydrate malabsorption – lactose, sucrose, DW xylose;[1] diagnosis of bacterial overgrowth – H_2 breath test is useful in conjunction with carbon-14 glycolate test; diagnosis of motility disorders such as irritable bowel and postgastrectomy syndromes by measurement of intestinal transit time. CONTRAINDICATIONS: Patient cannot drink liquids, active diarrhea may decrease response, severe pulmonary disease.

Patient Care/Scheduling PATIENT PREPARATION: NPO for at least 6-8 hours (preferably overnight) and during test (except for carbohydrate feeding). No smoking 15 minutes prior to test. No antibiotics 7 days prior to test. No grain cereals or foods 12 hours prior to test. Carbohydrate feeding: infants 2 g/kg low fiber, adults 20 g/kg low fiber. Lactulose is best feeding for bacterial overgrowth testing as it traverses the entire bowel unabsorbed.

Specimen Expired air CONTAINER: Haldane-Priestly tube for adults; for infants, Rahn-Otis end tidal sampler, nasal prongs, or postnasal catheter connected to bags fitted with 1-way stopcocks. Gas is then transported via an oiled syringe to a Vacutainer™. SAMPLING TIME: Up to 6 hours if interval sampling is used. Interval sampling is usually done every 30 min-

(Continued)

Breath Hydrogen Analysis *(Continued)*

utes for 2-4 hours. **COLLECTION:** Usually involves Haldane-Priestly tube into which the patient exhales with nose clamped **STORAGE INSTRUCTIONS:** Vacutainer™ for up to 3 weeks **TURNAROUND TIME:** 3-7 days.

Interpretation **NORMAL FINDINGS:** For lactose intolerance: if measured in rate of excretion, H_2 >0.5 mL/minute (nL <0.3); if measured as end tidal volume, H_2 >24 ppm or 20 ppm greater than fasting (nL <10). For intestinal overgrowth: two distinct H_2 peaks correspond to carbohydrate fermentation in the small bowel and then the colon.[1] For measurement of intestinal transit time: more than 95 minutes is normal. **LIMITATIONS:** If the test is performed during states of active diarrhea, transit time may not be long enough for sufficient fermentation. Significant bowel, pulmonary, or vascular disease may decrease H_2 absorption and secretion. Idiopathic or iatrogenic absence of intestinal flora makes the test worthless. Presence of normal flora that consume H_2 can give falsely low H_2 excretion. The test is useless in newborns prior to intestinal colonization.[2] The presence of acidic colonic milieu common in infants can give a falsely low H_2 excretion.[3] Exercise also lowers H_2 excretion.[4] Smoking and sleep may falsely elevate H_2 excretion.[5] **ADDITIONAL INFORMATION:** This test is based on the premise that the normal small bowel absorbs ingested carbohydrate, that the normal small bowel is sterile, and that undigested carbohydrate is then fermented by normal colonic flora with H_2 being the product of that fermentation. The predominence of H_2 produced in the colon is expelled rectally and the remainder is absorbed into the colonic circulation. It is then expelled into the pulmonary tree where it can be measured as exhaled H_2.

Footnotes

1. Bond JH and Levitt MD, "Use of Breath H_2 to Quantitate Small Bowel Transit Time Following Partial Gastrectomy," *J Lab Clin Med*, 1977, 90(1):30-6.
2. Barr RG, Hanley J, Patterson DK, et al, "Breath H_2 Excretion in Normal Newborn Infants in Response to Usual Feeding Patterns: Evidence for Functional Lactase Insufficiency Beyond the First Month of Life," *J Pediatr*, 1984, 104(4):527-9.
3. The Nutrition Foundation, "Influence of Colonic pH on the Hydrogen Breath-Analysis Test," *Nutr Rev*, 1982, 40(6):172-5.
4. Payne DL, Welsh JD, and Claypool PL, "Breath H_2 Response to Carbohydrate Malabsorption After Exercise," *J Lab Clin Med*, 1983, 102(1):147-50.
5. Rosenthal A and Solomons NW, "Time-Course of Cigarette Smoke Contamination of H_2 Breath-Analysis Tests," *Clin Chem*, 1983, 29(11):1980-1.

References

Caballero B, Solomons NW, and Torún B, "Fecal Reducing Substances and Breath H_2 Excretion as Indicators of Carbohydrate Metabolism," *J Pediatr Gastroenterol Nutr*, 1983, 2(3):487-90.

Newcomer AD, McGill DB, Thomas PJ, et al, "Prospective Comparison of Indirect Methods for Detecting Lactase Deficiency," *N Engl J Med*, 1975, 293(4):1232-6.

Breath Test *see* Breath Hydrogen Analysis *on previous page*

Carbohydrate Malabsorption Tests *see* Breath Hydrogen Analysis *on previous page*

Carbon-14 Glycine Cholate Test for Bacterial Overgrowth *replaced by* Breath Hydrogen Analysis *on previous page*

Carbon-14 Lactose Breath Test *replaced by* Breath Hydrogen Analysis *on previous page*

Carbon-14 Stool Excretion *replaced by* Breath Hydrogen Analysis *on previous page*

CCK Test *see* Biliary Drainage *on page 83*

Celioscopy *see* Peritoneoscopy *on page 114*

Colonoscopy

CPT 45378 (colonoscopy, fiberoptic, beyond the splenic flexure); 45379 (removal of foreign body); 45380 (biopsy and/or brushing); 45382 (control of hemorrhage); 45383 (tumor ablation); 45385 (removal of polyps)

Related Information

Anoscopy *on page 80*

Flexible Fiberoptic Sigmoidoscopy *on page 102*

Synonyms Full Colonoscopy; Lower Endoscopy

Abstract PROCEDURE COMMONLY INCLUDES: Direct visual examination of the colon, ileocecal value, and portions of the terminal ileum by means of a fiberoptic endoscope. Colonoscopy is best performed by a qualified gastroenterology specialist in a specialized endoscopy suite (occasionally may be carried out at the bedside in an intensive care unit). With the patient awake but sedated, a flexible endoscope is inserted per rectum and advanced through the various portions of the lower GI tract. Important anatomic landmarks are identified and mucosal surfaces are examined for ulcerations, polyps, friable areas, hemorrhagic sites, neoplasms, strictures, etc. Minor operative procedures may then be performed utilizing the standard colonoscope with appropriate accessories. These procedures include tissue biopsy for histopathology and/or microbiologic culture, polypectomy, electrocoagulation of bleeding sites, removal of foreign bodies, hot biopsy/fulguration of tumor, and others. INDICATIONS: In clinical practice, opinions differ regarding the appropriate indications for colonoscopy. Similarly, the precise role of related diagnostic tests, such as the barium enema and proctoscopy, has not been universally defined. A position paper issued by the American College of Physicians in 1987 outlines acceptable indications for colonoscopy as follows:[1]

- evaluation of potentially significant barium enema abnormalities, including ulcerations, filling defects, and strictures
- removal of colon polyps
- evaluation of lower GI bleeding of obscure origin; includes unexplained Hemoccult® positive stools, hematochezia with a negative proctoscopy, and persistent melena with a negative upper GI evaluation
- work-up of iron deficiency anemia of unknown etiology
- surveillance studies to rule out colon cancer, neoplastic polyps, or malignant degeneration (dysplasia) in the following situations: strong family history of colon cancer or familial polyposis; patients with treatable colon cancer or malignant polyps to rule out synchronous polyps; follow-up examination in patient's status postcolon cancer resection (or removal of neoplastic polyp), at 2-3 year intervals; follow-up examination in individuals with ulcerative colitis with left-sided involvement over 15 years or pancolitis over 7 years (surveillance every 1-2 years)
- diagnostic study of patients with inflammatory bowel disease to define the extent of disease involvement, to differentiate Crohn's disease from ulcerative colitis when barium enema or biopsy are nondiagnostic, or to assess the degree of disease activity if important in management
- discretionary follow-up of colonic lesions of unknown significance, noted on previous examination
- diagnosis and localization of lower GI hemorrhage, prior to possible electrocauterization or surgery
- therapeutic indications include colon decompression, removal of foreign bodies, dilatation of colonic strictures

These indications are not all-inclusive and are subject to physician discretion in individual cases.

Colonoscopy is generally **not** indicated in the following situations (as per the American College of Physicians):

- chronic irritable bowel syndrome
- acute, self-limited diarrhea
- routine surveillance of patients with stable inflammatory bowel disease (with the exception of cancer surveillance)
- melena with a clearly demonstrable upper GI source (eg, duodenal ulcer)
- hematochezia with a clearly demonstrable anorectal source on proctosigmoidoscopy (eg, anal fissure)

(Continued)

Colonoscopy *(Continued)*

- routine surveillance of patients with non-neoplastic polyps (hyperplastic polyps) or healed, nonmalignant disease
- surveillance of patients who have undergone curative resection of colon cancer, solely to rule out suture line recurrence
- routine evaluation of patients undergoing elective (noncolonic) abdominal surgery with no signs or symptoms referable to the colon

Again, exceptions to these guidelines may be made at physician discretion.

CONTRAINDICATIONS:

- toxic, fulminant colitis
- perforation of abdominal viscus; insufflation of the colon with air may worsen fecal contamination in the peritoneal cavity
- severe coagulopathy
- acute diverticulitis (unless carcinoma is high on the differential diagnosis)
- acute or recent myocardial infarction
- patient refusal

High risk situations (not necessarily contraindications) include:

- uncontrolled lower GI bleeding
- recent colon surgery
- multiple abdominal and pelvic surgeries in the past, with adhesions
- severe chronic obstructive pulmonary disease (COPD) or arteriosclerotic heart disease (ASHD)
- pregnancy in second or third trimester

Patient Care/Scheduling **PATIENT PREPARATION:** Technique and risks of the procedure are discussed with the patient, including the possibility of biopsy, polypectomy, or other operative procedure if applicable. Informed consent is obtained. In some medical centers formal consultation with gastroenterology staff is necessary to obtain a colonoscopy, whereas in other institutions the primary (ordering) physician arranges for the procedure directly with the endoscopy scheduling desk. Colonoscopy may be performed on either inpatients or outpatients. Customarily, inpatients are examined briefly by the endoscopist (or his representative) the day prior to colonoscopy to review the case, write orders, and answer remaining patient questions. Thorough bowel cleaning prior to colonoscopy is a critical first step in ensuring a technically adequate study. Even small amounts of retained fecal matter can obscure the distal lens of the endoscope. A standard bowel regimen is performed as follows: 48 hours prior to procedure patients are allowed a clear liquid diet only. This is limited to clear broth, tea, jello, fruit juices, ginger ale, and sherbet. Two nights before procedure, patient takes 60 mL milk of magnesia (optional) and one night beforehand (6 PM) patient takes either 2 oz of castor oil or 10 oz of magnesium citrate orally. On the morning of examination, mechanical cleansing of the sigmoid and left colon is carried out by two tap water enemas or until fluid return is clear. Alternatively, commercially-prepared solutions such as GoLYTELY® (Braintree Laboratories) may be used with equivalent results without the need for enemas. Again, patient is restricted to a clear liquid diet for 1-2 days beforehand. On the morning of colonoscopy, patient ingests at least 1 gallon of GoLYTELY® solution (200-250 mL orally/NG every 15 minutes). No further preparation is usually required unless patient is unable to tolerate the full volume. This method should not be used if bowel obstruction, perforation, or megacolon is suspected. Patients experiencing an acute flare of inflammatory bowel disease should receive a modified bowel prep prior to the colonoscopy. Often a clear liquid diet for 1-2 days and tap water enemas are sufficient, and cathartics may be avoided altogether, at physician discretion. Daily medications are allowed on the morning of colonoscopy with small sips of water. Iron compounds should be discontinued 1 week beforehand. Aspirin and aspirin-containing products should likewise be stopped 5 days prior to the procedure to minimize the risk of bleeding from polypectomy. Send hospitalized patients to the endoscopy suite on a cart along with medical record and relevant x-rays (include prior barium enema studies). For outpatients, arrangements for transportation home should be made in advance by the patient, since driving is not permitted postprocedure. Once patient has arrived in procedure room, a baseline set of vital signs is obtained. Premedication is given routinely, several minutes before examination. Meperidine (25-50 mg I.V.) and diazepam (starting at 1-3 mg I.V., or more) are commonly employed to decrease the discomfort of bowel stretching and insufflation and to produce a mild amnesia in some patients. **AFTERCARE:** Following procedure, patient is observed in the recovery area. Vital signs are recorded at least once postprocedure. Once sedation has worn off, patient may be discharged from the testing area. Driving is forbidden due to residual effects from sedatives. The patient is instructed to call physician if complications should develop. **SPECIAL INSTRUCTIONS:** Antibiotic prophylaxis for bacterial endocarditis is commonly administered for patients undergoing colonoscopy with prosthetic valves, a past history of endocarditis, rheumatic valvular disease, or other high risk cardiac lesions. Some authors, however, consider this unnecessary because of the low risk of bacteremia. (A definitive study is impractical and not likely to be performed.) Regimens recommended by the American Heart Association include:

- ampicillin 2 g I.M./I.V. and gentamicin 1.5 mg/kg given I.M./I.V. 30 minutes before and 8 hours after procedure
- if penicillin allergic, vancomycin and gentamicin can be administered
- if lower risk valvular condition, amoxicillin 3 g orally 1 hour prior and 1.5 g orally 6 hours later

COMPLICATIONS: Major complications include[2,3] : Perforation: estimated at 0.14% to 0.8% with diagnostic colonoscopy and 1% with polypectomy. This may be recognized immediately (intra-abdominal viscera directly visualized) or may be delayed for days. Perforation may be caused by mechanical trauma from the instrument tip, especially if the wall is weakened (from ischemia, diverticula, colitis), the colon is "tacked down" (previous pelvic surgery, tumor, adhesions), or an obstructive lesion is present. Less commonly, perforation may be noninstrumental, secondary to aggressive insufflation with air (serosal tears). Polypectomy-related perforation may result from a direct luminal laceration from a snare loop or hot forceps, or may be from delayed sloughing of necrotic bowel following thermal coagulation. This latter situation may lead to the "postpolypectomy coagulation syndrome" characterized by fever, evidence of peritoneal irritation (rebound tenderness), and leukocytosis. Radiographic evidence of perforation or free air is lacking, and patients recover without surgery. "Free" perforation from a large transmural laceration is less frequent (0.14% to 0.26%) and requires immediate surgery. Lesser degrees of perforation are more difficult to diagnose. If pneumoperitoneum is detected on KUB a Gastrografin™ (water-soluble) enema x-ray needs to be obtained. If leakage is not demonstrated, many cases can be managed conservatively. The profile of the high risk patient has been described previously. However, serious complications have been reported in routine cases.

Hemorrhage: incidence of serious bleeding from diagnostic colonoscopy without polypectomy is negligible, 0% to 0.5% of cases. Several large series have reported no incidents of this nature. With polypectomy the rate increases to 0.7% to 2.5% and may be immediate or delayed. Repeat colonoscopy may be necessary to coagulate a bleeding pedicle. In rare instances angiography and surgery have been required.

Respiratory depression: usually due to oversedation in the patient with chronic lung disease.

Bacteremia: incidence varies among series from 0% to 5%. Several large studies have reported no positive blood cultures (see Special Instructions).

Miscellaneous complications:

- vasovagal reactions
- explosion of combustible gases in the colon (H_2, methane) when in contact with an electric spark; this may occur with a grossly inadequate bowel prep
- splenic laceration
- transient EKG changes
- dehydration resulting from excessive use of laxatives and enemas for bowel cleansing
- volvulus

Method **EQUIPMENT:** The standard endoscope is 185 cm in length with a diameter of 12-13 mm. An intermediate length instrument of 135 cm is also available and examines up to the ascending colon. The endoscope is made up of numerous fiberoptic glass strands which transmit light along their entire length with minimal distortion. The multiple images are integrated at proximal eyepiece using a complex system of lenses. The image produced is

(Continued)

Colonoscopy *(Continued)*

thus reconstructed from multiple points. Newer instruments contain two channels within the endoscope which can accommodate two accessories at the same time, such as a snare wire and forceps. Air for insufflation and a water jet may also be introduced through these channels. The multidirectional tip is controlled at the endoscopist's end by two wheels, for either up-down or right-left deflection. The instrument head is connected to a variety of auxiliary devices via a separate cable, such as a suction box, an external cold light source, and water feed tank. **TECHNIQUE:** The procedure is performed by a qualified gastroenterologist in a properly equipped procedure room. At times, colonoscopy may be performed in an ICU, emergency room, or hospital bed using portable equipment. Following sedation, the patient is placed in left lateral decubitus position. A digital rectal examination is performed. After this the lubricated endoscope is inserted per rectum. Initially a "red-out" is seen in the rectum and insufflation is used as needed to optimally visualize the lumen. The instrument is advanced then only under direct vision. Landmarks are identified including the rectum (highly vascular, bluish vessels), sigmoid (ring-like valves), descending colon (narrow and tubular), transverse colon (triangular folds), hepatic flexure (dark blue hue from the liver), ascending colon (large lumen), ileocecal valve, and terminal ileum. Mucosal surfaces are reinspected as the endoscope is withdrawn. Minor operative procedures are performed as indicated.

Specimen All biopsy specimens and cytologic brushings are sent to Pathology Laboratory without delay. Any tissue for microbiological culture should be sent in a sterile container without fixative. Specimen collection, fixative, and transportation are usually the responsibility of the endoscopist. **TURNAROUND TIME:** Final pathology report on biopsy specimens is given within 2-3 days. Microbiologic stains, when performed, are available the same day, but cultures may be variably delayed.

Interpretation **NORMAL FINDINGS:** Preliminary report on colonoscopic findings written immediately by gastroenterologist, and placed in medical chart. Final typewritten report in 5-7 days. Important aspects of the examination frequently commented upon include:

- adequacy of bowel prep
- type of instrument used
- premedications used, antibiotic prophylaxis if given
- most proximal bowel segment examined
- mucosal abnormalities – polyps (size, appearance), pseudopolyps, hemorrhagic areas, ulcers, neoplastic or obstructing lesions, diverticula, friable areas, lipomas, telangiectasia, spasm, competence of ileocecal valve
- operative procedures performed during colonoscopy
- complications
- recommendations

LIMITATIONS: This is a relatively expensive procedure in comparison with the barium enema and other related endoscopic studies (EGD, proctoscopy, sigmoidoscopy). The quality of the study, and thus its interpretation, is highly dependent on the skill and experience of the endoscopist. It is also considered more technically difficult than upper endoscopy. Suboptimal studies are not uncommon and often are a result of inadequate bowel preparation.

Footnotes

1. Health Public Policy Committee, American College of Physicians, "Clinical Competence in Colonoscopy," *Ann Intern Med*, 1987, 107:772-4.
2. MacRae FA, Tan KG, and Williams CB, "Towards Safer Colonoscopy: A Report on the Complications of 5000 Diagnostic or Therapeutic Colonoscopies," *Gut*, 1983, 24:376-83.
3. Geenen JE, Schmitt WG, and Hoogan WJ, "Complications of Colonoscopy," *Gastrointest Endosc*, 1974, 66:812.

References

American Society for Gastrointestinal Endoscopy, *Appropriate Use of Gastrointestinal Endoscopy*, Manchester, MA: American Society for Gastrointestinal Endoscopy, 1986.
Grossman MB, "Gastrointestinal Endoscopy," *Ciba Found Symp*, 1980, 32(3):2-36.
Overholt BF, "Colonoscopy: A Review," *Gastroenterology*, 1975, 68:1308-20.
Ransohoff DF, Lang CA, and Kuo HS, "Colonoscopic Surveillance After Polypectomy: Considerations of Cost-Effectiveness," *Ann Intern Med*, 1991, 114(3):177-82.

Shinya H and Wolff WI, "Colonoscopy," *Surg Annu*, 1976, 8:257-95.
Rex DK, Lehman GA, Hawes RH, et al, "Screening Colonoscopy in Asymptomatic Average-Risk Persons With Negative Fecal Occult Blood Tests," *Gastroenterology*, 1991, 100(1):64-7.
Waye JD, "Colonoscopy," *Bockus Gastroenterology*, 4th ed, Chapter 43, Berk JE, ed, Philadelphia, PA: WB Saunders Co, 1985, 588-600.

Duodenal Aspirate *see* Biliary Drainage *on page 83*
Duodenal Drainage *see* Biliary Drainage *on page 83*
Duodenal Intubation and Aspiration *see* Small Bowel Biopsy *on page 120*
EGD *see* Upper Gastrointestinal Endoscopy *on page 126*
Endoscopic Biliary Drainage *see* Biliary Drainage *on page 83*
Endoscopic Retrograde Cannulation of Ampulla of Vater *see* Endoscopic Retrograde Cholangiopancreatography *on this page*
Endoscopic Retrograde Cannulation of Pancreas *see* Endoscopic Retrograde Cholangiopancreatography *on this page*
Endoscopic Retrograde Cannulation of Papilla of Vater *see* Endoscopic Retrograde Cholangiopancreatography *on this page*

Endoscopic Retrograde Cholangiopancreatography

CPT 43260 (with or without specimen collection); 43262 (for sphincterotomy/papillotomy); 43264 (for removal of stone(s) from biliary and/or pancreatic ducts); 43267 (for insertion of nasobiliary or nasopancreatic drainage tube); 43268 (for insertion of tube or stent into bile or pancreatic duct); 43271 (for balloon dilation); 43272 (for ablation of tumor or mucosal lesion)

Related Information
Sphincter of Oddi Manometry *on page 122*

Synonyms Endoscopic Retrograde Cannulation of Ampulla of Vater; Endoscopic Retrograde Cannulation of Pancreas; Endoscopic Retrograde Cannulation of Papilla of Vater; ERCP

Applies to Esophagogastroduodenoscopy (EGD); Percutaneous Transhepatic Cholangiogram (PTC)

Abstract PROCEDURE COMMONLY INCLUDES: Endoscopic visualization of the duodenum and papilla of vater, followed by radiologic assessment of the pancreatic duct and biliary tree. Procedure is performed on a conscious, but sedated patient. A specialized fiberoptic endoscope is introduced by mouth and advanced through the upper GI tract until the second portion of the duodenum is reached. Under direct visualization the papilla of vater is located and inspected. A small catheter is then advanced through the papilla of vater and into the pancreatic and biliary duct systems, all under fluoroscopic guidance. Contrast material is injected through the catheter, outlining the pancreatic duct (pancreatogram) and biliary ducts (cholangiogram). Forceps biopsies or cytologic brushings of the periampullary region and ducts may be taken. Endoscopically-guided therapeutic procedures are also possible, including endoscopic sphincterotomy and dissolution of stones. ERCP is a safe, nonsurgical means of assessing the anatomy of the ductal system and is successful in 80% to 90% of attempts. INDICATIONS: ERCP has emerged as a widely accepted, standard technique for diagnosing a variety of pancreaticobiliary tract disorders. However, several noninvasive radiologic procedures are also effective in diagnosing these disorders, including percutaneous transhepatic cholangiography (PTC), CT scan of the abdomen, ultrasound of the abdomen, and the radionuclide liver-spleen scan. These imaging techniques should be considered complementary (not competitive) with ERCP. The precise sequencing of studies must be individualized in each case, but generally the high-risk procedures (ERCP, PTC) are reserved for last. With these considerations in mind, the American Society for Gastroenterology (1986) published suggested guidelines for ERCP as follows:[1]

- evaluation of the patient with persistent jaundice in whom biliary obstruction is suspected (from retained stones, strictures, malignancy, etc)

(Continued)

Endoscopic Retrograde Cholangiopancreatography *(Continued)*

- evaluation of the nonjaundiced patient with suspected biliary tract disease, either intrahepatic or extrahepatic
- evaluation of the patient with signs or symptoms compatible with pancreatic cancer, when prior imaging studies (CT scan or ultrasound) are normal or equivocal
- evaluation of recurrent pancreatitis of unknown etiology
- diagnosis of pancreatic pseudocyst suspected on clinical grounds, when CT scan and/or ultrasound are normal or equivocal
- preoperative evaluation of a known pancreatic pseudocyst, known chronic pancreatitis, or pancreatic trauma prior to surgical repair or endoscopic therapy

ERCP may also be useful in:

- manometric study of the sphincter of Oddi (see separate entry)
- follow-up evaluation of endoscopic sphincterotomy or other relatively high-risk therapeutic procedures
- follow-up evaluation of nondiagnostic PTC studies
- situations where PTC is contraindicated (eg, severe coagulopathy)

ERCP is less useful in the following situations:[2]

- suspected gallbladder disease without evidence of bile duct abnormalities
- pancreatic cancer diagnosed clearly by CT scan

Therapeutic application of ERCP includes:

- endoscopic papillotomy for retained common duct stones, usually <1 cm diameter, to facilitate passage into the duodenum
- endoscopic sphincterotomy (using a sphincterotome) for retained common duct stones in the following situations: patients who have had their gallbladder removed (procedure of choice), patients who are poor surgical candidates and gallbladder is present; less commonly, endoscopic sphincterotomy may be indicated for papillary stenosis or the "sump syndrome"
- endoscopic extraction of retained stones from biliary or pancreatic ducts using a basket, snare, etc
- endoscopic placement of plastic stents or nasobiliary drainage tubes across biliary strictures
- balloon dilatations of biliary strictures
- laser ablation or fulguration of obstructing tumor

CONTRAINDICATIONS:

- patient refusal or poor cooperation
- recent attack of acute pancreatitis, within the past several weeks; one exception is the patient with known choledocholithiasis who will be undergoing endoscopic sphincterotomy or surgery
- recent myocardial infarction
- inadequate surgical back-up
- history of contrast dye anaphylaxis

Relative contraindications include:

- poor surgical candidacy; in general patients should be able to tolerate laparotomy if complications arise
- pseudocyst, due to an increased risk of infection (this has been debated)
- ascites
- severe cardiopulmonary background disease
- overlying residual barium in the GI tract from recent abdominal CT scan, lower GI series, etc

Patient Care/Scheduling **PATIENT PREPARATION:** Technique and potential complications of the procedure are discussed with the patient. Informed consent is obtained for ERCP, including likely therapeutic interventions. Formal consultation with gastroenterology staff is required prior to approval and scheduling. Patient is informed whether overnight hospitalization is necessary (most cases) or whether "same day" outpatient ERCP is feasible. On the day prior to the procedure, inpatient candidates are routinely seen by the endoscopist (or his representative) to briefly examine the patient, review details of the case, write orders, and answer remaining patient questions. Patient is made NPO after midnight (or at least 8 hours prior to study). Daily oral medications are permitted on the morning of ERCP with physician approval. Exceptions include antacids and Carafate® which may interfere with visualization of the mucosa. Aspirin products and nonsteroidal agents must be discontinued well in advance (at least 5 days for aspirin), especially if biopsy or sphincterotomy/papillotomy is anticipated. For hospital inpatients, dentures are removed and patient is transported to endoscopy suite on cart, accompanied by medical chart and relevant x-rays. For outpatients, procedure is the same except that transportation home must be arranged in advance if a "same day" procedure (driving not permitted due to sedative effects). Once patient is in the procedure room, baseline vital signs are recorded and an intravenous line started. Antibiotic prophylaxis may be given at this time (see Special Instructions). Premedications are routinely given including parenteral meperidine, diazepam, and often atropine (0.4 mg). A topical anesthetic agent such as Cetacaine® spray is applied to the pharynx. **AFTERCARE:** The patient is placed at strict bedrest and observed carefully in the recovery area. Vital signs are monitored frequently and physician contacted if any complications arise. If the patient has tolerated the procedure well, he may be discharged from the testing area once sedatives have worn off. NPO until gag reflux has returned, then clear liquids for 24 hours. Any patient undergoing a therapeutic procedure should be observed overnight in the hospital. If a "same day" outpatient procedure (not allowed in all institutions), patient must have ready access to the hospital emergency room should complications develop. **SPECIAL INSTRUCTIONS:** Prior to ERCP, if bile duct obstruction is suspected, antibiotic coverage is usually indicated. If high grade bile duct or pancreatic duct obstruction is confirmed during ERCP, antibiotics should be continued (or begun). Individuals at risk for infective endocarditis are often given antibiotic prophylaxis prior to ERCP, particularly if a therapeutic maneuver such as sphincterotomy is planned. High risk cardiac lesions include rheumatic valvular disease, prosthetic valves, and prior endocarditis. However, ERCP is considered a relatively low risk procedure for the development of endocarditis, in comparison with invasive dental procedures and genitourinary tract instrumentation. Some authorities feel that prophylactic antibiotics are not warranted. A controlled clinical trial to answer this question is unlikely and liberal use of prophylactic antibiotics will probably continue. **COMPLICATIONS:** In the hands of a skilled endoscopist, diagnostic ERCP is associated with a 3% incidence of morbidity and 0.2% mortality, based on nationwide statistics.[3] Complication rate is considerably higher with an inexperienced endoscopist. If endoscopic sphincterotomy or papillotomy is performed, overall morbidity rate increases to 8% and mortality 1% to 1.5%. Emergent surgical repair is necessary in 2%; it should be noted that these figures are superior to those documented for elective surgical exploration of the common bile duct.

Complications of ERCP may be classified as follows,

- Painless hyperamylasemia: May occur in ≤75% of cases with sometimes striking elevations of serum and urine amylase levels. This is **not** accompanied by abdominal pain, nausea, or other stigmata of pancreatitis and is clinically inconsequential. Within 4 days, amylase decreases to normal without treatment.
- Acute pancreatitis: Develops in 0.7% to 7.4% of cases and represents a small fraction of patients with elevated amylase levels. Pathogenesis is unclear. Implicated factors include the type of contrast used, the rate and volume of injection, the underlying condition of the pancreas, and the experience of the endoscopist. Management is the same as for gallstone or alcoholic pancreatitis.
- Sepsis: A rare complication but associated with a high mortality. The incidence of bacteremia has been variously estimated at 0% to 14%. Both cholangitis (incidence of 0.65% to 0.8%) and pancreatic sepsis (0.3% incidence) have been reported. The former is almost exclusively associated with ductal obstruction. Biliary stasis predisposes patients to infection of bile fluid, and gram-negative bacteria probably remain dormant behind the obstruction until ERCP. Pancreatic sepsis appears more likely if a pseudocyst is present. Injection of nonsterile contrast into the pseudocyst may lead to abscess if drainage is sluggish. Some authorities consider the presence of pseudocyst a contraindication to ERCP but others feel the statistical risk is unproven.
- Complications of upper endoscopy: Nonspecific complications common with upper gastrointestinal endoscopy (EGD) (see entry) including esophageal perfo-

(Continued)

Endoscopic Retrograde Cholangiopancreatography *(Continued)*

ration, hypoxia, adverse drug reactions, arrhythmias. Drug toxicity may play a more significant role with ERCP due to lengthier procedure time requiring multiple drug administrations.

- Instrumental injury: Uncommon with diagnostic ERCP alone unless anatomy is surgically distorted. Common therapeutic injuries are hemorrhage, laceration, and perforation.

Method EQUIPMENT: The duodenoscope used for ERCP is similar to the fiberoptic endoscope used for EGD with several modifications. The viewing lens and light window at the instrument tip are arranged for side viewing. Within the duodenoscope is a channel which can accommodate a polyethylene contrast-filled catheter, which can be advanced past the tip of the instrument; this separate catheter is used for cannulating the papilla of vater. Other devices may be passed through the endoscope including biopsy forceps, electrocautery devices, sphincterotome, cytology brush, etc. A teaching head may be used for additional viewing or the endoscopic images may be videotaped on a television monitor. TECHNIQUE: ERCP is performed with the patient on an x-ray table with radiologic equipment and fluoroscopy at hand. Following premedication the patient is placed in the left lateral decubitus position. The duodenoscope is passed by mouth through the anesthetized pharynx, and into the esophagus, stomach, and duodenum. A rapid visual examination of these segments may be made. Once the instrument has reached the second (descending) portion of the duodenum, the ampulla of vater is located, often on the medial wall. The periampullary region is carefully inspected. Often glucagon is given (0.2 mL doses) to decrease duodenal motility and facilitate visualization. The inner catheter (containing contrast dye) is then advanced from the lateral port of the endoscope and guided into the orifice. Once the ampulla has been engaged, the catheter is advanced several millimeters into the duct and a small volume of contrast injected. The dye filling pattern is observed under fluoroscopy ("the test shot") to determine orientation. In this manner the pancreatic duct and the bile duct may be selectively cannulated and imaged separately with contrast. Fluoroscopy is used as needed to assure proper catheter orientation. Formal spot radiographs are taken of contrast-filled ducts for the permanent record. At times x-ray table adjustments and patient repositioning may be necessary particularly if the gallbladder is imaged. Delayed films are also obtained following removal of the duodenoscope since contrast material normally remains in the ductal system for minutes. In addition, suspicious periampullary or ductal lesions may be biopsied and cytologic brush samples obtained. "Blind" biopsies of the ducts and/or pancreas may be taken at physician discretion. A variety of therapeutic procedures, mentioned earlier, may be performed.

Specimen Biopsy specimens and cytologic brushings are placed in appropriate containers and fixatives and sent to pathology laboratory without delay. Tissue for Gram stain and culture is placed in a sterile jar without fixative and hand carried to the Microbiology Laboratory. Details of specimen collection, fixative, and transportation are handled by the gastroenterology team. TURNAROUND TIME: Final report on biopsy and cytology specimen histology is given within 2-3 days (or longer in some cases).

Interpretation NORMAL FINDINGS: Preliminary written report on endoscopic and radiologic findings immediately completed by gastroenterology staff. Final typewritten report is added to the chart in several days. A "normal cholangiogram" implies a normal radiographic appearance of the following structures: common bile duct (CBD), common hepatic duct, left and right hepatic duct (and subdivisions), cystic duct, and gallbladder. Maximum diameter of the normal CBD is approximately 9 mm (range 4-9 mm) providing the gallbladder is present. If the patient has had prior cholecystectomy, diameters may be somewhat increased. The CBD normally will have a tapered appearance at its distal end, the so-called "vaterian segment" where it is surrounded by the papilla and sphincter of Oddi. A "normal pancreatogram" implies a smooth, patent main pancreatic duct which gradually tapers from the body (diameter 3.4 mm) to the tail (1.7 mm). With optimal filling of the pancreatic duct, approximately 15-30 secondary branches will be outlined with contrast. These are straight in appearance and of fine caliber. There is variability in the anatomy of the pancreatic ducts. For example, the duct of Santorini is present in 80% of normal individuals and its communication with the duodenum or main pancreatic duct is variable. CRITICAL VALUES: In formulating the diagnostic impression, information is obtained from three sources: direct visual examination, radiologic imaging, and biopsy specimens. Endoscopic examination of the papilla of vater may reveal a mucosal mass if carcinoma of the pancreatic head is present. Other malignancies may involve this region including ampullary carcinoma, cholangiocarcinoma, and rarely duodenal cancers. The endoscopic appearance of the papilla may be highly suggestive in other disease states, such as papilla "bulging" (possible impacted stone), edema, erythema, and patency (recently passed stone), visible purulent drainage (suppurative cholangitis), bright red blood through the orifice (hemobilia). Radiologic abnormalities in the cholangiogram may be specific and diagnostic. Certainly, retained stones in the common bile duct are easily recognized by discrete filling defects. Other deviations include biliary strictures, irregular filling defects or mass lesions beyond endoscopic visualization (carcinoma), ductal dilatation (obstruction of any cause), irregular intrahepatic ducts with strictures and ectasia (sclerosing cholangitis), cystic duct narrowing with cholelithiasis (acute cholecystitis). The pancreatogram may reveal congenital abnormalities (such as pancreas divisum), small pancreatic pseudocysts (not seen on CT scan), and pancreatic duct calculi. The radiologic appearance of carcinoma of the pancreas includes:

- single, irregular abrupt stricture of the pancreatic duct (probably the best criteria[4])
- gradual occlusion of the main duct
- alterations in the side branches near the tumor such as fragmentation and cystic destruction
- displacement of Wirsung's duct
- pooled contrast material in an irregular manner (within necrotic tumor)
- strictured CBD and pancreatic duct ("double duct" sign)

The radiologic appearance of chronic pancreatitis may closely resemble pancreatic cancer. However, the main pancreatic duct in chronic pancreatitis is classically irregular, tortuous, and with **multiple** stenoses – the "chain of lakes" appearance. Single smooth stenosis is also more consistent with chronic pancreatitis.[4] The yield of biopsy in pancreatic cancer is >90% in most large series. Nearly all pancreatic malignancies are ductal carcinomas; thus even small lesions are likely to cause stenosis or occlusion of the main pancreatic duct. In cases where tumor invades the pancreatic duct region or ampulla without entering the lumen, cytology specimens of pancreatic juice may be diagnostic.

LIMITATIONS: ERCP is relatively expensive and hazardous in comparison with other endoscopic procedures. Results are highly operator dependent, as demonstrated in large series. For both physician and patient there may be nontrivial radiation exposure if fluoroscopy time is prolonged. This procedure is technically difficult, particularly in patients who have had a Billroth II gastrectomy and gastrojejunostomy.

Footnotes

1. American Society for Gastrointestinal Endoscopy, Utilization Committee, *Appropriate Use of Gastrointestinal Endoscopy*, Manchester, MA: American Society for Gastrointestinal Endoscopy, 1986.
2. Vennes JA, "Gastrointestinal Endoscopy," *Cecil Textbook of Medicine*, 18th ed, Chapter 96, Wyngaarden JB and Smith LH, eds, Philadelphia, PA: WB Saunders Co, 1988, 668-74.
3. Shahmir M and Schuman BM, "Complications of Fiberoptic Endoscopy," *Gastrointest Endosc*, 1980, 26:86-91.
4. Cello JP, "Carcinoma of the Pancreas," *Gastrointestinal Disease: Pathophysiology, Diagnosis, Management*, 4th ed, Chapter 99, Sleisenger MH and Fordtran JS, eds, Philadelphia, PA: WB Saunders Co, 1989, 1872-80.

References

Bilbao MK, Dotter CT, Lee TG, et al, "Complications of ERCP: A Study of 10,000 Cases," *Gastroenterology*, 1976, 70:314-20.

Dutta SK, Cox M, Williams RB, et al, "Prospective Evaluation of the Risk of Bacteremia and the Role of Antibiotics in ERCP," *J Clin Gastroenterol*, 1983, 5:325-9.

Geenen JE and Venu RP, "Endoscopic Retrograde Cholangiopancreatography," *Bockus Gastroenterology*, 4th ed, Chapter 44, Berk JE, ed, Philadelphia, PA: WB Saunders Co, 1985, 601-11.

Sivak MV and Sullivan BH, "Endoscopic Retrograde Pancreatography: Analysis of the Normal Pancreatogram," *Am J Dig Dis*, 1976, 21:263-9.

Stewart ET, Vennes JA, and Geenen JE, *Atlas of Endoscopic Retrograde Cholangiopancreatography*, St Louis, MO: CV Mosby Co, 1977.

(Continued)

Endoscopic Retrograde Cholangiopancreatography *(Continued)*

Venu RP, Geenen JE, Toouli J, et al, "Endoscopic Retrograde Cholangiopancreatography Diagnosis of Cholelithiasis in Patients With Normal Gallbladder X-ray and Ultrasound Studies," *JAMA*, 1983, 249:758-61.

Endoscopic Retrograde Cholangiopancreatography (ERCP) With Pressure Measurement of Sphincter of Oddi *see* Sphincter of Oddi Manometry *on page 122*

ERCP *see* Endoscopic Retrograde Cholangiopancreatography *on page 91*

Esophageal Bougienage *see* Esophageal Dilation *on this page*

Esophageal Dilation

CPT 43220 (direct dilation under endoscopic guidance); 43450 (dilation of esophagus by unguided sound or bougie); 43455 (dilation under fluoroscopic guidance)

Related Information

Upper Gastrointestinal Endoscopy *on page 126*

Synonyms Bag Dilation of Esophagus; Esophageal Bougienage; Mechanical Dilation of the Esophagus; Peroral Esophageal Dilation; Pneumatic Esophageal Dilation

Abstract **PROCEDURE COMMONLY INCLUDES:** Forceful dilation of a pathologically narrowed esophagus in a patient with symptomatic dysphagia. Esophageal dilation is a therapeutic procedure performed only after a diagnosis has been clearly established. The procedure may be performed using a variety of instruments, the choice of which depends on the nature and sensitivity of the narrowing. One common method, called bougienage, is carried out by passing flexible, cylindrical dilators (bougies) of increasing diameter into the esophagus and across the area of constriction. Bougienage is safely performed in an endoscopy suite with the patient awake but mildly sedated. More forceful esophageal dilation may be accomplished using pneumatic or hydrostatic dilators. This latter technique has a higher complication rate and is performed in an endoscopy suite or an operating room. In general, esophageal dilation can be done in an unguided ("blind") fashion, under fluoroscopic guidance, or under direct visualization with an endoscope. Although this procedure is invasive by nature it is considered a medical (nonsurgical) approach. **INDICATIONS:** Esophageal dilation may be useful in the following disease states:

- benign esophageal strictures (usually arising from severe gastroesophageal reflux, caustic ingestions, radiation therapy to the thorax, etc)
- esophageal cancer; procedure is performed for palliation of dysphagia in advanced cases
- achalasia (a motor disorder of the esophagus); patients are considered candidates for forceful dilation only after medical therapy has failed (ie, failure of nitrates and calcium channel blockers)
- esophageal webs or rings

CONTRAINDICATIONS: Absolute contraindications include:

- severe bleeding diathesis
- active upper gastrointestinal bleeding
- agitated or uncooperative patient
- recent myocardial infarction
- active esophageal infection

Relative contraindications include:

- dilated, tortuous esophagus
- hiatal hernia
- previous myotomy
- variant achalasis

Patient Care/Scheduling **PATIENT PREPARATION:** The risks and benefits of the procedure are explained to the patient and informed consent is obtained. The procedure is performed by a gastroenterology specialist and the details of scheduling are usually handled by the operating team. The patient is made NPO (nothing by mouth) after midnight on the evening prior to the procedure. Small amounts of sedation may be used with bougienage, such as meperidine or a benzodiazepine; however, an awake and cooperative patient is preferred. Antibiotic prophylaxis for endocarditis may be considered in patients with high-risk cardiac lesions (see Special Instructions). **AFTERCARE:** Vital signs are monitored frequently postprocedure, usually every hour for at least 4 hours. The patient is made NPO for 4-6 hours after dilation. Following this, liquids may be attempted. The patient is observed for development of fever, pleuritic chest pain, hematemesis, and subcutaneous emphysema. In some hospitals, patients are routinely observed overnight. However, there is a trend towards "short-stay" units where patients are monitored for several hours and discharged to home if stable. Some physicians routinely prescribe an H_2-blocker (eg, ranitidine, cimetidine) or antacid after dilation due to the incidence of gastroesophageal reflux complicating the procedure. **SPECIAL INSTRUCTIONS:** Due to the small risk of bacteremia during esophageal dilation,[1] antibiotics may be useful for the prevention of bacterial endocarditis in patients with high-risk heart lesions. Patients who are at increased risk for endocarditis include those with prosthetic heart valves, rheumatic valvular disease, previous history of endocarditis, and others. Antibiotic prophylaxis is **not** recommended on a routine basis for patients without such heart lesions, according to the American Heart Association in 1990.[2] **COMPLICATIONS:**

- severe substernal pain
- esophageal perforation; the rate depends in part on the type of instrument used (simple bougies 0.04% to 0.40%, metal olives 0.4% to 0.6%, pneumatic dilators 1.0% to 1.3%)
- hemorrhage; small amounts of bleeding are common but clinically significant bleeding is rare
- aspiration
- esophageal reflux of gastric contents
- fever, sepsis, and mediastinitis are possible but unusual

Method **EQUIPMENT:** A number of different dilating instruments are available. Cylindrical instruments called bougies, may be mercury-filled tubes (Maloney, Hurst bougies) or woven silk. Another popular instrument is the "metal olive," a device often used in conjunction with a guide wire or swallowed string. Pneumatic (bag) dilators are used for more forceful dilation. These instruments apply force at right angles to the stricture and avoid the shear forces associated with bougienage. **TECHNIQUE:** Bougienage: With the patient in a sitting position, the rubber dilator is passed through the oropharynx with the patient swallowing. It is advanced gently across the stricture and the tip is passed into the stomach. The bougie is left in place several minutes. Fluoroscopy may be used during this procedure. The bougie is removed and the process is repeated using larger diameter instruments. The goal in most cases is a luminal diameter of 16-17 mm which allows passage of solid food. Bougienage is effective for benign and malignant esophageal strictures and some esophageal webs. It may be attempted in achalasia also but tends to be temporary (ie, for several days only) and pneumatic dilation may be indicated.

Forceful dilation: The patient is positioned on the fluorotable and the pneumatic dilator passed so that it lies across the lower esophageal sphincter (for achalasia), or the area of constriction (for benign esophageal strictures). Proper positioning is important and fluoroscopy is commonly employed to confirm this. The bag is inflated enough to open the constriction (usually 12 psi for achalasia) and held inflated for 30-60 seconds. Various techniques are available for ensuring that the stricture is obliterated. The goal of pneumatic dilation in achalasia is to produce a tear in the lower esophageal sphincter. The goal in the treatment of benign strictures is to increase the luminal size to about 16 mm.

Interpretation **NORMAL FINDINGS:** Esophageal dilation is a therapeutic procedure. When performed with upper endoscopy, there will be diagnostic information as well (see Upper Gastrointestinal Endoscopy). **LIMITATIONS:**

- failure rate may be high in achalasia, particularly for bougienage (2% to 30% failure rate in 1-20 years)
- pneumatic dilation for achalasia may be unsuccessful
- esophageal spasm may respond poorly to bougienage
- complications may be severe

ADDITIONAL INFORMATION: Bougienage is performed effectively in most patients with benign esophageal strictures. It is also useful in palliation of patients with obstructing esophageal

(Continued)

Esophageal Dilation *(Continued)*

tumors. The role of bougienage and pneumatic dilation in cases of esophageal spasm, achalasia, and refractory strictures is less clear. After failures for achalasia, a short Heller myotomy with an antireflux procedure may be attempted. A full Heller myotomy may be necessary in patients with difficult esophageal spasm. In many instances, the exact role of surgery versus conservative medical management (ie, repeated bougienage) is still controversial.

Footnotes

1. Welsh JD, Griffiths WJ, McKee J, et al, "Bacteremia Associated With Esophageal Dilation," *J Clin Gastroenterol*, 1983, 5(2):109-12.
2. Dajani AS, Bisno AL, and Chung KJ, "Prevention of Bacterial Endocarditis: Recommendations by the American Heart Association," *JAMA*, 1990, 264(22):2919-22.

Esophageal Manometric Study *see* Esophageal Motility Study *on this page*

Esophageal Manometry *see* Esophageal Motility Study *on this page*

Esophageal Motility Study

CPT 91010; 91011 (with mecholyl or similar stimulant); 91012 (with acid perfusion studies); 91020 (esophagogastric manometric studies)

Related Information

Bernstein Test *on page 81*
Standard Acid Reflux Test *on page 124*

Synonyms Esophageal Manometric Study; Esophageal Manometry

Abstract **PROCEDURE COMMONLY INCLUDES:** Passage of a multilumen manometry catheter into the esophagus and stomach. This device is connected to at least three separate pressure transducers and is capable of sensing squeeze pressures at different sites within the esophageal lumen. Quantitative data is obtained regarding the amplitude (mm Hg) and duration (seconds) of contractions of the upper esophageal sphincter (UES), lower esophageal sphincter (LES), and several sites within the esophageal body. A number of distinct esophageal motility disorders may be diagnosed. Provocative agents may also be employed to induce manometric abnormalities in patients with chest pain of obscure etiology. This procedure has become widely used and is considered the standard of diagnosis for most motor diseases of the esophagus. **INDICATIONS:** To evaluate the patient with suspected primary esophageal motor dysfunction. This includes (but is not limited to) the following:

- primary achalasia
- diffuse esophageal spasm
- chronic idiopathic intestinal pseudo-obstruction (manometry may aid in the initial diagnosis of this entity)
- nutcracker esophagus
- idiopathic LES incompetence

To evaluate the patient with suspected secondary esophageal motility disorder due to systemic disease, including:

- scleroderma
- polydermatomyositis
- systemic lupus erythematosus
- amyloidosis
- Chagas' disease
- primary skeletal muscle disease (eg, myotonia dystrophica)
- multiple sclerosis, amyotrophic lateral sclerosis

To evaluate the patient with chest pain of unclear etiology, in order to determine whether symptoms are of an esophageal origin. This usually follows a negative cardiac work-up. To assess the competence of the LES, in difficult cases of reflux esophagitis, where the diagnosis is still in doubt or where standard medical therapy has failed. To evaluate the success of various surgical procedures on the esophagus, such as esophageal dilatation, LES myotomy in achalasia, and antireflux surgery. To ensure proper placement of pH probes (used to diagnose acid reflux) by accurately locating the LES.

CONTRAINDICATIONS: Few contraindications exist for this procedure. In general, the patient should be alert, able to swallow on command, and capable of verbalizing symptoms. This is particularly true if provocative studies to elicit chest pain are planned. Manometry should not be performed on a patient with tenuous cardiopulmonary status in whom vagal stimulation is hazardous.

Patient Care/Scheduling **PATIENT PREPARATION:** Technique and goals of the procedure are discussed with the patient and informed consent is obtained. No antacids, nitrates, calcium channel blockers, pain medications, or anticholinergic agents are permitted for 24 hours prior to procedure (if possible). If study is scheduled for the AM, the patient is made NPO after midnight. NPO for 8 hours beforehand if scheduled for PM. Patient is sent to procedure room with medical record. No premedications are given prior to manometry and sedatives are not permitted. **AFTERCARE:** There are no specific restrictions postprocedure. The previous level of activity may be resumed if no complications have arisen. **SPECIAL INSTRUCTIONS:** Requisition from ordering physician should state if additional studies such as pH probe testing, acid perfusion (Bernstein) testing, or pharmacologic provocation are desired. Otherwise, decision will be left to the discretion of the operator. **COMPLICATIONS:** Esophageal manometry is considered a safe procedure with little morbidity. Potential complications are those common to any nasogastric (NG) intubation, such as gagging, epistaxis, vasovagal reactions, etc. More serious adverse reactions may result from medications given for provocative testing. In particular, ergonovine is used in some centers to provoke esophageal contraction and spasm. This agent is also used to induce coronary artery spasm during cardiac catheterization in patients with possible variant (Prinz metal's) angina. Thus, there are potential cardiac complications if ergonovine is used. Other agents have come into favor recently, such as edrophonium, which have little cardiac effects. Abdominal cramps and nausea of a transient nature have been reported with edrophonium.

Method **EQUIPMENT:** The manometry probe is a polyvinyl catheter with multiple lumens (from 3-8). Each lumen has a separate orifice. Probe diameter ranges from 1.1-5 mm, depending on the model. There are usually three or more side holes spaced approximately 5 cm apart which act as pressure sensors. Each catheter lumen is independently perfused with water from a multichannel pneumohydraulic infusion device (with low compliances). A separate pressure transducer is also attached to each lumen and pressures are recorded on a multichannel polygraph. A swallowing sensor is also used in some centers. **TECHNIQUE:** The procedure is performed in a fully-equipped GI Laboratory. Patient assumes a supine position and a swallowing sensor is placed around patient's neck. The catheter assembly is calibrated and pressures rechecked with a sphygmomanometer. The device is introduced via the nares using standard nasogastric intubation technique (alternatively, per mouth) and advanced until all sensing orifices are recording gastric (cardia) pressures. The station pull-through technique is commonly used. With the recorder on, the catheter is slowly withdrawn until the proximal channel is within the LES. Resting LES tone is measured first. Patient is given water via a 50 mL syringe and is asked to swallow and the relaxation response of LES is noted. The catheter is then pulled out slowly at 0.5 cm increments until the most distal orifice is sensing the LES (all channels having passed through the LES). The catheter is taped into position and patient performs a series of wet swallows (5 mL H_2O) over several minutes. Information is obtained regarding the LES, peristalsis, and esophageal body contractions. The catheter is then withdrawn approximately 3 cm and retaped, so that all sensing orifices are within the esophageal body. Wet swallows are repeated and contractions recorded. Next, pull-through is continued until the proximal orifice is surrounded by the UES; perfusion is stopped in this channel to prevent aspiration. Catheter is withdrawn until the proximal orifice is within the pharynx, the middle is in the UES, and the distal in the upper esophageal body. Ten dry swallows are performed. This concludes the standard procedure. When indicated, provocative testing is carried out once standard manometry is completed. The catheter is repositioned and edrophonium is injected (10 mg I.V. usually) or a placebo. Again, patient performs wet swallows and esophageal contractions are recorded at different catheter positions. Subjective complaints of chest pain are carefully recorded and correlated temporally with any new manometric findings. The acid perfusion (Bernstein) test may also be performed at this time.

Interpretation **NORMAL FINDINGS:** Preliminary written report on manometric findings and provocation testing is completed immediately by gastroenterology staff and placed in medical chart. This includes both selected numerical data and an overall diagnostic interpretation. Normal values are established for each individual testing center, and are depen-

(Continued)

Esophageal Motility Study *(Continued)*

dent to some degree on the equipment system selected. An example of a normal motility and provocation study as reported by one laboratory is shown in the table. **CRITICAL VALUES:** A wide variety of esophageal contraction abnormalities is possible. However, several "classic" patterns of manometric readings have been described, and may be diagnostic for a particular motor disorder. Selected patterns are shown in the following figure. As shown, a normal control subject experiences a short duration wave in the upper esophagus following a wet swallow. (In general, the upper esophagus is composed of striated muscle, and the middle and lower portions contain smooth muscle.) The wave progresses down the esophagus in a characteristic, timed fashion, that is, a peristaltic wave. The LES appropriately relaxes to accommodate the anticipated food bolus. In achalasia, however, the initial striated muscle contraction following a swallow may be normal but smooth muscle contractions (mid and lower esophagus) are of low amplitude and prolonged duration. Characteristically, the LES maintains a high

Esophageal Manometry	
1. Catheter (lumen)	4
2. LES	
Location (cm from nares)	38
Resting pressure (mm Hg)	27
Mean pressure (mm Hg)	15
Relaxation	Complete
3. Esophageal body	
Peristalsis	Normal
Amplitude, mean (mm Hg)	124
Amplitude, peak (mm Hg)	224
Duration, mean (sec)	3.5
Duration, max (sec)	5
4. UES	
Location (cm from nares)	16
Resting pressure (mm Hg)	33
Relaxation	Normal
Coordination with hypopharynx	Normal
Diagnosis: normal motility study	
Edrophonium provocation (1 mg IU)	No chest pain
Bernstein test	Negative

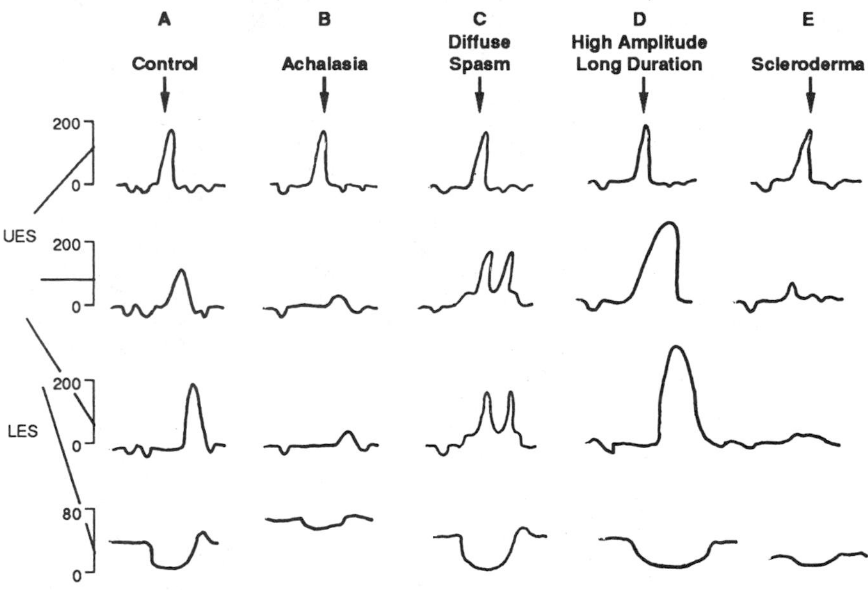

basal pressure and fails to relax after a swallow. In a condition known as diffuse esophageal spasm, there is an increase in the baseline pressure in the mid and lower esophagus after a swallow. In addition to this, multiple repetitive high amplitude (short duration) contractions are seen in smooth muscle. These are "aperistaltic" contractions, ie, not coordinated with the initial skeletal muscle contraction. LES pressures may be normal or high and relaxation is variable. The "nutcracker esophagus" is characterized by smooth muscle contractions of very high amplitude and long duration. Peristalsis is maintained, although propagation may be slowed. LES tone and relaxation are relatively normal. In scleroderma, a unique pattern is seen. Upper esophageal contraction is normal but all smooth muscle contractions are markedly diminished in amplitude or even absent. Unlike achalasia, the

LES pressure is low. In polymyositis (not shown) there is potential involvement of any striated muscle, including the pharynx and UES. Decreased amplitude contractions may be seen in the pharynx along with hypotension in the UES, but smooth muscle contractions remain normal. Milder variants of the idealized patterns in the figure may be seen. Also, mixtures of these contraction abnormalities are possible. In patients with chest pain of obscure etiology, esophageal manometry is often considered to rule out an unspecified motor disorder. If a patient experiences typical chest pain symptoms during the course of a standard examination **and** a classic motility disorder is recorded during the same time interval, an esophageal origin of symptoms is likely. Appropriate treatment of the motility disorder should be initiated. However, if typical chest discomfort occurs during standard manometry but pressure tracings are normal, then motility dysfunction is less likely as the cause of symptoms. It is not, however, entirely excluded. Conversely, if manometry is clearly abnormal but the patient denies any chest discomfort, the test is inconclusive. Some clinicians elect to treat the underlying motor disorder empirically. This is based on data which shows that the majority of patients who experience chest pain secondary to an esophageal motor disorder display continuous manometric abnormalities but only intermittent symptoms. In addition, ≤80% of patients with such continuous contraction abnormalities have reported significant chest discomfort. The proper management of this group is still evolving. Various pharmacologic agents have been used to induce abnormal contractions in selected patients with chest pain of obscure origin. This may be attempted in difficult cases where barium enema, upper endoscopy, and standard manometry are nondiagnostic. A cholinergic agonist, edrophonium chloride, is popular because of its specificity and favorable safety profile. If following injection of edrophonium there are symptoms of typical chest pain and manometric abnormalities, the test is considered positive. If either chest pain or contraction abnormalities are induced (but not both), test is inconclusive. Commonly, the acid perfusion test is included as a provocative test (see Bernstein Test). The finding of a hypotensive LES on manometry and a positive Bernstein test is strongly suggestive of symptomatic reflux esophagitis.

References

Benjamin SB, Richter JE, Cordova CM, et al, "Prospective Manometric Evaluation With Pharmacologic Provocation of Patients With Suspected Esophageal Motility Dysfunction," *Gastroenterology*, 1983, 84:893-901.

Clouse RE, "Motor Disorders," *Gastrointestinal Disease: Pathophysiology, Diagnosis, Management*, 4th ed, Chapter 33, Sleisenger MH and Fordtran JS, eds, Philadelphia, PA: WB Saunders Co, 1989, 559-95.

Clouse RE, Stenson WF, and Avioli LV, "Esophageal Motility Disorders and Chest Pain," *Arch Intern Med*, 1985, 145:903-6.

Cohen S, "Motor Disorders of the Esophagus," *N Engl J Med*, 1979, 301:184-92.

Orlando RC, "Esophageal Manometry," *Manual of Gastroenterologic Procedures*, 2nd ed, Chapter 4, Drossman DA, ed, New York, NY: Raven Press, 1987, 30-44.

Pope CE, "Diseases of the Esophagus," *Cecil's Textbook of Medicine*, 18th ed, Chapter 98, Wyngaarden JB and Smith LH, eds, Philadelphia, PA: WB Saunders Co, 1988, 679-89.

Esophagogastroduodenoscopy *see* Upper Gastrointestinal Endoscopy *on page 126*

Esophagogastroduodenoscopy (EGD) *see* Endoscopic Retrograde Cholangiopancreatography *on page 91*

Esophagoscopy (if Esophagus Alone Studied) *see* Upper Gastrointestinal Endoscopy *on page 126*

Esophagus Acid Reflux Test With Intraluminal pH Electrode for Detection of Reflux *see* Standard Acid Reflux Test *on page 124*

Esophagus Acid Reflux Test With Intraluminal pH Electrode (Prolonged Recording) *see* pH Study, 12- to 24-Hour *on page 117*

Flexible Fiberoptic Sigmoidoscopy

CPT 45330 (diagnostic); 45331 (biopsy)

Related Information

Anoscopy *on page 80*
Colonoscopy *on page 87*

Synonyms Flexible Proctosigmoidoscopy; Sigmoidoscopy, Flexible

Abstract PROCEDURE COMMONLY INCLUDES: Direct examination of the rectum, sigmoid colon, and proximal portions of the colon (≤60 cm) by means of a flexible fiberoptic endoscope. Flexible sigmoidoscopy is readily performed in a physician's office with minimal bowel preparation. In comparison with other endoscopic procedures, flexible sigmoidoscopy allows visualization of more proximal colonic segments than either anoscopy or rigid proctosigmoidoscopy, but is more limited than colonoscopy. INDICATIONS: Although the precise indications are still being debated, common uses include:

- screening of healthy, asymptomatic adults for colorectal cancer[1]
- evaluation of the patient with suspected lower gastrointestinal pathology in combination with a barium enema study (by itself, the barium radiographs may be insensitive in the distal colon)
- management of lower gastrointestinal bleeding; in selected patients this procedure can detect bleeding polyps, fissures, etc
- evaluation of the patient with suspected inflammatory disease of the colon, such as inflammatory bowel disease, infectious colitis, sigmoid diverticulitis, and others

More controversial indications include:

- temporary decompression of sigmoid volvulus (recurrence of the volvulus is common without prompt surgery)
- cancer surveillance in patients who have undergone surgical resection of a sigmoid colon neoplasia (to rule out recurrence at the anastomosis)

CONTRAINDICATIONS: Few absolute contraindications exist for this procedure. However, the procedure should best be avoided in the following high-risk situations:

- severe diverticulitis
- acute peritonitis
- toxic megacolon
- severe underlying cardiac or pulmonary disease
- uncorrectable coagulopathy
- acute intestinal perforation
- massive GI bleeding

In addition, flexible sigmoidoscopy should not be performed in situations where colonoscopy is indicated (see Colonoscopy). This includes polypectomy which should be performed by colonoscopy.

Patient Care/Scheduling PATIENT PREPARATION: Details of the procedure are discussed with the patient, including goals, technique, and risks. Informed consent is obtained. A number of preparative bowel regimens have been proposed. One popular and effective regimen is administration of a single phosphosoda (Fleet®) enema several minutes before sigmoidoscopy. This results in an adequate bowel prep in nearly 90% of patients. Other bowel regimens are: two phosphosoda enemas immediately prior to procedure, and oral laxative followed by a single enema. These alternative regimens are also effective. In the majority of cases, premedications such as sedatives, narcotics, or anesthetics are not necessary. (An occasional patient may benefit from a short-acting benzodiazepine.) AFTERCARE: In general, patients may resume their prior level of activity after sigmoidoscopy. Since sedatives are not administered in most cases, patients may drive home postprocedure. SPECIAL INSTRUCTIONS: Due to the risk of bacteremia during sigmoidoscopy, antibiotics may be useful for prevention of bacterial endocarditis in patients with high-risk heart disease. Patients who are at risk for endocarditis include those with prosthetic heart valves, rheumatic valvular disease, previous history of endocarditis, and others. Such patients may benefit from antibiotic prophylaxis, although the risk of endocarditis is low. According to the American Heart Association in 1990,[2] antibiotic prophylaxis is **not** recommended on a routine basis for patients without such heart lesions. COMPLICATIONS: Flexible sigmoidoscopy is a safe procedure in skilled hands. Complications that have been reported in the literature include: local pain, bleeding, bacteremia, cardiac arrhythmias, and bowel perforation. The incidence of perforation is quite low, estimated at 0.01% of cases.[3]

Method TECHNIQUE: The patient is placed in the left lateral decubitus position on an examination table. Digital rectal examination is performed first. Some physicians routinely perform anoscopy prior to flexible sigmoidoscopy, since the former allows superior visualization of the rectum and anal canal (see Anoscopy). Following this, the sigmoidoscope is lubricated and gently inserted into the rectum. The instrument is then advanced under direct visualization. The physician can direct the tip of the scope using handheld controls and guide the shaft of the instrument with torque. Only a minimal amount of insufflation of the bowel is necessary (unlike colonoscopy). The flexible sigmoidoscope is advanced to its full length, either 35 or 60 cm depending on the model. Areas of pathology are noted. Invasive procedures can be performed as needed, such as biopsy, fulguration, stool sampling, etc. As the instrument is withdrawn, all areas of the intestinal mucosa are inspected again. The rectum is well visualized during withdrawal by retroflexing the sigmoidoscope tip 180° in the final 10 cm.

Specimen All biopsy specimens and cytologic brushings are sent to the Pathology Laboratory promptly. Any tissue or stool samples for microbiological culture should be sent in sterile containers **without** fixative. TURNAROUND TIME: Final report on biopsy specimens is usually given within 2-3 days. Microbiologic stains, when performed, are often available the same day but bacterial and viral cultures require more time.

Interpretation NORMAL FINDINGS: Preliminary report on sigmoidoscopic findings is immediately completed by the physician and charted. Final report is given in several days. Important aspects of the examination often commented on include:

- indications for procedure
- type of instrument used
- adequacy of bowel prep
- depth of visualization (eg, 35 cm, 60 cm)
- appearance of the mucosa
- abnormalities such as polyps (size, appearance), pseudopolyps, fissures, neoplasms, ulcers, friable regions, blood, pus, diverticula, and others
- therapeutic procedures performed
- sites of biopsies
- sites of cultures
- complications
- recommendations

ADDITIONAL INFORMATION: The flexible sigmoidoscope is now routinely used in the surveillance of neoplasia-polyps in the asymptomatic patient. The procedure is well-tolerated and safe. It is estimated that about 55% of colon cancers and adenomas are within the theoretic reach of the 60 cm instrument. In reality, most but not all such lesions are detected during sigmoidoscopy. The sensitivity of the 60 cm instrument is about 85% (within its 60 cm range). The 35 cm scope is more comfortable and less expensive than its larger counterpart. Of course, the yield of this instrument is somewhat less, with only 40% of malignant or premalignant colonic lesions within its theoretic range. Again, the sensitivity of this device within its range of 35 cm is about 85%. Recommendations on the use of sigmoidoscopy for cancer surveillance have not been agreed upon.[1] The American College of Physicians recommends screening all adults older than 50 years of age at 3- to 5-year intervals. The following groups also agree with this recommendation: American Cancer Society, National Cancer Institute, and American College of Obstetrics and Gynecology. However, the Canadian Task Force on the Periodic Health Examination refrained from making a specific recommendation on routine screening sigmoidoscopy (although it was considered). The U.S. Preventive Services Task Force also made no specific recommendations for this procedure in adults older than 40 years of age, but felt that sigmoidoscopy should be excluded from routine preventive care in healthy adults from 18-39 years of age. Thus, there is a certain amount of discretion involved on the part of individual physicians regarding the utilization of this procedure.

Footnotes

1. Hayward RSA, Steinberg EP, Ford DE, et al, "Preventive Care Guidelines 1991," *Ann Intern Med*, 1991, 114(9):758-83.

(Continued)

Flexible Fiberoptic Sigmoidoscopy *(Continued)*

2. Dajani AS, Bisno AL, and Chung KJ, "Prevention of Bacterial Endocarditis: Recommendations by the American Heart Association," *JAMA*, 1990, 264(22):2919-22.
3. Traul DG, Davis CB, Pollock JC, et al, "Flexible Fiberoptic Sigmoidoscopy. The Monroe Clinic Experience. A Prospective Study of 5000 Examinations," *Dis Colon Rectum*, 1983, 26:161.

References

American Society for Gastrointestinal Endoscopy, "Appropriate Use of Gastrointestinal Endoscopy," Manchester, MA: American Society for Gastrointestinal Endoscopy, 1986.
Hocutt JE, Jaffe R, Owens GM, et al, "Flexible Fiberoptic Sigmoidoscopy," *Am Fam Physician*, 1982, 26:133-41.
Manier JW, "Flexible Sigmoidoscopy," *Gastroenterologic Endoscopy*, MV Sivak, ed, Chapter 49, Philadelphia, PA: WB Saunders Co, 1987, 975-91.

Flexible Proctosigmoidoscopy *see* Flexible Fiberoptic Sigmoidoscopy *on page 102*

Full Colonoscopy *see* Colonoscopy *on page 87*

Gallbladder Stimulation *see* Biliary Drainage *on page 83*

Gastric Acid Titration *see* Hollander Test *on next page*

Gastric Intubation *see* Hollander Test *on next page*

Gastric Saline Load Test

CPT 91060

Synonyms Saline Load Test for Gastric Emptying

Abstract PROCEDURE COMMONLY INCLUDES: The infusion of 750 mL saline into the stomach by means of a nasogastric (NG) tube which is followed by aspiration of the stomach contents 30 minutes later. Returned volumes ≥400 mL are suggestive of impaired gastric emptying.

INDICATIONS:

- objectively demonstrate delayed gastric emptying including suspected gastric outlet obstruction
- follow the clinical course of patients with known gastric outlet obstruction in order to assess effectiveness of treatment and possibly predict the need for surgical intervention
- follow the course of patients with acute or chronic gastric retention due to gastric motor dysfunction (eg, diabetic gastroparesis)

CONTRAINDICATIONS:

- any condition that prohibits standard nasogastric intubation – nasal obstruction, facial trauma, basilar skull fracture, etc
- active upper GI bleeding
- uncooperative, agitated patient
- severe "free" gastroesophageal reflux usually from an incompetent lower esophageal sphincter
- poorly compensated congestive heart failure in which absorption of infused saline would cause clinical deterioration.

Patient Care/Scheduling PATIENT PREPARATION: Technique and risks of the procedure are explained and consent is obtained. Patient should be NPO for at least 4 hours prior to testing; in formal studies involving the saline load test an overnight fast is often required. Requisition should include a list of current medications, particularly those known to inhibit gastric motility (narcotics, tricyclic antidepressants, anticholinergics, levodopa). AFTERCARE: If no complications have occurred, patient may be dismissed from GI procedure room. No specific postprocedure restrictions are necessary and activity status should be determined by primary physician, based in part on test results. COMPLICATIONS: Complications associated with nasogastric intubation in general (eg, nasal trauma, laryngeal trauma, accidental tracheal intubation, etc); pulmonary aspiration of saline, especially if free GE reflux exists; nausea and vomiting with gastric distention; exacerbation of congestive heart failure due to salt load. The exact incidence of major complications is unknown but probably diminishingly rare. These represent theoretical concerns for the most part and this procedure is considered relatively risk-free.

Method EQUIPMENT: Nasogastric tube (#16 F), 50 mL syringe, basin, lubricant, gloves, 750 mL normal saline (0.9% NaCl solution); I.V. tubing optimal TECHNIQUE: Procedure may be performed by either a GI specialist or generalist. Patient is placed in a sitting position and nasogastric tube inserted approximately 60 cm. If location of NG tube is in doubt, obtain KUB film. Gastric contents are thoroughly aspirated using the 50 mL syringe, and amount recorded. Following this, 750 mL saline is infused via the NG tube, by means of an I.V. setup suspended 120 cm above the stomach (or manually using the 50 mL syringe). The entire 750 mL is dripped in over 3-5 minutes. Various patient positions have been advocated during the saline infusion, including supine, left lateral, and sitting. After 30 minutes gastric contents are again aspirated thoroughly. In order to maximize return, aspirate with patient in several positions – supine, sitting, left and right lateral decubitus. DATA ACQUIRED: Measurement of total gastric aspirate volume (in milliliters).

Interpretation NORMAL FINDINGS: Volume of gastric residue <300 mL. In Goldstein's original description of this procedure the average gastric residue in normal controls following saline loading was 60 mL.[1] However, normal values were as high as 385 mL, although this was distinctly unusual, and 63 of 69 controls were <200 mL. CRITICAL VALUES: Volume of gastric residue >400 mL. In Goldstein's study the average gastric residue in patients with clinical gastric retention was 640 mL, although a few values in the 300-400 range were reported.[1]

Footnotes

1. Goldstein H and Boyle JD, "The Saline Load Test – A Bedside Evaluation of Gastric Retention," *Gastroenterology*, 1965, 49:375-80.

References

Graham DY, "Complications of Peptic Ulcer Disease and Indications for Surgery," *Gastrointestinal Disease: Pathophysiology, Diagnosis, Management*, 4th ed, Chapter 50, Sleisenger MH and Fordtran JS, eds, Philadelphia, PA: WB Saunders Co, 1989, 925.

Meeroff JC, Go VLW, and Phillips SF, "Control of Gastric Emptying by Osmolality of Duodenal Contents in Man," *Gastroenterology*, 1975, 68:1144-51.

Nuzum CT, "The Saline Load Test," *Manual of Gastroenterologic Procedures*, 2nd ed, Chapter 2, Drossman DA, ed, New York, NY: Raven Press, 1987, 18-20.

Pelot D, Dana ER, Berk JE, et al, "Comparative Assessment of Gastric Emptying by the "Barium-Burger" and Saline Load Tests," *Am J Gastroenterol*, 1972, 58:411-6.

Hollander Test

CPT 91052

Applies to Acid pH Measurement; BAO (Basal Acid Output); Gastric Acid Titration; Gastric Intubation; I-PAO (Insulin Induced Peak Acid Output)

Replaces Isolated Basal Acid Output Measurements

Abstract PROCEDURE COMMONLY INCLUDES: Intubation of the stomach and suction collection of gastric contents for basal acid output determination. This is followed by insulin injection and scheduled monitoring of blood glucose and potassium, in addition to continued collection of gastric contents. Following collection, gastric contents undergo pH, acid concentration, and volume measurements. INDICATIONS: The test is not a suitable predictor of ulcer recurrence. However, with a positive test, risk of recurrence is increased and recurrence is rare if the response is negative. Hollander tests have been used to assess the completeness of vagotomies, especially the selective rather than truncal varieties. A negative test suggests an effective procedure (see Limitations). CONTRAINDICATIONS: This test is contraindicated in patients with known coronary arterial disease or EKG changes prior to test, elderly patients or those prone to serious arrhythmia. It has been suggested that insulin infusion rather than injection may be a safer way of performing the test (0.05 units/kg/hour).[1]

Patient Care/Scheduling PATIENT PREPARATION: Discontinue all anticholinergics, tranquilizers, and mood elevators 24-48 hours prior to procedure. NPO after midnight. No antacids, cimetidine, Inderal®, alcohol, tobacco, Zantac®. AFTERCARE: Observe for symptoms of sore throat, bleeding perforation (as outlined under upper endoscopy procedures). While

(Continued)

Hollander Test *(Continued)*

the effect of insulin administration should be diminished, the patient must be observed for continued hypoglycemic reaction and fed as soon as possible on return to the nursing unit. **SPECIAL INSTRUCTIONS:** The patient should undergo constant EKG monitoring and an amp of P_{50} should be readily available as patient is prone to hypoglycemia and hypokalemia.

Method **TECHNIQUE:** Gastric contents are measured for volume. pH of contents is measured with a pH meter. Blood glucose and potassium are measured by standard technique. BAO is calculated in mmol of acid secreted/hour. I-PAO is calculated in mmol acid secretion/hour using the two consecutive 15-minute aspirates with the highest acid output. BAO and I-PAO are compared.

Specimen Gastric aspirate **CONTAINER:** Glass container **SAMPLING TIME:** 3-4 hours **COLLECTION:** An I.V. is started. A #16 Levine tube is placed in the stomach with the drainage holes in the most dependent part of the stomach. Position is checked by fluoroscopy. With the patient in the supine position, continuous suction is applied, and the stomach is emptied every 10 minutes, and the contents discarded. Suction is continued and four samples are collected over 15 minutes each. This is used to determine BAO (in mmol HCl produced per hour). Regular insulin is injected I.V. in a dose of 0.2 units/kg. Blood sugars are then drawn at 15, 30, 45, 60, 90, and 120 minutes after injection. Following insulin injection, gastric suction is continued and eight samples of gastric aspirate are collected over 15 minutes each. This is used to determine the I-PAO. **CAUSES FOR REJECTION:** Failure to drop blood glucose by at least 45 mg/100 mL. Failure to fast or abstain from medications as under preparation. **TURNAROUND TIME:** 24 hours.

Interpretation **NORMAL FINDINGS:** The test is positive if acid concentration rises >20 mmol/L over the basal acid concentration. If the basal secretion is achlorhydric, a rise ≥10 mmol/L is considered significant. **LIMITATIONS:** It is a potentially dangerous exam in patients with known heart disease or the elderly. In addition, its prognostic value in regards to ulcer recurrence is doubtful. There is high incidence of negative tests becoming positive months after vagotomy. This happens to a lesser degree if antral resection is also done.[2] Therefore, the test may not assess completeness of vagotomy, but rather amount of acid secreting tissue.[3] Also, patient may have a potassium or hypoglycemic reaction, or the blood sugar may not drop sufficiently. **ADDITIONAL INFORMATION:** This test is based on the premise that drops in blood sugar stimulate the vagus nerve which in turn induces gastric acid secretion. The main use for the test is the evaluation of the effectiveness of vagotomy. It should be remembered, however, that the recurrence of ulcer requires a failure of vagotomy, but that not all vagotomies that are considered failures following Hollander Test give rise to a recurrent ulcer.

Footnotes

1. DeVries BC, Holtkamp HC, Leeuwerik PJ, et al, "The Insulin Infusion Test: A Safe Procedure?" *Br J Surg*, 1978, 65(2):121-2.
2. Nylamo EI, Inberg MV, and Nelimarkka OI, "The Insulin Test After Vagotomy and Antral Resuction or Drainage - Stability and Referral of Test Response in Repeated Tests," *Acta Chir Scand*, 1979, 145(8):549-54.
3. Nylamo EI, Inberg MV, and Nelimarkka OI, "Insulin Test After Selective Gastric and Truncal Vagotomy. Test Response and Acid Secretion Is the Early and Late Postoperative Phase," *Ann Chir Gynaecol*, 1979, 68(5,6):160-4.

References

Haukland HH, Waldum HL, and Johnson JA, "Effect of Proximal Gastric Vagotomy on Insulin-Induced Gastric H+ and Pepsin Secretion and Serum Group I Pepsinogens," *Scand J Gastroenterol*, 1982, 17(4):555-9.

Hydrogen Breath Test *see* Breath Hydrogen Analysis *on page 85*

Hydrogen Exhalation Test *see* Breath Hydrogen Analysis *on page 85*

Intestinal Biopsy (for Disaccharidase Deficiency) *replaced by* Breath Hydrogen Analysis *on page 85*

Intestinal Intubation for Culture *replaced by* Breath Hydrogen Analysis *on page 85*

Intestinal Perfusion and Lactose Barium Radiography *replaced by* Breath Hydrogen Analysis *on page 85*

I-PAO (Insulin Induced Peak Acid Output) *see* Hollander Test *on page 105*

Isolated Basal Acid Output Measurements *replaced by* Hollander Test *on page 105*

I.V. Secretin Gastrin Levels

CPT 91052

Synonyms Secretin Test for Gastrinoma

Applies to Basal Serum Gastrin Determination; Secretin Stimulated Serum Gastrin Determination; Serum Radioimmunoassay for Gastrin

Abstract **PROCEDURE COMMONLY INCLUDES:** I.V. injection of secretin and blood sampling at specific intervals for serum gastrin. A basal specimen is drawn and then, 5, 10, 15, 20, 25, and 30 minutes after injection. Radioimmunoassay is used to measure serum for gastrin. **INDICATIONS:** To rule out gastrinoma (Zollinger-Ellison syndrome) in patients with appropriate symptoms (recurrent peptic ulcer unresponsive to appropriate medical or surgical therapy, diarrhea or steatorrhea, multiple endocrine neoplasia (MEN) type I symptomatology) who have acid secretion and a fasting hypergastrinemia that is <1000 pg/mL (>1000 pg/mL with acid secretion and appropriate symptoms is diagnostic of Zollinger-Ellison syndrome). This test, if negative, may suggest a diagnosis of G-cell hyperplasia if the appropriate symptomatology is present (see Additional Information). **CONTRAINDICATIONS:** Allergic to secretin.

Patient Care/Scheduling **PATIENT PREPARATION:** May consider applying a secretin skin test before proceeding. **SPECIAL INSTRUCTIONS:** NPO after midnight.

Method **TECHNIQUE:** The secretin test for Zollinger-Ellison syndrome is possible because of an unknown mechanism by which there is a paradoxical increase in serum gastrin following secretin injection. In the normal patient and in the patient with G-cell hyperplasia, the gastrin response is decreased. In the patient with duodenal ulcer, there may be no change, a decrease, or a slight increase in serum gastrin.

Specimen Blood **SAMPLING TIME:** 35 minutes **COLLECTION:** Basal serum gastrin is drawn at 5 minutes preceding and then immediately before secretin injection.[1] Pure porcine GIH secretin 2 units/kg is injected over 30 seconds. Serum gastrins are drawn at 5-minute intervals for 30 minutes. **TURNAROUND TIME:** 48 hours.

Interpretation **NORMAL FINDINGS:** <200 pg/mL increase in serum gastrin **LIMITATIONS:** Five percent false-negative (often seen in the presence of hypocalcemia[2]) **ADDITIONAL INFORMATION:** Elevated serum fasting gastrins may be elevated >1000 pg/mL in pernicious anemia, achlorhydria, hypochlorhydria, chronic gastritis, gastric cancer, rheumatoid arthritis, vitiligo, and diabetes mellitus. However, most of the patients with these maladies are not acid hypersecretory or do not have refractory peptic ulcer disease. After Zollinger-Ellison has been excluded by the secretion test, a meal stimulated gastrin test may be performed. If it causes excess gastrin release, a diagnosis of G-cell hyperfunction is likely. A combined secretion calcium test has been devised which may be a more potent stimulant to gastrin secretion.[3] Following diagnosis of Zollinger-Ellison, an abnormal CT is the most helpful means of locating the potentially malignant gastrinoma.

Footnotes

1. Sleisenger MH and Fordtran JS, *Gastrointestinal Disease – Pathophysiology, Diagnosis, Management*, Philadelphia, PA: WB Saunders Co, 1983, 696-701.
2. Jansen JB and Lamers CB, "Effect of Changes in Serum Calcium on Secretin-Stimulated Serum Gastrin in Patients With Zollinger-Ellison Syndrome," *Gastroenterology*, 1982, 83:173-8.
3. Romanus ME, Neal JA, Dilley WG, et al, "Comparison of Four Provocative Tests for the Diagnosis of Gastrinoma," *Ann Surg*, 1983, 197:608-17.

References

McGuigan JE and Wolfe MM, "Secretin Injection Test in the Diagnosis of Gastrinoma," *Gastroenterology*, 1980, 79:1324-31.

Lactose (Sucrose and d-Xylose) Tolerance Test *replaced by* Breath Hydrogen Analysis *on page 85*

Laparoscopy *see* Peritoneoscopy *on page 114*

Laparotomy in Selected Cases *replaced by* Peritoneoscopy *on page 114*

Liver Biopsy

CPT 47000

Related Information

Peritoneoscopy *on page 114*

Synonyms Blind Liver Biopsy; Needle Biopsy of the Liver; Percutaneous Liver Biopsy

Applies to Percutaneous Needle Aspiration Biopsy Under Fluoroscopic, CT, or Ultrasound Guidance; Transjugular Needle Biopsy of the Liver

Abstract **PROCEDURE COMMONLY INCLUDES:** Percutaneous biopsy of liver parenchyma in a "blind" fashion (ie, not under radiologic guidance). This is carried out at the bedside under local anesthesia. A specialized, thin-bore needle is advanced between the ribs overlying the region of hepatic dullness. Several 2 cm cores of deep liver tissue are excised. Fresh specimens may be sent for gross pathologic inspection, routine light microscopy, special stains for liver storage diseases, transmission and immune electron microscopy, immunohistochemistry (using monoclonal antibodies), DNA hybridization studies, and microbiologic culture. Liver biopsy is a valuable and time-honored means of diagnosing diffuse liver parenchymal disease as well as disseminated focal disease. **INDICATIONS:** Candidates for liver biopsy must be carefully selected. This procedure, by nature, is invasive and histologic findings may often be reported as "consistent with" a particular disease (without being pathognomonic) or simply "nondiagnostic". In most cases, noninvasive imaging studies such as CT scan or ultrasound are now obtained first. With these considerations in mind, indications for liver biopsy include:

- suspected cases of liver cirrhosis, in order to confirm the diagnosis pathologically; establish etiology if possible (alcohol, alpha$_1$-antitrypsin deficiency, primary biliary cirrhosis, Wilson's disease, hemochromatosis, etc); assess and stage level of activity; assess complications
- chronic hepatitis, with or without cirrhosis, to identify cases of chronic activity hepatitis (liver biopsy mandatory for diagnosis) and differentiate this entity from chronic persistent hepatitis and lobular hepatitis
- suspected liver disease in the known alcoholic patient, to confirm alcoholic liver disease, exclude alternative causes of liver disease (which may be present in ≤20% of cases), stage and assess disease activity
- diagnosis of hepatoma or metastatic neoplasms
- suspected multisystem disease with liver involvement, where traditional diagnostic techniques have not been fruitful (eg, sarcoidosis, amyloidosis, tuberculosis, glycogen storage disease)
- staging of lymphoma
- unexplained hepatomegaly
- cholestasis of unknown etiology, where prior studies for biliary obstruction are negative
- persistently elevated liver enzyme tests
- selected cases of fever of unknown origin
- selected cases of hepatitis of unknown etiology, in order to differentiate viral from drug-induced etiologies (not always possible) or to assess complications, such as cholestasis
- evaluation of response to treatment

Liver biopsy is less useful in:

- acute hepatitis A or B infection, unless the diagnosis is in question
- extrahepatic biliary obstruction, where percutaneous transhepatic cholangiography and ERCP are considered first-line procedures
- fluid-filled liver cysts detected on ultrasound or CT scan, probably more amenable to guided thin needle aspiration first

CONTRAINDICATIONS: Mahal et al (1979) noted that failure to heed accepted contraindications led directly to 22 bleeding episodes in 3800 percutaneous liver biopsies.[1] Contraindications include:

- impaired hemostasis, accepted as prothrombin time more than 3 seconds over control, PTT more than 20 seconds over control, thrombocytopenia, and markedly prolonged bleeding time
- severe anemia (Hgb <9.5 g/dL)
- local infection near needle entry site, such as right sided pleural effusion or empyema, right lower lobe pneumonia, local cellulitis, infected ascites or peritonitis
- tense ascites (low yield technically, risk of leakage)
- high-grade extrahepatic biliary obstruction with jaundice (increased risk of bile peritonitis)
- septic cholangitis
- possible hemangioma
- possible echinococcal (hydatid) cyst
- lack of compatible blood for transfusion
- uncooperative patient

Patient Care/Scheduling **PATIENT PREPARATION:** Procedures and risks of the procedure are explained and consent is obtained. Formal consultation with gastroenterology staff is usually required. Procedure entails overnight hospitalization in most cases but some patients may be candidates for a "same day" outpatient biopsy. This latter group is in good general health, not jaundiced, and displays no signs of liver failure (ascites, encephalopathy). They need to stay within several minutes of the hospital for 1-2 days postbiopsy and must have supervision from family or friends. Scheduling arrangements for both in-hospital and outpatient liver biopsies are handled by gastroenterology team. All aspirin products and nonsteroidal agents must be discontinued at least 5 days beforehand. If taking oral anticoagulants (Coumadin®), hospitalization is required to convert to heparin therapy before biopsy. Patient is NPO after midnight the evening prior. Daily medications may be taken on the day of procedure pending physician approval. In some hospitals, patient drinks 1-2 glasses of milk in the early AM on procedure day to empty the gallbladder. Screening laboratory studies ordered 24-48 hours in advance commonly include CBC, PT/PTT, BUN, bleeding time, and type and crossmatch for possible transfusion. Electrolytes and liver function tests are optional. If pneumonia or pleural effusion suspected on examination, PA and lateral chest x-ray is obtained. Premedication with meperidine and/or diazepam may be administered at physician discretion. This is not routine in some centers due to possible toxicity. **AFTERCARE:** Protocols are individualized for each hospital. In general, patient is monitored in a recovery area with frequent vital signs postbiopsy. If no complications are apparent, patient is transferred back to hospital room by cart. Strict bedrest is enforced for 24 hours; for the first 2 hours patient is positioned on his right side. After 5 hours, patient may be allowed to sit up. Vitals (blood pressure, pulse) are checked every 15-30 minutes for 2 hours, every 30 minutes for the next 2 hours, and then every hour for 8 hours. Following this, vitals every 4 hours are permissible. Physician should be immediately notified if hypotension, tachycardia, fever, or uncontrolled pain occurs. Diet is restricted to clear liquids for several hours, then full liquids as tolerated. Acetaminophen is usually sufficient for pain control. Some physicians recheck hematocrit 24 hours after procedure before approving hospital discharge. **SPECIAL INSTRUCTIONS:** In the appropriate high-risk patient, antibiotic prophylaxis for infective endocarditis may be considered. Little data exists regarding the risk of bacteremia, however, much less endocarditis. **COMPLICATIONS:** Based on several large series, serious morbidity has been estimated at 0.1% to 0.2%. Fatality rates have ranged from 0% to 0.17%, both figures being derived from studies involving >20,000 biopsies each. The more commonly seen complications are:

- pain – the most common adverse event, noted in ≤50% of cases. Usually it is confined to the right shoulder, probably referred pain from diaphragmatic pleura. Analgesia is required in approximately 20% of patients with acetaminophen sufficient in most cases. Symptoms resolve in 1-2 days.
- hemorrhage – minor episodes are common. Self-limited oozing from the puncture site may persist for approximately 1 minute, but with loss of only 5-10 mL blood. Significant hemorrhage is less frequent but is the most common cause of death from liver biopsy. Several series have estimated an incidence of approximately 0.2%, but Sherlock (1984) reported 40 patients out of 6379 required transfusion for intraperitoneal bleeding.[2] She felt these statistics may even underestimate the

(Continued)

Liver Biopsy *(Continued)*

incidence since those with severe coagulopathies were excluded. Bleeding usually results from a tear of a distended portal or hepatic vein. Specific sites include the abdominal cavity (hemoperitoneum), liver capsule (capsular hematoma), liver parenchyma (intrahepatic hematoma), or biliary tree (hemobilia). Postulated risk factors are coagulopathy, amyloid liver, hepatocellular injury, hemangioma, and vascularized tumor. However, bleeding may be massive when no risk factors are present. Not all episodes require surgery. In a study 4 of 7532 patients needed surgical intervention while 12 others with severe hemorrhage were transfused and observed.

- bile leakage with peritonitis – associated with severe obstruction of the larger bile ducts. This is felt to result from laceration of a small, distended duct or from puncture of the gallbladder. With the widespread use of noninvasive imaging, the size of the bile ducts is known prebiopsy and the complication rate has declined.
- laceration of internal organs and viscera – right kidney, gallbladder, colon, pancreas, and others
- others: right-sided pneumothorax, arteriovenous fistula – 5.4% of all biopsies, drug toxicity

Method **EQUIPMENT:** Several biopsy needles are available.

- Menghini needle – 1.9 mm diameter steel shaft with sharpened beveled tip and syringe; specimen is obtained using suction/aspiration into a 10 mL syringe. Requires only 1 second within the liver ("1-second technique") and patient need not hold his breath. Disadvantages are small samples and fragmentation of biopsy specimens.
- "Trucut" needle – disposable 2.05 mm diameter needle designed to cut out cores of tissue. Specimens are less fragmented, even in the cirrhotic liver, and thus a high success rate. However, dwell time in liver is longer (5-10 seconds), patient must cooperate more, and several steps are necessary.
- Vim-Silverman needle – sheath with inner cutting blade (similar to a "punch" biopsy). Trucut needle is a modernized Vim-Silverman.

TECHNIQUE: Patient lies supine in bed with right hand behind his head. Liver margins are estimated by percussion. Two approaches are popular, transthoracic (intercostal) or subcostal (anterior). With the former, biopsy site is identified along the midaxillary line in the center of hepatic dullness, usually the eighth or ninth intercostal space. This approach avoids other abdominal organs but always penetrates the pleura. With the subcostal approach, the biopsy site lies below the bottom rib anteriorly, and is used when a liver mass is easily palpable below the right costal margin. The risk of visceral laceration is higher and this approach is infrequently used; fine needle aspiration under CT guidance has become more popular. A wide area is prepped and draped in sterile fashion with operators in gowns, gloves, and masks. The skin is anesthetized with 1% lidocaine, then deeper structures are infiltrated – subcutaneous tissue, intercostal muscles, and diaphragm. Some operators make a small superficial incision with a No 11 blade at the needle entry site to facilitate needle insertion. Techniques differ with the type of biopsy needle selected. In general, the biopsy needle is advanced as far as the diaphragm (depth estimated by a finder needle). If a Menghini needle is used, suction is applied to the syringe, the needle is pushed rapidly through the pleura and into the liver parenchyma. A 2.5 cm core of liver is aspirated and needle withdrawn, all within 1 second. If other needles are used, patient may need to hold his breath at end expiration to decrease the risk of pneumothorax. Several passes of the biopsy needle are performed to minimize sampling bias.

Specimen At least 2-3 liver cores, each >2 cm in length. Initial specimen processing and transportation handled by gastroenterology team. A typical protocol would be as follows:

- tissue fixation – for light microscopy, specimen is routinely fixed in 10% buffered formalin within 1 minute. For transmission electron microscopy, 1 mm cubes of specimen are fixed immediately in glutaraldehyde with further processing in Pathology Laboratory.
- routine tissue stains including: H & E – general liver histology stain; reticulin stain – for connective tissue, especially cirrhosis, fibrosis, bridging necrosis; trichrome – fibrosis; iron stain – useful for hemosiderosis, hemochromatosis, bile pigments;

diastase PAS stain – useful for $alpha_1$-antitrypsin globules, bile ducts, iron; orcein – for hepatitis B surface antigen (if present, fine granular brown material stains in hepatocytes). Also for copper-binding protein in Wilson's disease.

- cytologic preparation – fluid from aspirating syringe may be smeared on clean microscope slide, fixed, and sent to Cytology Laboratory
- microbiological culture – specimen sent without fixative in sterile container. Special stains (AFB, KOH, etc) and cultures (tuberculosis, viral, *Brucella*, parasites, fungi) as needed
- optional special stains, ie, congo red for amyloidosis, immunohistochemistry

Footnotes

1. Mahal AS, Knauer CM, and Gregory PB, "Bleeding After Liver Biopsy: How Often and Why?" *Gastroenterology*, 1979, 76:1192.
2. Sherlock S, Dick R, and van Leeuwen DJ, "Liver Biopsy Today. The Royal Free Hospital Experience," *J Hepatol*, 1984, 1:75.

References

Lefkowitch JH, "Pathologic Diagnosis of Liver Disease," *Hepatology: A Textbook of Liver Disease*, 2nd ed, Chapter 29, Zakim D and Boyer TD, eds, Philadelphia, PA: WB Saunders Co, 1990, 711-32.

Perrault J, McGill DB, Ott BJ, et al, "Liver Biopsy: Complications in 1000 Inpatients and Outpatients," *Gastroenterology*, 1978, 78:103-6.

Schaffner F, "Needle Biopsy of the Liver," *Bockus Gastroenterology*, 4th ed, Chapter 49, Berk JE, ed, Philadelphia, PA: WB Saunders Co, 1985, 657-66.

Sherlock S, "Needle Biopsy of the Liver," *Diseases of the Liver and Biliary System*, 7th ed, Chapter 3, Oxford, England: Blackwell Scientific Publications, 1985, 28-37.

Van Ness MM and Diehl AM, "Is Liver Biopsy Useful in the Evaluation of Patients With Chronically Elevated Liver Enzymes?" *Ann Intern Med*, 1989, 111(6):473-8.

Long-Interval Distal Esophageal pH Monitoring *see* pH Study, 12- to 24-Hour *on page 117*

Lower Endoscopy *see* Colonoscopy *on page 87*

Measurement of Intestinal Transit Time *see* Breath Hydrogen Analysis *on page 85*

Mechanical Dilation of the Esophagus *see* Esophageal Dilation *on page 96*

Needle Biopsy of the Liver *see* Liver Biopsy *on page 108*

Open Small Bowel Biopsy, Laparotomy *replaced by* Small Bowel Biopsy *on page 120*

Paracentesis

CPT 49080 (initial); 49081 (subsequent)

Synonyms Abdominal Paracentesis; Ascites Fluid Tap

Abstract **PROCEDURE COMMONLY INCLUDES:** At the bedside, physician introduces a needle into the peritoneal space of a patient with free ascites, and samples the fluid for diagnostic and/or therapeutic purposes. **INDICATIONS:** Diagnostic indications include:

- patients with new onset of ascites
- ascites fluid of unknown etiology
- patients with clinically suspected ascites fluid infections (abdominal pain, unexplained fever, leukocytosis, declining mental status)

Therapeutic paracentesis is indicated when ascites fluid has accumulated enough to cause respiratory compromise, abdominal pain, or worsening of existing inguinal or umbilical hernias. Paracentesis should not be performed to diagnose the presence of ascites fluid. This should be known prior to the procedure (by physical examination or radiological imaging).

CONTRAINDICATIONS: Severe coagulopathy not correctable by vitamin K, fresh frozen plasma, etc; inability of physician to demonstrate ascites fluid on physical examination; lack of patient cooperation. Recent literature suggests the following factors are **not** contraindications for paracentesis: morbid obesity, low grade coagulopathy, multiple abdominal surgical scars, and bacteremia.[1]

(Continued)

Paracentesis *(Continued)*

Patient Care/Scheduling **PATIENT PREPARATION:** Technique and risks of the procedure are explained. Premedications (eg, sedatives or narcotics) are not routinely required. Laboratory requisitions are completed in advance to avoid delay in fluid processing later. Prothrombin and partial thromboplastin times prior to paracentesis are ordered at physician discretion (some elect to transfuse fresh frozen plasma immediately prior to procedure if PT/PTT are prolonged). **AFTERCARE:** No special limitations exist for the patient postprocedure. If large amounts of ascites are removed (several liters), frequent blood pressure measurements are needed to monitor possible hypotension. Patients may ambulate postprocedure if vital signs remain stable. Occasionally, ascites fluid may leak persistently from the puncture site; in this instance, the patient should remain supine with the site angled directly upwards, until the leak stops spontaneously. **SPECIAL INSTRUCTIONS:** In clinical practice, paracentesis is at times performed on patients with significant hepatic encephalopathy. Additional personnel may be required for conferring with family members and for proper patient positioning during the procedure. **COMPLICATIONS:** The medical literature is divided on the incidence of complications from paracentesis. Earlier literature was more negative and tended to emphasize the possible complications, based on retrospective analysis.[2,3] Some authors suggested that paracentesis itself was the cause of many cases of ascites fluid infection.[4] A recent prospective study concluded that paracentesis is a safe procedure, carrying <1% risk of major complications and <1% risk of minor complications.[1] No deaths or bowel perforations were seen in 229 consecutive attempts. The most feared complication is needle perforation of an abdominal viscus or solid organ such as liver or spleen. Others include: intraperitoneal hemorrhage from laceration of an umbilical vein, scrotal or penile edema, abdominal wall hematoma, contamination of ascites by nonsterile technique. Hypotension can be seen when large amounts of ascites (>1500 mL) are removed rapidly.

Method **EQUIPMENT:** Sterile gloves, drapes (optional), and adequate local anesthesia (26-gauge subcutaneous needle, 2% lidocaine). In clinical practice, various needles and angiocatheters are used. A 22-gauge, 1.5" metal needle with a plastic catheter is recommended. If a thick panniculus is encountered, a 3" to 5" 22-gauge needle may be substituted. Also required are a sterile 50 mL syringe and, if large volumes of ascites are to be removed, a sterile 1 L vacuum bottles with connecting tubing. **TECHNIQUE:** Patient empties bladder prior to procedure. Physician confirms presence of ascites by physical examination with patient in a semirecumbent position. Preferred site of entry is in the midline, inferior to the umbilicus. If a midline scar is present from prior surgery or if percussion is not reliable, an area near the flank is selected. At times, physician may request patient to assume the hand-knees position if small amounts of ascites are present. The entry site is then caudad to the umbilicus. The site is prepped with iodine solution and skin and deeper tissues are infiltrated with lidocaine. The skin is retracted caudally and the 22-gauge needle (attached to syringe) is inserted into the anesthetized area and advanced while aspirating. When ascites fluid returns freely, the needle is held in position and not advanced further (avoiding bowel trauma). Multiple aliquots (50 mL) may be obtained in this manner. For larger volumes, the syringe is removed and connecting tubing is directly attached to the 22-gauge needle to allow drainage into vacuum bottles. Once the desired amount is collected, the needle is withdrawn quickly and the caudal skin retraction is released, allowing the skin to return to its normal position. This causes the entrance and exit needle sites to form a "Z-tract" which minimizes ascites leakage. **DATA ACQUIRED:** Ascites fluid is routinely analyzed for cell count and differential, chemistries including LD, albumin and protein, Gram stain, bacterial culture, and cytology. Additional tests include special cultures for tuberculosis or fungi, ascites fluid pH, amylase, lipase, glucose, triglycerides, lactate, CEA, and hyaluronic acid.

Specimen When the procedure is performed therapeutically, the maximum volume of ascites that can be removed safely depends on the presence or absence of peripheral edema.[5] It is recommended that in patients without edema, the upper limit should be 1500 mL. Patients with peripheral edema may tolerate larger volumes without hypotension (in one study, ≤5 L).[6] When performed for diagnostic purposes, smaller volumes (50-100 mL) are adequate for routine studies. If malignancy or fastidious infection is suspected, larger volumes (>100 mL) will improve laboratory yield. **CONTAINER:** Purple top tube for cell count; red top tube for routine chemistries; aerobic and anaerobic culture media bottles for bacteriology. For cytology, send sterile vacuum bottles with 5000 units of heparin added. If ascites fluid pH desired, send specimen in anaerobic syringe (gas bubbles removed) on ice to acute care laboratory. **COLLECTION:** Some authorities recommend inoculating the bacterial culture media with ascites fluid immediately at bedside.[7] The average concentration of bacteria in ascites fluid is very low in most cases of spontaneous peritonitis. In addition, a significant number of organisms may not survive in the time needed for specimen transport and plating in the Microbiology Laboratory. Bedside inoculation of appropriate media (standard blood culture bottles) may improve the chances of obtaining a positive bacterial culture several fold.

Interpretation **NORMAL FINDINGS:** Ascites fluid is traditionally categorized as either "exudative" or "transudative" based on laboratory analysis.[8] Transudative ascites is caused for the most part by cirrhosis physiology; that is, increased portal venous pressure or decreased portal venous colloid osmotic pressure. Examples of transudates include hepatic cirrhosis, congestive heart failure, constrictive pericarditis, Budd-Chiari syndrome, inferior vena caval obstruction, and nephrotic syndrome. Exudative ascites is generally noncirrhotic in its pathophysiology and may be due to peritoneal membrane permeability defects. Examples of exudates include malignancy, spontaneous bacterial peritonitis (SBP), or other ascites infections (such as tuberculosis), vasculitis, pancreatitis, myxedema. **CRITICAL VALUES:** Transudates are characteristically "low-protein" ascites and have been defined by ascites protein <3 g/dL; exudates >3 g/dL. Exceptions are common and other laboratory tests are often used in conjunction with the protein concentration. These include (for transudates): LD <200 units/L, protein ascites/serum ratio <0.5, LD ascites/serum ratio <0.6. Values outside these ranges support the diagnosis of an exudate. The "albumin gradient," defined as serum albumin minus ascites albumin, has recently been shown to accurately identify ascites caused by portal hypertension physiology (eg, cirrhosis).[9] An albumin gradient >1.1 is considered transudative and is due to an oncotic (albumin) pressure gradient between the systemic arterial pressure and ascites fluid, as seen with elevated portal pressures. Exudates tend to have gradients <1.1. The early diagnosis of spontaneous bacterial peritonitis (SBP) prior to bacterial culture results can frequently be made on routine analysis of ascites fluid.[10] Patients with SBP, or other ascites fluid infections, have ascites WBC count >500/mm^3 along with many polymorphonuclear (PMN) cells on the differential (>250/mm^3). In addition, two other laboratory indices suggestive of SBP are ascites pH <7.35 and ascites lactate <25 ng/dL.[11] The clinical utility of these last two criteria has not been as well established as the standard PMN count. Many physicians will begin empiric antibiotics on the basis of PMN >250/mm^3 alone. Gram stain of ascites fluid has low sensitivity for detecting SBP due to the low bacterial concentration, even on a centrifuged sample. Malignant ascites can be expected to have abnormal cytology in >50% of the cases. Indirect evidence of neoplasm include: grossly hemorrhagic fluid (may also be traumatic); ascites CEA >10 ng/mL with adenocarcinoma; ascites hyaluronic acid >0.25 mg/mL with mesothelioma; high ascites triglyceride levels with chronic chylous ascites (>80% of cases are lymphoma); ascites WBC count >500/mm^3 with peritoneal carcinomatosis (but PMN count low, <250/mm^3), pH <7.35, lactate <25 mg/dL. None of these values are considered diagnostic of malignancy and should be used only as supportive evidence. **LIMITATIONS:** As described previously, the strict use of the ascites protein concentration alone in differentiating exudate from transudate has considerable potential for error. Multiple criteria should be considered, including the albumin gradient and relevant clinical findings. **ADDITIONAL INFORMATION:** Paracentesis is a safe procedure when ascites is easily demonstrable on physical examination. When small amounts of ascites are present, a fluid wave may be difficult to demonstrate even when ≤1.5 L ascites are present. CT scan or abdominal ultrasound guided needle aspiration is particularly useful in these cases. Patients with ascites from cirrhosis may develop SBP and yet have minimal evidence of infection; some patients may be completely asymptomatic.[12] A low threshold for performing paracentesis is recommended in this setting, despite the low-grade coagulopathy that frequently is seen.

Footnotes

1. Runyon BA, "Paracentesis of Ascitic Fluid: A Safe Procedure," *Arch Intern Med*, 1986, 146:2259-61.
2. Liebowitz HR, "Hazards of Abdominal Paracentesis in the Cirrhotic Patient," *N Y State J Med*, 1962, 62:1822-6, 1997-2004, 2223-9.

(Continued)

Paracentesis *(Continued)*

3. Mallory A and Schaefer JW, "Complications of Diagnostic Paracentesis in Patients With Liver Disease," *JAMA*, 1978, 239:628-30.
4. Conn HO, "Bacterial Peritonitis: Spontaneous or Paracentric?" *Gastroenterology*, 1979, 77:1145-6.
5. Rocco VK and Ware AJ, "Cirrhotic Ascites: Pathophysiology, Diagnosis, and Management," *Ann Intern Med*, 1986, 105:573-85.
6. Kao HW, Rakov NE, Savage E, et al, "The Effect of Large Volume Paracentesis on Plasma Volume – A Cause of Hypovolemia?" *Hepatology*, 1985, 5:403-7.
7. Runyon BA, Umland ET, and Merlin T, "Inoculation of Blood Culture Bottles With Ascitic Fluid; Improved Detection of Spontaneous Bacterial Peritonitis," *Arch Intern Med*, 1987, 147:73-5.
8. Bender MD and Ockner RK, "Ascites," *Gastrointestinal Disease*, 4th ed, Sleisenger MH and Fordtran JS, eds, Philadelphia, PA: WB Saunders Co, 1988.
9. Pare P, Talbot J, and Hoefs JC, "Serum Ascites Albumin Concentration Gradient: A Physiologic Approach to the Differential Diagnosis of Ascites," *Gastroenterology*, 1983, 85:240-4.
10. Hoefs JC and Runyon BA, "Spontaneous Bacterial Peritonitis," *Dis Mon*, 1985, 31:1-48.
11. Yang C-Y, Liaw Y-F, Chu C-M, et al, "White Count, pH, and Lactate in Ascites in the Diagnosis of Spontaneous Bacterial Peritonitis," *Hepatology*, 1985, 5:85-90.
12. Pinzello G, Simonetti RG, and Craxi A, "Spontaneous Bacterial Peritonitis: A Prospective Investigation in Predominantly Nonalcoholic Cirrhotic Patients," *Hepatology*, 1983, 3:545-9.

Pecoral Jejunal Biopsy *see* Small Bowel Biopsy *on page 120*

Percutaneous Liver Biopsy *see* Liver Biopsy *on page 108*

Percutaneous Needle Aspiration Biopsy Under Fluoroscopic, CT, or Ultrasound Guidance *see* Liver Biopsy *on page 108*

Percutaneous Transhepatic Cholangiogram (PTC) *see* Endoscopic Retrograde Cholangiopancreatography *on page 91*

Peritoneal Endoscopy *see* Peritoneoscopy *on this page*

Peritoneoscopy

CPT 49300 (without biopsy); 49301 (with biopsy)

Related Information

Liver Biopsy *on page 108*

Synonyms Celioscopy; Laparoscopy; Peritoneal Endoscopy

Replaces Laparotomy in Selected Cases

Abstract **PROCEDURE COMMONLY INCLUDES:** Direct visualization of anterior intra-abdominal structures by means of a rigid laparoscope. This is performed in an endoscopy suite under local anesthesia or in an operating room under general anesthesia. The technique involves insertion of a Veres needle into the peritoneal cavity, followed by insufflation with gas (either CO_2 or nitrous oxide). Once this pneumoperitoneum has been created, the laparoscope is advanced into the peritoneal cavity through a small periumbilical incision. The following structures can be readily visualized: omentum, surface of the liver, peritoneum, gallbladder, portions of the spleen, diaphragm, and the serosal surfaces of the small bowel and colon. In female patients, the ovaries, Fallopian tubes, and uterus are also accessible. The areas of pathology are noted and visually-directed biopsies may be obtained.

INDICATIONS: The more common diagnostic indications include:

- ascites of unknown etiology. In the majority of cases, bedside paracentesis should be performed first. If the ascites fluid is found to be exudative (but otherwise nondiagnostic), peritoneoscopy may be used to rule out occult malignancy, fungal peritonitis, tuberculosis, and other conditions.
- diffuse or focal liver disease of unknown etiology. Direct inspection of the liver combined with a visually-directed liver biopsy can increase diagnostic accuracy. This may be particularly helpful in suspected cases of hepatocellular carcinoma,

lymphoma metastatic to liver, granulomatous hepatitis, and tuberculosis. Even when diffuse liver disease is present, as in cirrhosis, laparoscopic liver biopsy and visual inspection of the liver appears to be more sensitive than "blind" liver biopsy.
- suspected peritoneal carcinomatosis
- cancer staging; peritoneoscopy may be used to determine the stage of malignancies such as ovarian cancer and Hodgkin's disease when formal surgical laparotomy is contraindicated.

Additional indications for peritoneoscopy include:

- evaluation of chronic abdominal pain syndromes. This procedure may occasionally be useful in diagnosing abdominal adhesions or endometriosis in patients with chronic pain. Some physicians may use laparoscopy as a means of avoiding a formal laparotomy in difficult cases. The precise role and efficacy of peritoneoscopy in this setting is unclear.
- suspected ectopic pregnancy
- suspected pelvic inflammatory disease
- primary or secondary amenorrhea
- fever of unknown origin; in selected cases to rule out lymphoma or granulomatous diseases
- infertility evaluation (eg, diagnosis of tubal defects)
- suspected appendicitis
- emergency evaluation of abdominal trauma

Therapeutic uses for peritoneoscopy include:

- tubal ligation
- pancreatic biopsy by laparoscope through lesser sac
- therapeutic wedge resection of the ovaries in polycystic ovary syndrome
- lysis of adhesions
- removal of foreign bodies (eg, intrauterine device which has perforated into the Cul-de-sac)
- treatment of endometriosis with electrocautery or laser
- laparoscopic cholecystectomy

CONTRAINDICATIONS: Absolute contraindications to peritoneoscopy include:

- acute peritonitis, particularly when surgical intervention is warranted
- unstable cardiac or pulmonary status
- acute intestinal obstruction; the presence of multiple dilated loops of bowel increases the risk of perforation by the needle or trocar
- uncorrectable, severe coagulopathy
- uncooperative patient

Relative contraindications are as follows:

- presence of abdominal adhesions, usually from multiple abdominal surgeries or severe peritonitis. This increases the risk of bowel perforation. In each case, the risk-benefit ratio should be carefully considered (some authors consider this an absolute contraindication)
- presence of an abdominal hernia. On rare occasions, a hernia can become incarcerated during peritoneal insufflation
- infection involving the abdominal wall, such as cellulitis
- history of multiple abdominal surgeries (increased likelihood of dense adhesions)

Patient Care/Scheduling **PATIENT PREPARATION:** Patients who are candidates for peritoneoscopy must be referred to the appropriate specialist in gastroenterology, obstetrics and gynecology, or surgery. A complete medical history and physical is required. The technique, risks, and benefits of the procedure are discussed with the patient and informed consent is obtained. The details of scheduling are usually the responsibility of the subspecialist performing the procedure (such as date, time, operating area, etc). If peritoneoscopy is to be performed under general anesthesia, preoperative medical clearance may be necessary. The following laboratory studies are routinely obtained: complete blood count (including platelet count), electrolytes, prothrombin time (PT), and partial thromboplastin time (PTT). An electrocardiogram and chest X-ray are usually indicated if general anesthesia is planned. NPO (nothing by mouth) for at least 8 hours before procedure. Usu-

(Continued)

Peritoneoscopy *(Continued)*

ally nothing after midnight the day before. Preoperative enemas are not necessary unless the patient complains of fecal impaction. Laxatives should be avoided. Prescription medications normally taken by the patient must be reviewed in advance by the physician, and explicit instructions provided. This is particularly relevant if the patient is on insulin, antiarrhythmic agents, or antianginals. Patient should avoid taking aspirin products or nonsteroidal anti-inflammatory agents for several days before procedure. On the day of the procedure, the patient is shaved and prepped by the medical team. Premedication is usually with Demerol® and a benzodiazepine. The bladder should be emptied prior to the procedure. **AFTERCARE:** Following procedure, the patient is observed in the endoscopy recovery area or postanesthesia care unit. Vital signs are obtained frequently. The length of time for observation depends on the general medical condition of the patient. It is not mandatory to hospitalize patients overnight, unless a liver biopsy was performed or the procedure was complicated. **SPECIAL INSTRUCTIONS:** NPO after midnight. **COMPLICATIONS:** Laparoscopy is considered a safe procedure, especially when candidates are carefully selected. Certainly, the presence of a relative contraindication (eg, multiple surgeries in the past) increases the risk. The incidence of death associated with this procedure has been estimated at 1 in 2000, and severe complications in an additional 1 in 500.[1] A wide variety of adverse outcomes have been reported. Most often these appear related to incorrect placement of the needle used to create the pneumoperitoneum, although complications can occur during any phase. These include:

- injury or perforation of bowel, liver, spleen, ovary, gallbladder
- subcutaneous emphysema, pneumomediastinum
- bleeding, especially at biopsy sites or within the abdominal wall
- vasovagal reactions, myocardial infarction
- fever, infection, peritonitis
- pain, especially in the shoulder from diaphragmatic irritation
- aortic rupture

Method **TECHNIQUE:** As indicated previously, the procedure may be performed under local anesthesia (with sedation) or under general anesthesia. For most gastroenterologic indications, local anesthesia is preferable. The patient may be required to perform certain simple maneuvers during laparoscopy. The patient is placed supine on a standard operating room table. The table is equipped with stirrups. The buttocks are extended 4" to 5" over the edge of the table, which is tilted in Trendelenburg position for gynecologic procedures. Table may be tilted in any direction as needed to visualize any area of peritoneum required. The site of needle entry is identified and anesthetized. This is often the inferior rim of the umbilicus, although other areas are acceptable. A small skin incision is made and a Veres needle is advanced into the peritoneal cavity. Approximately 2 L of gas is then instilled into the peritoneal cavity (either CO_2 or nitrous oxide). The Veres needle is then removed. The skin incision previously made is enlarged and the laparoscopic trocar and sleeve are inserted. A twisting motion is used until the trocar is within the gas-filled peritoneal cavity. The laparoscope is then inserted through the sleeve and advanced under direct visualization. Additional volumes of gas may be introduced into the abdomen through the sleeve. The various internal structures are observed directly and pathologic areas biopsied as indicated. In some cases, accessory trocars may be required for introduction of instruments for suction, biopsy, fulguration, hemostasis, etc.

Specimen Liver biopsy, tumor biopsy, peritoneal biopsy, ovarian wedge biopsy, ascitic or peritoneal fluid aspiration and washing. Specimens for histopathologic examination should be placed in a clean container with appropriate fixative. Samples for microbial culture should be placed in a sterile container (or syringe) **without** fixative. Cultures for anaerobic organisms should be inoculated into anerogic media or transported immediately to the Microbiology Laboratory. For cytologic samples, peritoneal fluid samples should be promptly spread on a clean microscope slide and fixed. **CONTAINER:** Clean container with fixative for tissue specimens for histology. Sterile syringes for peritoneal aspirates for culture. Syringes for peritoneal aspirates for cytology. Fluid should be immediately spread on slide and fixed in 95% alcohol. **SAMPLING TIME:** 1-2 hours **TURNAROUND TIME:** 2-3 days.

Interpretation **NORMAL FINDINGS:** Preliminary report on gross laparoscopic findings written in patient's chart immediately by operating physician. Final typewritten report is attached to chart within several days. Specifically, the laparoscopist usually comments on the following aspects of the case:

- premedications administered
- type of instrument used
- gross appearance of omentum, peritoneal surfaces
- size and appearance of the liver, gallbladder, spleen, diaphragm, small bowel, colon, female reproductive organs, appendix
- presence or absence of ascites
- areas of pathology including malignancy, endometrial implants, adhesions, vascular abnormalities, abscesses, ectopic pregnancies, foreign bodies, as appropriate
- biopsies, brushings, ascites fluid aspirations
- other operative procedures performed
- complications

The laparoscopist also includes an overall clinical impression, based on the clinical history and visualized abnormalities.

ADDITIONAL INFORMATION: Despite the safety and efficacy of peritoneoscopy, it is an infrequently performed gastroenterologic procedure. It is, however, well-established in the field of obstetrics and gynecology, due to the accessibility of the female pelvic organs. From a GI standpoint, peritoneoscopy appears of most benefit in evaluating the patient with ascites of unknown etiology, where malignancy or tuberculosis are possibilities. Clinical trials comparing the diagnostic yield of laparoscopy versus laparotomy are lacking. Until such studies are performed for different clinical indications, the selection of laparoscopy will depend in part on physician familiarity and confidence with the procedure.

Footnotes

1. Vilardell F and Marti-Vicente A, "Laparoscopy," *Bockus Gastroenterology*, 4th ed, Berk JE ed, Philadelphia, PA: WB Saunders Company, 1985, 612-21.

References

Boyce HW Jr, "Laparoscopy," *Diseases of the Liver*, 5th ed, Schiff L and Schiff ER, eds, Philadelphia, PA: JB Lippincott, 1982, 333-48.

Lightdale CJ, "Indications, Contraindications, and Complications of Laparoscopy," *Gastroenterologic Endoscopy*, Sivak MV Jr, ed, Philadelphia, PA: WB Saunders Company, 1987, 1030-44.

Nord HJ, "Technique of Laparoscopy," *Gastroenterologic Endoscopy*, Sivak MV Jr, ed, Philadelphia, PA: WB Saunders Company, 1987, 994-1029.

Peroral Endoscopy *see* Upper Gastrointestinal Endoscopy *on page 120*

Peroral Esophageal Dilation *see* Esophageal Dilation *on page 96*

pH Study, 12- to 24-Hour

CPT 91033

Related Information

Standard Acid Reflux Test *on page 124*

Synonyms Esophagus Acid Reflux Test With Intraluminal pH Electrode (Prolonged Recording); Long-Interval Distal Esophageal pH Monitoring

Abstract **PROCEDURE COMMONLY INCLUDES:** Placing a pH probe into the distal esophagus for a 12- to 24-hour period in order to generate a graph depicting continuous pH readings. Information is obtained regarding quantity and pattern of gastroesophageal (GE) reflux events, the correlation with symptoms, and the efficiency of esophageal acid clearance.

INDICATIONS:

- quantify the number of acid reflux episodes which occur over 12-24 hours under physiologic conditions; particularly useful in patients with suspected reflux esophagitis (based on the history and physical) who have failed empiric therapy, or whose symptoms are atypical
- further evaluate patients with typical symptoms of reflux esophagitis but whose upper endoscopy is normal

(Continued)

pH Study, 12- to 24-Hour *(Continued)*

- evaluate difficult cases of nocturnal pulmonary aspiration or noncardiac chest pain, particularly to see if subjective complaints correlate temporally with episodes of acid reflux
- monitor, in selected cases, the effectiveness of medical or surgical antireflux therapy

CONTRAINDICATIONS:

- any condition that prohibits standard nasogastric intubation – nasal obstruction, maxillofacial trauma, basilar skull fracture, severe coagulopathy, etc
- active upper GI bleeding
- refractory nausea and vomiting
- uncooperative patient, especially in terms of diet, compliance, cigarette use, and coffee intake since these factors are carefully regulated during the procedure
- agitated or confused patient, since an accurate record of reflux events must be kept, including time of day and nature of symptoms

Patient Care/Scheduling **PATIENT PREPARATION:** Technique and risks of the procedure are explained in detail and consent is obtained. Patient must understand beforehand that cigarettes, alcohol, and coffee will not be permitted and that a special diet will be prescribed. Requisition should include a list of current medications and length of monitoring desired. **AFTERCARE:** Patient may be discharged if no complications have arisen. Activity may be *ad libitum* or as determined by referring physician. No specific postprocedure restrictions are necessary. **SPECIAL INSTRUCTIONS:** Prolonged pH monitoring currently is performed as an in-hospital procedure in that the patient is confined to the facility for the duration of the study. Thus, all administrative arrangements must be handled well in advance, usually in conjunction with a GI specialist. In some tertiary care centers, equipment for ambulatory 24-hour pH monitoring is now available (patient not confined to facility). If this is desired, arrange with the GI specialist or laboratory directly. **COMPLICATIONS:** This procedure is considered safe and no significant attendant morbidity has been reported. Potential complications are mainly those related to any nasogastric (NG) intubation (eg, nasal trauma, vasovagal reaction, tracheal intubation, etc).

Method **EQUIPMENT:** In GI procedure room: pH electrode, separate glass reference electrode, pH meter, potentiometric strip chart recorder with isolation module, reference pH solutions. In most cases an esophageal manometry system with transducer equipment is needed initially. Also required are tape, electrocardiographic paste, and a form in which the patient records time of symptoms and daily activities. **TECHNIQUE:** Performed by GI specialist in adequately equipped procedure room. Esophageal manometry is carried out in most cases to locate the exact position of the lower esophageal sphincter (LES). Following this, a pH probe is passed through the nose, using standard nasogastric intubation technique, and is positioned 5 cm above the LES. The separate reference electrode is taped to the arm. Both pH probe and reference electrode are connected to the pH meter and chart recorder (by means of the isolation module). The system is calibrated against reference pH solutions to ensure accuracy. Patients are placed on a restricted diet in which the pH of all food and beverage is >5. No coffee or cigarettes are permitted due to potential effects on lower esophageal sphincter tone. Patients are instructed to carefully record the time of symptoms, changes in body position (standing, sitting, lying, etc), and time of meals. If the full 24-hour examination is carried out, patient is kept in the "upright phase" during working hours (standing or sitting only), and in the "recumbent phase" during sleep (lying flat without elevation of the head of bed). Once the recumbent period is completed the procedure is terminated and equipment removed. Ambulatory pH monitors are available in some tertiary centers. These devices are portable and patients are permitted to leave the testing center to assume usual daily activities. **DATA ACQUIRED:** Graphic recording strip of intraesophageal pH over a 12- to 24-hour period. Printout graph paper plots "pH" on the vertical axis against "time" on the horizontal axis. Patient submits log book for comparison analysis.

Interpretation **NORMAL FINDINGS:** Individual composite reflux score within two standard deviations of the mean score of a reference group, using the criteria of Johnson and DeMeester. Other definitions may be used and are mentioned in the following information. Data is analyzed and final interpretation is provided by a GI specialist. Basic principles of interpretation are as follows. From the 24-hour pH recording, six variables are analyzed:

- percent of total recording time with intraesophageal pH <4

- percent of time in upright position with pH <4
- percent of time in recumbent position with pH <4
- total number of reflux episodes requiring ≥5 minutes to clear
- average number of reflux episodes per hour
- duration of longest period of esophageal acid exposure (single episode)

A "reflux episode" is defined as a fall in pH to ≤4 for at least 5 seconds. Several methods of interpreting the raw data have been proposed. Johnson and DeMeester described a weighted scoring system utilizing these six variables.[1] A total "reflux score" is calculated and this is compared with reflux scores from an asymptomatic control group. If the reflux score calculated for a patient is more than two standard deviations (SD) above the mean score of 15 control volunteers, the degree of reflux is considered "abnormal". This system has come under some criticism because of complexity and length of time required for calculation. Some researchers advocate independent analysis of each of the six variables, without weighing certain variables more heavily. Schlesinger suggests another, more simple grading system based on a prospective study of 64 patients undergoing 24-hour pH monitoring. Discrimination from asymptomatic controls was best achieved by analyzing only two variables – (1) number of reflux events requiring ≥5 minutes to clear and (2) total exposure time of the esophagus to acid.

CRITICAL VALUES: Abnormal reflux defined as reflux score more than two standard deviations above reference group. Again, other definitions may be used, based on the interpreting physician's preference. **LIMITATIONS:**

- Test is relatively expensive and work intensive for both physician and patient.
- Interpretation is still under some debate.
- In-hospital monitoring is usually required unless ambulatory equipment available.
- Volume of gastric acid reflux is not measured (ie, 1 mL reflux versus 25 mL). The significance of this is not clear.
- Bile or alkaline reflux is not measured.
- False-negative rate may be higher in certain subgroups than originally estimated (see following information).

ADDITIONAL INFORMATION: The patient who presents with symptoms consistent with GE reflux disease is commonly encountered in clinical practice. The majority of cases do not require laboratory testing. Those individuals with typical retrosternal burning pain are usually treated empirically for presumed reflux esophagitis. Diagnostic testing is neither indicated nor economically feasible in this large group of patients. Patients who present with atypical symptoms, who have persistent pain despite aggressive medical treatment, or who may have complications of reflux disease (eg, nocturnal asthma, esophageal strictures) are candidates for additional diagnostic testing. However, no single test for reflux esophagitis is clearly superior. In fact, no sequence of testing or combination of tests has been generally agreed upon. The 24-hour pH test was designed to quantitate exposure of the distal esophagus to acid. Initial studies suggested superior sensitivity (88%) and specificity (98%) for this test, but later studies suggested these figures were inflated. Schlesinger et al demonstrated a 29% false-negative rate in patients with endoscopically proven erosive esophagitis.[2] In the subgroup of patients with typical reflux symptoms but normal endoscopies, a sensitivity of only 21% was reported. Despite these caveats, this procedure is gaining increasing importance and popularity. No other procedure examines patients over a prolonged period or under near-physiologic conditions. It is based, in part, on the rationale that symptomatic GE reflux is not an "all or none" phenomenon, unlike the rationale underlying the standard acid reflux test. An important clinical application of this test is the temporal correlation of subjective symptoms with objective pH measurements. The occurrence of typical symptoms in the absence of pH changes argues strongly against reflux esophagitis as the etiology of symptoms.

Footnotes

1. Johnston LF and DeMeester TR, "Twenty-Four Hour pH Monitoring of the Distal Esophagus," *Am J Gastroenterol*, 1974, 62:325-32.
2. Schlesinger PK, Donahue PE, Schmid B, et al, "Limitations of 24-Hour Intraesophageal pH Monitoring in the Hospital Setting," *Gastroenterology*, 1985, 89:797-804.

References

DeMeester TR, Wang C, Wernly JA, et al, "Technique, Indications, and Clinical Use of 24-Hour Esophageal pH Monitoring," *J Thorac Cardiovasc Surg*, 1980, 79:656-70.

(Continued)

pH Study, 12- to 24-Hour *(Continued)*

Johnson LF, "24-Hour pH Monitoring in the Study of Gastroesophageal Reflux," *J Clin Gastroenterol*, 1980, 2:387-99.

Pneumatic Esophageal Dilation *see* Esophageal Dilation *on page 96*

Proctoscopy *see* Anoscopy *on page 80*

Rectosphincteric Manometry *see* Anorectal Manometry *on page 77*

Saline Load Test for Gastric Emptying *see* Gastric Saline Load Test *on page 104*

SART *see* Standard Acid Reflux Test *on page 124*

SBB *see* Small Bowel Biopsy *on this page*

Secretin Stimulated Serum Gastrin Determination *see* I.V. Secretin Gastrin Levels *on page 107*

Secretin Test for Gastrinoma *see* I.V. Secretin Gastrin Levels *on page 107*

Serum Radioimmunoassay for Gastrin *see* I.V. Secretin Gastrin Levels *on page 107*

Sigmoidoscopy, Flexible *see* Flexible Fiberoptic Sigmoidoscopy *on page 102*

Small Bowel Biopsy

CPT 44100 (biopsy of intestine by capsule, tube, peroral)

Related Information

Upper Gastrointestinal Endoscopy *on page 126*

Synonyms Pecoral Jejunal Biopsy; SBB; Small Intestinal Biopsy

Applies to Duodenal Intubation and Aspiration

Replaces Open Small Bowel Biopsy, Laparotomy

Abstract **PROCEDURE COMMONLY INCLUDES:** Obtaining specimens of small bowel tissue by means of a suction tube (Rubin tube) or a gravity-directed capsule (Carey capsule). The procedure is performed under fluoroscopic guidance, but biopsy samples are obtained in a "blind" fashion. A similar procedure may be performed under direct visualization of the intestinal mucosa using an upper gastrointestinal endoscope. Fresh specimens of small bowel are sent for histologic analysis and/or other specialized studies (microbiologic culture, enzyme assay, immunocytochemistry). **INDICATIONS:** Small bowel biopsy (SBB) is useful in diagnosing diseases of the duodenum and jejunum safely and rapidly. SBB is an invaluable means of diagnosing primary diseases of the small intestine. In certain cases, it may also be used to diagnose systemic diseases which involve the small bowel secondarily. The clinical utility of the SBB depends largely on the diagnoses being considered in an individual case.

SBB is definitely useful in the following diseases (histologic abnormalities are distinctive)[1]:

- Whipple's disease
- abetalipoproteinemia
- agammaglobulinemia

SBB is probably useful in the following diseases (mucosal lesions are patchy and may be missed):

- giardiasis
- amyloidosis
- small bowel lymphoma
- eosinophilic gastroenteritis
- intestinal lymphangiectasia
- systemic mastocytosis

SBB is possibly useful in the following diseases (histologic abnormalities may be nonspecific):

- celiac sprue (however, a normal biopsy excludes this disease)
- tropical sprue
- vitamin B_{12} as folate deficiency

- scleroderma
- radiation enteritis

In clinical practice, this procedure is most commonly performed to evaluate malabsorption of uncertain etiology, or diarrhea from the small intestine. SBB may also be used to monitor response to therapy, particularly when the clinical improvement is limited.

CONTRAINDICATIONS: Tight stricture, pyloric obstruction, uncorrectable coagulopathy, uncooperative or comatose patient.

Patient Care/Scheduling **PATIENT PREPARATION:** Technique and risks of the procedure are explained to the patient and informed consent is obtained. In some medical centers, formal consultation with gastroenterology staff is mandatory before obtaining a SBB. In other institutions, the procedure may be arranged directly by the ordering physician with the gastroenterology procedure laboratory. Patient should be fasting for 6-8 hours prior to SBB. If a morning procedure is planned, patient is NPO after midnight. If SBB is scheduled for later afternoon, some centers allow a light breakfast that morning. Daily medications are permitted with small sips of water. Due to the risk of bleeding, aspirin products and nonsteroidal anti-inflammatory agents should be discontinued well in advance (at least 5 days for aspirin). This procedure may be performed in combination with upper gastrointestinal endoscopy. Such requests must be clearly stated in advance by the primary physician (see Upper Gastrointestinal Endoscopy for details). If a bleeding disorder is suspected, a complete blood count, prothrombin time (PT), and partial thromboplastin time (PTT) should be drawn. **AFTERCARE:** Patient should remain NPO until the topical anesthetic has worn off (usually 1-2 hours). If intravenous sedatives were administered during the procedure, patient should not drive for the remainder of the day. Prior to discharge, patient should be carefully instructed to contact a physician if severe abdominal pain occurs or rectal bleeding is seen. **COMPLICATIONS:** In the great majority of cases, SBB is a safe procedure. The most serious complication is bleeding. In one reported series, only three bleeding episodes occurred after 4200 small bowel biopsies, and none were severe enough to warrant blood transfusion. Other complications include abdominal pain, bacteremia, and aspiration during passage of the tube or capsule.

Method **TECHNIQUE:** A topical anesthetic such as Cetacaine® spray is applied to the pharynx. Intravenous sedation may be given at physician direction but is not mandatory. Several devices may be used for biopsy. If the Carey capsule or Rubin's tube methods are used, the instrument is introduced into the hypopharynx and advanced under fluoroscopy into the stomach. The patient is then placed on his right side and the instrument tip is allowed to advance across the pylorus by gravity and peristalsis. Metoclopramide may be helpful in facilitating passage of the tube or capsule. If a directable biopsy instrument is used, the technique is similar except that the catheter tip may be redirected by a control stick for ease in passing the pylorus. The instrument tip is advanced to the ligament of Treitz rapidly under fluoroscopy. Biopsies of the small bowel are obtained by manipulation of the instrument's cutting edge with a wire. To increase diagnostic yield, multiple biopsies are usually taken. Biopsies taken in this fashion are considered "blind biopsies." The entire procedure may be completed in minutes. The endoscopic method allows advancement of the endoscope under direct visualization without the need for fluoroscopy. Several pinch biopsies of small bowel are obtained using large endoscope forceps. Samples obtained are visually-directed but may be small or distorted by crush artifact. Only the second or third portions of the duodenum is reached by the standard endoscope (and not the jejunum).

Specimen Fresh duodenal or jejunal tissue. All biopsy specimens are sent to the Pathology Laboratory without delay in appropriate containers and fixatives. The details of specimen collection, fixation, and transportation are usually supervised by the gastroenterology team.

Interpretation **NORMAL FINDINGS:** No abnormalities seen on gross examination or light microscopy. However, a "normal" biopsy may also be a result of sampling error, especially in small bowel diseases which are "patchy." A formal report is issued by pathologist. **CRITICAL VALUES:** Abnormalities are as noted by the pathologist. Examples of histologic patterns in specific disease states include:

- Whipple's disease – clusters of periodic acid-Schiff (PAS)-positive macrophages in the lamina propria
- abetalipoproteinemia – vacuolated epithelial cells secondary to fat stores

(Continued)

Small Bowel Biopsy *(Continued)*

- intestinal lymphoma – characteristic lymphoma cells in lamina propria and submucosa
- eosinophilic enteritis – mucosa invaded by numerous eosinophils, often patchy
- amyloidosis – amyloid fibrils present on Congo red staining
- giardiasis – parasites visibly adhering to the mucosa
- Crohn's disease – noncaseating granulomas identified
- celiac sprue – almost complete absence of villi, hypertrophy, and elongation of crypts, infiltration of mononuclear cells

ADDITIONAL INFORMATION: Small bowel biopsy is done in adults as well as children if malabsorption is suspected. Usually these patients exhibit symptoms of chronic diarrhea or steatorrhea, weight loss, failure to thrive, as well as hematologic or laboratory evidence of malabsorption.

Footnotes

1. Greenberger NJ and Isselbacher KJ, "Disorders of Absorption," *Harrison's Principles of Internal Medicine*, 11th ed, Chapter 237, Braunwald E, Isselbacher KJ, Petersdorf RG, et al, eds, New York, NY: McGraw-Hill, 1987, 1260-76.

References

Heizer WD, "Intubation for Small Bowel Biopsy and Duodenal Aspiration," *Manual of Gastroenterologic Procedures*, 2nd ed, Chapter 10, Drossman DA, ed, New York, NY: Raven Press, 1987, 71-9.

Martin DM and Nasrallah SM, "Small Intestinal Capsule Biopsy Under Endoscopic Guidance," *Gastrointest Endosc*, 1983, 29:37-8.

Perea DR, Weinstein WM, and Rubin CE, "Small Intestinal Biopsy," *Hum Pathol*, 1975, 6:157-217.

Weinstein WM and Hill TA, "Gastrointestinal Mucosal Biopsy," *Bockus Gastroenterology*, 4th ed, Chapter 47, Berk JE, ed, Philadelphia, PA: WB Saunders Co, 1985, 626-44.

Small Intestinal Biopsy *see* Small Bowel Biopsy *on page 120*

Sphincter of Oddi Manometry

CPT 43263

Related Information

Endoscopic Retrograde Cholangiopancreatography *on page 91*

Synonyms Endoscopic Retrograde Cholangiopancreatography (ERCP) With Pressure Measurement of Sphincter of Oddi; Sphincter of Oddi Pressure Measurement or Profile

Abstract **PROCEDURE COMMONLY INCLUDES:** Placement of a manometry catheter within the sphincter of Oddi to diagnose abnormalities in motor function. Performed during the course of ERCP as an optional, adjunctive test. Baseline sphincter pressures are measured by means of a water-filled, pressure-sensitive catheter. A continuous graph of sphincter of Oddi pressure (mm Hg) versus time (seconds) is generated. This procedure is useful in evaluating patients with "idiopathic" pancreatitis, and is based on the concept that intermittent biliary obstruction (and pancreatitis) may result from sphincter of Oddi dysfunction. **INDICATIONS:** This procedure has only recently gained clinical acceptance, and thus applications are still evolving. Sphincter manometry may be indicated in patients with recurrent pancreatitis with normal ERCP examinations. Recent studies suggest that a subgroup of patients with "idiopathic" recurrent pancreatitis (no structural lesions on ERCP) will demonstrate abnormally elevated resting pressures of the sphincter of Oddi. **CONTRAINDICATIONS:** If a formal ERCP is planned in addition to sphincter of Oddi manometry, contraindications include:

- patient refusal or poor cooperation
- recent attack of acute pancreatitis within the past several weeks
- recent myocardial infarction
- inadequate surgical back-up
- history of contrast dye anaphylaxis

Relative contraindications include:

- poor surgical candidacy; in general patients should be able to tolerate laparotomy if complications arise

- pseudocyst, due to an increased risk of infection (has been debated)
- ascites
- severe cardiopulmonary background disease
- overlying residual barium in the GI tract from recent abdominal CT scan, lower GI series, etc

Patient Care/Scheduling PATIENT PREPARATION: Since this procedure is performed in conjunction with ERCP the same considerations apply.

Method EQUIPMENT: A triple lumen water-perfused manometry catheter is commonly used. This catheter contains side-hole orifices for pressure sensing and are spaced approximately 2 mm apart. Each catheter lumen is separately perfused with a low compliance hydraulic system. TECHNIQUE: After completion of the standard ERCP, contrast dye is allowed to drain from the ducts. The manometry catheter is then advanced through the biopsy channel within the endoscope. Under direct visualization, the catheter is introduced into the papilla of vater and advanced into either the common bile duct or pancreatic duct. Baseline ductal pressures are recorded. The catheter is then withdrawn at 2 mm intervals while continuous pressure measurements are being taken. This has been termed the "station pull-through technique". Pressures within the sphincter of Oddi are obtained, including a baseline resting tone and superimposed phasic contractions. Depending on results, a variety of pharmacologic interventions may be attempted, including:

- cholecystokinin-octapeptide (CCK-OP), which abolishes phasic activity of sphincter of Oddi and increases duodenal contractions
- glucagon, which also eliminates sphincter phasic activity
- pentagastrin, which increases both basal and phasic pressures
- bethanechol, which stimulates sphincter phasic activity and others.

Interpretation NORMAL FINDINGS: Preliminary report is written in chart by the gastroenterologist before the patient leaves the procedure area. Final typewritten report of manometry accompanies final ERCP report.

- baseline (resting) sphincter of Oddi pressure: 15-25 mm Hg
- superimposed phasic pressure waves at sphincter of Oddi: 50-200 mm Hg (3-5 cycles/minute)
- pancreatic duct pressure: 10 mm Hg

CRITICAL VALUES: Abnormalities in either resting pressures and/or phasic pressures. Most common abnormality is increased resting pressure >30 mm Hg (without pharmacologic provocation). LIMITATIONS:

- reliability and validity of procedure still under study
- clinical indications and applications are limited
- technically difficult procedure
- not available in all gastroenterology laboratories

ADDITIONAL INFORMATION: Despite the clinician's best efforts, a small number of patients with recurrent bouts of pancreatitis will continually defy diagnosis. In this problematic group no clues regarding etiology can be found on clinical examination, noninvasive imaging studies, or ERCP. The syndrome is characterized by recurrent abdominal pain, abnormal liver function tests (often despite prior cholecystectomy), hyperamylasemia, and delayed drainage of contrast material from the biliary tree. Through the years, this clinical presentation has been variously called biliary dyskinesia, papillary stenosis, or sphincter of Oddi spasm. More recently, researchers have found that roughly 20% of such patients with "idiopathic" recurrent pancreatitis manifest significant motor abnormalities in the sphincter of Oddi. Dysfunction of this sphincter may be due to either fixed stenosis (from inflammation or fibrosis) or "functional" abnormalities (motor). Sphincter of Oddi manometry has become the standard means of evaluating the latter condition, supplanting previous criteria such as the Nardi test, sphincter of Oddi biopsy, and delayed drainage of contrast material. Preliminary work suggests that some patients with sphincter of Oddi abnormalities may benefit from surgical intervention. Both sphincteroplasty (with septectomy) and endoscopic sphincterotomy have eliminated attacks of pancreatitis in certain patients. Further study is needed of this new, but promising, technology.

References

Bar-Meir S, Geenen JE, Hogan WJ, et al, "Biliary and Pancreatic Duct Pressures Measured by ERCP Manometry in Patients With Suspected Papillary Stenosis," *Dig Dis Sci*, 1979, 24:209.

(Continued)

Sphincter of Oddi Manometry *(Continued)*

Geenen JE, "New Diagnostic and Treatment Modalities Involving Endoscopic Retrograde Cholangiopancreatography and Esophagogastroduodenoscopy," *Scand J Gastroenterol*, 1982, 77(suppl):93-106.

Moody FG, Calabuig R, Vecchio R, et al, "Stenosis of the Sphincter of Oddi," *Surg Clin North Am*, 1990, 70(6):1341-54.

Soergel KH, "Acute Pancreatitis," *Gastrointestinal Disease: Pathophysiology, Diagnosis, Management*, 4th ed, Chapter 97, Sleisenger MH and Fordtran JS, eds, Philadelphia, PA: WB Saunders Co, 1989, 1814-42.

Toouli J, Roberts-Thomson IC, Dent J, et al, "Sphincter of Oddi Motility Disorders in Patients With Idiopathic Recurrent Pancreatitis," *Br J Surg*, 1985, 72:859-63.

Venu RP, Geenen JE, Hogan WJ, et al, "Idiopathic Recurrent Pancreatitis: Diagnostic Role of ERCP and Sphincter of Oddi Manometry," *Gastrointest Endosc*, 1985, 31:141, (abstract).

Sphincter of Oddi Pressure Measurement or Profile *see* Sphincter of Oddi Manometry *on page 122*

Standard Acid Reflux Test

CPT 91032

Related Information

Bernstein Test *on page 81*
Esophageal Motility Study *on page 98*
pH Study, 12- to 24-Hour *on page 117*

Synonyms Esophagus Acid Reflux Test With Intraluminal pH Electrode for Detection of Reflux; SART; Tuttle Test

Abstract **PROCEDURE COMMONLY INCLUDES:** Placement of a pH probe and manometer into the esophagus to objectively demonstrate the presence of gastroesophageal (GE) reflux. With the patient in a supine position, an abrupt fall in esophageal pH at rest, following strain maneuvers, or after exogenous gastric acid loading indicates acid reflux. This serves as a convenient, introductory test for suspected reflux esophagitis. **INDICATIONS:**

- objectively demonstrate the presence of GE reflux under controlled conditions; particularly useful when the diagnosis of reflux esophagitis is still somewhat in doubt
- evaluate cases of noncardiac chest pain, in which acid reflux is a reasonable possibility
- monitor, in selected cases, the effectiveness of antireflux interventions, both surgical and medical

CONTRAINDICATIONS: SART requires an alert, cooperative subject who, at the minimum, can perform Valsalva maneuvers, Mueller maneuvers, and leg raises. Thus, for the obtunded, agitated, or critically ill patient this test should be deferred. Other contraindications include active upper GI bleeding, nausea and vomiting, and possibly active peptic ulcer disease. In addition, since passage of the probe/manometer via a nasogastric (NG) approach often engenders a vagal response, patients with malignant cardiac arrhythmias or unstable hemodynamics should be tested with caution, if at all.

Patient Care/Scheduling **PATIENT PREPARATION:** Technique and risks of the procedure are explained and consent is obtained. Patient should be kept NPO at least 8 hours prior to testing, and preferably overnight. Avoid antacids and H_2 blockers prior to procedure (check with the GI Laboratory if there are questions regarding medications). **AFTERCARE:** Patient may be discharged from GI procedure room providing no complications have occurred. Activity may be *ad libitum* as tolerated and no specific postprocedure restrictions are necessary. If patient experiences pyrosis after the acid-loading step of the procedure, give 30-60 mL antacid. If SART is positive, inform patient that he will be contacted by the referring physician for specific antireflux instructions. **COMPLICATIONS:** SART is considered quite safe and no significant morbidity or mortality has been reported. Minor complications include nausea, eructation, vagal reactions, and transient dyspepsia (if acid load test is positive), with little long-term clinical significance.

Method **EQUIPMENT:** In GI procedure room: pH electrode probe (eg, Beckman glass electrode or MI-506 flexible microelectrodes), pH meter (eg, Beckman Laboratory model), reference electrode, pen recording device, reference pH solutions, esophageal manometry catheter with transducer equipment (see Esophageal Motility Study for details), and solutions of 0.1 N HCl **TECHNIQUE:** Performed by GI specialist in adequately equipped procedure room. Initially, pH meter and probe are calibrated against standard reference pH solutions. Afterwards, the pH probe may be threaded through the lumen of certain manometry catheters, so that the distal tip of the probe protrudes 1 cm. The probe and catheter assembly are advanced into the stomach, using a nasogastric approach. With the patient in a supine position, gastric pH is recorded (expected value <4). The probe is then slowly withdrawn, crossing the lower esophageal sphincter (LES); location of LES is verified by pressure tracings from the manometer. By convention, the probe is then fixed into position 5 cm above the LES. Intraesophageal pH is recorded and compared with gastric pH. If no difference in pH is found between stomach and esophagus, free GE reflux is suspected. If such is the case, instruct patient to make frequent swallows. Failure to raise intraesophageal pH ≥6 despite multiple swallows confirms free GE reflux. Procedure may be stopped at this point. If, however, intraesophageal pH is normal on the initial reading (ie, pH >6), four types of straining maneuvers are carried out. In the supine position, patient performs Valsalva maneuvers, Müller maneuvers, and leg raises. In the fourth maneuver, the examiner compresses patient's abdomen by hand. Each maneuver is performed twice. Intraesophageal pH is recorded during and immediately after each event. An abrupt fall in luminal pH may indicate GE reflux (see Critical Values). Eructation, wretching or belching at this stage may require repetition of some maneuvers since each lowers LES tone. If esophageal pH stays >6 despite these straining maneuvers, the acid-loading step may be performed, especially if clinical suspicion of reflux is still high. The probe and catheter are readvanced into the stomach and 200-300 mL 0.1 N hydrochloric acid infused. The pH probe is then withdrawn and, as before, positioned 5 cm above the LES. Again, patient performs two sets of the four straining maneuvers (Valsalva, Müller, etc), with frequent pH recordings. **DATA ACQUIRED:** Various pH measurements, as described. Subjective complaints of pyrosis may be noted but are not a part of the SART per se.

Interpretation **NORMAL FINDINGS:** pH in esophagus remains >6 despite straining maneuvers and acid loading. **CRITICAL VALUES:**

- If pH in esophagus equals pH in stomach (and both <4) when patient is supine, acid reflux is present, probably "free" reflux. Failure to raise pH with swallowing saliva further confirms free reflux.
- If the criteria for "free" reflux are not met, positive test for GE reflux may also be defined as an abrupt fall in intraesophageal pH <4 during or immediately following any **two** straining maneuvers.
- If the first two criteria are not met, a positive test may still be seen if intraesophageal pH falls to 4 during or immediately after two straining maneuvers during the acid-loading step

LIMITATIONS: Severe nausea, emesis, inability to pass catheter back to stomach.

References

Benz LJ, Hootkin A, Margulies S, et al, "A Comparison of Clinical Measurements of Gastroesophageal Reflux," *Gastroenterology*, 1972, 62:1-5.

Orlando RC, "pH Probe for Reflux (Turtle Test)," *Manual of Gastroenterologic Procedures*, 2nd ed, Drossman DA, ed, New York, NY: Raven Press, 1987, 51-4.

Tuttle SG, DeHarello A, and Grossman MI, "Esophageal Acid Perfusion Test and a Gastroesophageal Reflux Test in Patients With Esophagitis," *Gastroenterology*, 1960, 38:861-72.

Standard Duodenal Intubation Method of Biliary Drainage *see* Biliary Drainage *on page 83*

Stool pH Test *replaced by* Breath Hydrogen Analysis *on page 85*

Tests for Fecal Reducing Substances *replaced by* Breath Hydrogen Analysis *on page 85*

Transduodenal Drainage With CCK *see* Biliary Drainage *on page 83*

Transjugular Needle Biopsy of the Liver *see* Liver Biopsy *on page 108*

Tuttle Test *see* Standard Acid Reflux Test *on previous page*

Upper Endoscopy *see* Upper Gastrointestinal Endoscopy *on this page*

Upper Gastrointestinal Endoscopy

CPT 43200 (esophagoscopy, rigid or flexible); 43202 (for biopsy); 43234 (upper GI endoscopy, simple primary examination); 43235 (upper GI endoscopy including esophagus, stomach, duodenum, and/or jejunum); 43239 (for biopsy)

Related Information

Esophageal Dilation *on page 96*
Small Bowel Biopsy *on page 120*

Synonyms EGD; Esophagogastroduodenoscopy; Esophagoscopy (if Esophagus Alone Studied); Peroral Endoscopy; Upper Endoscopy

Abstract **PROCEDURE COMMONLY INCLUDES:** Direct visual examination of the upper gastrointestinal tract by means of a flexible fiberoptic endoscope. Typically, the procedure is carried out on an awake, but sedated, patient either in a specially equipped endoscopy suite or at the bedside in an intensive care unit. The endoscope is advanced (by mouth) through the oropharynx, esophagus, stomach, and duodenum. Important anatomic landmarks are identified and mucosal surfaces are examined for suspicious lesions such as ulcers, erosions, polyps, strictures, malignancies, varices, bleeding sites, etc. Biopsy specimens are easily obtained, and may be sent for histopathology, cytology, and/or microbiological culture. Other minor operative procedures may be performed utilizing the standard endoscope, including polypectomy, cytologic brushings, sclerotherapy of esophageal varices, extraction of foreign bodies, and electrocautery of bleeding sites. **INDICATIONS:** The precise indications for esophagogastroduodenoscopy (EGD) are still evolving and physician discretion still plays a major role.[1,2] Practice patterns amongst physicians vary considerably. Controversy exists regarding the use of EGD as a first-line diagnostic procedure for suspected upper GI disease. Some clinicians have virtually abandoned the standard upper GI barium swallow in favor of endoscopy. This approach addresses the problem of the false-negative upper GI series but is quite expensive and not without risk. In each case, a number of factors must be individually weighed, such as the risk of complications, cost of the procedure (versus upper GI series), expected diagnostic benefits, and probability of a normal (negative) examination. Diagnostic indications may be grouped as follows.

High yield indications:

- acute upper GI bleeding, to establish the exact location of hemorrhage prior to endoscopic cautery, surgery, etc
- dysphagia, especially if esophageal strictures or ulcerations are seen on a previous upper GI series. Note that EGD may still be indicated if the barium swallow is normal but clinical suspicion of esophageal disease remains high
- dyspepsia, if refractory to standard medical antireflux therapy. EGD is also indicated whenever a surgical antireflux procedure is planned
- odynophagia, when inflammation or infection is clinically suspected, especially if esophagitis from *Candida*, cytomegalovirus, or herpes simplex virus is likely
- surveillance endoscopy for known premalignant conditions, such as Barrett's esophagus, lye-induced strictures, Plummer-Vinson syndrome
- abnormalities seen on upper GI series which require visual confirmation and tissue biopsy (eg, polyps, gastric ulcers, redundant gastric folds, strictures)
- suspected gastric outlet obstruction

Lower yield indications (procedure not always appropriate):

- atypical chest pain
- abdominal pain of unknown etiology
- routine, uncomplicated cases of gastroesophageal reflux
- uncomplicated cases of duodenal ulcer demonstrated by upper GI series

Therapeutic indications for EGD are numerous and include:

- sclerotherapy of bleeding esophageal varices
- management of upper GI bleeding using electrocautery, photocoagulation, etc
- laser ablation of esophageal cancer
- endoscopic placement of esophageal stints

- placement of permanent feeding tubes under endoscopic guidance (PEG tubes)
- dilatation of esophageal strictures
- polypectomy
- dissolution of bezoars

CONTRAINDICATIONS:

- acute myocardial infarction
- hypoxemia with respiratory distress
- hypotension and shock, regardless of etiology
- massive upper GI bleeding with hypotension where emergency surgery is clearly appropriate (EGD may needlessly delay surgery and visualization is often obscured by copious amounts of blood.)
- uncontrolled hypertension
- patient refusal

Relative contraindications (high risk situations) include:

- noncorrectable coagulopathy
- recent myocardial infarction (within weeks)
- severe coronary artery disease
- recent upper GI tract surgery where anastomotic sites may still be "fresh"
- active peritonitis
- subluxation or instability of the cervical spine
- anterior cervical spine osteophytes
- perforated viscus
- Zenker's diverticulum (possibly)

Patient Care/Scheduling **PATIENT PREPARATION:** Technique and risks of the procedure are explained to the patient and informed consent is obtained. In some medical centers formal consultation with gastroenterology staff is mandatory before obtaining an EGD. In other institutions procedure is arranged directly with the endoscopy scheduling desk by the primary physician. EGD may be performed on either inpatients or outpatients. Customarily, inpatients are examined briefly by the endoscopist (or his representative) the day prior to EGD in order to review details of the case, write orders, and answer patient questions. It should be emphasized that patients frequently experience apprehension and fear regarding choking on the endoscope. Careful and thoughtful reassurances from the medical team may be quite effective in allaying these anxieties. Patient is kept strictly NPO for 8 hours prior to EGD. If a morning procedure is planned, patient is NPO after midnight. If EGD is scheduled for later in the afternoon, some centers allow a light breakfast that morning. Daily medications are permitted with small sips of water. Medicines which potentially interfere with visualization of the mucosa, such as antacids or Carafate®, should be discontinued beforehand. If a tissue biopsy is anticipated, aspirin products, and nonsteroidal agents are discontinued well in advance (at least 5 days for aspirin). If gastric outlet obstruction is clinically suspected, nasogastric suction is performed prior to EGD in order to remove retained luminal contents. This also applies to the patient with known or suspected impairment of gastric motility. For inpatients, dentures are removed and patient is transported to endoscopy suite on a cart, along with medical chart and relevant x-rays. For outpatients, arrangements for driver transportation home must be made in advance by patient, since driving is not permitted after procedure. Once patient is in the procedure room, baseline vital signs are obtained (pulse, blood pressure, etc). Intravenous sedation is routinely given, commonly diazepam (or another short-acting benzodiazepine) and meperidine several minutes prior to examination. A topical anesthetic agent such as Cetacaine® spray (benzocaine and tetracaine hydrochloride) is often applied to the pharynx. **AFTERCARE:** Immediately postprocedure the patient is observed in the recovery area. Vital signs are usually recorded at least once, and prn in the "high risk" patient. If no complications have occurred and sedation has worn off, patient may be discharged from the testing area. A normal diet may be resumed once gag reflex has returned. Driving is not allowed due to residual sedative effects. **COMPLICATIONS:** Morbidity and mortality of upper endoscopy is relatively low, but should not be overlooked. Statistics compiled from several large clinical series suggest an incidence of adverse outcomes of 0.1% to 0.2%. Death has been reported between 0.14-0.65/1000 endoscopies. Major complications, as described by Shamir and Schuman, are as follows.[3]

(Continued)

Upper Gastrointestinal Endoscopy *(Continued)*

- Perforation of esophagus or stomach: Up to 0.1% of all EGDs (some large centers report no cases of perforation). The upper esophagus above the cricopharynx appears most vulnerable. Other risk factors are esophageal cancer, strictures, or cervical osteophytes.
- Bleeding: Considered rare even after biopsies, at 0.3/1000 cases. In most cases, bleeding is not due to a coagulation defect, rather it results from biopsy of friable tissue.
- Cardiopulmonary complications: Significant cardiac arrhythmias are distinctly unusual. If a Holter monitor is placed, transient rhythm disturbances such as sinus tachycardia, premature ventricular contractions (PVCs), premature atrial contractions (PACs), and rarely ischemic changes may be recorded in <22% of cases. Few adverse clinical outcomes have been reported.

Other complications include the following.

- Pulmonary aspiration has been estimated at 0.8/1000 cases, but carries a mortality rate of 10%. Prout demonstrated that some degree of aspiration occurs in as many as 25% of cases, using iodinated oil as a marker. No cases of clinical pneumonia developed.[4]
- Toxicity of premedications: Minor complications are fairly common but usually inconsequential. Diazepam may cause a local phlebitis and meperidine may induce transient nausea. More importantly, the patient with severe COPD or liver cirrhosis may experience respiratory depression from this combination. In one series from England, 0.67 out of 1000 EGDs were followed by respiratory arrest requiring mechanical ventilation.[5]
- Infection: Prospective studies have shown a bacteremia rate of 3% to 8% (positive blood cultures). Some centers routinely use antibiotic prophylaxis in patients with valvular heart disease, although the risk of endocarditis is probably extremely low.[6]
- Miscellaneous: Parotid swelling, abdominal pain from air insufflation, transient megacolon, transient fever with pulmonary infiltrates (following sclerotherapy of varices).

Method **EQUIPMENT:** The fiberoptic endoscope has replaced the rigid endoscope as the instrument of choice. This device has a length of approximately 1200 mm and diameter of 9.5-12.5 mm. The instrument shaft is composed of numerous specialized glass fibers (>30,000) which allow the transmission of light down the length of each thin fiber with minimal distortion. The multiple fiberoptic images are integrated at the proximal eyepiece unit, by means of a complex system of lenses. The endoscopist thus views a reconstructed, mosaic image at the proximal eyepiece (similar to a television image). Also within the instrument shaft are several separate channels designed for passage of optional devices such as biopsy forceps, polyp snare, cytology brush, cautery or laser device, and suction. Air may also be introduced for insufflation of the stomach. For clearing of debris from the viewing area, a jet stream of water from a separate reservoir can be flushed through one channel. At the head or handle of the endoscope are two control devices ("wheels") which maneuver the instrument tip as it is advanced, an up-down angle wheel (deflection of almost 180°) and a right-left angle wheel (deflection of 100°). The instrument head is connected with a separate cold light source (usually a halogen lamp) by means of a cable comprised of incoherent fiberoptic bundles (the "umbilical cord"). The water feed tank and automatic suction box also attach to this cable. Optional accessories include an additional eyepiece for simultaneous viewing by a second operator (the "teaching head"), an ultrasound probe for real time imaging of the stomach wall, pancreas, etc, and photographic or videotape recording devices. **TECHNIQUE:** Performed only by an experienced gastroenterologist in a properly equipped endoscopy suite. At times, it may be necessary to carry out this procedure in an emergency room or ICU bed. Following sedation, patient is placed in the left lateral decubitus position (although successful intubation is possible in other positions). A hollow mouthpiece is inserted to protect the patient's teeth and facilitate instrument passage. The endoscope is slowly advanced orally and is "swallowed" by the patient. Once past the cricopharyngeal region the instrument is guided only under direct visualization. An important landmark is the Z-line at the gastroesophageal junction, approximately 40 cm from the teeth. The tip is then advanced into the cardia, with gentle insufflation of air. The various portions of the stomach are inspected – cardia, fundus, greater and lesser curvature, antrum. Following thus, the tip is then passed through the pylorus, into the duodenal bulb, and sometimes as far as the descending portion of the duodenum. Mucosal surfaces are reinspected as the instrument is withdrawn. Biopsies, cytologic brushings, polypectomy, cauterization of bleeding lesions, etc, are performed as indicated. Sclerotherapy of esophageal varices is not considered part of the routine EGD. This is a separate therapeutic procedure requiring additional equipment and somewhat more involved patient preparation.

Specimen All biopsy specimens and cytologic brushings are sent to the Pathology Laboratory without delay in appropriate containers and fixatives. Tissue for Gram stain, KOH prep, and culture should be sent in sterile containers without fixative to the Microbiology Laboratory. The details of proper specimen collection, fixation, and transportation are usually supervised by the gastroenterology team. **TURNAROUND TIME:** Final report on biopsy specimen histopathology is given within 2-3 days. Gram stain and KOH prep are known immediately (within minutes if necessary) but culture results may require several days (or more than 1 week if viral culture requested).

Interpretation **NORMAL FINDINGS:** No upper GI tract pathology encountered. Preliminary written report on endoscopic findings is completed immediately by gastroenterology staff and placed in medical chart before the patient is discharged from the endoscopy suite. A final typewritten report is added to the chart in 5-7 days. In general, the endoscopist comments in detail on all findings, normal and abnormal, and concludes with an overall clinical impression. **CRITICAL VALUES:** No grading schemes or numerical "cutoffs" per se. Subjective interpretation of visual findings by an experienced gastroenterologist constitutes the data base. Important aspects of the endoscopic examination frequently commented upon include:

- location of the Z-line
- presence or absence of hiatal hernia
- appearance of mucosal surfaces, with attention to ulcerations, erosions, strictures, masses, streaks, polyps, Barrett's-type epithelium, redundant tissue, etc
- location and appearance of bleeding site(s) or varices
- abnormalities in tone (spasm) of the lower esophageal sphincter or pylorus
- miscellaneous abnormalities
- operative procedure(s) performed during endoscopy
- complications
- technical adequacy of the study

In some centers, instant photographs of suspicious lesions are taken during endoscopy and included in the medical chart. In our institution, many endoscopic examinations are recorded on real time videotape for later review by the referring physician and endoscopist.

LIMITATIONS: Quality of study and its interpretation are highly dependent on the expertise of the endoscopist. Recognition of subtle abnormalities and visualization of all portions of the upper GI tract require a high degree of clinical competence. A variety of technical factors may lead to a suboptimal study. Endoscopists refer to "blind spots" – regions difficult to visualize in most cases – which include the superior aspect of the duodenal bulb, portions of the fundus, and the lesser curvature below the incisura. Active uncontrolled bleeding, retained blood in the stomach, and retained food or antacids may also lead to an inadequate study. EGD should not be used for the diagnosis of esophageal motility disorders. The procedure of choice for this entity is esophageal manometry. Similarly, EGD is not a first-line test for the diagnosis of reflux esophagitis (although characteristic histologic changes may be found on mucosal biopsy).

Footnotes

1. Gibb SP, Laney JS, and Tarshis AM, "Use of Fiberoptic Endoscopy in Diagnosis and Therapy of Upper Gastrointestinal Disorders," *Med Clin North Am*, 1986, 70:1307-24.
2. Grossman MB, "Gastrointestinal Endoscopy," *Ciba Found Symp*, 1980, 32:2-36.
3. Shahmir M and Schuman BM, "Complications of Fiberoptic Endoscopy," *Gastrointest Endosc*, 1980, 26:86-91.
4. Prout BI and Metreweli C, "Pulmonary Aspiration After Fiberendoscopy of the Upper Gastrointestinal Tract," *Br Med J [Clin Res]*, 1972, 4:269-71.
5. Schiller KFR, Cotton PB, and Salmon PR, "The Hazards of Digestive Fiberendoscopy: A Survey of British Experience," *Gut*, 1972, 13:1027.

(Continued)

Upper Gastrointestinal Endoscopy *(Continued)*

6. Durack DT, "Prophylaxis of Infective Endocarditis," *Principles and Practices of Infectious Diseases*, 3rd ed, Chapter 63, Mandell GL, Douglas RG, and Bennett JE, eds, New York, NY: Churchill-Livingstone, 1990, 716-21.

References

Botet JF and Lightdale C, "Endoscopic Sonography of the Upper Gastrointestinal Tract," *AJR*, 1991, 156(1):63-8.

Kahn KL, Kosecoff J, Chassin MR, et al, "The Use and Misuse of Upper Gastrointestinal Endoscopy," *Ann Intern Med*, 1988, 109(8):664-70.

Morrissey JF and Reichelderfer M, "Medical Progress: Gastrointestinal Endoscopy," *N Engl J Med*, 1991, 325(16):1142-9.

Rubin CE, Silverstein FE, and McDonald GB, "Indications for Fiberoptic Endoscopy," *Viewpoints Digestive Dis*, 1978, 10:5.

Schrock TR, "Complications of Gastrointestinal Endoscopy," *Gastrointestinal Disease: Pathophysiology, Diagnosis, and Management*, 4th ed, Chapter 13, Sleisenger MH and Fordtran JS, eds, Philadelphia, PA: WB Saunders Co, 1989, 216-21.

Schuman BM, "Upper Gastrointestinal Endoscopy," *Bockus Gastroenterology*, 4th ed, Chapter 41, Berk JE, ed, Philadelphia, PA: WB Saunders Co, 1985, 564-80.

Sugawa C and Schuman BM, *Primer of Gastrointestinal Fiberoptic Endoscopy*, Boston, MA: Little, Brown and Co, 1981.

NEPHROLOGY, UROLOGY, AND HEMATOLOGY

Carlos M. Isada, MD

In the following section, procedures related to Nephrology and Urology are detailed. These related medical-surgical fields are an integral part of general medical practice. Procedures such as the simple and complex cystometrogram are discussed in some detail. Given the advancing age of the American population, issues such as urinary incontinence in the elderly are becoming a major part of office practice. More invasive procedures such as the kidney biopsy are also discussed in depth. Although it is performed by a subspecialist, the basics of the procedure (including risk/benefit analysis) should be known by the generalist. Other techniques evaluating the genitourinary system are included in other sections. These include the intravenous pyelogram, renal ultrasound, renal flow scan, and others.

In this section, invasive procedures related to hematology are also included. The field of hematology is primarily one of the laboratory diagnosis. These tests are outlined in the companion *Laboratory Test Handbook*. The bone marrow biopsy is addressed in detail since this technique is commonly performed by general physicians, resident house staff, and trained nurse clinicians.

Arteriogram *replaced by* Penile Blood Flow *on page 152*

Bone Marrow *see* Bone Marrow Aspiration and Biopsy *on this page*

Bone Marrow Aspiration and Biopsy

CPT 85095 (aspiration); 85097 (smear interpretation); 85100 (aspiration, staining and interpretation); 85101 (aspiration and staining only); 85102 (needle biopsy); 85103 (staining and interpretation); 85105 (interpretation only); 85109 (staining and preparation only)

Applies to Bone Marrow; Bone Marrow Iron Stain; Bone Marrow Sampling; Bone Marrow Trephine Biopsy; Iron Stain

Abstract PROCEDURE COMMONLY INCLUDES: Aspiration and/or biopsy of bone marrow (BM) for microscopic analysis. Both procedures are carried out under local anesthesia at the patient's bedside. For aspiration, a specialized hollow needle is advanced into the intramedullary cavity (usually iliac crest). Approximately 0.4 mL liquid marrow and bone fragments are aspirated into a syringe, then smeared onto a slide. Frequently, a bone marrow biopsy is performed as a complementary, but separate, procedure (different equipment and site). A specialized biopsy needle (eg, Jamshidi needle) is used to obtain a core of solid cortical bone. This technique preserves the normal marrow architecture of the biopsy sample and allows for formal for histologic analysis. INDICATIONS: Bone marrow sampling is indicated in the evaluation of a wide variety of hematologic disorders, usually noted first on the CBC or peripheral smear. It is also useful in the diagnosis of systemic diseases which may potentially involve the marrow, such as infectious or granulomatous processes. Bone marrow aspiration and biopsy should be considered separate procedures, although indications often overlap. Indications for bone marrow **aspiration** include:

- evaluation of severe anemia, especially when etiology is in doubt and reticulocyte count is low
- evaluation of macrocytic anemia, to confirm the presence of megaloblastic anemia or to exclude sideroblastic anemia and normoblastic erythropoiesis
- leukopenia and/or thrombocytopenia, to differentiate excessive consumption from decreased production
- persistent leukocytosis of unknown etiology
- suspected myelodysplastic syndrome
- suspected leukemia, to confirm diagnosis and to classify subtype (FAB categorization)
- suspected immunoglobulin disorders, such as multiple myeloma, for diagnosis and staging
- evaluation of lipid storage diseases
- evaluation of suspected iron storage abnormalities
- acquisition of marrow for chromosomal analysis
- acquisition of tissue for microbiological culture (fungi, bacteria, mycobacteria, parasites)
- evaluation of response to therapy for hematologic malignancies

Bone marrow biopsy preserves the marrow architecture and is useful in evaluating systemic diseases secondarily involving the marrow. Bone marrow **biopsy** indications include:

- evaluation of pancytopenia
- evaluation of possible myelophthisic anemia (bone marrow infiltrated with leukemic cells, metastatic tumor, lymphoma, granulomas, etc)
- diagnosis and staging of solid tumors or lymphoma
- evaluation of selected cases of fever of unknown origin
- diagnosis of systemic amyloidosis when other methods have failed
- suspected cases of myelofibrosis
- evaluation of myeloproliferative syndromes (polycythemia vera, essential thrombocythemia, etc)
- failed bone marrow aspiration attempts (the so-called "dry tap")

Authorities differ on the exact indications for both bone marrow aspiration and biopsy. Some believe that most hematologic abnormalities are adequately evaluated by bone marrow aspiration alone (without biopsy). Bone marrow biopsy should not be routinely performed with aspiration, it is argued, due to the following reasons:

- diagnosis can often be made by aspiration
- significant patient discomfort accompanies biopsy
- there is needless expense and patient risk

Thus, bone marrow biopsy should only be performed if specific indications are present (as listed).

Other experts routinely include a biopsy whenever aspiration is performed. The following reasons are cited.

- Bone marrow biopsy may be diagnostic in cases where aspiration is negative or equivocal.
- It is nearly impossible to predict in advance which aspiration attempts will be technically difficult.
- Bone marrow biopsy actually causes less discomfort than aspiration in some cases.
- Cost-benefit analysis may favor the combined approach. The cost to physician, technologist, and patient may be doubled if patient is forced to undergo a separate bone marrow biopsy at a later date.

CONTRAINDICATIONS:

- uncooperative patient
- cellulitis, osteomyelitis, or radiation therapy involving the proposed site of needle entry
- severe, noncorrectable coagulopathy
- thoracic aortic aneurysm if a sternal approach is used
- Paget's disease involving the iliac bone represents a high risk situation, due to excessive bleeding at trephine biopsy site (but not necessarily a contraindication).

Patient Care/Scheduling **PATIENT PREPARATION:** Technique and risks of the procedure are explained to the patient and consent is obtained. Considerable patient apprehension often accompanies this procedure and requires thorough, step-by-step explanation beforehand. If coagulopathy is known or suspected, a recent CBC and PT/PTT should be drawn. Requisition must state in advance any special studies to be performed on specimen, such as AFB stain, Congo red stain for amyloid, cytogenetics studies, etc. Contact referring physician if any questions arise or contact appropriate laboratories directly. Patients are commonly premedicated with a short-acting benzodiazepine or analgesic such as meperidine. **AFTERCARE:** Needle puncture site(s) are covered with a dry sterile dressing. If the bone marrow biopsy is performed from the posterior iliac crest, patient must lie on back for a full 30 minutes before being discharged. In the presence of a low-grade coagulopathy or mild thrombocytopenia, direct pressure should be applied by operator (not patient) to puncture sites until local bleeding ceases. Instruct patient to keep dressings dry. Ideally, puncture sites should be examined approximately 24 hours later by nurse or physician, but this is not always feasible. **SPECIAL INSTRUCTIONS:** This procedure requires at least two operators. The first obtains the aspiration and/or biopsy specimen in a sterile fashion (usually a physician or specialized nurse clinician) and the second immediately examines and prepares the specimen (usually a nurse or technologist from the Hematology Laboratory). **COMPLICATIONS:** Bone marrow sampling is considered a relatively safe but invasive procedure. Minor complications include local bleeding, hematoma, and discomfort at the needle puncture site. Local infection is rarely seen if proper aftercare is followed. Major complications have been reported with sternal biopsy (Bahir 1963), including fatal puncture of mediastinal structures. Historical reports of fistula formation, osteomyelitis, and profuse bleeding were associated with biopsy of what are now considered nonstandard sites, such as the tibia. Minimal complications are associated with sampling of the iliac crest, the preferred site.

Method **EQUIPMENT:** Commercially assembled trays for aspiration and biopsy are widely available. These prepackaged kits typically contain a bone marrow biopsy needle (usually Jamshidi needle), aspiration needle (usually Illinois needle), various syringes (5 mL, 10 mL, 20 mL), assorted needles (18-gauge, 25-gauge), and 1% lidocaine with epinephrine for local anesthesia. Also included are gauze, sterile gloves, drapes and towels, No 11 scalpel blade, and alcohol and iodine prep. The Jamshidi needle is a large-bore (usually 11-

(Continued)

Bone Marrow Aspiration and Biopsy *(Continued)*

gauge), hollow needle with a tapered tip, thin metal stylet, and wide plastic grip to allow easy needle rotation. The Illinois needle is somewhat smaller, but likewise comes with a stylet and plastic sheath for improved grip. Smaller gauge needles are available for use in the pediatric population. **TECHNIQUE:** The procedure is performed by experienced operators only. May be carried out at the bedside if adequate lighting is available, otherwise done in a procedure room.

Aspiration: Preferred site is the posterior superior iliac spine (PSIS), alternatively the sternum. Patient is placed on his side or lies prone. Landmarks are identified by palpation – the PSIS primarily, but the anterior superior iliac spine also. A wide circular area (approximately 5" in diameter) overlying the PSIS is prepped with povidone-iodine in the usual sterile fashion. Using the 25-gauge needle and lidocaine, the skin directly over the PSIS is anesthetized. Following this, deeper structures are liberally anesthetized with the 18-gauge needle, including a several centimeter area of the periosteum. A 4 mm long skin incision is made over the PSIS by means of the No 11 scalpel blade, then extended deeper through fatty tissues down to the anesthetized periosteum. The Illinois aspiration needle (with stylet in place) is advanced through this soft tissue incision and firmly into the cortex of the PSIS, using a constant rotary motion of the needle ("drilling"). Once the needle has penetrated approximately 1 cm into the marrow cavity, the stylet is removed and a 10 mL syringe is attached to the open (distal) end of the aspiration needle. At least 4-5 mL marrow is aspirated using firm suction. This volume is adequate for most routine hematologic studies, but larger volumes are usually needed for fungal or tuberculous cultures, cytogenetics, cell markers, etc. This step often causes the most patient discomfort. After aspiration, the syringe is detached and immediately handed over to the technologist in order to prevent the specimen from clotting (aspiration needle is still in the PSIS). The technologist examines the specimen grossly for marrow particles, which may be visible to the naked eye. If present, this signifies that an adequate marrow specimen has likely been obtained; if absent, the aspiration needle is redirected slightly and the previous listed steps repeated. After completion, the needle is removed and direct pressure applied.

Biopsy: May be carried out immediately following aspiration, while patient is still under local anesthesia. Preferred site is again the PSIS; however, unlike bone marrow aspiration, biopsy is never obtained from the sternum. A Jamshidi biopsy needle is passed through the same skin and soft tissue incision used for aspiration (alternatively, a completely new site may be used). However, a separate hole in the PSIS must be made. Once into the cortical bone, the needle is advanced using a pronounced clockwise/counterclockwise rotary motion. The needle is oriented along an imaginary line connecting the PSIS and the anterior superior iliac spine, forcing a slight angle of the needle with respect to the skin. The needle should **not** be advanced perpendicular to the skin; this results in poor quality biopsies (often with mostly cartilage). The stylet is then removed. The "drilling" is continued until the needle is at least 2 cm deep into the cortex. This may be estimated by periodically replacing the stylet into the needle and noting the distance the stylet protrudes. The biopsy core is subsequently "sheared off" by the following maneuvers:

- needle is rotated a full 10 turns clockwise then 10 turns counterclockwise
- needle is withdrawn slightly and redirected at a different angle
- needle is readvanced
- steps 1-3 are repeated (until the core is sheared off). The needle is withdrawn, again using rotary motions so as not to lose the core. The blunt obturator or "push wire" is passed through the sharp tip of the Jamshidi needle and the specimen pushed gently out of the needle base and onto a sterile gauze. The technologist immediately makes imprints of the core then places the specimen in fixative.

The techniques for aspiration and biopsy outlined are generally agreed upon in major textbooks. However, some clinicians strongly believe that bone marrow biopsy should always **precede** aspiration, despite the "textbook" recommendations. They argue that artifacts in the core biopsy may be induced by aspiration.

Specimen The bone marrow aspirate is immediately examined for visible bone spicules. The presence of these small spicules suggests an adequate specimen. Direct smears of the aspirate fluid are prepared by the technologist at the bedside. These smears consist of marrow particles and free marrow cells spread onto coverslips. This technique helps to preserve the cytologic appearance of individual blood cells. Bone marrow biopsy samples are handled differently. In many institutions, touch preparations are made first, before specimen fixation. The marrow specimen is touched gently to a clean glass slide in several places, without smearing. These "touch preps" are allowed to air-dry and subsequently undergo routine staining. This technique also helps preserve cytologic detail. Once the touch preparations are completed, the remainder of the specimen is placed in a fixative such as formalin or Zenker's solution. The specimen is then processed according to individual laboratory protocol (for example, overnight fixation, decalcification, wash steps, dehydration, and serial sectioning). Routine stains are performed on processed specimens. These include hematoxylin and eosin (H & E), Wright-Giemsa stain, and iron stain. Optional studies may be obtained at physician request such as cytogenetic analysis, flow cytometry, electron microscopy, and amyloid stains. The Hematology Laboratory must be notified in advance for these studies. Bone marrow specimens may also be submitted for microbiological analysis. Cultures may be obtained for aerobic and anaerobic bacteria, fungi (eg, *Histoplasma capsulatum*), acid-fast bacilli (eg, *Mycobacterium tuberculosis* or *Mycobacterium avium-intracellulare*), and viruses (cytomegalovirus). Fixatives should **not** be added to specimens submitted for culture. Again, it is important to notify the Microbiology Laboratory in advance for these cultures.

Interpretation **NORMAL FINDINGS:** The bone marrow aspirate and biopsy are reviewed by a staff pathologist or hematologist. The preliminary report on the bone marrow aspirate may often be available several hours after the procedure, on request. Normal values for bone marrow cell lines in the adult are as follows:

Granulocytes

- blasts: 0% to 1 %
- promyelocytes: 1% to 5%
- neutrophil myelocytes and metamyelocytes: 7% to 25%
- neutrophil bands and segs: 20% to 60%
- eosinophils: 0% to 3%
- basophils: 0% to 1%
- monocytes: 0% to 2%
- lymphocytes: 5% to 15%
- plasma cells: 0% to 2%

Erythrocytes

- proerythrocytes: 0% to 1%
- early erythrocytes: 1% to 4%
- late erythrocytes: 10% to 20%
- normoblasts: 5% to 10%

The above bone marrow differential cell counts are calculated from the bone marrow aspirate specimen. Other useful data provided by the bone marrow aspirate include:

- myeloid/erythroid ratio (normal ratio 3-4:1)
- total cells counted
- overall cellularity
- erythropoiesis
- granulopoiesis

The bone marrow biopsy provides additional information on marrow architecture (which cannot be obtained from the aspirate). When examining the biopsy specimen, the pathologist may comment on:

- gross description including size of sample
- overall cellularity
- presence of granulomas
- infiltrative marrow processes such as lymphoma, carcinoma, granulomas
- iron stores
- results of special stains

References

Batjer JP, "Preparation of Optimal Bone Marrow Samples," *Lab Med*, 1979, 10:101-6.

Beckstead JH, "The Bone Marrow Biopsy: A Diagnostic Strategy," *Arch Pathol Lab Med*, 1986, 110:175-9.

(Continued)

Bone Marrow Aspiration and Biopsy *(Continued)*

Brynes RK, McKenna RW, and Sundberg RD, "Bone Marrow Aspiration and Trephine Biopsy: An Approach to a Thorough Study," *Am J Clin Pathol*, 1978, 70:753-9.
Williams WJ and Nelson DA, "Examination of the Marrow," *Hematology*, 4th ed, Chapter 3, WJ Williams, E Beutler, AJ Erslev, et al, eds, New York, NY: McGraw-Hill, 1990, 24-31.

Bone Marrow Iron Stain *see* Bone Marrow Aspiration and Biopsy *on page 132*

Bone Marrow Sampling *see* Bone Marrow Aspiration and Biopsy *on page 132*

Bone Marrow Trephine Biopsy *see* Bone Marrow Aspiration and Biopsy *on page 132*

Closed Kidney (Renal) Biopsy *see* Kidney Biopsy *on page 145*

CMG *see* Cystometrogram, Complex *on this page*

CMG *see* Cystometrogram, Simple *on page 139*

Complex Urodynamic Testing of Bladder Function *see* Cystometrogram, Complex *on this page*

Cystometrogram, Complex

CPT 51726

Related Information

Cystometrogram, Simple *on page 139*

Synonyms CMG; Complex Urodynamic Testing of Bladder Function; Multichannel Cystometrogram

Abstract **PROCEDURE COMMONLY INCLUDES:** Graphic recording of the pressure-volume characteristics of the urinary bladder. Performed in a Urodynamics Laboratory, the bladder is passively filled with water or gas by means of a transurethral catheter. Simultaneous intra-abdominal (rectal) pressure is obtained. Intravesical pressures are measured as the bladder is being filled by means of a microtip transducer or a fluid-filled catheter attached to a transducer. Information regarding bladder sensation, capacity, compliance, tone, and contractility may be obtained along with a cystometrogram (graphic plot of bladder pressure versus volume). **INDICATIONS:** The exact indications are controversial, as with simple cystometry. Most would agree that complex cystometry is useful in evaluating persistent urinary incontinence or retention felt secondary to bladder pathology. Clinical settings include:[1]

- overflow incontinence, to differentiate a flaccid bladder from an obstructed bladder
- urgency incontinence, to document detrusor instability
- bladder sensory or motor dysfunction associated with diabetes, Parkinson's disease, multiple sclerosis, or stroke
- postprostatectomy incontinence
- spinal cord injury with voiding disorders
- failed surgery for incontinence

Cystometry is less useful in evaluating:

- stress urinary incontinence
- psychogenic incontinence
- urinary obstruction in the male with retention

CONTRAINDICATIONS:

- patient refusal
- demented patient with severe cognitive deficits
- inability to pass Foley catheter
- active urinary tract infection

Patient Care/Scheduling **PATIENT PREPARATION:** Technique and risks are explained to the patient and consent is obtained. Patient should understand that a rectal probe will be inserted. Requisition to Urodynamics Laboratory should specify current medications. All sedatives, cholinergics, and anticholinergics should be discontinued prior to procedure. No anxiolytics or pain medications are given as premedications. If patient complains of dysuria (along with other voiding problems), obtain urinalysis at physician discretion. In all cases, patient is requested to void immediately prior to procedure. Remove indwelling Foley, if applicable, well in advance. **AFTERCARE:** No specific activity restrictions are necessary and previous level of activity may be resumed. At physician discretion, a urinalysis may be ordered 48-72 hours later to exclude procedure-induced infection. **COMPLICATIONS:** Complex cystometry is felt to be quite safe. Minor complications are similar to those associated with any bladder catheterization and include urethral pain, microscopic hematuria, and urinary tract infection (estimated at <8%).

Method **EQUIPMENT:** Basic equipment includes multilumen catheter for bladder catheterization (or two separate catheters), rectal balloon catheter with transducer, microtip transducers for bladder pressure measurement (or fluid-filled catheter attached to Statham transducer), multichannel recorder, sterile water reservoir (or carbon dioxide gas reservoir), and an adjustable infusion pump. **TECHNIQUE:** Complex cystometry may be performed in several ways. The basic procedure is described as follows. After normal voiding, the patient is placed in a supine position. A bladder catheter is inserted transurethrally and residual volume is measured. This catheter may be a triple or double lumen Foley catheter. (Some urologists prefer using two catheters per urethra, one for bladder filling, usually 14F, and a smaller one for pressure measurement.) With the bladder empty, patient is asked to relax completely and avoid all bladder or abdominal contractions. One channel of the catheter is connected with the infusion pump and the other channel is connected with a microtip transducer or fluid-filled catheter/transducer system. The anal probe is inserted and intra-abdominal pressures are continuously recorded. Using the infusion pump, the bladder is filled with sterile, room temperature water through one channel. The rate of filling is clearly documented: whether "slow fill" at 10 mL/minute, "medium fill" at 10-100 mL/minute, or "rapid fill" at >100 mL/minute. In general, the infusion pump allows continuous filling at a constant rate. (If not available, filling may be performed incrementally with gravity drainage.) Intravesical pressures are continuously recorded through the separate channel in the catheter, along with simultaneous anorectal pressures. Patient subjectively reports the first perceived sensation of bladder fullness and the first strong urge to void. Filling is continued until patient reports discomfort or until an involuntary bladder contraction is seen. The described technique is termed "filling cystometry". In some centers, the study is continued past this point and the examiner proceeds with "voiding cystometry". Patient is asked to void as vigorously and completely as possible while the catheter measuring intravesicular pressure is still in place. Pressures within the bladder are recorded as before, throughout bladder emptying. If two separate urethral catheters were used originally, the larger catheter (used for filling) is removed prior to voiding. A number of provocative maneuvers, including the following, may be employed at physician discretion.[2]

- Rapid fill cystometry: After standard cystometry is performed, flow is increased to >100 mL/minute of fluid (or 300 mL CO_2 if gas cystometry used). This is done to provoke detrusor contraction. If these are seen, the diagnosis detrusor areflexia is ruled out.
- Changes in patient position (sitting, standing) and maneuvers such as coughing, heel jouncing. As with rapid fill cystometry, these techniques attempt to overcome the inhibition of the detrusor reflex, which is normally present. If a bladder contraction is recorded, the peripheral nerve supply to the detrusor is intact.
- Saline infusions at temperatures above or below body temperature: This helps in further evaluating bladder sensation in equivocal cases and may also provoke a detrusor contraction.
- Bethanechol (Urecholine®) supersensitivity test: Bethanechol, a parasympathomimetic agent, is injected 2.5 mg subcutaneously and cystometry is repeated 10, 20, and 30 minutes afterwards. In the normal individual, small increases in bladder pressure are seen when cystometry is repeated. A marked increase in bladder pressure 15-20 cm H_2O over baseline indicates a lower motor neuron (LMN) lesion, the "supersensitive bladder". This is based on Cannon's law of denervation – when an end-organ is deprived of its nerve supply it becomes hypersensitive to normal excitatory neurotransmitters. Complete lack of response to bethanechol suggests technical error or myogenic bladder damage.
- Trial of anticholinergics or muscle depressants: If uninhibited detrusor contractions are seen on initial cystometry, the efficacy of specific drugs may be tested by repeating cystometry after drug administration.

(Continued)

Cystometrogram, Complex *(Continued)*

In addition, gas cystometry using CO_2 may be used instead of water for filling. Gas cystometry has the advantage of being more convenient and less time-consuming. Disadvantages include inaccuracy of bladder volume measurements (controversial), difficulties reproducing values, and inability to assess voiding cystometry (obviously only fluid may be voided). Tanagho suggests using gas cystometry only as an initial screen, if at all, with equivocal or abnormal results repeated with a liquid medium.[3]

DATA ACQUIRED:

- residual volume (mL)
- threshold for sensation of bladder fullness (mL)
- maximum cystometric capacity (mL) – volume where patient reports strong urge to void; usually less than true bladder capacity measured during normal, physiologic filling
- bladder contractility
- cystometrogram – bladder pressure (ordinate) plotted against volume (abscissa) on a multichannel recorder
- bladder compliance – Δ volume divided by Δ pressure (ΔV/ΔP) at any point on the cystometrogram
- provocative maneuver results, if performed.

Interpretation **NORMAL FINDINGS:** Official is report issued from the Urodynamics Laboratory. Normal values are identical to those listed for simple cystometry (see following entry). Normal values for provocative testing are described under Technique. With complex cystometry, voluntary or involuntary voiding contractions may be more precisely defined as sustained increases in intravesical pressure, usually 20-40 cm H_2O, with minimal increases in intra-abdominal pressure. The measurement of intra-abdominal pressure serves only as a reference point to ensure that apparent bladder pressure increases are not due to abdominal muscle contraction. This provides an important advantage over simple cystometry. **CRITICAL VALUES:** Identical to those listed for simple cystometry (see Cystometrogram, Simple). The graphic recording of pressure-volume characteristics is presumably more accurate than simple cystometry. Direct comparison of the shape of the test curve (as well as the absolute pressure values) may be made with normal CMG tracings and tracings of known pathologic entities. This is depicted in the following figure.

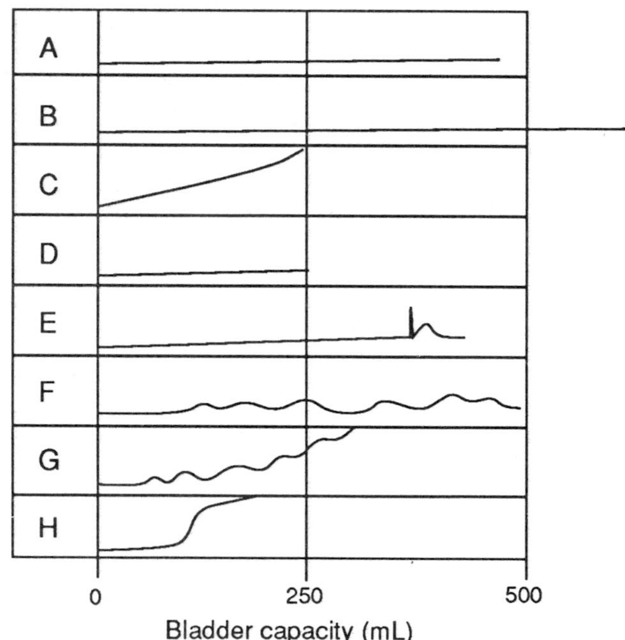

This chart represents idealized adult cystometrograms for the following conditions:

A. normal filling curve, normal compliance, no contractions
B. large capacity bladder
C. bladder with decreased compliance
D. small-capacity bladder, no involuntary contractions
E. bladder contraction from a cough
F. detrusor contractions, low-amplitude
G. involuntary bladder contractions in a bladder with decreased compliance
H. early onset involuntary bladder contractions (high amplitude)

LIMITATIONS:

- Complex cystometry is of questionable utility in diagnosis of structural abnormalities, such as prostatic hypertrophy or stress urinary incontinence.
- Passive filling of bladder with water is unphysiologic and with CO_2, is even more unphysiologic.
- Complex cystometry does not measure urine flow, force, urethral function, and myoneural coordination. These parameters require other forms of synchronous urodynamic testing.
- Technical factors may still lead to false-positive or false-negative results. Although considered the "gold standard" for clinical bladder function testing, complex cystometry is far from perfect and more experimental techniques (eg, continuous ambulatory urodynamic monitoring) have been developed.
- Cost and inconvenience are more significant than with simple cystometry. Patient must travel to Urodynamics Laboratory.

ADDITIONAL INFORMATION: The role of complex cystometry in the evaluation of the patient with a voiding disorder (incontinence, retention, bladder discomfort) has not been agreed upon. Clearly, it provides information concerning bladder function which cannot be obtained from cystoscopy or radiographic studies. These latter two procedures examine only structural abnormalities. Some authors rely on the history and physical examination to yield a likely diagnosis and then begin a trial of empiric medical therapy to confirm this diagnosis. Only a small subset of patients undergo complex urodynamic testing. Other experts believe that voiding histories are often inaccurate and cystometry is necessary to identify the neuropathic or unstable bladder. Medical or surgical therapies may then be pursued with confidence.

Footnotes

1. Leach GE and Yip CM, "Urologic and Urodynamic Evaluation of the Elderly Population," *Clin Geriatr Med*, 1986, 2:731-55.
2. Wein AJ, English WS, and Whitmore KE, "Office Urodynamics," *Urol Clin North Am*, 1988, 15(4):609-23.
3. Tanagho EA, "Urodynamic Studies," *Smith's General Urology*, Tanagho EA and McAninch JW, eds, 12th ed, Chapter 21, Norwalk, CT: Appleton and Lange, 1988, 452-72.

References

Blaivas J, "Multichannel Urodynamic Studies," *Urology*, 1984, 23:421-38.
Hinman F, "Office Evaluation of Urodynamic Problems," *Urol Clin North Am*, 1979, 6:149-54.
International Continence Society, "First Report on the Standardization of Terminology of Lower Urinary Tract Function," *Br J Urol*, 1976, 48:39-42.
Massey A and Abrams P, "Urodynamics of the Female Lower Urinary Tract," *Urol Clin North Am*, 1985, 12:231-46.

Cystometrogram, Simple

CPT 51725

Related Information

Cystometrogram, Complex *on page 136*

Synonyms CMG; Cystometry; Filling Cystometrogram; Simple CMG; Urodynamic Testing of Bladder Function

(Continued)

Cystometrogram, Simple *(Continued)*

Abstract **PROCEDURE COMMONLY INCLUDES:** Bedside evaluation of urinary bladder function in selected patients with urinary incontinence or retention. The bladder is passively filled with sterile water through a transurethral Foley catheter. Intravesical pressures are measured with an open manometer as bladder volume increases. Information regarding bladder sensation, capacity, and contractility is obtained. **INDICATIONS:** The exact indications for simple cystometry are controversial. Even amongst urologists, considerable debate exists in the medical/surgical literature considering the optimal role of this procedure. Simple cystometry is useful in the patient with persistent urinary incontinence or retention felt to be secondary to impaired bladder filling or storage. Common clinical indications for this test include:

- suspected "neurogenic bladder"
- suspected detrusor motor instability, the hyperreflexive bladder
- suspected abnormalities in bladder sensation, capacity, or contractility
- the geriatric patient with persistent urinary incontinence of unclear etiology (controversial)

Simple cystometry is less useful in evaluating the following conditions:[1]

- suspected stress urinary incontinence in the female
- suspected psychogenic urinary incontinence in the male
- suspected urinary obstruction in the male

CONTRAINDICATIONS:

- patient refusal
- the demented patient with severe cognitive impairment; this procedure requires the patient to accurately report sensations of bladder filling
- inability to pass transurethral Foley catheter
- active urinary tract infection

Patient Care/Scheduling **PATIENT PREPARATION:** Technique and risks of the procedure are explained to the patient and consent is obtained. Ideally, patient should be off sedatives, cholinergics, or anticholinergics prior to testing. Indwelling Foley catheters should be removed well in advance so that residual volume may be measured. No pain medications or anxiolytics are routinely necessary. Patient is asked to void, if possible, immediately prior to procedure. **AFTERCARE:** No specific postprocedure restrictions are required and previous activity level may be resumed. At physician discretion, a urinalysis (and possibly urine culture) may be ordered on follow-up, 48-72 hours later. **SPECIAL INSTRUCTIONS:** Simple cystometry may be easily performed by a trained nurse or physician assistant and in most cases does not require direct physician supervision. This is a considerable advantage over complex cystometry which is usually performed in the Urodynamics Laboratory. **COMPLICATIONS:** This procedure is considered relatively safe. The vast majority of patients tolerate simple cystometry with minimal problems. Reported complications are similar to those seen with straight catheterization, such as local urethral discomfort, hematuria, and urinary tract infection. The precise complication rate is not known, but in one study involving 171 incontinent geriatric patients, <8% developed new urinary symptoms consistent with infection and <2% required antibiotic therapy.[2]

Method **EQUIPMENT:** Standard Foley catheter or 14F red rubber catheter required. Alternatively, a 3-channel Foley catheter (often used for bladder irrigation) may be used. Also needed are a urinary catheterization tray (drapes, lubricant, iodine, gloves, syringes, etc), Y-connector, 50 mL syringe, sterile water in graduated container, sterile tubing, nonsterile measuring basin. An open manometer, such as a spinal manometer, is commonly used. **TECHNIQUE:** Numerous minor variations in technique have been described with the choice depending on physician preference and patient logistics. In its simplest form, a manometer is not used. After voiding, patient is placed in supine position and a Foley catheter (or 14F red rubber straight catheter) is inserted transurethrally into the bladder. Residual urine volume is measured and the catheter is left in place. With the bladder empty, the patient is requested to relax completely and avoid all bladder or abdominal contractions for the remainder of the procedure. The inner piston of a 50 mL syringe is removed and the syringe tip inserted into the distal (open) end of the catheter. Using the syringe as a funnel, room temperature sterile water is infused through the syringe and catheter in 50 mL increments. The syringe is elevated so the highest level of the fluid column is always 15 cm above the symphysis pubis. Thus, fluid enters the bladder by gravity drainage and not forcibly by syringe pressure. After each 50 mL water, the height of the water column is observed. Patient subjectively reports first perceptible sensation of bladder fullness and first strong urge to void. When patient notes a strong voiding urge, additional volume is added in 25 mL increments until discomfort is reported or an involuntary bladder contraction occurs. A bladder contraction appears as a sharp and sustained rise in the water column despite attempted voluntary bladder relaxation (and may be seen at any time during the procedure). The procedure is terminated at this stage. This brief sequence of maneuvers has been described in several formal studies comparing simple and complex multichannel cystometry.[2,3] A common and time-honored variation of this procedure requires the use of a spinal manometer. Initial steps are identical. After residual volume is measured, a Y-connector is attached to the distal end of the Foley. Through one arm of the Y-connector, sterile water in a calibrated reservoir is instilled by gravity drainage. The other arm is connected to an open spinal manometer via sterile connecting tubing. An anaeroid manometer (Lewis cystometer) may also be used. Pressure within the tubing system is "bled off" into the manometer port. As water incrementally fills the bladder, increasing intravesicular pressure is transmitted back through the tubing and is crudely estimated by the height of the water column in the manometer. A plot of bladder pressure versus volume may be constructed in this manner. Alternatively, a 3-channel Foley may be used. Again, fluid is introduced through 1-catheter channel, but in this technique the spinal manometer is connected to a physically separate channel. This allows more accurate intravesical pressure estimations. When bladder pressure is measured in the fluid in the flow channel (as in the Y-connector arrangement), several confounding variables are introduced, such as the internal resistance to fluid in the catheter. Some of these variables are eliminated by this simple maneuver. **DATA ACQUIRED:**

- residual volume (mL)
- threshold for sensation of bladder fullness (mL) – the volume at which patient reports first sensation of fullness
- maximum cystometric capacity (mL) – the volume at which patient describes a strong urge to void, or the volume just prior to an involuntary contraction
- bladder contractility (presence and number of involuntary bladder contractions, as defined)

If a manometer is used, additional data includes:

- pressure-volume characteristics of the bladder during filling, this is termed the cystometrogram – bladder pressure (ordinate) plotted against volume (abscissa)
- bladder compliance, defined as $\Delta V/\Delta P$ and is derived from the cystometrogram.

Interpretation **NORMAL FINDINGS:** Approximated as follows:

- residual volume – usually minimal or no urine obtained
- threshold for sensation of bladder fullness, 100-200 mL
- maximum capacity, 400-500 mL
- bladder contractility, no involuntary contractions noted
- cystometrogram[4], normally divided into the following four phases: (see figure on the following page)

  Phase 1: Initial pressure rise, stabilizes at the initial filling pressure or "resting pressure," normally approximately 10 cm H_2O.

  Phase 2: The tonus limb, where compliance is high; pressure normally is low and remains constant as volume increases.

  Phase 3: The limit of bladder elastic properties; increasing volume causes marked pressure increases. Patient normally can still voluntarily control micturition, even though maximum bladder capacity has almost been reached.

  Phase 4: Voluntary voiding (not tested with simple cystometry).

- compliance – normally very high in phase two of the cystometrogram (approaching infinity)

CRITICAL VALUES: Residual volume: Significant postvoid residual may result from sensory neuropathy, lower motor neuron (LMN) disease, or bladder outlet resistance (functional or mechanical).[5]

(Continued)

Cystometrogram, Simple *(Continued)*

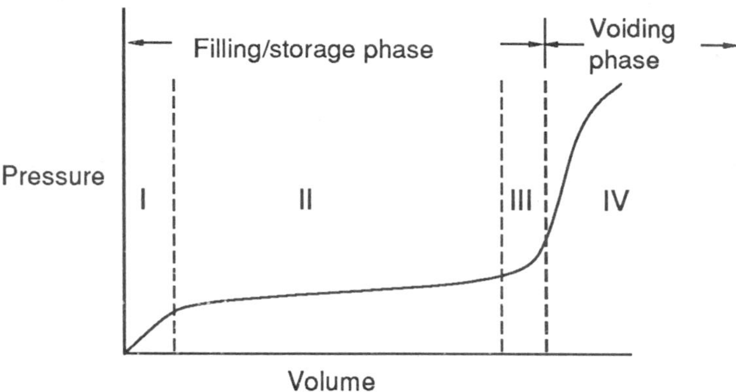

Idealized cystometrogram. Note that the voiding phase is only assessed with complex cystometry. Reproduced with permission from Wein AJ, et al, *Urol Clin North Am*, 1988, 15(4):613.

Threshold of sensation: Decreased sensation (ie, threshold >200 mL) is seen with sensory neuropathies such as diabetes mellitus, tabes dorsalis, cauda equina syndrome, or normal variant.

Maximum capacity: Decreased in a variety of disorders including upper motor neuron (UMN) disease, fibrotic bladder (eg, tuberculous interstitial cystitis), dysfunctionalized bladder, etc. Increased capacity (>500 mL) is seen with sensory neuropathy, LMN disease, chronic obstruction, bladder "training".

Contractility: Involuntary contractions at volumes less than capacity are abnormal. This condition has been called "detrusor hyperreflexia" and "uninhibited" or "unstable" bladder. Increased contractility is found in various stroke syndromes, UMN lesions, hypertrophic bladder. Contractility is absent or weak in LMN lesions, sensory neuropathies, or voluntary inhibition.

Cystometrogram: Both the pattern of the tracing (pressure vs volume) and the absolute values should be compared against a standard normal curve. Some cystometrogram patterns may be diagnostic but tracings generated from simple cystometry are crude and may be difficult to interpret. (See figure in Cystometry, Complex.)

Compliance: A noncompliant bladder may result from a variety of disorders, including bladder wall fibrosis, bladder contraction, idiopathic male enuresis.

LIMITATIONS: Procedure has questionable utility in the diagnosis of voiding disorders due to structural abnormalities, such as stress urinary incontinence or prostatic hypertrophy with retention, or complex voiding disorders. By nature, passive filling of the bladder is nonphysiologic and may potentially alter measured variables (eg, bladder capacity) in yet-to-be-understood ways. Only urologic function related to the bladder is assessed. Urine flow, force, urethral function, and myoneural coordination are not tested. Numerous technical factors may lead to false-positive or false-negative results. As previously mentioned, intravesical pressure is only crudely estimated by spinal manometry and is limited by confounding factors, such as inflow tubing resistance. Phase 4 of the standard cystometrogram is not evaluated (ie, the voiding phase of micturition). Complex cystometry is required for this. Increases in intra-abdominal pressure will alter pressure readings. This is not controlled for adequately in this procedure. Increases in manometric pressure readings may be due to increased intravesical pressure, increased abdominal wall pressure, or both. Thus, any abdominal muscle contraction may be misinterpreted as a bladder contraction. Although the examiner may simply observe the patient's abdomen for signs of muscle contraction, this is imprecise. With complex cystometry this is avoided by simultaneously recording intravesical and anorectal pressures (which estimate intra-abdominal pressure). The cystometrogram generated by manometer readings is discontinuous and crude. Provocative measures (position changes, medications, etc) are not routinely performed. These are usually reserved for complex cystometry. **ADDITIONAL INFORMATION:** The main advantage of simple cystometry is its convenience and low cost in comparison with more complex urodynamic testing. It may be performed by a trained nurse in less than minutes and need not be done in a hospital setting. Thus, it has been advocated for the evaluation of the nursing home patient or the elderly clinic patient. Several studies have compared simple and complex cystometry directly. Sutherst and Brown (1984) found that simple cystometry achieved a sensitivity of 100% for bladder instability with 89% specificity (when compared with complex cystometry as a gold standard). Ouslander (1988) also showed a high degree of correlation between the two tests in terms of bladder capacity and stability. However, the role of cystometry has not been clearly defined. Some authorities believe that only a small percentage of patients with voiding disorders need to undergo cystometry. This subpopulation may be identified using statistically derived algorithms based primarily on historical and physical examination findings.[6] Others feel that the urologic history is misleading often enough (or inaccurate in the demented geriatric patient) to justify frequent use of simple cystometry. In many cases, it is argued, management of a voiding disorder will be influenced by the objective results from cystometry. In all cases, test results must be interpreted in conjunction with the clinical suspicion.

Footnotes

1. Hinman F, "Office Evaluation of Urodynamic Problems," *Urol Clin North Am*, 1979, 6:149-54.
2. Ouslander J, Leach G, Abelson S, et al, "Simple Versus Multichannel Cystometry in the Evaluation of Bladder Function in an Incontinent Geriatric Population," *J Urol*, 1988, 140(6):1482-6.
3. Sutherst JR and Brown MC, "Comparison of Single and Multichannel Cystometry in Diagnosing Bladder Instability," *Br Med J [Clin Res]*, 1984, 288:1720.
4. Wein AJ, English WS, and Whitmore KE, "Office Urodynamics," *Urol Clin North Am*, 1988, 15(4):609-23.
5. Tanagho EA, "Urodynamic Studies," *Smith's General Urology*, Tanagho EA and McAninch JW, eds, 12th ed, Chapter 21, Norwalk, CT: Appleton and Lange, 1988, 452-72.
6. Hilton P and Stanton SL, "Algorithmic Method for Assessing Urinary Incontinence in Elderly Women," *Br Med J [Clin Res]*, 1981, 282:940.

Cystometry *see* Cystometrogram, Simple *on page 139*

Filling Cystometrogram *see* Cystometrogram, Simple *on page 139*

Injection of the Corpora Cavernosa With Pharmacologic Agents (Papaverine, Phentolamine)

CPT 54235

Related Information

Nocturnal Penile Tumescence Test *on page 150*
Penile Blood Flow *on page 152*

Synonyms Intracavernous Injection of Papaverine; Papaverine Test

Abstract **PROCEDURE COMMONLY INCLUDES:** Injection of a vasoactive compound such as papaverine into the corpora cavernosa of the penis in order to produce an erection. Papaverine is a phosphodiesterase inhibitor which relaxes smooth muscle (both vascular and nonvascular) and stimulates venous congestion. The cavernous tissue of the penis becomes filled with blood and a pharmacologic erection is induced. This procedure is useful in evaluating men with erectile dysfunction. It has been used to differentiate organic (biologic) impotence from psychogenic impotence. Papaverine injection produces a full erection in healthy males as well as individuals with psychogenic impotence. In patients with vasculogenic impotence, however, papaverine injection is unlikely to produce an erection. Thus, if a full erection results from papaverine injection, vascular insufficiency is probably excluded as the cause of impotence. **INDICATIONS:** The Papaverine Test is useful in identifying patients whose erectile dysfunction is secondary to vascular insufficiency. It may also be used to confirm results obtained from nocturnal penile tumescence testing, particularly

(Continued)

Injection of the Corpora Cavernosa With Pharmacologic Agents (Papaverine, Phentolamine) *(Continued)*

when unsupervised home testing is performed (see Nocturnal Penile Tumescence Test). **CONTRAINDICATIONS:** Relative contraindications to testing include:

- prior adverse reaction to papaverine
- uncorrectable coagulopathy
- orthostatic hypotension
- hemoglobinopathies (sickle cell trait, sickle cell disease, etc)

Patient Care/Scheduling **PATIENT PREPARATION:** A medical history and physical examination is required for all patients with erectile failure. Screening laboratory studies such as prolactin, follicle stimulating hormone (FSH), luteinizing hormone (LH), and testosterone are often ordered prior to any procedures. If the patient is a good candidate, the technique of papaverine injection is discussed with the patient along with potential complications. Informed consent is obtained. Special scheduling for this procedure is not necessary since injection is performed quickly in a physician's office. **AFTERCARE:** All patients should remain in the testing center until the erection has completely subsided. In the majority of patients this occurs spontaneously within hours or minutes, but a few may require pharmacologic reversal. Reversal is performed either by aspiration alone or by injection of epinephrine plus aspiration. **COMPLICATIONS:** Intracavernous injection is a safe procedure. Minor adverse reactions include priapism, lightheadedness, and penile hematoma. As noted above, priapism can be reversed if necessary.

Method **TECHNIQUE:** Papaverine injection may be carried out in conjunction with objective measurements of penile tumescence, such as Snap-Gauge or Rigiscan (see Nocturnal Penile Tumescence Test). These devices are optional. The penis is examined immediately prior to testing. The flaccid penis is injected with papaverine hydrochloride and, if desired, phentolamine mesylate also. Phentolamine decreases adrenergic tone and facilitates smooth muscle relaxation. A fine hypodermic needle is commonly used, such as a 26-gauge, 3/8" needle. No local anesthesia is required. A tourniquet is not necessary and the injection is made directly into the corpora cavernosa. Usual doses employed are 50 mg of papaverine and 1-6 mg of phentolamine in a volume of 2 mL. After injection, the patient is asked to stand next to the examination table and penile response is then observed. **DATA ACQUIRED:**

- time elapsed from injection to maximal penile response
- observer's subjective rating of erection quality: absent, partially rigid, full tumescence, and rigidity
- objective measurement of penile tumescence (in millimeters) and/or rigidity (from 0% to 100%) if formal monitoring devices are used
- duration of erection.

Interpretation **NORMAL FINDINGS:** Healthy individuals with normal sexual function achieve full erections after papaverine injection. Studies also suggest that men with psychogenic impotence also respond with full erections after papaverine. Most erections are produced within 10 minutes of injection and may last several hours. **CRITICAL VALUES:** Absent or partial erections after papaverine injection suggest a vascular cause for impotence. An incomplete erectile response may also be secondary to other factors such as excessive patient anxiety, incorrect technique, etc. Thus, some authors regard an incomplete response as "inconclusive" and not diagnostic of vascular insufficiency. A normal erectile response makes vasculogenic impotence unlikely. **ADDITIONAL INFORMATION:** Intracavernous injection with papaverine was first introduced in the early 1980s. Since then it has grown in popularity, due to its safety, convenience, and speed. It is easier to perform than formal, overnight nocturnal penile tumescence monitoring. It also is a dynamic assessment of erectile function, unlike the penile brachial index (PBI) which measures blood flow in the flaccid penis. More research is required for this promising technique.

References

Abber JC, Lue TF, and Orvis BR, "Diagnostic Tests for Impotence: A Comparison of Papaverine Injection With the Penile-Brachial Index and Nocturnal Penile Tumescence Monitoring," *J Urol*, 1986, 135:923-5.

Buvat J, Buvat-Herbaut M, DeHaene JL, et al, "Is Intracavernous Injection of Papaverine a Reliable Screening Test for Vascular Impotence?" *J Urol*, 1986, 135:476-8.

Lakin MM and Montague DK, "Intracavernous Injections of Papaverine and Phentolamine: Correlation With Penile Brachial Index," *Urology*, 1989, 33(5):383-6.

Virag R, Frydman D, Legman M, et al, "Intracavernous Injection of Papaverine as a Diagnostic and Therapeutic Method in Erectile Failure," *Angiology*, 1984, 35:79-87.

Intracavernous Injection of Papaverine *see* Injection of the Corpora Cavernosa With Pharmacologic Agents (Papaverine, Phentolamine) *on page 143*

Iron Stain *see* Bone Marrow Aspiration and Biopsy *on page 132*

Kidney Biopsy

CPT 50200 (renal biopsy, needle); 88304 (surgical pathology); 88312 (special stains); 88346 (immunofluorescence); 88348 (electron microscopy)

Related Information

Ultrasound, Kidney Biopsy *on page 402*

Synonyms Closed Kidney (Renal) Biopsy; Renal Biopsy

Abstract **PROCEDURE COMMONLY INCLUDES:** Biopsy of the renal parenchyma for diagnostic purposes. In most cases this is performed percutaneously under local anesthesia, either as a "blind" procedure or under ultrasound guidance. Fresh kidney specimens are sent for gross and microscopic analysis, including H & E stain, PAS/PAMS stain, immunofluorescence staining, and in selected cases, scanning electron microscopy. Kidney biopsy is useful in diagnosing primary (intrinsic) renal disease, assessing the nature and severity of renal involvement in various systemic disorders, and (less commonly) establishing the diagnosis of certain systemic diseases (eg, amyloidosis). **INDICATIONS:** The exact indications for performing a renal biopsy are not universally agreed upon and opinions vary widely amongst nephrologists, despite almost four decades of experience. There continues to be lively debate in the medical literature over these indications. Glassock and Massry classify their procedural indications as follows:[1]

"Most useful" indications include:

- idiopathic nephrotic syndrome in the adult (prior to empirical glucocorticoid therapy)
- non-nephrotic range proteinuria (1-2 g/day) of unknown cause accompanied by an abnormal urinary sediment
- proteinuria with glomerular hematuria (ie, urinary tract infections and neoplasms have been excluded)
- acute renal failure of unknown cause, when obstruction has been ruled out the diagnosis of acute tubular necrosis cannot be established clinically, both kidneys are of normal size
- suspected cases of rapidly progressive glomerulonephritis (RPGN) or the acute nephritic syndrome
- suspected cases of active lupus nephritis, characterized by hematuria (>6 RBCs/hpf), proteinuria (>200 mg/day), and elevated serum creatinine
- suspected cases of renal vasculitis, particularly polyarteritis nodosa and Wegener's granulomatosis (which often requires aggressive combination therapy)
- evaluation of the renal allotransplant patient with possible graft rejection, acute tubular necrosis (ATN), drug-induced interstitial nephritis, infarction, or recurrence of original disease in the graft

"Possible useful" indications include:

- persistent glomerular hematuria without proteinuria
- proteinuria >1 g/day with normal urinary sediment
- evaluation of suspected inherited glomerular diseases such as Alport's or Fabry's disease
- evaluation of the known diabetic with rapid, unexpected deterioration of renal function, sudden development of nephrotic syndrome, or early development of azotemia in the absence of diabetic retinopathy

Renal biopsy is "not useful" in evaluating:

- malignant hypertension
- polycystic kidney disease

(Continued)

Kidney Biopsy *(Continued)*

- hepatorenal syndrome
- pyelonephritis
- chronic renal failure with shrunken kidneys
- routine cases of diabetic nephropathy
- clinically silent lupus nephritis (controversial)

Proponents of kidney biopsy believe that a definitive histologic diagnosis of a specific renal disease should be made prior to any empirical trial of immunosuppressives (ie, cases of nephrotic syndrome, RPGN, etc). Opponents of early kidney biopsy believe that empirical steroids should be attempted first with careful monitoring of renal function. Usually kidney biopsy is unnecessary whether or not the renal disease is steroid-responsive. This latter opinion is based primarily on group statistical studies and decision analysis theory. Certainly, the details of each individual case must be reviewed prior to decision-making regarding biopsy. The costs and potential complications of the procedure should be weighed against the probability of altering patient management based on the biopsy results.

CONTRAINDICATIONS: Absolute contraindications:

- uncorrectable and clinically severe bleeding diathesis
- patient refusal

Relative contraindications:

- severe thrombocytopenia, $<50,000/mm^3$ (usually correctable by platelet infusion)
- solitary kidney (except with a renal allograft)
- renal artery aneurysm
- active pyelonephritis or perinephric abscess
- hydronephrosis
- uncontrolled severe hypertension
- uncorrected volume depletion

A prolonged Ivy bleeding time is commonly seen in patients with renal failure, due in part to platelet dysfunction. This does **not** represent a contraindication to kidney biopsy.[1] At the worst, it should be considered a high risk situation. Experience in several centers has demonstrated the safety of kidney biopsy in this setting. In some centers, however, desmopressin (DDAVP®) is infused prior to biopsy in order to normalize the bleeding time in azotemic patients but this practice has not been widely accepted. Other potentially high risk situations (not contraindications) include:

- moderate thrombocytopenia, $100,000\text{-}150,000/mm^3$
- moderate hypertension
- BUN >100 mg/dL (considered a contraindication in the 1950s)

Patient Care/Scheduling **PATIENT PREPARATION:** Procedure and risks of the procedure are explained and informed consent is obtained. Patient should understand that kidney biopsy usually requires a 24-hour hospital stay postprocedure. All administrative issues related to the planned hospitalization should be completed in advance. If patient is on antihypertensive medications he should be instructed to continue these up to and including the day of admission (unless directed otherwise by physician). Some nephrologists customarily obtain a platelet count, PT, and PTT on the day of the procedure, while others order these tests only when coagulopathy is suspected. As previously mentioned, the Ivy bleeding time has limited clinical utility in this setting and need not be routinely ordered for the azotemic patient. A hematocrit and urinalysis are often obtained as a baseline reference for later comparison with postprocedure values. Except in unusual, high risk situations, it is not necessary to type and crossmatch blood for transfusion. Premedication with a short-acting benzodiazepine may be helpful in the anxious patient. In some centers, I.V. access is routinely established (heparin lock and D_5W at a maintenance rate). Vital signs are recorded beforehand and physician is informed if blood pressure is elevated. **AFTERCARE:** Immediately after biopsy is completed, vital signs are obtained. If stable, patient should lie supine in bed for at least 12 hours. Pulse and blood pressure are monitored four times at 15-minute intervals, two times at 30-minute intervals, three times at 1-hour intervals, then every 4 hours until discharge (usual total hospital time is 24 hours). Hematocrits are obtained at 12 and 24 hours after procedure routinely or prn if gross hematuria or hypotension develops. Commonly, all voided urine samples are collected by nursing staff, saved in labeled plastic containers at the bedside, and serially examined for gross and microscopic hematuria. Physician should be contacted if gross hematuria occurs, hematocrit drops significantly, severe pain at biopsy site persists, or blood pressure falls. These may be indicative of an enlarging hematoma. After hospital discharge, patient should avoid heavy lifting, strenuous exercise, and contact sports for 1-2 weeks. **SPECIAL INSTRUCTIONS:** Special handling of the specimen may be necessary when certain diseases are suspected. Standard tissue processing is usually insufficient for analyzing glycogen, uric acid crystals, and other crystal diseases. The Pathology Laboratory should be contacted in advance in these special circumstances. **COMPLICATIONS:** The precise complication risk for an individual patient is difficult to predict, since this figure is heavily influenced by the skill of the operator and the presence of relative contraindications.

Common complications include:

- microscopic hematuria, present in nearly every case (thus, some authorities do not consider this a complication)
- perirenal hematoma, also very common; usually self-limited and asymptomatic, but may be seen on ultrasound or CT scan
- postbiopsy pain, usually described as a dull ache. More pronounced pain may signify expanding hematoma.

Less common complications:

- aggravation of hypertension
- persistent perirenal bleeding and gross hematuria. Blood transfusion is required in approximately 1 out of 500 biopsies; surgical intervention in 1 out of 1000.[1]
- arteriovenous fistula formation; reported in ≤10% of biopsies, usually asymptomatic but sometimes may cause hematuria
- kidney rupture
- calyceal fissure
- puncture of pancreas, bowel, spleen, liver
- laceration of aorta or renal artery
- death (1:1000 to 1:3000)

In one large series, overall complication rate was estimated at 2.1%, out of 5500 reported biopsies.[2] Complications included expanding hematoma and bleeding requiring blood transfusion or nephrectomy. Mortality was approximately 1 in 1000. In another recent survey, 94 complications were reported from 1000 consecutive biopsies (gross hematuria accounted for 73%).[3] Thus, textbook estimates of complications range from 2% to 10%.

Method **EQUIPMENT:** Kidney biopsy is obtained using either a Travenol Trucut needle or a Vim-Silverman needle. The former is a one-piece, disposable apparatus 11.4 cm long (≤15 cm), consisting of a needle with cannula and obturator. The Vim-Silverman needle is also commonly employed and is composed of three separate pieces: obturator, cannula with sharpened end, and two semicircular cutting blades. A 23-gauge finder needle is used by some nephrologists. Various needles and syringes are used for local anesthesia, with some preferring a long needle (6" – 20-gauge) for deep tissue anesthesia. Other standard equipment includes a scalpel blade, lidocaine, sterile drapes, Betadine®, gauze, gowns and masks, specimen containers. **TECHNIQUE:** The procedure is performed by an experienced nephrologist. This procedure requires subspecialty training and is outside the realm of the generalist. Briefly, the patient is placed in a prone position with a pad or rolled towel under the abdomen. Either the right or left kidney may be biopsied and individual physician preferences differ. The ideal site is the outer aspect of the lower pole of the selected kidney where there is less risk of vascular puncture. This is located by using either bedside ultrasound or anatomic landmarks (lower portion of the 12th rib and spinous processes of the lumbar vertebrae) and usually lies approximately 2 cm inferior to the 12th rib. Using formal sterile technique (masks, caps, gowns, etc), the desired area is prepped with Betadine® and draped. Skin is anesthetized with lidocaine in the usual manner. A small cutaneous incision is made with the scalpel blade and then carried several centimeters deeper into subcutaneous tissues. Lidocaine is liberally injected along this incision using a long (6") anesthesia needle, infiltrating down to the kidney. (At this point, some physicians opt to use a "finder needle" in order to estimate the depth of the kidney below the skin.) The biopsy needle is then advanced slowly through this incision with the patient holding

(Continued)

Kidney Biopsy *(Continued)*

his breath each time the needle is pushed forward. Once the renal capsule has been penetrated, the patient is asked to breathe normally. If the needle apparatus is in proper position, the distal (visible) end of the needle will move in a pendulous fashion with inspiration and expiration in a characteristic "arc". The patient holds his breath in inspiration and the biopsy core is obtained. Details regarding biopsy trocar manipulation differ for the Vim-Silverman and the Travenol Trucut needles. The biopsy needle is withdrawn from the patient and the specimen is removed. In most instances, a second (and sometimes third) pass is made with the biopsy needle, using identical technique, so that several tissue cores are obtained. **DATA ACQUIRED:** Biopsy tissue for laboratory analysis.

Specimen Fresh renal parenchymal tissue (not yet placed in fixative). Usually has a somewhat cylindrical appearance and may be up to 2 cm long, although often smaller (ie, 4-8 mm). To date, no one single method of tissue fixation has been devised for light microscopy, electron microscopy (EM), and immunofluorescence (IF) staining. Thus, if only a single biopsy core has been obtained it must be physically sectioned, usually into three portions along the short axis. At the minimum, pathology laboratories require 6-12 glomeruli for light microscopy, 4-6 glomeruli for IF, and 2-3 for EM. Of course, larger numbers of glomeruli are always preferred so as not to overlook focal renal disease, but technically this is not always possible. Three separate biopsy cores from three separate needle passes is ideal from the pathologist's viewpoint. **CONTAINER:** Sterile jar or Petri dish, sterile towels, or gauze moistened with saline are sometimes used for transport of specimen for frozen sectioning. **COLLECTION:** For light microscopy, specimen is placed in buffered formalin. Alternative fixatives include Zenker's and Bouin's solutions, among others. Later, the fixed specimen undergoes dehydration prior to being embedded (usually in paraffin), then is sectioned and mounted on slides. Commonly used tissue stains include H & E, PAS, and PAMS (periodic acid-methanamine silver); optional stains include congo red for amyloid. For electron microscopy, the specimen is placed in glutaraldehyde solution. All further specimen processing takes place in a specialized EM laboratory. For immunofluorescence microscopy, the specimen needs to be immediately frozen then cryosectioned. Subsequently, the specimen is stained for the presence of IgG, IgM, IgA, C_3, C_1q, and other serum proteins. Either monoclonal antibodies or fluorescent antisera directed against these proteins is used. **CAUSES FOR REJECTION:** Initial specimen allowed to dry out before fixing, incorrect fixative, inadequate specimen size, delay in transit time to laboratory (especially for frozen sections).

Interpretation **NORMAL FINDINGS:** No abnormalities seen on gross, histologic, IF microscopy, or EM. However, a "normal" biopsy in a patient with clinically suspected renal disease (elevated serum creatinine, active urinary sediment, etc) may be solely a result of sampling error. In other words, some disease processes may be focal (eg, focal segmental glomerulosclerosis), variable (lupus nephritis), or early. A typical biopsy section may sample only 10 glomeruli, out of >1,000,000 glomeruli found in each kidney. Final report is issued by pathologist. **CRITICAL VALUES:** The specimen is examined by the pathologist in a step-wise, systematic manner. Any abnormal finding is reported along with pertinent normal structural findings.[4]

Gross examination: specimen size, color, and consistency noted. Proportion of cortex and medulla estimated. Pale areas with surrounding hyperemia may be suggestive of necrosis, infarction, infectious inflammation.

Light microscopy: H & E, PAS, PAMS sections systematically studied. Features such as sample size (number of glomeruli), integrity of renal architecture, and acute vs chronic nephron loss noted. The following structures are examined.

- Glomeruli: Attention paid to important abnormalities such as glomerulosclerosis, crescents, thickened or disrupted glomerular basement membrane (GBM), mesangial expansion
- Renal tubules: Rule out ischemic or toxic tubular damage, tubular atrophy, epithelial abnormalities, inflammatory infiltrates, intraluminal casts and RBCs, etc
- Interstitium: Rule out interstitial fibrosis, extracellular crystals, edema, inflammatory cells (ie, perivascular or peritubular inflammation), granulomas
- Vasculature: Rule out emboli, thrombi, arteriosclerosis, hyaline deposits, necrotizing vasculitis

When present, glomerular disease is conventionally reported as "focal" (some glomeruli diseased but most are normal), "generalized" (only a few glomeruli spared), "segmental" (only a portion of an individual glomerulus effected), "diffuse" (entire glomerulus diseased).

Electron microscopy: Typically only a few nephrons are scanned in detail. Of the different components of the nephron, EM is most useful in detecting glomerular pathology. Anatomic structures within the glomerulus can be examined with high resolution, including Bowman's capsule, the glomerular basement membrane (GBM), endothelium, and mesangium. Some structural abnormalities can only be demonstrable by EM. In minimal change disease, diffuse foot process effacement is detectable on EM but not light microscopy. Also, immune complex deposition disease may sometimes be evident by EM when light microscopy and IF microscopy are negative or equivocal. Immune complexes typically appear as "election dense deposits" on EM. Of clinical importance, these deposits may be accurately localized to the subendothelium, subepithelium, mesangium, or basement membrane. The location and pattern of these deposits may be diagnostic of specific renal disease. Other pathologic conditions that may be evident on EM are amyloidosis, microangiopathic injury (as in thrombotic thrombocytopenia purpura), and various storage diseases (Gaucher's).

Immunofluorescence microscopy: Frozen sections are analyzed for the presence and distribution of serum proteins in kidney tissue, particularly immune complexes, or antibodies to GBM. After "staining" with monoclonal antibodies directed against immunoglobulins and complement, the specimen is studied under a fluorescence microscope. Four staining patterns are common:

- linear deposits along the GBM
- granular deposits in subepithelium, coarse (as in poststreptococcal glomerulonephritis) or fine (as in membranous glomerulonephritis)
- granular subendothelial deposits, coarse or fine
- mesangial deposits

Data acquired separately from histologic inspection, IF microscopy, and EM are integrated to form the final interpretation. As mentioned, a combination of findings may be pathognomonic. For example, Goodpasture's syndrome is characterized by linear deposits of specific anti-GBM antibody with C_3 deposition on immunofluorescence, but light microscopy is variable (from nearly normal glomeruli to many crescents) and EM findings are negative for dense deposits. For a discussion of typical biopsy findings in the many primary and secondary renal diseases see Schrier's textbook, *Diseases of the Kidney*.[4]

LIMITATIONS: When primary (intrinsic) renal disease is present, kidney biopsy is in many instances diagnostic. Exceptions to this include advanced glomerular disease where pathologic findings become nonspecific, technical error, and sampling bias (diseased glomeruli not present on small biopsy sample). Primary glomerular disease is also one cause of rapidly progressive glomerulonephritis (RPGN), a syndrome characterized by extracapillary crescent formation. However, a long list of diseases is associated with crescent formation and this often becomes a nonspecific finding. Unless other clues are present in such cases, the precise nature of the underlying renal disease (whether primary or not) will remain obscure. When the kidney is secondarily involved by systemic disease, biopsy findings are often nondiagnostic. Pathologic changes may be reported as "typical of" or "consistent with" a particular systemic disease, but findings are seldom pathognomonic. For example, biopsy results are usually nonspecific in Wegener's granulomatosis, diabetes mellitus, TTP, and multiple myeloma.[5] These multisystem diseases are more easily diagnosed by alternative methods of testing. **ADDITIONAL INFORMATION:** Kidney biopsy is valuable in diagnosing primary renal disease and in assessing the severity of renal disease in known systemic disorders. In addition, prognostic information and response to medical therapy may be gained from biopsy. Despite the controversy surrounding the exact indications for this procedure, it is often clinically important to define the nature and extent of kidney pathology, in order to guide therapy in a rational manner and predict the natural course of disease. This becomes particularly important in the renal transplant candidate. On occasion, a high risk patient may undergo an open surgical kidney biopsy instead of a closed needle biopsy. The former is performed by a urologist in a formal operative suite and is usually reserved for the patient with a significant coagulopathy which might require direct tamponade of bleeding sites.

(Continued)

Kidney Biopsy *(Continued)*

Footnotes

1. Glassock RJ and Massry SG, "Renal Biopsy," *Textbook of Nephrology*, 2nd ed, Chapter 92, Baltimore, MD: Williams & Wilkins, 1989, 1577-80.
2. Hlatky MA, "Is Renal Biopsy Necessary in Adults With Nephrotic Syndrome?" *Lancet II*, 1982, 2:1264-7.
3. Diaz-Buxo JA and Donadio JV, "Complications of Percutaneous Renal Biopsy: An Analysis of 1000 Consecutive Biopsies," *Clin Nephrol*, 1975, 4:223-7.
4. Tisher CC and Croker BP, "Indications for and Interpretation of the Renal Biopsy: Evaluation by Light, Electron, and Immunofluorescence Microscopy," *Diseases of the Kidney*, 4th ed, Chapter 15, Schrier RW and Gottschalk CW, eds, Boston, MA/Toronto: Little, Brown and Co, 1988, 527-56.
5. Dennis VW, "Investigations of Renal Function," *Cecil Textbook of Medicine*, 18th ed, Chapter 76, Wyngaarden JB and Smith LH, eds, Philadelphia, PA: WB Saunders Co, 1988, 527-8.

Multichannel Cystometrogram *see* Cystometrogram, Complex *on page 136*

Nocturnal Erection Monitoring *see* Nocturnal Penile Tumescence Test *on this page*

Nocturnal Penile Tumescence Test

CPT 54250

Related Information

Injection of the Corpora Cavernosa With Pharmacologic Agents (Papaverine, Phentolamine) *on page 143*

Penile Blood Flow *on page 152*

Synonyms Nocturnal Erection Monitoring; NPT; Sleep Erection Monitoring

Abstract PROCEDURE COMMONLY INCLUDES: Objective measurement of penile tumescence and/or rigidity during sleep to document the presence of sleep-associated erections. Nocturnal penile tumescence (NPT) testing may be performed in a formal Sleep Laboratory under electroencephalographic monitoring or at the patient's home using inexpensive portable devices. A variety of these screening devices are available, such as the mercury-filled strain gauge (records maximal changes in penile circumference), the Snap-Gauge (records penile rigidity), and the Rigiscan (records continuous rigidity and tumescence). NPT monitoring is a frequently used ancillary test of erectile dysfunction and is based on the assumption that men with psychogenic impotence have normal erections during sleep, whereas men with organic impotence have impaired erections during sleep. INDICATIONS: NPT testing is indicated when the etiology of erectile failure is unclear after a complete medical history and physical. This procedure may be useful in differentiating organic impotence (ie, from diabetes, medications) from psychogenic impotence. It should be noted that NPT testing is based on a number of assumptions which have recently come under some scrutiny. Important limitations exist. CONTRAINDICATIONS: There are no absolute contraindications to NPT testing. However, the following are several situations where home NPT monitoring may be inappropriate. In these instances, the results of unsupervised home NPT monitoring are unreliable. Formal sleep monitoring in a laboratory may be more accurate and reliable.

- patient with dementia
- patient with poor vision or poor hand coordination who is unable to apply penile loops
- patient with suspected malingering behavior

Patient Care/Scheduling PATIENT PREPARATION: The details of NPT testing are discussed with the patient and consent is obtained. If the procedure is to be performed at home, several guidelines are useful. Patient should maintain his normal sleeping hours as much as possible. Interruptions should be minimized. Heavy alcohol or narcotic use should be avoided due to the potential suppressive effects on erectile function. Similarly, sleeping medications should be avoided unless under a physician's specific instructions. Patient should take his usual prescription medications unless otherwise directed by physician. In certain cases, NPT testing is best performed in a Sleep Laboratory with all night polygraphic sleep monitoring. This form of testing is valid, reliable, and expensive. Testing may need to be repeated on a second night (and sometimes a third night) if there is evidence of erectile dysfunction on the first night. Similar caveats regarding alcohol and narcotic use also apply. The details of scheduling are handled by the referring physician in conjunction with the Sleep Laboratory. **AFTERCARE:** No specific activity restrictions are necessary. **COMPLICATIONS:** None. NPT testing is a safe, noninvasive procedure.

Method **TECHNIQUE:** Several devices are available for home NPT monitoring and are briefly described below. Other similar devices are also available.

- NPT stamp test: This simple screening test uses adhesive paper stamps 1 1/4" x 1" similar to postage stamps. A strip of four stamps is snugly wrapped around the penis with the overlying stamp wetted and sealed. The following morning the stamp ring is examined for breaks along the perforations. This may be repeated over a three night period.
- Strain-Gauge: This device measures changes in penile circumference. An elastic loop is placed around the shaft of the penis. The loop contains a conductive medium such as mercury. An increase in penile circumference causes a stretching of the loop and a change in electrical signal. This is recorded on a portable monitor.
- Snap-Gauge (Dacomed Corp, Minneapolis, MN): This measures penile rigidity, unlike the previous techniques which measure only penile circumference. Three plastic elements are arranged in parallel on a Velcro fastener which is wrapped around the penis. Each plastic film breaks at a predetermined rigidity of the penis (ie, 10 oz, 15 oz, 20 oz).
- Rigiscan (Dacomed Corp, Minneapolis, MN): This device consists of two loops surrounding the penis, attached to a small computer with memory capacity. The Rigiscan measures both penile tumescence and rigidity on a continuous basis.

Interpretation **NORMAL FINDINGS:** Data acquired by home NPT testing is reviewed by physician. The definition of a positive or normal test is highly dependent on the type of monitoring technique employed. For example, a normal Stamp Test consists of a stamp ring broken at the perforations. This indicates that at least one nocturnal erection has occurred, but it provides no data regarding rigidity of erection, movement artifact, frequency, and duration of erections. For the Snap-Gauge, a normal test is defined as rupture of all three plastic elements. Again, this device does not assess erection duration or frequency. More complex instruments such as the mercury-filled Strain-Gauge and the Rigiscan provide continuous data over an extended time period. Normal values for penile tumescence and rigidity have been generated from healthy individuals. For the Rigiscan, penile tumescence is measured in millimeters at the base and the tip of the penis and penile rigidity is reported on a relative scale (0% to 100%) and is also measured at the base and tip. A 60% rigidity value by Rigiscan corresponds to the lowest intracorporeal pressure necessary for an erection. Although normative values have been established, the criteria for diagnosing organic impotence are variable and not well established. The precise cut-points for diagnosing organic impotence have not been agreed upon. **LIMITATIONS:**

- basic assumptions underlying NPT have been challenged by some
- home NPT devices have a significant false-positive and false-negative rate
- supervised NPT testing with polysomnogram recording is expensive and labor intensive
- specific criteria used to diagnose organic impotence has not been standardized
- few studies have addressed the diagnostic accuracy of home NPT devices
- patients with the penile-steal syndrome may have normal NPT results
- motion artifact may be misleading and significant

ADDITIONAL INFORMATION: As reviewed by Schiavi,[1] NPT testing is based on several assumptions:

- NPT is normal in men with psychogenic impotence
- normal NPT excludes organic impotence
- NPT is abnormal in men with organic impotence

The weight of the data available supports these three assumptions. However, each has been challenged and it is likely that exceptions exist to each of these "rules." Thus, if NPT

(Continued)

Nocturnal Penile Tumescence Test *(Continued)*

testing is normal in a patient in whom vasculogenic impotence is strongly suspected, further diagnostic evaluation may be warranted. Nevertheless, this procedure is safe, well-tolerated and often valid. Effective therapeutic interventions are available for men with either vasculogenic or psychogenic impotence, and thus this differentiation becomes important clinically. An abnormal NPT result often prompts further investigative studies of a more invasive nature. Formal NPT testing in a sleep laboratory is considered by some experts to be the best (and perhaps the only) test capable of differentiating organic from psychogenic impotence.

Footnotes

1. Schiavi RC, "Nocturnal Penile Tumescence in the Evaluation of Erectile Disorders: A Critical Review," *J Sex Marital Ther*, 1988, 14(2):83-97.

References

Barry JM, Blank B, and Boileau M, "Nocturnal Penile Tumescence Monitoring With Stamps," *Urology*, 1980, 15(2):171-2.

Bohlen JG, "Sleep Erection Monitoring in the Evaluation of Male Erectile Failure," *Urol Clin North Am*, 1981, 8(1):119-34.

Bradley WE, "New Techniques in Evaluation of Impotence," *Urology*, 1987, 29(4):383-8.

Melman A, "Evaluation and Management of Erectile Dysfunction," *Surg Clin North Am*, 1988, 68(5):965-81.

Schiavi RC, "Nocturnal Penile Tumescence in the Evaluation of Erectile Disorders: A Critical Review," *J Sex Marital Ther*, 1988, 14(2):83-97.

Schmidt HS and Wise HA, "Significance of Impaired Penile Tumescence and Associated Polysomnographic Abnormalities in the Impotent Patient," *J Urol*, 1981, 126:348-52.

NPT *see* Nocturnal Penile Tumescence Test *on page 150*

Papaverine Test *see* Injection of the Corpora Cavernosa With Pharmacologic Agents (Papaverine, Phentolamine) *on page 143*

Penile Blood Flow

CPT 76999 (unlisted procedure)

Related Information

Injection of the Corpora Cavernosa With Pharmacologic Agents (Papaverine, Phentolamine) *on page 143*

Nocturnal Penile Tumescence Test *on page 150*

Ultrasound, Penile *on page 408*

Synonyms Penile Doppler Studies

Applies to Penile Blood Pressure as Compared to Brachial Blood Pressure

Replaces Arteriogram

Abstract PROCEDURE COMMONLY INCLUDES: Compression of penis with pneumatic cuff and measurement of systolic blood pressure. Brachial blood pressure is also recorded. INDICATIONS: To determine if the cause of impotence is vasculogenic. It is also used in postoperative evaluation of penile blood flow following lower abdominal and pelvic surgeries.

Method EQUIPMENT: A 9.5 MHz directional ultrasound volcimeter is used to locate the cavernous artery. If this cannot be accomplished, the dorsalis penis or the frenucar artery may be used. A 1-2.5 cm pneumatic cuff attached to an aneroid manometer is placed around the base of the penis and inflated to suprasystolic pressure. The cuff is then slowly deflated until the Doppler shifted arterial signal is resumed. This pressure is recorded. The steps listed are repeated three times and the average penile blood pressure is calculated. Obtain a brachial systolic pressure three times and calculate the mean systolic blood pressure. Calculate the ratio of the penile systolic blood pressure to the brachial systolic blood pressure to yield the penile-brachial index (PBI) or penile flow index. If the PBI is normal, this procedure should be repeated following a 3-minute exercise of the buttocks and legs such as running in place or bicycling. If the difference between the exercise PBI (EPBI) and the resting PBI (RPBI) is >0.15, this is consistent with pelvic steal syndrome.

Specimen SAMPLING TIME: 1-2 hours CAUSES FOR REJECTION: Patient with Texas catheter TURNAROUND TIME: Immediate.

Interpretation NORMAL FINDINGS: Penile-brachial index <0.8 LIMITATIONS: It may be technically difficult to detect the cavernous artery pulse because it is not a superficial artery. It is adequate blood flow to this artery, not the dorsalis penis, that is necessary for erection. Also, these studies are performed on the flaccid not the the erect penis. The test may be found to be objectionable to patient or technician. ADDITIONAL INFORMATION: In the work-up of impotence, one should obviously start with a good sexual as well as medical history (including medication) and physical. Such clues as a slow onset of symptoms, evidence of claudication, and the presence of decreased pulses and bruits suggest a vascular etiology. In addition, baseline blood work should be done before any procedures are performed. This should include electrolytes, blood glucose, urinalysis, CBC, liver, renal and thyroid functions, serum FSH, LH prolactin, and testosterone. Penile Doppler studies are commonly performed following nocturnal penile tumescence monitoring (NPTM) that is suggestive of organic disease. It should be remembered that normal NPTM do not necessarily mean that impotence is psychogenic as only changes in penile circumference are measured not necessarily the degree of rigidity or duration of erection. In addition, patients with penile steal syndrome may have completely normal NPTMs. Therefore Doppler studies should probably be performed even if NPTMs are normal and there is suspicion of vasculogenic impotence. If the preliminary H & P suggests diffuse vascular disease, abdominal x-ray, and aortoiliac arteriograms may have to be performed to rule out Leriche syndrome as a cause of impotence. Supplementary tests may be performed such as plethysmography, cavernosography, and arteriogram. If Doppler studies are borderline, a penile hyperemic study may be performed. If there is strong evidence of organic etiology with normal blood work and vascular studies, neurologic etiology should be considered especially if suggested by the H & P. Bulbocavernosus latency times may be performed. It is important to remember that evidence of neurologic dysfunction does not rule out vascular disease as neuropathies are commonly a result of poor vascular supply. Finally, if no organic basis is found, an MMPI (Minnesota multiphasic personality inventory) may be helpful in finding psychogenic causes of impotence. In regards to treatment, successful surgical treatment is seen with aortofemoral bypasses. However, local small vessel or corporeal revascularizations have show high failure rates. Usually penile implants must be performed. In situations of marginal penile perfusion, performance may be improved with vasodilators and cessation of smoking.

References

Bell D, Lewis R, and Kerstein MD, "Hyperemic Stress Test in Diagnosis of Vasculogenic Impotence," *Urology*, 1983, 22(6):611-3.

Depalma RG, "Impotence in Vascular Disease: Relationship to Vascular Surgery," *Br J Surg*, 1982, 69(suppl):14-6.

Lane RJ, Appleberg M, and Williams W, "A Comparison of Two Techniques for the Detection of the Vasculogenic Component of Impotence," *Surg Gynecol Obstet*, 1982, 155:230-4.

Sacks SA, "Evaluation of Impotence, Comprehensive Compassionate Approach," *Postgrad Med*, 1983, 74(4):182-97.

Zorgniotti AW, "Practical Diagnostic Screening for Impotence," *Urology*, 1984, 23(5):98-102.

Penile Blood Pressure as Compared to Brachial Blood Pressure *see* Penile Blood Flow *on previous page*

Penile Doppler Studies *see* Penile Blood Flow *on previous page*

Renal Biopsy *see* Kidney Biopsy *on page 145*

Simple CMG *see* Cystometrogram, Simple *on page 139*

Sleep Erection Monitoring *see* Nocturnal Penile Tumescence Test *on page 150*

Urodynamic Testing of Bladder Function *see* Cystometrogram, Simple *on page 139*

NEUROLOGY

Carlos M. Isada, MD

The proper approach to the patient with neurologic disease is based upon the history and physical examination. In recent years, however, this simple but fundamental principle has become obscured. With the proliferation of neurodiagnostic tests (readily available in both university and community hospitals), there has been a tendency to obtain these "objective" studies early on. At times, this is done in lieu of a careful neurologic examination. It is in this spirit that the following neurologic procedures are presented. Neurodiagnostic tests should only be sought after formulation of an adequate differential diagnosis.

In general practice, commonly ordered neurodiagnostic tests include the electroencephalogram, electromyogram, lumbar puncture, and audiometry. These specific procedures are thus discussed in some detail. Other procedures likely to be considered by the internist or resident physician are also described, but certainly the neurologist has a wide range of specialized tests at his disposal which are not covered in this section.

Within each entry there has been an attempt to emphasize clinical applications for a given diagnostic test. This is admittedly a difficult task since specific indications for many procedures are physician dependent and no consensus opinion exists. Whenever possible, important controversies regarding clinical applicability have been mentioned. Less emphasis has been placed on the technicalities of interpretation.

Few well-controlled clinical trials have been conducted to assess the sensitivity and specificity of many of these procedures. To complicate matters, much of the published literature regarding indications, contraindications, and complications is based on anecdotal experience. Thus, an individual entry should not be regarded in a dogmatic fashion, but rather as an outline of general test characteristics.

Audiogram *see* Pure Tone Audiometry *on page 175*

Audiologic Assessment *see* Pure Tone Audiometry *on page 175*

BAEP *see* Brainstem Auditory Evoked Responses *on this page*

BAER *see* Brainstem Auditory Evoked Responses *on this page*

Basic Comprehensive Audiometry *see* Pure Tone Audiometry *on page 175*

Brainstem Auditory Evoked Potentials *see* Brainstem Auditory Evoked Responses *on this page*

Brainstem Auditory Evoked Responses

CPT 92585

Related Information

Electroencephalography *on page 158*

Synonyms BAEP; BAER; Brainstem Auditory Evoked Potentials

Abstract PROCEDURE COMMONLY INCLUDES: Activation of brainstem auditory pathways by means of brief click stimuli are presented to each ear separately. Electrical potentials are produced by auditory neurons in response to these stimuli. These are called auditory evoked responses (potentials). This electrical activity is detected and recorded by EEG electrodes on the scalp. Immediately after each click stimulus is presented, seven consecutive potentials are normally recorded, waves I through VII. Each of these waveforms corresponds closely to a specific brainstem relay station. For example, wave I corresponds to the acoustic nerve, wave II the cochlear nucleus in the pons, wave III the superior olivary nucleus, and so on. This relationship between electrical potential and anatomic structure allows localization of auditory lesions to within several millimeters. BAER testing is a safe, objective means of diagnosing and localizing early, subclinical lesions of the auditory system. INDICATIONS: BAER is helpful in the following clinical situations:

- diagnosis of acoustic neuromas; BAER is extremely sensitive in detecting these extrinsic lesions and plays an important role in many "textbook" algorithms designed to diagnose acoustic neuromas
- diagnosis of intrinsic brainstem lesions, including: multiple sclerosis (BAER is less sensitive than visual evoked potentials); brainstem infarctions, when auditory pathways are involved; brainstem gliomas; various degenerative disorders of the central nervous system (eg, olivopontocerebellar degeneration); Charcot-Marie-Tooth disease, Wilson's disease and others

Note: Results obtained on BAER testing are not pathognomonic for the disorders listed.

- evaluation of the comatose patient; BAER results are not significantly influenced by barbiturates or anesthetics. Thus, BAER may have a role in the confirmation of brain death when conventional EEG is inconclusive.
- continuous monitoring of brainstem function in patients undergoing general anesthesia
- intraoperative assessment of cranial nerve VIII function in patients undergoing removal of an acoustic neuroma
- evaluation of hearing loss in the child or neonate, since BAER testing does not require verbal responses
- assessment of hysterical or factitious hearing loss
- BAER is generally **normal** (or minimally abnormal) in the following: trigeminal neuralgia; brainstem transient ischemic attacks (TIAs); "locked-in" syndrome; lateral medullary infarcts; factitious hearing loss

CONTRAINDICATIONS: Absolute contraindications to BAER testing have not been reported. BAER may be performed in patients with mild to moderate degrees of peripheral hearing loss (eg, otosclerosis). Patients with severe peripheral hearing loss may still undergo BAER testing but there is a possibility that the acoustic nerve may not be sufficiently activated by click stimuli (this can be quickly determined by the examiner). Impacted cerumen represents a relative contraindication and should be removed prior to the study. Similarly, BAER testing should be postponed in the patient with acute (serous) otitis media. Patient cooperation, while helpful, is not absolutely necessary. This procedure may be performed

(Continued)

Brainstem Auditory Evoked Responses *(Continued)*

on the deeply comatose patient. Severe spasms of the head and neck musculature may interfere with EEG tracings. BAER testing may still be attempted after appropriate medications.

Patient Care/Scheduling PATIENT PREPARATION: Procedural details are explained and verbal consent is obtained. Routine medications, including ear drops, may be taken on the morning of the procedure. Patient should wash hair the night beforehand. An overnight fast is not necessary and the patient may eat a breakfast or lunch before the examination. AFTERCARE: No specific restrictions are necessary. Patient may resume previous level of activity. Since sedatives are not used, outpatients may drive themselves home. SPECIAL INSTRUCTIONS: Requisition form from the ordering physician should include brief clinical history, pertinent neurologic findings, and diagnostic impression. Inform laboratory in advance if children or neonates are to be tested.

Method EQUIPMENT:

- scalp electrodes, the same as for conventional EEG
- earphones
- tone stimulator, capable of producing "clicks" (white noise) at different decibel levels and polarities
- signal amplifier and filter
- computer system for signal averaging

TECHNIQUE: BAER is performed with the patient comfortably seated in a sound-dampened room. Surface electrodes are placed on the scalp at the vertex (top of head) and the earlobe of the testing ear. Each ear is tested separately with continuous white noise presented to the nontest ear. The threshold for perceiving click stimuli is quickly determined and intensity is increased 70 dB above this. Click stimuli are then presented through the earphones to the test ear. This stimulus is a brief (100 msec) electrical square wave and is repeated at 10 Hz. Electrical activity in the auditory pathways is detected by the scalp electrodes and recorded for a 10 msec interval following each click. Since the evoked responses are typically low in amplitude, amplification is necessary. Computer signal averaging is used to diminish random, background electrical noise from surrounding neurons. In total, >500 clicks are presented to each ear amounting to >1000 consecutive trials. The evoked potentials for each trial are transmitted to a computer and the signals are averaged. The composite waveform generated appears as seven discernible waves, numbered I-VII. The entire procedure requires 1 to 1 1/2 hours. DATA ACQUIRED: Auditory evoked responses for each ear, signal averaged by the computer. These responses appear graphically as a plot of electrical potential on the Y axis versus time on the X axis.

Interpretation NORMAL FINDINGS: The normal auditory evoked response consists of a tracing with seven distinct waves. Test results are interpreted by an experienced neurologist (turnaround time depends on the institution). A normal BAER is depicted in the figure on the following page with electrical potential on the vertical axis and time on the horizontal axis. From this computer-generated wave several important parameters are studied:

- absolute latency – the time interval from stimulus presentation to the wave peak
- interpeak latency – the time interval between the peaks of any two waves
- wave amplitude
- wave duration

Normal values have been published based on studies of healthy individuals. However, precise cutoffs are determined by each laboratory depending on equipment, technique, etc. The seven waves of a normal BAER tracing correspond to discrete anatomical structures as follows:

- wave I – acoustic nerve
- wave II – cochlear nucleus (pons)
- wave III – superior olivary nucleus
- wave IV – lateral lemniscus
- wave V – inferior colliculus (midbrain)
- wave VI – medial geniculate (hypothesis only)
- wave VII – auditory radiations (hypothesis only)

The precise origin of waves VI and VII is unclear at the present time. They play a minor role in the routine interpretation of a BAER test.

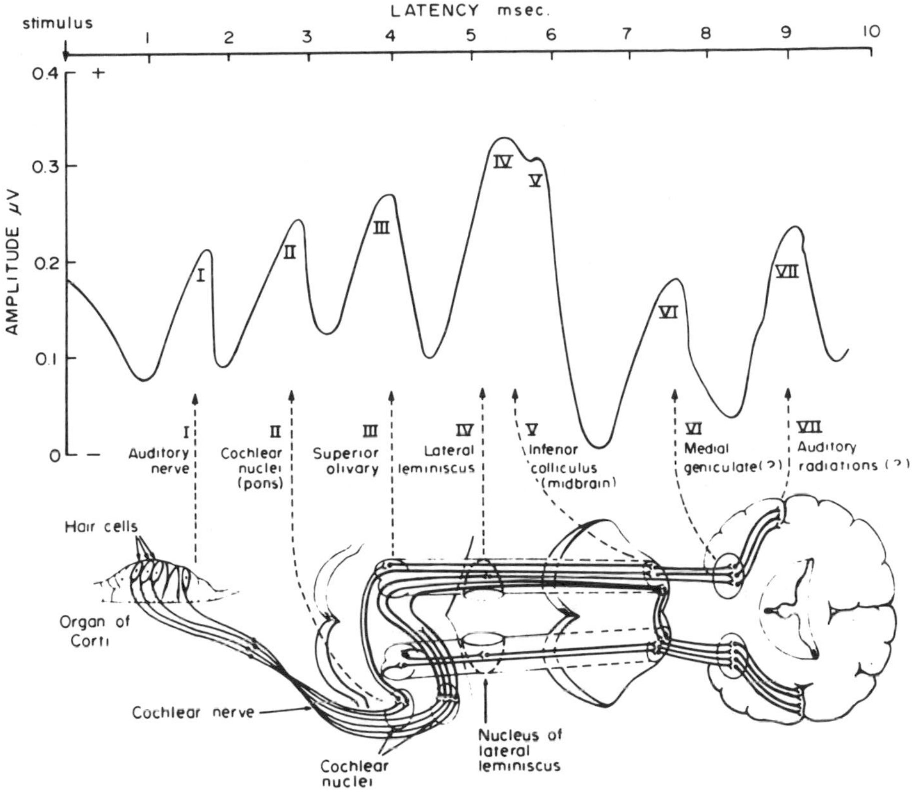

Far-field brainstem auditory evoked responses (BAER). Diagram of the proposed electrophysiologic-anatomic correlations in humans. Reproduced with permission from Adams RD and Victor M, *Principles of Neurology*, 3rd ed, "Part 1/Approach to the Patient With Neurologic Disease," New York, NY: McGraw-Hill Book Co, 1985, 28.

CRITICAL VALUES: In general, an abnormality in a specific wave (eg, wave II) suggests a lesion in the corresponding "relay station" (eg, cochlear nucleus). For purposes of interpretation, abnormalities in interpeak latency are the most helpful (although in some cases, a wave may be absent altogether). A prolongation of the interpeak latencies involving waves I-III, for example, is suggestive of an acoustic neuroma. In contrast, prolongation of the absolute latency is less useful diagnostically and usually represents a disorder of the peripheral auditory apparatus. Idealized evoked responses in various conditions are listed in the following table.

Brainstem Auditory Evoked Responses

Lesion	BAER Abnormality
Acoustic neuroma	↑ interpeak latency, especially waves I–III, ipsilateral
Multiple sclerosis	↓ amplitude wave V and/or ↑ interpeak latency
Elevated intracranial pressure	Absent wave V
Brain death	Waves II–VII absent or waves I–VII absent, bilaterally (difficult to interpret when wave I is absent)
Traumatic damage to the cochlea	Waves I–VII absent, ipsilateral

(Continued)

Brainstem Auditory Evoked Responses *(Continued)*

References

Adams RD and Victor M, *Principles of Neurology*, 4th ed, New York, NY: McGraw-Hill Book Co, 1989.

Cassvan A, Ralescu S, Moshkovski FG, et al, "Brainstem Auditory Evoked Potential Studies in Patients With Tinnitus and/or Vertigo," *Arch Phys Med Rehabil*, 1990, 71(8):583-6.

Chiappa KH, *Evoked Potentials in Clinical Neurology*, New York, NY: Raven Press, 1983.

Chiappa KH, Harrison JL, Brooks EB, et al, "Brainstem Auditory Evoked Responses in 200 Patients With Multiple Sclerosis," *Ann Neurol*, 1980, 7:135-43.

Chiappa KH and Ropper AH, "Evoked Potentials in Clinical Medicine," *N Engl J Med*, 1982, 306:1140-50.

Kveton JF, "The Efficacy of Brainstem Auditory Evoked Potentials in Acoustic Tumor Surgery," *Laryngoscope*, 1990, 100(11):1171-3.

Starr A and Achor J, "Auditory Brainstem Responses in Neurological Disease," *Arch Neurol*, 1975, 32:761-8.

Calorics *see* Electronystagmography *on page 164*

Cerebrospinal Fluid Tap *see* Lumbar Puncture *on page 165*

Diagnostic Audiometry *see* Pure Tone Audiometry *on page 175*

EEG *see* Electroencephalography *on this page*

Electrodiagnostic Study *see* Electromyography *on page 160*

Electroencephalogram *see* Electroencephalography *on this page*

Electroencephalography

CPT 95819 (EEG including recording awake, drowsy, asleep, with hyperventilation and/or photic stimulation); 95822 (sleep only); 95823 (physical or pharmacological activation only); 95824 (cerebral death evaluation only)

Related Information

Brainstem Auditory Evoked Responses *on page 155*

Visual Evoked Responses *on page 187*

Synonyms EEG; Electroencephalogram

Applies to Somatosensory Evoked Potentials

Abstract **PROCEDURE COMMONLY INCLUDES:** Analysis of the electrical activity of the brain using scalp electrodes. This procedure is based on the principle that neurons within the cerebral cortex will normally generate low-amplitude electrical potentials. Electrodes positioned over specific regions of the cortex are able to detect these signals. Brain rhythms are then amplified and transmitted to a multichannel polygraph which records waveforms with automatic ink pens on moving paper. This written document, often more than 100 pages, is called the electroencephalogram. It is a continuous plot of voltage (vertical axis) versus time (horizontal axis). Abnormalities in the EEG brain wave pattern may be diagnostic of specific neurologic diseases. EEG is an indispensable means of evaluating gray matter disease and it is the only electrophysiologic measure of ongoing cortical function.

INDICATIONS: Common indications for EEG in general practice include:

- evaluation of the patient with a suspected seizure disorder; EEG is unique in its ability to objectively document the presence of seizure activity. In addition, EEG is crucial in localizing the site of a seizure focus and classifying the nature of epileptiform discharges. EEG is nearly always abnormal during an acute generalized seizure (eg, grand mal, petit mal), and frequently abnormal during an acute focal seizure (eg, Jacksonian). The EEG may also have diagnostic utility during the interictal period with abnormal discharges seen in 80% of patients with petit mal and 60% of patients with grand mal seizures.
- assessment of coma and other impairments in mental status; the EEG is abnormal in nearly every case of metabolic encephalopathy or ischemic encephalopathy, but is normal in most psychiatric conditions. In some instances, EEG may reveal

important etiologic data not suspected clinically. For example, when coma is caused by hepatic encephalopathy, barbiturate overdose, or subclinical status epilepticus, distinctive and diagnostic EEG waveforms may be seen.
- diagnosis of certain infections of the central nervous system (CNS); characteristic EEG patterns may be seen in herpes simplex encephalitis, Creutzfeldt-Jakob disease, and subacute sclerosing panencephalitis.

Additional roles for EEG include:
- diagnosis of intracranial mass lesions; EEG is capable of diagnosing and localizing lesions such as brain tumors, abscesses, meningiomas, etc. However, this test cannot reliably distinguish between these entities. In recent years, the CT scan and MRI scan have supplanted the EEG in the evaluation of space occupying lesions.
- evaluation of cerebrovascular disease; in a patient who has suffered a recent cortical stroke, EEG can demonstrate regional electrical abnormalities in the distribution of the thrombosed vessel. In the patient who has suffered a subcortical stroke ("lacunar stroke"), the EEG is usually normal even though the patient is hemiplegic. Thus, EEG may play a role in distinguishing cortical from subcortical stroke syndromes. In addition, EEG has been used in the past to diagnose and localize subarachnoid hemorrhage. However, CT scan or MRI scan have become the diagnostic tests of choice for stroke and subarachnoid hemorrhage.
- assessment of head injury; following a cerebral concussion, EEG is usually normal, but after a cerebral contusion, EEG is usually abnormal (although nonspecific). EEG has also been used to predict the subset of patients with head trauma who will go on to develop a seizure disorder.
- evaluation of persistent sleep disorders; overnight EEG recording is included as part of the polysomnogram (along with other monitoring techniques).
- intraoperative monitoring of cerebral activity; EEG may be used during certain neurosurgical procedures, carotid endarterectomies, and some non-neurologic surgeries as well (eg, cardiothoracic surgery). It is also useful in assessing depth of anesthesia.
- evaluation of suspected pseudoseizures; the EEG is normal despite generalized clonic movements
- EEG is characteristically **normal** in the following: multiple sclerosis (in severe cases some nonspecific changes may be seen); delirium tremens; Wernicke-Korsakoff's syndrome; Alzheimer's disease; cryptococcal meningitis; cerebral concussion; psychiatric disturbances, including bipolar disorder; tension headache; pseudoseizures

CONTRAINDICATIONS: No absolute contraindications exist for EEG.

Patient Care/Scheduling **PATIENT PREPARATION:** Details of the procedure are discussed with the patient. When possible, sedative medications should be discontinued well in advance. This includes benzodiazepines, barbiturates, ethanol, etc. Fasting prior to EEG is not necessary, in fact, relative hypoglycemia has been reported to alter the EEG. The patient should also be reasonably rested beforehand since sleep deprivation has been known to cause alpha-rhythm abnormalities. If the patient has already been receiving anticonvulsant agents (eg, phenytoin (Dilantin®), carbamazepine) the management is more complex. The decision to withdraw or continue anticonvulsants prior to EEG testing should be handled by the physician. When approaching the patient with a new-onset seizure disorder (witnessed or suspected), many clinicians will obtain the initial EEG while the patient is still on an anticonvulsant agent. If results are negative, the EEG may be repeated later after discontinuing anticonvulsants for 1-2 days. Although this approach is admittedly cautious, it reduces the chance of seizure "breakthrough". Patient should wash hair the night before the test. Hair cream, oils, spray, and lacquer should not be applied after washing. **AFTERCARE:** If an overnight sleep study has been performed, patient is not permitted to drive home afterwards. Otherwise, if a routine (wake) EEG is performed no specific post-procedure restrictions are necessary. If anticonvulsant medications were discontinued specifically for the EEG, the patient is instructed to restart medications until notified by physician. **SPECIAL INSTRUCTIONS:** Requisition for EEG from the ordering physician should state patient's age, brief clinical history, overall impression, and reason for EEG. Special

(Continued)

Electroencephalography *(Continued)*

requests can be made for overnight study, sleep study, nasopharyngeal leads, activation procedures, evoked response testing, etc. **COMPLICATIONS:** EEG is considered a safe procedure and is well tolerated. The following "activation" techniques may be successful in inducing a seizure, but this is a desired "complication".

Method **TECHNIQUE:** At the start of the procedure, surface electrodes are placed on the scalp over designated areas. From 8-20 electrodes may be used, each approximately 0.5 cm in diameter. The patient is asked to rest comfortably on the examining table, first with eyes open, then closed. The underlying electrical activity of the cerebral cortex is measured (deeper structures are more difficult to measure). The signals are amplified, filtered, and transmitted to a polygraph. The electrical signals detected at each electrode move a separate ink writing pen on the polygraph. Thus, activity within anatomically different areas of the brain (temporal lobe, occipital, frontal, etc) are recorded on separate "channels". A continuous graph is produced on moving paper plotting voltage (vertical axis) versus time (horizontal axis). The written record may be several hundred pages long. Testing requires approximately 1 hour. Several "activation" measures may be attempted in order to induce a seizure under controlled laboratory conditions. These include:

- hyperventilation (leads to acute respiratory alkalosis and cerebral vasoconstriction)
- stroboscopic stimulation
- sleep EEG (for suspected temporal lobe epilepsy).

References

Adams RD and Victor M, *Principles of Neurology*, 4th ed, New York, NY: McGraw-Hill Book Co, 1989, 19-31.

Aminoff MJ, *Electrodiagnosis in Clinical Neurology*, 2nd ed, New York, NY: Churchill-Livingstone, 1986.

Chusid JG, *Correlative Neuroanatomy and Functional Neurology*, 18th ed, Los Altos, CA: Lange Medical Publications, 1982, 223-44.

Davis TL and Freemon FR, "Electroencephalography Should Not Be Routine in the Evaluation of Syncope in Adults," *Arch Intern Med*, 1990, 150(10):2027-9.

Kiloh LG, McComas AJ, and Osselton JW, *Clinical Electroencephalography*, 4th ed, London, England: Butterworth's Publishers, 1981.

Niedermeyer E and DaSilva FL, *Electroencephalography*, 2nd ed, Baltimore, MD: Urban and Schwarzenberg, 1987.

Spehlmann R, *EEG Primer*, Elsevier, North Holland: Biomedical Press, 1981.

Wee AS, "Is Electroencephalography Necessary in the Evaluation of Syncope?" *Arch Intern Med*, 1990, 150(10):2007-8.

Electromyography

CPT 95860 (1 extremity and related paraspinal areas); 95861 (2 extremities); 95863 (3 extremities); 95864 (4 extremities); 95867 (cranial nerve supplied muscles)

Related Information

Nerve Conduction Studies *on page 169*
Neuromuscular Junction Testing *on page 173*
Single Fiber Electromyography *on page 179*

Synonyms Electrodiagnostic Study; EMG

Abstract **PROCEDURE COMMONLY INCLUDES:** Insertion of a needle electrode into skeletal muscle to measure electrical activity and assess physiologic function. In this procedure, percutaneous, extracellular needle electrodes are placed into a selected muscle group. Muscle action potentials (AP) are detected by these electrodes, amplified, and displayed on a cathode ray oscilloscope. In addition, fluctuations in voltage are heard as "crackles" over a loudspeaker, permitting both auditory and visual analysis of the muscle APs. Testing is performed with the muscle at rest, with a mild voluntary contraction, and with maximal muscle contraction (where recruitment pattern and interference are noted). Unlike nerve conduction studies, EMG does not involve external electrical stimulation. Muscle APs (normal or abnormal) are physiologically generated. In various diseases of the motor system, typical electrical abnormalities may be present: increased insertional activity, abnormal motor unit potentials, fibrillations, fasciculations, positive sharp waves, decreased recruitment pattern, and others. EMG assesses the integrity of upper motor neurons, lower motor neurons, the neuromuscular junction, and the muscle itself. However, EMG is seldom diagnostic of a particular disease entity. Its major use lies in differentiating between the following disease classes: primary myopathy, peripheral motor neuron disease, and disease of the neuromuscular junction. As with nerve conduction velocity studies (with which EMG is usually paired), EMG should be considered an extension of the history and physical examination. **INDICATIONS:** In the neurologic literature, EMG has been performed in a wide variety of clinical situations, many of which are experimental or highly specialized in nature. Common indications for EMG in general practice include:

Evaluation of the patient with clinical features of primary muscle disease (symmetric and proximal weakness, muscle atrophy, intact sensory system, etc). Examples include:

- muscular dystrophy
- glycogen storage disease
- myotonia
- inflammatory myopathies (systemic lupus, sarcoidosis, infectious myopathies)
- polydermatomyositis
- alcoholic myopathy
- endocrine myopathies, and others

Evaluation of the patient with lower motor neuron disease, including:

- suspected peripheral nerve lesions, such as diffuse peripheral neuropathies, spinal root lesions, and trauma
- suspected disease of the anterior horn cells (characterized by asymmetric weakness, muscle atrophy, fasciculations), as in amyotrophic lateral sclerosis or poliomyelitis

Assessment of the patient with suspected upper motor neuron disease, when prior imaging studies are inconclusive. This includes occult lesions of the corticospinal tract (syringomyelia, tumor) and, less commonly, lesions of the cerebral tract (tumor, CVA). Evaluation of the patient with suspected neuromuscular junction disease (NMJ). This includes myasthenia gravis and the paraneoplastic Eaton-Lambert syndrome. Conventional EMG, as described here, is not the diagnostic test of choice for myasthenia gravis. However, other forms of EMG such as single fiber EMG and repetitive stimulation tests are highly specific for NMJ disease. Assessment of the patient with severe and persistent muscle cramps. Serial documentation of response to therapy for known cases of myopathy or neuropathy. Identification of significantly diseased muscle groups to help guide muscle biopsy (if clinical examination is not inconclusive). EMG is less useful in:

- the restless legs syndrome
- transient, self-resolving muscle cramps
- uncomplicated cases of polymyalgia rheumatica unless the diagnosis is in doubt or underlying myositis is suspected
- routine cases of fibrositis/fibromyalgia (EMG abnormalities have recently been documented in the medical literature but needle examination is not routinely indicated)

CONTRAINDICATIONS: The following situations represent relative contraindications:

- severe coagulopathy, including hemophilia and marked thrombocytopenia. It should be noted that EMG has been performed safely with platelet counts as low as 20,000/mm^3, but this is not recommended.
- systemic anticoagulation (eg, intravenous heparin, oral Coumadin®)
- patients with an unusual susceptibility to systemic infections (EMG has been known to cause transient bacteremia)
- patients undergoing a muscle biopsy after EMG require special consideration. It is well known that needle insertion and manipulation during EMG may cause local microscopic tissue damage on a traumatic basis. Histologically, this damage may be confused with a focal myopathy. Thus, some experts avoid detailed needle examinations of the specific muscle group which will be biopsied (although EMG testing of surrounding muscle groups is frequently performed).

Patient Care/Scheduling **PATIENT PREPARATION:** Details of procedure are reviewed with the patient. Considerable patient apprehension often accompanies "needle tests" and

(Continued)

Electromyography *(Continued)*

calm reassurance from the medical team will go far in allaying such anxieties. Aspirin products should be discontinued 5-7 days beforehand. Nonsteroidal agents should also be stopped several days in advance. Routine medications may be taken on the morning of the examination. If coagulopathy is suspected, appropriate hematologic tests should be ordered (PT/PTT, CBC, bleeding time, etc). If a primary muscle disease is suspected, creatine phosphokinase (CPK) level should be drawn prior to needle examination. Routine EMG testing may cause minor elevations in CPK up to one and one-half times baseline. However, striking elevations in CPK, as seen with polymyositis or muscular dystrophy, are not associated with EMG testing. **AFTERCARE:** No specific activity restrictions are necessary. Patient may resume previous activity level. **SPECIAL INSTRUCTIONS:** Requisition from ordering physician should include brief clinical history, tentative neurologic diagnosis, and the specific limb(s) or muscle group(s) in question. Physician should also state whether nerve conduction studies are desired, although in some centers these may be added at the neurologist's discretion. **COMPLICATIONS:** Local discomfort at the site of needle insertion is common. This is often mild in severity and has no significant sequelae. Pneumothorax has been rarely documented in the literature. This was associated with needle examination of paraspinal muscles. Transient bacteremia has been reported, but routine antibiotic prophylaxis for patients with high-risk cardiac lesions is not generally recommended.

Method **EQUIPMENT:** EMG is performed in a specially equipped procedure room, usually reserved for electrodiagnostic studies. Basic instrumentation includes:

- needle electrodes; these may be monopolar (sharpened, coated steel wires), coaxial, or bipolar (two wires within a needle). These needles record electrical activity from muscle fibers directly contacting the tip, as well as fibers within a several millimeter radius.
- amplifier with filters
- cathode ray oscilloscope with the vertical axis measuring voltage, the horizontal axis measuring time. This device usually has an audio amplifier and loudspeaker, which converts APs to sound energy.
- data storage apparatus (eg, magnetic tape recorder)

TECHNIQUE: A brief neurologic examination is performed prior to the start of the procedure. For EMG of the extremities, patient lies recumbent on the examination table. When paraspinal muscles are tested, the patient adopts a prone position. No intravenous sedatives or pain medications are used. Local anesthesia is also not required despite the generous number of needle insertions. The skin is cleansed thoroughly with alcohol pads, as necessary. Patient is instructed to relax as much as possible. The following steps are carried out.

- Recording needle electrode is inserted percutaneously into the muscle under consideration. The initial electrical activity of the muscle, as seen on the oscilloscope screen and heard over the loudspeaker, is termed the **insertional activity**.
- Next, the needle is held stationary and the muscle action potentials during voluntary relaxation are recorded.
- Patient performs a mild, submaximal contraction of the test muscle. The summed muscle action potentials - the motor unit potential - are observed on the oscilloscope.
- Finally, a maximal muscle contraction is carried out. The compound action potentials generated during this maneuver are studied for **interference** and **recruitment pattern**.

Needle examination is, by nature, a slow and labor-intensive process. Numerous muscles must be tested individually including both symptomatic and clinically asymptomatic muscles. Within a specific muscle, several independent sites may need to be examined, particularly when the muscle has a large surface area. A number of myopathic processes are focal and sampling errors even within an individual muscle are possible (ie, disease process may effect proximal portion of a muscle, sparing distal fibers).

Interpretation **NORMAL FINDINGS:** Results are interpreted by neurologist or physiatrist with preliminary impression written in chart immediately. A formal, typed report is completed several days later. The fundamental principles underlying test interpretation are as follows.

- Insertional activity: Immediately upon needle insertion, there is a brief burst of electrical activity lasting <300 msec. This "insertional activity" is heard over the loudspeaker and may be increased or decreased in various disease states.
- Electrical activity at rest: Muscle tissue is normally silent at rest. No action potentials are seen on the oscilloscope.
- Minimal muscle contraction: When a minimal contraction is performed, several motor unit potentials (MUPs) are activated. Several individual APs are normally visible on the oscilloscope at a rate of 4-5/second. The idealized configuration of a single MUP is depicted in the following figure (see normal column).
- Full voluntary contraction: As the strength of the muscle contraction increases, further muscle units are "recruited". On the oscilloscope the APs appear more disorganized and individual APs can no longer be recognized. At the peak of a contraction the "complete recruitment pattern" is seen, which represents a compilation of motor unit potentials firing asynchronously. The normal interference pattern is considered "full," that is, the amplitude of APs is high ($\leq$5 mV) and firing rate is fast (40/second).

EMG FINDINGS

	EMG Steps (Lesion)	Normal	Neurogenic Lesion: Lower Motor	Neurogenic Lesion: Upper Motor	Myogenic Lesion: Myopathy	Myogenic Lesion: Myotonia	Myogenic Lesion: Polymyositis
1	Insertional Activity	Normal	Increased	Normal	Normal	Myotonic Discharge	Increased
2	Spontaneous Activity	—	Fibrillation / Positive Wave	—	—	—	Fibrillation / Positive Wave
3	Motor Unit Potential	0.5-1.0 mV / 5-10 ms	Large Unit / Limited Recruitment	Normal	Small Unit / Early Recruitment	Myotonic Discharge	Small Unit / Early Recruitment
4	Interference Pattern	Full	Reduced / Fast Firing Rate	Reduced / Slow Firing Rate	Full / Low Amplitude	Full / Low Amplitude	Full / Low Amplitude

Idealized EMG findings; normal, neurogenic lesions, and myogenic lesions. Reproduced with permission from Kimura J, Chapter 13, "Types of Abnormality," *Electrodiagnosis in Diseases of Nerve and Muscle: Principles and Practice*, 2nd ed, Philadelphia, PA: FA Davis, 1989, 263.

CRITICAL VALUES: Abnormalities in one or more of the previously stated parameters may be seen.

Insertional activity: Increased in both neurogenic disorders (eg, lower motor nerve disease) and myogenic disorders (eg, polymyositis), and thus is considered nonspecific. Decreased insertional activity is less common, but may be associated with far advanced denervation or myopathy, especially when muscle is replaced by fat or collagen. A distinctive insertional pattern is seen with myotonia, an unusual neurologic disorder, and is termed "myotonic discharge".

Abnormal activity at rest: Instead of the electrical silence which characterizes the muscle at rest, spontaneous action potentials in single muscle fibers ("fibrillation potentials") may be observed in several disease states.

Fibrillations are seen 1-3 weeks after destruction of a lower motor neuron. Denervated muscle fibers develop heightened chemosensitivity and individual muscle fibers contract spontaneously. The phenomenon of "positive sharp waves" may also be seen. Fibrillations may also occur with severe polymyositis when extensive areas of necrosis interrupt nerve innervation. The naked eye is unable to perceive fibrillations.

(Continued)

Electromyography *(Continued)*

Fasciculations represent random contractions of a full motor unit, often visible through the skin. (A motor unit is comprised of an anterior horn cell, axon, neuromuscular junction, and the numerous muscle fibers supplied by the axon.) Fasciculations may be benign, with no other EMG abnormalities observed. They may also be associated with amyotrophic lateral sclerosis, other anterior horn cell diseases, nerve root compression, herniated nucleus pulposus syndrome, acute polyneuropathy, and others.

Abnormalities in the motor unit potential (MUP): Individual motor unit potentials are distinguishable during a submaximal muscle contraction. Abnormalities in amplitude, shape (number of phases, serrations, configuration), and duration are possible. Increased MUP amplitude is seen in lower motor neuron disease but is normal in upper motor neuron disease. Decreased MUP amplitude is characteristic of polymyositis and other myopathies and duration of the MUP is also decreased.

Abnormalities in interference pattern: The normal "full recruitment" pattern seen during maximal muscle contraction is often compromised in disease states. In myogenic lesions, such as polymyositis and myotonia, the amplitude of the MUPs is significantly decreased but the recruitment pattern is normal (ie, the number of activated motor units is normal but the number of muscle fibers per motor unit is diminished). In LMN lesions, the number of motor units recruited is decreased. In severe cases of neuropathy, the maximum interference pattern resembles that of a single MUP, with individual potentials visible. Amplitude of MUPs may be normal. These findings are summarized in the previous figure.

References

Adams RD and Victor M, *Principles of Neurology*, 4th ed, New York, NY: McGraw-Hill Book Co, 1989, 1009-27.

Aminoff MJ, *Electromyography in Clinical Practice*, 2nd ed, New York, NY: Churchill-Livingston, 1987.

Goodgold J and Eberstein A, *Electrodiagnosis of Neuromuscular Diseases*, 3rd ed, Baltimore, MD: Williams & Wilkins, 1983.

Griggs RC, Bradley WG, and Shahani B, "Approach to the Patient With Neuromuscular Disease," *Harrison's Principles of Internal Medicine*, 12th ed, Wilson JD, Braunwald E, Isselbacher KJ, et al, eds, New York, NY: McGraw-Hill Book Co, 1991, 2088-96.

Johnson EW and Wiechers D, "Electrodiagnosis," *Krusen's Handbook of Physical Medicine and Rehabilitation*, 3rd ed, Kottke FJ, Stillwell GK, and Lehmann JF, eds, Philadelphia, PA: WB Saunders Co, 1982, 56-85.

Kimura J, *Electrodiagnosis in Diseases of Nerve and Muscle: Principles and Practice*, 2nd ed, Philadelphia, PA: FA Davis Co, 1989.

Electronystagmography

CPT 92541 (spontaneous nystagmus test); 92542 (positional); 92543 (caloric vestibular test); 92544 (optokinetic); 92545 (oscillating tracking test); 92546 (torsion swing test)

Synonyms Calorics; ENG; Vestibular Test

Abstract **PROCEDURE COMMONLY INCLUDES:** Vertical and horizontal occular recording of saccades, gaze, optokinetics, pendulum pursuit, head positions, Hallpike maneuvers, spontaneous nystagmus, calorics, and fixation suppression. **INDICATIONS:** Provide information to aid in the diagnosis of disorders of the auditory and vestibular systems.

Patient Care/Scheduling **PATIENT PREPARATION:** Patient's ear canals must be free of excessive cerumen, irritation, and tympanic membrane perforation. Sedatives and tranquilizers are to be withheld for 48-72 hours prior to testing if approved by attending physician. Patient must be alert and cooperative to instructions and should bring eyeglasses and hearing aids. Patient may have breakfast or lunch prior to testing.

Specimen **CAUSES FOR REJECTION:** Uncooperativeness or refusal by patient, excessive cerumen, tympanic membrane perforation or irritated auditory canal, blindness or severely impaired visual acuity, uncontrollable muscle artifact, nausea and emesis **TURNAROUND TIME:** Final report is given within 24 hours.

Interpretation **LIMITATIONS:** Patient's failure to understand test instructions, nausea and vomiting following caloric stimulation.

EMG *see* Electromyography *on page 160*

ENG *see* Electronystagmography *on previous page*

Hearing Test *see* Pure Tone Audiometry *on page 175*

Latency Studies *see* Nerve Conduction Studies *on page 169*

LP *see* Lumbar Puncture *on this page*

Lumbar Puncture

CPT 62270

Related Information

Myelogram *on page 323*

Synonyms Cerebrospinal Fluid Tap; LP; Spinal Tap

Abstract PROCEDURE COMMONLY INCLUDES: Collection of cerebrospinal fluid (CSF) for chemical, cellular, and microbiological analysis. Performed as a bedside procedure under local anesthesia, a needle is passed into the L4-L5 vertebral interspace and subarachnoid fluid is withdrawn. INDICATIONS: Practitioners vary in their threshold for performing an LP. This procedure is clearly indicated in the following clinical settings[1]:

- clinically suspected meningitis, either acute (where procedure is emergent), subacute, or chronic; also, suspected encephalitis or meningoencephalitis
- suspected central nervous system syphilis in clearly symptomatic patients (tertiary neurosyphilis)
- evaluation of potential CNS lymphoma, meningeal leukemia, and meningeal carcinomatosis
- staging of lymphoma, previously diagnosed from another site
- clinically suspected demyelinating disease such as multiple sclerosis or Guillain-Barré syndrome
- possible cases of subarachnoid hemorrhage

CSF findings in each of these indications is fairly distinctive and LP substantially aids in clinical diagnosis. In contrast, several diseases have abnormal, but nonspecific, CSF findings and LP has low sensitivity and specificity. These include brain abscess or subdural empyema, primary brain tumor, tumors metastatic to brain, subdural or epidural hematoma, connective tissue diseases with CNS involvement (such as CNS lupus or Sjögren's syndrome). Additional studies (such as head CT scan) are necessary to confirm each of these conditions. LP should usually be delayed in favor of other more accurate and less invasive tests. Controversial indications for LP include suspected spinal epidural abscess, evaluation of the acute stroke to identify those which are hemorrhagic, evaluation of dementia (arguably to exclude neurosyphilis or chronic meningitis), evaluation of the asymptomatic patient with a positive serologic test for syphilis (to exclude asymptomatic neurosyphilis).

CONTRAINDICATIONS: Procedure is contraindicated if there is a local infection at the proposed site of needle entry due to the potential for infectious seeding of meninges (several literature case reports). The presence of a severe bleeding diathesis is a relative contraindication to LP and an increased risk of spinal subdural hematoma has been demonstrated. Elevated intracranial pressure is an absolute contraindication to LP because of the risk of uncal herniation (see Complications). The presence of septicemia is **not** considered a contraindication. Retrospective studies have failed to show an increased incidence of meningitis in septic patients undergoing LP compared with septic patients who do not undergo the procedure.[2]

Patient Care/Scheduling PATIENT PREPARATION: Procedure and risks are explained and consent is obtained. If patient is confused or obtunded, obtain consent from guardians. If a coagulopathy is suspected, obtain platelet count and prothrombin/partial thromboplastin time if time permits. No intravenous pain medications such as meperidine are required routinely. Likewise, sedatives or anxiolytics may serve to confuse later assessments of mental status. AFTERCARE: Patient should be kept at strict bedrest for a minimum of 3 hours postprocedure to minimize post-LP headache. Regarding the optimal patient positioning, opinions vary. Some authors recommend the prone position post-LP based on a study involving >1000 subjects which demonstrated a 0.5% incidence of headache in pa-

(Continued)

Lumbar Puncture *(Continued)*

tients kept prone versus 36.5% in the supine group.[3] The frequency of obtaining vital signs and neurologic checks after the procedure should be based on the patient's overall status. Nursing staff should be familiar with potential LP complications, especially acute deteriorations in mental status (possible tonsillar herniation), sensory deficits, leg muscle weakness, and bladder and bowel incontinence (possible expanding spinal subdural hematoma). If no complications arise, activity may later be upgraded to *ad lib* as tolerated, with physician's approval. **COMPLICATIONS:** Although a wide range of complications has been reported, LP should generally be considered a safe procedure. The most common complication is "spinal headache" with an estimated incidence of 10% to 25%. This may be minimized by using a small gauge spinal needle and placing the patient in the prone position after the procedure. Another common complication is local bleeding, the "traumatic tap," which results from needle rupture of venous plexuses surrounding the spinal sack. Incidence may be as high as 20%. As long as no coagulation defect exists, the traumatic tap is clinically insignificant and rarely leads to spinal hematoma. Immediate painful paresthesias due to nerve root irritation is another common complication (≤13%), but usually resolves upon repositioning the spinal needle. Rare complications (<1%) include persistent pain or leg paresthesias; spinal epidural, subdural or subarachnoid hematomas; arachnoiditis from tracking in povidone-iodine on the needle; local infection (epidural or subdural empyema); transient cranial nerve palsies (especially CN VI when large volumes of CSF removed); rupture of nucleus pulposus; delayed formation of intraspinal epidermoid tumors (when stylet is not used); and vagal cardiac arrest. Note that the use of anticoagulants or presence of a coagulopathy significantly increases the risk of spinal hematoma formation (≤7%). Tonsillar herniation is an infrequent but potentially lethal complication of LP which occurs in patients with increased intracranial pressure. The exact incidence is not clear. In one series of patients with papilledema and increased intracranial pressure from a variety of causes, tonsillar herniation occurred after LP in <1.2% of cases.[4] A particularly high risk group appears to be the patient with brain abscess or subdural empyema, with an estimated 10% to 20% incidence of LP-induced herniation and death.[5] The herniation risk in patients with brain tumor is not known, although one study (which predated head CT scans) reported neurologic deterioration following LP in only 1 of 400 brain tumor cases.[6] In general, due to incomplete data, a variety of clinical approaches have been adopted to avoid this fatal complication (see Additional Information).

Method **EQUIPMENT:** Commercial LP trays are available. Common items include iodine, alcohol pads, sterile gloves and drapes, local anesthesia (usually 1% lidocaine) with appropriate needles and syringes, four sterile collecting tubes, 3-way stopcock with connecting tubing, manometer, and spinal needle with stylette. In general, a small bore spinal needle should be used, such as a 25-gauge, due to a lower incidence of spinal headache compared with a 20- or 22-gauge needle. **TECHNIQUE:** In all cases, perform a careful fundoscopic and neurologic exam to rule out papilledema or a focal neurologic deficit. LP is then performed in one of two ways. In the standard method, patient is placed on a firm surface in the lateral recumbent position, curled with knees down in towards the chest and neck maximally flexed. The lumbar region should be close to the edge of the bed, with the plane of the back and shoulders as perpendicular to the bed as possible. Proper positioning is by far the most important step to ensure success and may require several assistants. The L4-L5 interspace is identified by drawing an imaginary line between the two posterior iliac crests. This area is cleaned, prepped, and draped. Skin and deeper subcutaneous tissues are infiltrated with lidocaine. The spinal needle with stylette is then passed into the L4-L5 interspace along the midline, bevel upwards. Angle the needle slightly cephalad along an imaginary line between the site of entry and the umbilicus. As the needle is advanced, the stylette should be frequently withdrawn and replaced every 1-2 mm in order to identify the first drop of CSF (and avoid overpenetration). Once CSF fluid is seen in the needle hub, the manometer is immediately attached to the needle via connecting tubing. Opening pressure should be measured promptly (do not wait more than 1 minute) with the patient's legs and hips extended. If the opening pressure is elevated (>180 mm CSF), try to eliminate factors that may cause false elevations. Instruct patient to straighten his legs, breathe evenly, avoid Valsalva maneuvers, and relax his abdominal muscles. If the opening pressure remains markedly elevated, close the 3-way stopcock, collect only the CSF already in the manometer, disconnect all the tubing, reinsert stylette, and consider neurosurgical consultation. If opening pressure is normal, CSF is then collected in tubes 1-4 in sequence. Manometer is reconnected afterwards and a closing pressure recorded. Stylette is replaced and both needle and stylette removed together. Pressure is held over the puncture site. An alternate approach may be needed in the patient whose vertebral landmarks are difficult to palpate. Initially, patient is placed in a seated position with neck and spine maximally flexed, arms resting on a bedside table. The L4-L5 interspace is identified as before and the remainder of the procedure is identical. This may be used with the obese patient or the patient with ankylosing spondylitis or severe scoliosis. Variations of this procedure have been described including: a lateral approach through the paravertebral muscles, the "hanging drop" technique used by anesthesiologists for identifying entry into the subdural space, and suboccipital puncture of the cisterna magna. These techniques are not necessary in the majority of cases. **DATA ACQUIRED:** Estimation of spinal fluid pressure as described. CSF fluid analytic tests are ordered based on clinical suspicion. Routine tests include cell count and CSF glucose level. Optional tests (not all samples): protein, VDRL, bacterial antigen detection battery, fungal antigens (such as *Cryptococcus*), culture (bacterial, fungal, viral, tuberculous), India ink preparation for *Cryptococcus*, infectious antibody titers, Gram stain, acid-fast bacilli smear, and cytology. Specialized tests include oligoclonal bands and myelin basic protein (for multiple sclerosis). The interested reader should refer to the *Laboratory Test Handbook* for further details.

Specimen 10-12 mL maximum removed from the adult. Smaller volumes are sufficient for most routine tests (confirm with laboratory). **CONTAINER:** Sterile tubes, numbered 1 to 4 **COLLECTION:** Tube 1: CSF protein and glucose; tube 2: cell count and differential; tube 3: Gram stain and cultures; tube 4: save for optional studies **STORAGE INSTRUCTIONS:** Specimen should be sent to laboratory immediately, preferably hand carried by physician.

Interpretation **NORMAL FINDINGS:** (Adults) opening pressure: 80-180 mm of CSF in lateral recumbent position, somewhat higher in sitting position. Respiratory variation of 5-10 mm normal. Clarity: normally very clear. CSF glucose: 60% to 70% of blood glucose. This estimation does not hold for blood glucose levels >300 mg/dL where CSF glucose empirically fails to rise. CSF protein: 15-55 mg/dL. CSF cell count and differential: 0-5 mononuclear white blood cells/mm^3 (lymphocytes and monocytes). The presence of even 1 or 2 polymorphonuclear cells (PMNs) is abnormal. Red blood cells: 0. Gram stain and culture: negative. **CRITICAL VALUES:** Interpretation of CSF findings have been reviewed in detail elsewhere.[7] As a rule, interpretation of abnormal CSF values must always be made in close conjunction with the individual patient's clinical presentation. Considerable overlap exists among the "classic" CSF patterns which are meant to characterize different disease entities. No constellation of CSF findings is entirely specific for a given disease. LP has its greatest value in the diagnosis of bacterial meningitis. A classic CSF "purulent profile" has been described for bacterial meningitis, characterized by elevated WBCs in CSF (often >500/mm^3), predominance of PMN cells on CSF differential (>5/mm^3, presumed high sensitivity, low specificity), depressed CSF glucose levels (<40 mg/dL, 58% sensitivity), low CSF glucose to blood glucose ratio (<0.3, sensitivity 70%). Gram stain of CSF is positive in most cases (60% to 90%) as is the culture (80%). However, even acute bacterial meningitis may present in an atypical fashion, with predominant CSF lymphocytosis (10%), negative Gram stain, or, rarely, normal CSF leukocyte counts. In addition, the "purulent profile" may also be seen in noninfectious conditions such as subarachnoid hemorrhage (≤20% of cases). In contrast, CSF findings in viral meningitis typically reveal <100 WBCs/mm^3, predominantly mononuclear cells on differential, normal glucose levels, normal or elevated protein levels, and negative Gram stain. However, some overlap exists with the profile for bacterial meningitis and 10% of patients with viral meningitis may have mostly PMNs, especially early in the course. Viral cultures are positive in <50% of the cases at best and may be as low as 5% for herpes simplex virus. Thus, viral cultures have a limited role and LP is most useful clinically in ruling out bacterial meningitis. Viral meningitis rarely presents with WBC counts in CSF >1000/mm^3, CSF protein levels >100 mg/dL, or glucose <40 mg/dL. Such patients should be treated as bacterial meningitis until proven otherwise. Fungal meningitis rarely presents a normal CSF picture but the abnormalities are very nonspecific (elevated protein, depressed glucose, and lymphocytic pleocytosis). For the diagnosis of cryptococcal meningitis, the cryptococcal antigen detection test is accurate very early on. Similar nonspecific CSF profiles are seen in tuberculous meningitis and sometimes may mimic bacterial meningitis. The acid-fast smear has notoriously low sensitivity (<25%) but

(Continued)

Lumbar Puncture *(Continued)*

acid-fast bacilli culture has a 90% sensitivity. Malignancy involving the meninges (primary or metastatic) often results in a CSF picture mimicking infectious meningitis.[8] Typically, there is a CSF leukocytosis, elevated protein, and glucose may range from normal to markedly decreased. A completely normal CSF exam essentially rules out CNS malignancy. Sensitivity of CSF cytology varies considerably among studies and varies from 60% to 90%, independent of such factors as tumor type, metastases, or primary brain site. A significant 3% false-positive rate has been reported which has limited its role as a routine staging screen for patients with malignancy. LP may be useful in diagnosing selected cases of subarachnoid hemorrhage (SAH), especially those in which head CT scan is equivocal. Interpretation of LP results may be problematic since RBCs in CSF commonly arise from a traumatic tap. The presence of xanthochromia in CSF has traditionally been associated with SAH, but has also been found in nearly one-third of traumatic taps. Similarly, a decreased RBC count from tube 1-4 has usually meant a traumatic tap but studies have shown a specificity of only 56%. Because of these limitations and potential LP complications, head CT scan has supplanted LP as the major diagnostic test in cases of suspected SAH. The diagnosis of multiple sclerosis may be supported by special CSF studies including oligoclonal banding and myelin basic protein, but sensitivity and specificity are variable. Another demyelinating condition, Guillain-Barré syndrome, is characterized by an isolated CSF protein value >200 mg/dL, with the remainder of CSF parameters normal. The absence of an elevated protein level practically excludes Guillain-Barré. In general, LP is more useful in Guillain-Barré syndrome than multiple sclerosis. **LIMITATIONS:** When a "traumatic tap" occurs (iatrogenic trauma), white blood cells may be passively transferred to the CSF. In general, for every 700 RBCs found in the CSF, 1 WBC is also expected (applies to the traumatic tap **only**). **ADDITIONAL INFORMATION:** Because of the risk of tonsillar herniation following LP, controversy exists concerning the routine use of head CT scan prior to LP. Data is incomplete and several clinical approaches are available. The conservative approach is to always perform a head CT prior to LP regardless of neurologic findings, so as never to overlook an intracranial mass lesion. Other clinicians follow a more flexible approach and argue that tonsillar herniation only occurs with demonstrable papilledema or focal neurologic deficits; thus, when both of these physical signs are absent LP may be safely performed without prior head CT. A middle ground approach has been advocated where head CT scan is performed prior to LP in the following situations: papilledema, focal neurologic deficits, recent history of sinusitis or otitis media, severe and progressive headache, and deterioration of mental status. In our institution, we generally adopt the conservative approach (acute meningitis is treated empirically prior to CT and LP).

Footnotes

1. Marton KI and Gean AD, "The Spinal Tap: A New Look at an Old Test," *Ann Intern Med*, 1986, 104:840-8.
2. Eng RHK and Seligman SJ, "Lumbar Puncture-Induced Meningitis," *JAMA*, 1981, 245:1456-9.
3. Brocker RJ, "Technique to Avoid Spinal Tap Headache," *JAMA*, 1958, 68:261-3.
4. Korein J, Cravisto H, and Leicach M, "Re-evaluation of Lumbar Puncture: A Study of 129 Patients With Papilledema or Intracranial Hypertension," *Neurology*, 1959, 9:290-7.
5. Chun CH, Johnson JD, Hofstetter M, et al, "Brain Abscess: A Study of 45 Consecutive Cases," *Medicine*, 1986, 65:415.
6. Lubic LG and Marotta JT, "Brain Tumor and Lumbar Puncture," *Arch Neurol Psychiatry*, 1954, 72:568.
7. Dougherty JM and Roth DO, "Cerebrospinal Fluid," *Emerg Med Clin North Am*, 1986, 4:281-97.
8. Reik L, "Disorders That Mimic CNS Infections," *Neurol Clin*, 1986, 4:223-48.

References

Fishman RA, *Cerebrospinal Fluid in Diseases of the Nervous System*, Philadelphia, PA: WB Saunders Co, 1980.

Keroak MA, "The Patient With Suspected Meningitis," *Emerg Med Clin North Am*, 1987, 5:807-26.

Simon R and Brenner B, "Neurosurgical Procedures," *Emergency Medicine*, Chapter 149, Baltimore, MD: Williams & Wilkins, 1982, 156-67.

NCV *see* Nerve Conduction Studies *on this page*

Nerve Conduction Studies

CPT 95900 (nerve conduction, velocity and/or latency, motor nerve); 95904 (sensory nerve)

Related Information

Electromyography *on page 160*

Synonyms Latency Studies; NCV; Nerve Conduction Velocity

Abstract **PROCEDURE COMMONLY INCLUDES:** Electrical stimulation of a peripheral nerve and recording of the evoked action potentials. Nerve conduction studies may be performed on either sensory nerves or mixed sensorimotor nerves. Following percutaneous electrical stimulation of an axon, a physiologic action potential (AP) is generated. This signal propagates down the axon, where it is detected at a distant site by surface electrodes. If a motor nerve is tested, the AP of the corresponding muscle is recorded. If a sensory nerve is examined, the AP of the identical nerve is recorded. In either case, the evoked AP is displayed on an oscilloscope screen where amplitude (in mV) and duration (in msec) are read directly. From this, several important parameters are calculated including the **latency time** (the time interval between stimulus presentation and initiation of action potential) and maximum **nerve conduction velocity** (speed of impulse propagation). This technique provides objective information regarding nerve function not obtainable from conventional electromyography alone. NCV testing is considered the procedure of choice in evaluating the patient with peripheral nerve dysfunction and should be considered an extension of the history and physical examination. **INDICATIONS:** NCV testing is useful in the following situations:

- confirm the presence of a sensory deficit in an objective manner, especially when the physical examination is inconclusive (or malignancy is suspected)
- evaluate the patient with diffuse polyneuropathy to determine severity and extent of disease and to distinguish demyelinating from axonal processes
- assess the patient with muscle weakness in order to distinguish a neuropathic process from primary muscle disease
- evaluate the patient with acute ascending paralysis to confirm the diagnosis of Guillain-Barré syndrome rapidly prior to plasmapheresis
- confirm the diagnosis of mononeuritis multiplex
- assess nerve entrapment syndromes (mononeuropathies) such as carpal tunnel syndrome; to determine the lesion site, differentiate entrapment from diffuse neuropathy, assess severity, and evaluate response to surgical interventions

Conventional NCV testing may often be **normal** in the following:

- primary muscle disease
- radiculopathies
- disease involving very proximal segments of a peripheral nerve (if suspected clinically, "H reflex" testing is indicated)
- most axonal-type neuropathies, unless the so-called "fast-fibers" are severely damaged
- anterior horn cell disease, such as any atrophic lateral sclerosis, NCVs are typically normal, or only marginally abnormal
- peripheral nerve lesions of any type, if examined early in the disease course. For example, in the first 1-2 weeks of acute Guillain-Barré syndrome, NCVs are usually normal. Even with complete transection of a peripheral nerve (eg, trauma), NCVs distal to the lesion remain normal for several days.

Despite these potentially "normal" test results, NCV testing may still provide valuable information. For example, in the patient with possible amyotrophic lateral sclerosis, it is important to document a normal NCV study in addition to the more typical EMG abnormalities.

CONTRAINDICATIONS: Relative contraindications include:

- the agitated, uncooperative patient
- presence of a cardiac pacemaker (or implantable cardiac defibrillation device). The pacemaker may be effected by the electrical current delivered to the skin.
- presence of an indwelling cardiac catheter, such as Swan-Ganz or central venous line. See Complications.

(Continued)

Nerve Conduction Studies *(Continued)*

Patient Care/Scheduling PATIENT PREPARATION: Risks and benefits of the procedure are discussed with the patient and informed consent is obtained. As a general rule, patient should be seen and evaluated by physician prior to this procedure. The accuracy of this test depends in part on the accuracy of the clinician's impression. Patient may take usual medications on the morning of examination including pain medications as needed. AFTERCARE: No specific activity restrictions are required postprocedure. Patient may resume prior level of activity. SPECIAL INSTRUCTIONS: Requisition from ordering physician should include brief clinical history, pertinent neurologic findings, specific disease conditions sought, and specific limbs to be tested. Ordering physician should also state if electromyography (or other electrophysiologic testing) is desired. COMPLICATIONS: NCV testing is safe and well tolerated in nearly all patients. Since surface electrodes are preferred over needle electrodes in most instances, the patient who refuses "needle tests" may accept and tolerate this procedure. Kimura (1983) argued that NCV testing is contraindicated in the patient with a cardiac pacemaker. He acknowledged that this was a theoretical concern. An electrical stimulus delivered to the skin in close proximity to the pacemaker site may interfere with pacemaker function. In addition, the patient with an indwelling cardiac catheter may also be "electrically sensitive." The current generated by NCV testing may be directed towards cardiac tissue because of these devices, presumably increasing the risk of arrhythmias. Again, there is little experimental (or clinical) data available to support this and these concerns remain hypothetical.

Method EQUIPMENT: NCV testing is performed with commercial EMG equipment adaptable to a nerve stimulator. Surface electrodes are round silver plates (0.5-1 cm diameter) placed directly on the skin for nerve stimulation. When two electrodes are contacted by the nerve stimulator, one will act as the cathode and the other as the anode, and current will flow between these negative and positive poles respectively, depolarizing the underlying nerve. The nerve stimulator itself is available in a variety of designs. Commonly it is a bipolar device with two metal prongs, 2-3 cm apart, attached to an insulated handle. The electrical impulse produced is a square wave of short duration (0.5-1 msec) and variable intensity (0-600 V). All stimulators are capable of generating either a threshold stimulus (evoked action in potential in a few axons) or a supramaximal stimulus (all axons in a nerve stimulated). Stimuli may be delivered in pairs or as a constant train. The stimulation and cathode ray oscilloscope are coordinated so that the "sweep" on the oscilloscope precedes the stimulus by a variable delay. In this way, a marker indicating the precise moment of stimulus delivery is always visible. The evoked action potentials, whether muscle or nerve, are preferably recorded on surface electrodes. (Occasionally, needle electrodes may be needed, especially when evaluating small, atrophic muscle fibers.) The compound action potentials detected by the recording electrodes are amplified 1000 times for muscle action potentials and approximately 100,000 times for sensory action potentials. Due to this magnitude of amplification, surrounding "noise" must be reduced, primarily through the use of high frequency, low-pass filters and amplifiers with a high signal-to-noise ratio (100,000:1) and high impedance (megaohm range). The amplified action potential is displayed on a cathode ray oscilloscope (frequency range 10 Hz to 10 kHz). Action potentials may be photographed using a synchronized shutter mechanism and/or stored onto magnetic tape. The oscilloscope is also capable of displaying multiple, serial action potentials on the screen for simultaneous comparison (each succeeding AP is placed on a higher baseline). The oscilloscope screen is calibrated for electric potential on the vertical axis (eg, 1 cm = 1 volt) and time on the horizontal axis (in msec). Some devices calculate the values for latency automatically and provide an automatic digital readout. TECHNIQUE: Technique differs somewhat amongst laboratories. The following outlines common principles only. A brief neurologic examination is conducted by the examiner prior to the procedure. Patient is asked to rest comfortably with muscles relaxed. For evaluation of a motor nerve, the axon must be stimulated at two (or more) sites, ie, a distal and proximal site. For example, when testing the median nerve the electrical stimulus is delivered to the wrist (distal site) and the antecubital fossa (proximal site); each site is tested separately. The cathodic lead of the bipolar stimulator depolarizes the nerve and the resultant action potential propagates down the axon in one direction (the anode hyperpolarizes the nerve and blocks conduction in the opposite direction). Recording electrodes located over the innervated muscle (eg, thenar muscle with median nerve testing) sense the compound muscle action potential which eventually results. This entire sequence (or "sweep") is displayed on the oscilloscope, starting from the original stimulus presentation (indicated by a "stimulus artifact" marker), followed by a delay prior to the start of the muscle action potential. Paired stimuli or a train of stimuli are presented. These steps are repeated at separate sites along the same axon. The **latency** (in msec) is defined as the time delay between the stimulus artifact and the first (negative) deflection of the muscle action potential. Values for latency are determined for both the proximal and distal stimulation sites with the recording electrode sites kept constant. Latency in motor nerve testing reflects the sum of pure nerve conduction time and the delay at the neuromuscular junction (NMJ). Since conduction velocity for the nerve alone is desired, the delay at the NMJ must be factored out. This is the basis for testing at both proximal and distal stimulating sites. Maximum NCV is calculated by the following:

- NCV (motor nerve) = distance (in mm) between proximal and distal sites / proximal latency (msec) - distal latency (msec)

NCV is an estimation of action potential propagation between the two sites of electrical stimulation. It does not measure nerve function past the distal site (eg, the hand) or closer than the proximal site (eg, spinal root). The nerve conduction time from stimulus presentation at the distal electrode to the start of the muscle action potential, the **distal** or **terminal latency**, is often recorded separately from maximum NCV. Distal latency reflects both nerve conduction and NMJ transmission. Sensory nerves may be tested in an analogous fashion. NCVs may be obtained in two ways: (1) orthodromic testing - stimulating electrodes are placed distally (eg, over digital nerves) and sensing electrodes placed proximally (eg, forearm), or (2) antidromic testing - stimulating electrodes placed proximally and sensing electrodes distally; this mimics physiologic impulse propagation. **Latency** is the time delay between electrical stimulation and appearance of the nerve action potential at the sensing electrode. Testing of sensory nerves does not involve muscle action potentials or NMJ delays. Calculation of sensory nerve latencies is more simple than motor latencies, since stimulation is required at only one site along the axon:

- NCV (sensory) = distance (mm) between stimulation point and recording electrode / sensory latency (msec)

Other important variables are the **amplitude** of the action potentials (in mV), **dispersion** of the action potentials, and the presence of **conduction blocks**. NCV may be determined for any peripheral nerve accessible to surface electrical stimulation. Only a limited number of nerves can be tested, in practicality, and the examination must be tailored to the clinical impression. In most centers, nonaffected limbs are also screened for generalized neuropathy (or to serve as internal controls). Commonly evaluated nerves include:

- upper extremity - median, ulnar, radial nerves (both sensory and motor)
- lower extremity - peroneal, tibial, superficial peroneal, sural nerves

Less accessible nerves in the upper extremity include the brachial plexus and shoulder girdle nerves. In the lower extremity the lumbosacral plexus, saphenous nerve, and lateral femoral cutaneous nerve are relatively difficult to test and are not usually used for asymptomatic screening.

Interpretation **NORMAL FINDINGS:** Preliminary written impression is given by neurologist or physiatrist usually on the same day. Normal values for distal latency, conduction velocity, and amplitude of evoked action potential have been established. These values are dependent on age and gender. Since equipment and technique vary from one laboratory to another, each laboratory develops its own set of normal values. Published normal values for median nerve motor conduction are:

- distal latency, 3.7 msec
- conduction velocity, elbow to wrist, 58 msec
- amplitude (wrist stimulation), 13.2 mV.

Of course, normal values vary for each peripheral nerve.

CRITICAL VALUES: In addition to objectively confirming the existence of a peripheral neuropathy, NCV testing can usually distinguish between the two major pathologic forms of neuropathy - axonal and demyelinating neuropathy. It is difficult to distinguish these disorders on the basis of history and physical examination alone. In addition, management strategies for these disorders are quite divergent. NCV testing allows initial categorization of a

(Continued)

Nerve Conduction Studies *(Continued)*

neuropathic process as a mononeuropathy, mononeuritis multiplex, or polyneuropathy. Within these broad categories, the pathologic process may be further divided into axonal or demyelinating lesions. In general, demyelinating diseases are characterized by decreased conduction velocities, markedly prolonged distal latencies, and normal (or slightly decreased) AP amplitude. In addition, two may be variably present: (1) AP dispersion (temporal variability of APs), and (2) conduction block (markedly decreased or absent AP amplitude with proximal nerve stimulation but not with distal site stimulation). NCV testing is often effective in diagnosing demyelinating disorders. Polyneuropathies due to demyelinating diseases include Guillain-Barré syndrome, diphtheric polyneuritis, demyelinating neuropathy associated with carcinoma, and several rare genetic neuropathies, Dejerine-Sottas disease, metachromatic leukodystrophy, and others. Axonal neuropathies are characterized by normal conduction velocity but decreased AP amplitude. Usually only a fraction of the axons in a nerve undergo degeneration. The fastest conducting axons in a nerve may be relatively spaced (unless disease is severe). Since nerve conduction velocities reflect only the fast fibers, and not the slow or medium velocity fibers, conduction velocities are typically normal despite extensive axonal degeneration. Polyneuropathies due to axonal degeneration are common and include neuropathies due to systemic disease (uremia, porphyria, vitamin B_{12} deficiency, systemic amyloidosis, severe hypothyroidism, chronic liver disease), medications (cis-Platinum, vincristine, metronidazole), toxins (alcohol, arsenic, lead, and others), and hereditary neuropathies (ataxia-telangiectasia syndrome, Friedreich's ataxia). Many neuropathies are due to mixed axonal-demyelinating processes. Examples include diabetic neuropathy, neuropathy associated with multiple myeloma or lymphoma, and several drugs. Characteristic features of the neuropathies are shown in the following table. NCV testing is also useful in the diagnosis of mononeuropathy multiplex, a condition in which neuropathy develops in multiple, but noncontiguous nerves, either simultaneously or over a prolonged period of time. Individual nerve trunks appear to be afflicted in a random fashion. NCV testing can determine if mononeuritis multiplex is being caused by an axonal or demyelinating neuropathy. Axonal processes potentially leading to mononeuritis multiplex are polyarteritis nodosum and vasculitic syndromes associated with connective tissue diseases (systemic lupus erythematosus, rheumatoid arthritis, and others). Demyelinating mononeuritis multiplex is most often due to chronic inflammatory demyelinating polyradiculoneuropathy (CIDP). Again, the distinction between axonal and demyelinating processes is crucial in clinical decision making. Focal involvement of a single nerve or mononeuropathy is frequently encountered in general practice. This implies local nerve compression usually from trauma or entrapment. NCV testing reveals localized slowing of nerve conduction at the point of compression due to localized demyelination (which precedes distal axon degeneration). Carpal tunnel syndrome is a common entrapment syndrome involving the median nerve. Testing can localize the lesion, exclude polyneuropathy, and assess severity. The presence of axonal degeneration distal to the compression site may warrant surgical intervention.

Nerve Conduction Studies

	Axonal Neuropathy	Severe Axonal Neuropathy	Demyelinating Neuropathy
Conduction velocity	N	N or ↓	↓↓
Distal latency	N or ↑	↑	↑↑
Action potential amplitude	↓	↓↓	N
Dispersion of APs	—	—	Possible
Conduction blocks	—	—	Possible
Examples	Uremic, alcoholic		Guillain-Barré syndrome

References

Adams RD and Victor M, *Principles of Neurology*, 4th ed, New York, NY: McGraw-Hill Book Co, 1989, 1009-27.

Aminoff MF, *Electrodiagnosis in Clinical Neurology*, 2nd ed, New York, NY: Churchill-Livingstone, 1986.
Asbury AK, "Disease of the Peripheral Nervous System," *Harrison's Principles of Internal Medicine*, 12th ed, JD Wilson, ed, New York, NY: McGraw-Hill Book Co, 1991, 2096-107.
Johnson EW and Wiechers D, "Electrodiagnosis," *Krusen's Handbook of Physical Medicine and Rehabilitation*, 3rd ed, FJ Kottke, GK Stillwell, and JF Lehmann, eds, Philadelphia, PA: WB Saunders Co, 1982, 56-85.
Kimura J, *Electrodiagnosis in Diseases of Nerve and Muscle: Principles and Practice*, 2nd ed, Philadelphia, PA: FA Davis Co, 1989.

Nerve Conduction Velocity *see* Nerve Conduction Studies *on page 169*

Neuromuscular Junction Testing

CPT 95937

Related Information

Electromyography *on page 160*
Single Fiber Electromyography *on page 179*

Synonyms Neuromuscular Transmission Study; Repetitive Stimulation Testing

Abstract **PROCEDURE COMMONLY INCLUDES:** Stimulation of an individual motor nerve by means of repetitive electrical impulses with measurement of muscle electrical activity. Supramaximal electrical stimuli are delivered to the skin overlying a motor nerve. A percutaneous electrode, placed over the corresponding muscle, records the evoked muscle action potentials using standard EMG technique. This procedure is unique in that electrical stimuli are delivered in a repetitive train (1-4 Hz). In diseases of the neuromuscular junction, characteristic changes in the compound action potential may be seen upon repetitive stimulation. **INDICATIONS:** Evaluation of the patient with a disorder of the neuromuscular junction suspected on clinical grounds. This includes both postsynaptic disorders such as myasthenia gravis and presynaptic disorders such as the Eaton-Lambert myasthenic syndrome (associated with oat cell carcinoma) and botulism. **CONTRAINDICATIONS:** No absolute contraindications have been described for this procedure (except patient refusal).

Patient Care/Scheduling **PATIENT PREPARATION:** Procedure and risks are discussed in detail with the patient and informed consent is obtained. In practice, many patients express anxieties concerning "needle tests," particularly those procedures involving multiple needle stabs. A thorough explanation of the technique along with calm reassurance will help allay such fears. Patient may take all routine medications on the morning of the examination including anticholinesterase medications. **AFTERCARE:** No specific activity restrictions are necessary following this procedure. **SPECIAL INSTRUCTIONS:** Requisition form submitted by the ordering physician should state the clinical history, pertinent findings, overall neurologic impression, and all electrophysiologic test(s) desired (ie, neuromuscular testing with or without conventional EMG, nerve conduction velocity studies, etc). **COMPLICATIONS:** Neuromuscular junction testing is a safe procedure with no serious complications reported. With myasthenia gravis, patient may experience transient weakness in the tested muscles, but this procedure does not induce so-called myasthenic crisis. Minor discomfort may be associated with needle puncture and electrical stimulation but in general is well tolerated.

Method **EQUIPMENT:** Standard EMG equipment is employed, including surface recording electrodes, preamplifier, electrical stimulus generator, cathode ray oscilloscope, and loudspeaker. Procedure is carried out in a fully equipped electrodiagnostic testing room. **TECHNIQUE:** Patient assumes a comfortable sitting or recumbent position. Examiner selects the skeletal muscles to be tested based on historical clues; often muscles of the hand are tested first (eg, hypothenar muscles). The motor nerve innervating the selected muscle is stimulated with brief, supramaximal electrical pulses delivered through the skin. Initially, stimuli are presented slowly, from 1-10/second (optimally 2-4/second) and the evoked muscle action potentials are observed on the oscilloscope. If the muscle activity is felt to be normal, the rate may be increased (≤50/second). If testing remains normal, the procedure should be repeated on several other muscles, including a large proximal muscle such as the deltoid. Provocative measures have been employed in some centers to increase test sensitivity. These are optional and involve "priming" of the myoneural junction (exercise, curare).

(Continued)

Neuromuscular Junction Testing *(Continued)*

Interpretation NORMAL FINDINGS: When repetitive stimuli are delivered at 1-10/second, muscle action potentials appear uniform and amplitudes high. Even when stimuli are maintained for 60 seconds, amplitudes do not diminish significantly. The same holds true for rapid rates of stimulation. Normal muscle can tolerate 25 stimuli/second without fatiguing. Results of the procedure are interpreted by a neurologist and impression is recorded immediately in chart. CRITICAL VALUES: In myasthenia gravis, slow rates of nerve stimulation (2-3/second) produce a characteristic funnel-shaped decrement in muscle action potentials over time. As shown in the following figure, action potential amplitudes decrease over the first five stimuli, but not to zero. This is termed the "M response". This effect plateaus almost immediately and subsequent amplitudes may increase slightly. This pattern of early electrical decrement with subsequent stabilization is highly specific for myasthenia gravis. In presynaptic disorders (Eaton-Lambert syndrome, botulism), a nearly opposite pattern is seen. When stimuli are presented at a rapid rate (20/second), action potentials initially are of low amplitude. Subsequently, the voltage increases in a continuous fashion as seen in the following figure. Again, this finding is felt to be fairly specific for presynaptic disorders.

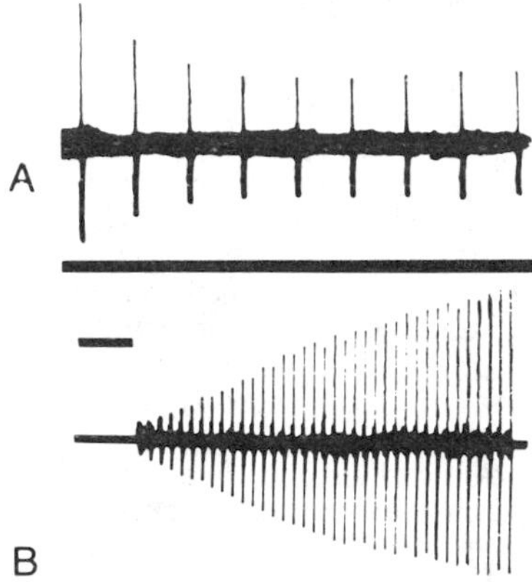

Action potentials obtained by neuromuscular junction testing in (A) myasthenia gravis and (B) Eaton-Lambert syndrome. Reproduced with permission from Adams RD and Victor M, "Part V/Diseases of Peripheral Nerve and Muscle," *Principles of Neurology*, 4th ed, New York. NY: McGraw-Hill, 1989, 956.

LIMITATIONS:

- Decremental response in the action potential is nonspecific. This has been described with myotonia, amyotrophic lateral sclerosis, and other diseases (however, the precise pattern of decrement-plateau, as seen in myasthenia gravis, is felt to be unique).
- Results may be falsely negative if minimally involved muscle groups are examined.
- Early in myasthenia gravis, the "M response" may not be seen.

References

Adams RD and Victor M, "Laboratory Aids in the Diagnosis of Neuromuscular Disease," *Principles of Neurology*, 4th ed, New York, NY: McGraw-Hill Book Co, 1989, 1009-27.

Johnson EW and Wiechers D, "Electrodiagnosis," *Krusen's Handbook of Physical Medicine and Rehabilitation*, 3rd ed, Kottke FJ, Stillwell GK, and Lehmann JF, eds, Philadelphia, PA: WB Saunders Co, 1982, 56-85.

Shahani BT and Young RR, "Clinical Electromyography," *Clinical Neurology*, Baker AB, ed, Philadelphia, PA: Harper and Row, 1985, 1-52.

Neuromuscular Transmission Study *see* Neuromuscular Junction Testing *on previous page*

Pattern-Shift Visual Evoked Responses *see* Visual Evoked Responses *on page 187*

Pure Tone Audiometry

CPT 92551 (screening test, pure tone, air only); 92552 (pure tone audiometry, air only); 92553 (air and bone)

Related Information

Speech Audiometry, Threshold Only *on page 181*
Speech Discrimination Audiometry *on page 184*

Synonyms Audiogram; Audiologic Assessment; Diagnostic Audiometry; Hearing Test

Applies to Basic Comprehensive Audiometry; Tympanometry

Abstract PROCEDURE COMMONLY INCLUDES: Assessment of overall hearing sensitivity by means of a standardized set of pure tones, electronically generated by an audiometer. A patient with clinically suspected hearing loss is presented with a series of pure tones over a range of frequencies. For each frequency the "auditory threshold" is determined, that is, the minimal intensity of sound required for audibility. Both air conduction (using earphones) and bone conduction (using a specialized bone vibrator) may be tested. Using this data, the threshold hearing level (in decibels) is plotted against frequency (in Hertz) for each pure tone. Four separate curves are generated – right ear air conduction (AC), right ear bone conduction (BC), left ear AC, and left ear BC. This comprises the pure tone audiogram. In addition to quantifying the degree of hearing loss, the pattern of the audiogram may point to the etiology of such loss, such as conductive hearing loss, sensorineural loss, or mixed deficits. Pure tone audiometry is regarded by some as the initial screening test of choice for audiologic dysfunction. INDICATIONS:

- evaluation of hearing loss, suspected from either the patient's self-report and/or abnormalities on bedside examination (eg, Weber and Rinne tuning fork tests)
- periodic screening for hearing loss during prolonged ototoxic drug therapy, eg, gentamicin treatment for enterococcal endocarditis
- periodic industrial screening for individuals at risk for noise-induced hearing loss
- selected cases of tinnitus, particularly when the neurologic examination is normal and entities such as acoustic neuroma, vascular compression, Ménière's syndrome, and others are suspected

CONTRAINDICATIONS: Although audiometry is essentially risk-free and no contraindications exist, the accuracy of this test hinges on truthful, voluntary responses from the patient. Diagnostic yield may be limited in the elderly patient with dementia as well as the very young child; however, both groups frequently require (and deserve) testing. Audiometry results must be carefully interpreted and more sophisticated audiologic testing may be required.

Patient Care/Scheduling PATIENT PREPARATION: In general, patients should undergo clinical examination by a physician prior to audiometry. Reversible or self-limited causes for hearing loss are ruled out first, such as impacted cerumen, acute otitis media, and labyrinthitis. The procedure is explained to the patient in general terms and consent is obtained. (This is repeated in a more detailed, step-by-step fashion by the audiologist.) No dietary or activity restrictions are necessary and patient may take usual medications on day of examination. Hearing aid (if applicable) should be brought to test area. AFTERCARE: No specific activity restrictions required. COMPLICATIONS: No significant complications reported.

Method EQUIPMENT: The audiometer is an electronic device capable of generating pure tones at a specific frequency, specific intensity, and duration, either singly or in series. As such, pure tones are nonenvironmental (ie, not heard outside the laboratory environment). For air conduction testing, tones are presented to each ear independently with specialized earphones. For bone conduction testing, a bone vibrator is placed onto the mastoid process of either right or left temporal bone; external auditory canals are not usually occluded. All equipment must be continually calibrated to conform with international standards. This ensures that a gradual loss of hearing noted on serial testing is truly valid and not due to machine error. Regarding parameters of the pure tone stimulus, the following are observed.

- Pulsed or intermittent pure tones are preferred to continuous tones. This avoids the phenomenon of "threshold adaptation."
- Optimal duration of each tone is from 200-500 msec based on signal theory.
- When tones are presented in rapid series, "off-time" intervals of 200 msec are generally maintained between stimuli.
- Characteristics of tones may be manually adjusted by audiologist.

Audiometry is performed in an isolated sound-dampened environment. As with other psychoacoustic testing, all audiometric equipment is discretely arranged so that visual (nonacoustic) cues are minimized.

(Continued)

Pure Tone Audiometry *(Continued)*

TECHNIQUE: At the outset, patient is instructed to signal the audiologist each time a tone is perceived. A variety of response signals may be employed – responding "yes" with each tone, tapping the rhythm of tones, or pointing to the ear where the tone is heard. For air conduction thresholds, earphones are comfortably positioned and the better ear tested first, if known. If not known, some audiologists will quickly screen each ear using the same initial frequency and the better ear tentatively determined. Tones are often presented in an ascending series, that is, from low to high frequency. Although the range of human hearing may span from 20-20,000 Hz, the frequencies of 200-6000 Hz appear most relevant for comprehension of speech. Standardized frequencies tested include 125, 250, 500, 1000, 1500, 2000, 3000, 4000, 6000, and 8000 Hz. This represents octave intervals, by convention, but intervening frequencies may also be tested. At a given frequency, tones are initially presented at a low intensity and incrementally increased by ≥5 dB steps. More than 50% of tones heard is conventionally accepted as the auditory threshold for that particular frequency. For example, a series of pure tones at 1000 Hz frequency is presented to the left ear at an initial intensity of 0 dB. The patient provides no response and the intensity is increased to 5 dB, then 10 dB, etc. At 25 dB, the patient responds to 50% of the tones and this is tentatively considered the auditory threshold. Often, tone intensities slightly above and below this auditory threshold are tested to verify and help "hone in" on the precise threshold value. If responses are consistent, the auditory threshold for left ear air conduction is taken as 25 dB at a frequency of 1000 Hz. Specific situations are as follows.

- If profound hearing loss is expected, frequencies from 125-500 Hz are tested first (some audiologists screen initially at 500 Hz then skip to 4000 Hz, if normal hearing expected).
- If a tone is not audible even at maximum audiometer output, "no response" is recorded.
- If 100% correct response occurs at a minimal intensity, testing below 0 dB is possible. The "0 dB" hearing level in audiometry is a modal value derived from a large population of normals. Thus, certain individuals may demonstrate greater hearing sensitivity and thresholds down to -20 dB are measurable.

In order to minimize the problem of tone perception in the nontest ear, sophisticated "masking" techniques have been developed. Continuous white noise of a narrow band width is channeled into the nontest earphone. Masking noise is designed to avoid distortion of pure tones in the test ear ("overmasking"), while decreasing the signal-to-noise ratio in the nontest ear. For bone conduction thresholds the technique is similar. A bone vibrator is placed over the mastoid process of the appropriate ear and pure tones are transmitted. Factors such as vibrator placement and pressure may influence results. Fewer frequencies are tested: 250, 500, 1000, 2000, 3000, and 4000 Hz. In addition, audiometer output is limited to approximately 80 dB due to distortion and other technical factors. Interrupted signals in an ascending series are again preferred. Masking of the nontest ear is even more significant with bone conduction testing. Each ear is tested separately for air and bone conduction yielding four independent sets of data.

Interpretation **NORMAL FINDINGS:** Normal values for auditory thresholds were defined by the International Standards Organization (ISO) in 1984. These values are derived from large population studies of normal adults 18-30 years of age. In most instances, a written interpretation is completed by a licensed audiologist or otologist on the same day. For both AC and BC, normal threshold levels at each pure tone frequency have been designated as "0 dB hearing level". Audiometers have been calibrated to this scale. The audiogram is a plot of tone intensity (dB) on the vertical axis against frequency (Hz) on the horizontal axis. A normal audiogram is illustrated in figure A, where most thresholds are approximately 0 dB (only AC and BC for the right ear is depicted). In normal individuals, a small discrepancy is often seen between air and bone conduction thresholds, the "AC-BC gap". At any given frequency the threshold for AC is somewhat lower than BC (ie, a stronger signal is needed for BC). **CRITICAL VALUES:** Abnormalities in the audiogram are characterized in terms of severity of hearing loss, specific frequencies most effected, unilateral or bilateral loss, and relative air versus bone conduction loss. From this analysis the audiologist may be able to quantify the general degree of loss and classify hearing loss in clinical terms – conductive hearing loss versus sensorineural loss (versus nonorganic loss). This is termed "site of lesion" testing. Several principles of interpretation deserve mention.

- For site of lesion testing, "conductive" loss implies a lesion in the external auditory meatus, tympanic membrane, and/or middle ear. "Sensorineural" loss usually implies a lesion in the cochlea or acoustic nerve (cranial nerve VII), but not the cortex. "Central" hearing loss refers to a lesion in the brainstem or auditory cortex. This cannot be adequately evaluated by pure tone audiometry. "Nonorganic" hearing loss implies an intact auditory circuit with deafness due to other factors (eg, malingering, psychosis).
- Mixed lesions are not uncommon.
- Normal AC thresholds imply normal auditory structures from external ear to acoustic nerve and BC thresholds are presumed normal as well.
- Loss of AC sensitivity is nonspecific and BC thresholds are necessary to differentiate conductive from sensorineural loss.

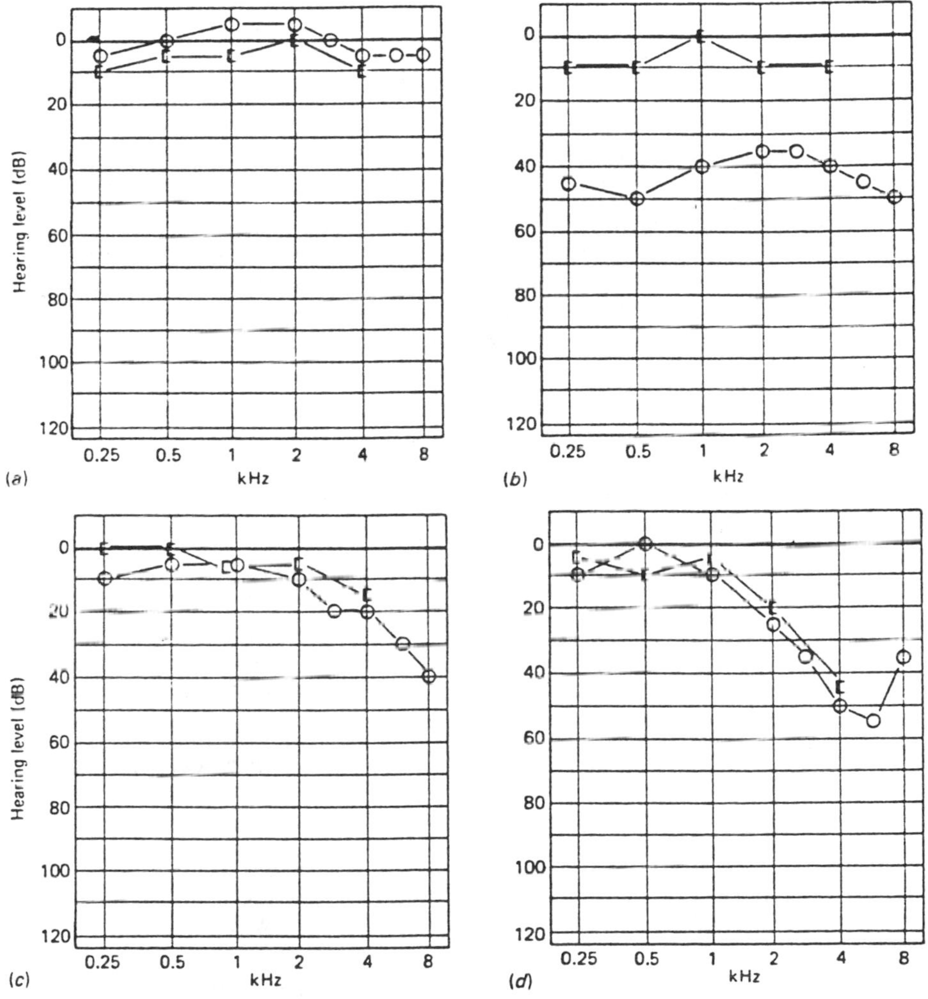

Idealized pure tone audiograms, right ear only. Symbols: o = air conduction, [= bone conduction. Figure a represents a normal audiogram. Figure b represents pure conductive hearing loss. Figure c depicts hearing loss associated with aging. Figure d depicts typical noise-induced hearing loss. Reproduced with permission from Lutman ME, "Diagnostic Audiometry," *Scott-Brown's Otolaryngology*, 5th ed, Chapter 7, Stephens D, ed, London, England: Butterworth's, 1987.

(Continued)

Pure Tone Audiometry *(Continued)*

- In theory, BC thresholds reflect events in the cochlea or acoustic nerve alone bypassing pathology in the external and middle ear (however, numerous exceptions exist).
- The difference between AC and BC thresholds at a given frequency reflects conductive hearing loss.
- The difference between BC thresholds and 0 dB reflects sensorineural loss.

Examples of idealized audiograms are shown in figures B, C, D. In figure B there is a marked decrease in sensitivity for AC thresholds with BC relatively spared. Both low and high frequencies are equally impaired in this example. This pattern is classically seen with pure conductive hearing loss. If a large mass component is playing a role (eg, serous otitis media), thresholds may be more impaired at higher frequencies. If conductive loss is due to stiffness of the stapes (eg, early otosclerosis), AC thresholds may be preferentially elevated at lower frequencies. Other examples of conductive hearing loss include eustachian tube dysfunction, otitis media, and impacted cerumen. With most cases of sensorineural loss, both AC and BC are significantly impaired and hearing loss is more pronounced as the frequency increases. Figure C depicts a constant loss of sensitivity for AC and BC, steadily worsening from low to high frequency. This pattern is often seen with the normal aging process. Figure D depicts the pattern seen with noise-induced hearing loss. Again, both AC and BC are impaired equally, but sensitivity appears to be most effected at 4000 Hz. Hearing loss declines steadily from 250-4000 Hz (typical of sensorineural loss) but then improves from 4000-8000 Hz (atypical). Another exception to the classic pattern of sensorineural loss is seen in early Ménière's disease where AC and BC thresholds are most elevated in the lower frequencies.

LIMITATIONS:

- Test is highly dependent on patient cooperation and reliability.
- Only nonenvironmental sounds are tested, not human speech.
- Only threshold levels of hearing are evaluated; there is no testing of suprathreshold sounds.
- Issues such as perceived clarity of sounds are not addressed.
- The effect of the stimulus on the listener's brain and auditory system cannot be measured directly and must be inferred (unlike brainstem auditory evoked potentials).
- Nonorganic hearing loss may be difficult to rule out.
- The assumption that BC thresholds are independent of external and middle ear pathology has been proven false. Tonndorf (1972) showed that disease in the external and middle ear may elevate BC thresholds, often unpredictably.
- The problem of cross-hearing may be quite significant, especially with BC thresholds where the skull readily transmits vibrations to both cochlea.
- If sensorineural loss is found, one cannot reliably differentiate cochlear from retrocochlear lesions.
- Only the site of lesion may be inferred, not any specific etiologies, ie, one cannot say whether conductive loss is due to middle ear effusion, otosclerosis, cerumen, etc.
- Technical limitations

ADDITIONAL INFORMATION: Pure tone audiometry, despite its limitations, is extremely useful in screening for loss of hearing sensitivity. The procedure is relatively simple, rapid (20-30 minutes), and has high reliability and reproducibility in most cases. Pure tones are easily generated and audiologist may individualize each case with ease.

References

Conijn EA, Van-der-Drift JF, Brocaar MP, et al, "Conductive Hearing Loss Assessment in Children With Otitis Media With Effusion. A Comparison of Pure Tone and BERA Results," *Clin Otolaryngol*, 1989, 14(2):115-20.

Lovrinic JH, "Pure Tone and Speech Audiometry," *Audiology for the Physician*, Chapter 2, Keith RW, ed, Baltimore, MD: Williams & Wilkins, 1980, 13-31.

Lutman ME, "Diagnostic Audiometry," *Scott-Brown's Otolaryngology*, 5th ed, Chapter 7, Stephens D, ed, London, England: Butterworth's Publishers, 1987, 244-71.

Single Fiber Electromyography

CPT 95872

Related Information

Electromyography *on page 160*

Neuromuscular Junction Testing *on page 173*

Synonyms SF-EMG; Single Fiber EMG

Applies to Repetitive Stimulation Tests

Abstract **PROCEDURE COMMONLY INCLUDES:** Recording the electrical activity of a single motor fiber using conventional electromyographic techniques. A specialized electrode is inserted percutaneously into a selected muscle (eg, extensor digitorum communis) and the electrical activity of the muscle fiber is displayed as an action potential wave on a cathode ray oscilloscope. Unlike conventional EMG, the electrode is small enough to pick up activity in only one or two muscle fibers, an almost "pure" action potential. SF-EMG is used to diagnose diseases of the neuromuscular junction, such as myasthenia gravis. This technique estimates **muscle jitter** (the electrical variability between two muscle fibers in the same motor unit) and **fiber density** (the number of individual muscle fibers in a single motor unit). SF-EMG is a sensitive means of confirming the diagnosis of myasthenia gravis; muscle jitter and fiber density may be abnormal even when the disease is subclinical. **INDICATIONS:** Diagnosis of diseases of the neuromuscular junction, including myasthenia gravis, Eaton-Lambert syndrome (myasthenic paraneoplastic syndrome associated with small cell carcinoma of the lung), and botulism. Some authorities advocate SF-EMG as a means of distinguishing neuropathy from myopathy, but this is controversial. **CONTRAINDICATIONS:** Although there are no absolute contraindications to SF-EMG, test results may be compromised in the patient with severe weakness, gross tremor, or uncontrolled movement disorder. Repetitive stimulation tests may be more appropriate in these situations.

Patient Care/Scheduling **PATIENT PREPARATION:** SF-EMG is often performed along with conventional EMG and the same considerations apply. **AFTERCARE:** No specific activity restrictions are necessary postprocedure. **SPECIAL INSTRUCTIONS:** The requisition from the ordering physician should include a brief clinical history, pertinent neurologic findings, and overall clinical impression. In many cases, SF-EMG is performed at the neurologist's discretion in conjunction with conventional EMG without an explicit order. **COMPLICATIONS:** This procedure is essentially risk-free and no significant complications have been reported. Patients tolerate this procedure well, possibly due to the low number of needle punctures required.

Method **EQUIPMENT:** A small, highly selective electrode is used for SF-EMG recording, usually a 25 micron diameter wire within a hollow cutting needle. This is equivalent to approximately 50% of the width of a single muscle fiber. Single fiber action potentials are recorded with minimal distortion and transmitted to a standard oscilloscope and a loudspeaker. A 500 Hz filter is often used to eliminate background noise from distant muscle fibers. **TECHNIQUE:** Any muscle accessible to conventional EMG may be studied using SF-EMG. Several authors advocate routine testing of the extensor digitorum communis due to its accessibility and the ease of voluntary patient control. Initially, the patient is trained to perform a minimal muscle contraction (eg, raising the third finger). Following this, the needle electrode is inserted percutaneously and electrical activity measured at rest and during a minimal contraction. A single fiber action potential is signified by a crisp "pop" on the loudspeaker and a uniform, reproducible waveform on the oscilloscope. The two major parameters obtained during SF-EMG are fiber density and muscle jitter. The former is based on the observation that a randomly inserted electrode will record the action potential from a single fiber approximately 70% of the time. In the remaining 30%, the electrode will pick up electrical activity of two or more fibers. The fiber density is determined by inserting the electrode randomly into the same muscle 20 separate times. The number of individual fibers sensed during each insertion is noted (ie, one, two, three or more fibers). In other words, the number of synchronous action potentials is counted at each of 20 different

(Continued)

Single Fiber Electromyography *(Continued)*

electrode positions; the average value (mean) of the 20 measurements is the fiber density. This parameter estimates the number of single muscle fibers in one motor unit. Muscle jitter represents the electrical variability between two single muscle fibers in the same motor unit. Although innervated by the same nerve (by definition) these two fibers may differ slightly with respect to impulse propagation and electrical potential. If the first fiber is held "still" in time on the oscilloscope, the action potential of the second fiber appears to vary in time with respect to the first fiber. The time difference between the appearance of the two action potentials (in microseconds) is recorded for 200 consecutive depolarizations. The mean value for these 200-time intervals is termed the mean consecutive difference and is the numerical value that estimates jitter.

Interpretation **NORMAL FINDINGS:** Single fiber action potentials resemble fibrillation potentials in terms of configuration and duration. Normal values for fiber density have been established from asymptomatic volunteers and vary for individual muscles. For the extensor digitorum communis the fiber density is normally 1.3-1.8. Normal values for muscle jitter have also been established. For the extensor digitorum communis jitter is normally approximately 55 msec (expressed as the mean consecutive difference). Interpretation is done by certified neurologist specially trained in this technique. **CRITICAL VALUES:** In disorders of the neuromuscular junction, such as myasthenia gravis, jitter is markedly increased. In addition, the phenomenon of "blocking" may be seen as well. When two single fibers are being tested for jitter, the second fiber may intermittently fail to fire. These blocked action potentials represent failure of impulse conduction. In normal individuals, the value for jitter stays constant even through repeated muscle contractions. With myasthenia gravis jitter continually increases with repetitive muscle contractions. With Eaton-Lambert syndrome, jitter is also increased when tested initially, but with repetitive muscle contraction jitter decreases over time. Fiber density is increased early on in neuropathic processes that are characterized by reinnervation. However, some authors have argued that fiber density is also increased in a variety of myopathic conditions, particularly when segmental muscle necrosis has occurred, with subsequent regeneration. Thus, some experts feel that fiber density lacks the diagnostic specificity to distinguish neuropathy from myopathy. Others point out that both fiber density and jitter are usually normal, or only slightly increased, in myopathic conditions. **LIMITATIONS:**

- Procedure requires some degree of patient training. Patient must perform a minimal muscular contraction.
- When a significant baseline tremor or movement disorder exists test results may be difficult to interpret.
- Increased jitter or fiber density cannot be used to reliably differentiate neuropathy from myopathy.
- SF-EMG should not be used as the sole diagnostic test in evaluating neurologic disorders.

ADDITIONAL INFORMATION: SF-EMG is a rapid and well-tolerated means of assessing neuromuscular junction disease. Although SF-EMG has limited diagnostic specificity, the sensitivity is outstanding for diseases such as myasthenia gravis. SF-EMG may be the first objective marker of neurologic disease when both physical examination and conventional EMG are normal.

References

Adams RD and Victor M, "Laboratory Aids in the Diagnosis of Neuromuscular Disease," *Principles of Neurology*, 4th ed, New York, NY: McGraw-Hill Book Co, 1989, 1009-27.

Johnson EW and Wiechers D, "Electrodiagnosis," *Krusen's Handbook of Physical Medicine and Rehabilitation*, 3rd ed, Kottke FJ, Stillwell GK, and Lehmann JF, eds, Philadelphia, PA: WB Saunders Co, 1982, 56-85.

Shahani BT and Young RR, "Clinical Electromyography," *Clinical Neurology*, Baker AB, ed, Philadelphia, PA: Harper and Row, 1985, 1-52.

Single Fiber EMG *see* Single Fiber Electromyography *on previous page*

Somatosensory Evoked Potentials *see* Electroencephalography *on page 158*

Speech Audiometry, Threshold and Discrimination *see* Speech Discrimination Audiometry *on page 184*

Speech Audiometry, Threshold Only

CPT 92555

Related Information

Pure Tone Audiometry *on page 175*
Speech Discrimination Audiometry *on page 184*

Synonyms Speech Reception Threshold (SRT); Speech Threshold; Spondee Threshold

Abstract **PROCEDURE COMMONLY INCLUDES:** Determining the lowest hearing level necessary for the detection and comprehension of human speech. The listener is presented with a series of selected test words, either disyllabic words (spondees) or running speech, using earphones in a sound-attenuated room. The speech reception threshold (SRT) is defined as the lowest hearing intensity (in audiometric decibels) at which the listener correctly repeats 50% of the words. The SRT for an individual is compared against population norms in order to grade the degree of relative hearing loss. This test is also useful in confirming hearing thresholds obtained using pure tone audiometry. SRT is considered a routine component of basic audiologic evaluation. **INDICATIONS:**

- screen for hearing impairment suspected on clinical grounds; some experts consider SRT the initial screening procedure of choice
- confirm hearing thresholds obtained by pure tone audiometry (normal or abnormal), primarily as a cross-check for test reliability
- follow-up on abnormal pure tone audiometry, usually as a prelude to speech discrimination testing

CONTRAINDICATIONS: SRT is essentially risk-free and no absolute contraindications have been reported.

Patient Care/Scheduling **PATIENT PREPARATION:** In most cases, patients should be examined by a physician prior to speech audiometry. Reversible or self-limited causes of hearing loss are ruled out (impacted cerumen, labyrinthitis, acute otitis media, etc). The procedure is explained to the patient in a step-by-step manner. No dietary or activity restrictions are necessary and the patient may take usual medications including nasal sprays, decongestants, etc. Hearing aid should be brought to test center (if applicable). **AFTERCARE:** No specific post-test restrictions. Follow-up is arranged by primary physician or audiologist as necessary. **SPECIAL INSTRUCTIONS:** Validity of procedure depends on patient accuracy and reliability. Diagnostic yield may be limited in the demented patient or very young child. In many clinical instances, however, testing is clearly indicated in these same individuals and SRT should not be withheld arbitrarily on the basis of age alone. **COMPLICATIONS:** None reported.

Method **EQUIPMENT:** As with pure tone audiometry, an electronic audiometer is utilized, a device capable of transmitting recorded speech via earphones. Alternatively, monitored live voice (MLV) may be employed with the audiometer in the "off" position. The audiometer is equipped with a separate voltage unit (VU) meter to monitor sound intensity. Regarding the speech stimuli, several protocols have been published and extensively reviewed. The majority of these auditory word lists are composed of disyllabic words called "spondees" (each syllable spoken with equal intensity). Word lists adhere to the following criteria.

- Words must be familiar to most listeners ("baseball").
- Words display phonetic variation.
- A normal sample of speech sounds is used.
- There is homogeneity of audibility.

Prerecorded lists of spondees are commercially available, such as the Psychoacoustic Laboratory (PAL) Test No 9 (two lists of 42 words each) and the Central Institute for the Deaf (CID) Tests W-1 and W-2 (36 spondaic words). In comparison with live speech, the recorded versions may contain psychoacoustic modifications including the following.

- "Difficult" spondees are presented at a higher intensity (2 dB louder).
- Spondees judged "simple" are 2 dB softer.
- The carrier phrase "say the word" is included before each spondee at a level 10 dB greater than the test spondee.

(Continued)

Speech Audiometry, Threshold Only *(Continued)*

- Word lists may be scrambled to provide multiple equivalent forms of the test (PAL No 9).
- Automatic attenuation is incorporated; for example, in the W-2 test the sound intensity is automatically decreased by 3 dB every third word.

As mentioned, monitored live voice (MLV) technique may be employed instead of recorded speech. Either standard spondee lists may be read, or less commonly, "running" speech presented. MLV allows modifications for children and other specialized groups. A widely-accepted Children's Spondee List has been published for MLV.

TECHNIQUE: Patient is seated in sound-dampened room with earphones comfortably placed. Some audiologists provide the listener with an alphabetized list of spondees to be tested in order to ensure word familiarity. The listener is instructed to simply repeat the word(s) heard through the earphones without a "penalty" for an incorrect response. Speech signals may be presented in either a descending or ascending fashion. Tillman and Olsen (1973) described a descending clinical protocol as follows.[1]

- A spondaic word is presented approximately 40 dB above the estimated speech threshold.
- If listener responds correctly, decrease by 10 dB and present a different spondaic word.
- Repeat step 2 until a word is repeated incorrectly, at which point a second spondaic word is presented at that same intensity. If this second word is correctly repeated, continue to decrease intensity by 10 dB until two consecutive spondaic words are incorrectly identified. If, however, an error is made on the second word, increase intensity by 10 dB and proceed to the next step.
- Once the intensity is increased, threshold exploration is begun. This entails a somewhat complex series of steps using longer spondee lists and smaller increments or decrements in intensity (2-5 dB steps). The SRT in this method must be calculated by the audiologist (using correction factors as well), and approximately the 50% correct response criteria traditionally used to define SRT. This protocol is popular, rapid, and avoids the redundancy of bracketing techniques. Speech signals may also be presented in an ascending protocol, as described by the American Speech and Hearing Association (1979).[2] This technique begins with a spondee at the lowest possible intensity; subsequent steps are analogous (but not identical) to those of the descending series. The former protocol does not require a prior estimation of auditory threshold (as does the Tillman protocol), but may be somewhat more time consuming. Both protocols are comparable, per Huff and Nerbonne (1982).[3]

SRTs are obtained for each ear independently. As with pure tone audiometry, masking techniques are necessary, that is, white noise is presented to the nontest ear. Contralateralization of speech stimuli may occur via bone conduction, especially when SRT of the test ear is greater than bone conduction threshold of the nontest ear by 40 dB or more, or when SRT differs by >40 dB between ears.

Interpretation **NORMAL FINDINGS:** Interpretation is done by licensed audiologist or otologist on the same day. Normal values for auditory thresholds have been derived from population studies of healthy adults. The average threshold level (for both pure tone and speech audiometry) within this population has been calculated and defines audiometric "0 dB". Thus, an average SRT would be 0 dB for both right and left ears in a young, healthy adult. This standard of audiometric zero has been accepted by the American National Standards Institute (ANSI-1969) and differs from the decibel measurement of sound pressure level (dynes/cm^2). "Normal" hearing thresholds vary somewhat depending on the author. Hearing level loss from 0-25 dB is considered normal in most classification systems. Such individuals display no difficulties in speech comprehension and hearing aid evaluation is not necessary. Note that negative SRT values (eg, -5 dB) are possible in some normal individuals since 0 dB represents only a population mean. Clinical trials have demonstrated that SRT correlates closely with threshold for pure tones. The threshold for pure tones should agree with the threshold for speech to within 5-6 dB, provided the pure tone curve is flat. (If the curve is sloping, the pure tone thresholds at 500 and 1000 Hertz may be averaged, and compared with SRT.) **CRITICAL VALUES:** The speech reception threshold in each ear

Hearing level (loss) in dB re:ANSI-1969

0 10 20 30 40 50 60 70 80 90 100 110 120

	Profoundly deaf						Clarke (1957)
	Slight deafness	Partial deafness	Severe deafness	Profound deafness			Dale (1962)
Class A: Not significant	Class B: Slight	Class C: Mild	Class D: Marked	Class E: Severe	Class F: Extreme		Davis & Silverman (1970)
Normal	Mild	Moderate	Severe	Profound			Pauls & Hardy (1953)
Normal	Mild	Moderate	Moderately severe	Severe	Profound		Goodman (1965)
Normal	Class 1: Mild losses	Class 2: Marginal losses	Class 3: Moderate losses	Class 4: Severe losses	Class 5: Profound losses		Streng et al (1955)
Normal	Hard of hearing	Educationally or partially deaf	Deaf				Streng et al (1955)

Hearing impairment scales, classifying degree of severity. Applies to both speech reception thresholds and pure tone thresholds. Reproduced with permission from Lloyd LL and Kaplan H, *Audiometric Interpretation: A Manual of Basic Audiometry*, Baltimore, MD: University Park Press, 1978, 16.

may be compared with established population norms. A variety of hearing impairment scales have been devised to classify the degree of loss: mild, moderate, severe, and profound. These scales are listed in the figure and apply to both speech reception thresholds and pure tone thresholds. Again, 0 dB is taken as an average hearing level. For example, by the Goodman scale, an individual with SRT values of 20 dB in the right ear and 45 dB in the left ear would have normal hearing in the right ear but moderate impairment in the left. SRT levels are elevated in both conductive and sensorineural types of hearing loss and do not discriminate. A discrepancy between SRT and pure tone threshold 12 dB or more is considered significant and deserves further evaluation. A discrepancy of this magnitude suggests a severe defect in speech discrimination as seen with the following:

- certain central nervous system lesions
- presbycusis
- inappropriate spondee selection (eg, unfamiliar words)

In addition, discrepancy may also be due to tinnitus (pure tone threshold more affected than speech), problems with equipment calibration, and patient artifacts including malingering.

LIMITATIONS:

- Speech signals are technically more difficult to calibrate than pure tones.
- Listener response is relatively complicated.
- Results may be influenced by familiarity of the patient with the specific word lists used.
- Speech comprehension at suprathreshold levels is not assessed.

ADDITIONAL INFORMATION: Lovrinic recommends SRT as the first test to be administered to patients with clinical hearing loss. Arguments include the following.

- The stimuli used with SRT (spondaic words) are more concrete and familiar for many patients than pure tones.
- Spondees are more clinically relevant than nonenvironmental tones since a day-to-day function (speech reception) is being evaluated.
- It is more difficult for the factitious (malingering) patient to consistently produce falsely elevated speech reception thresholds.
- Even less time is needed than pure tone audiometry.

(Continued)

Speech Audiometry, Threshold Only *(Continued)*

Footnotes

1. Tillman TW and Olsen WO, "Speech Audiometry," *Modern Developments in Audiology*, 2nd ed, Jerger J, ed, New York, NY: Academic Press, 1973, 37-74.
2. American Speech, Language and Hearing Association, Committee on Audiometric Evaluation, "Guidelines for Determining the Threshold Level for Speech," *ASHA*, 1979, 21:353-6.
3. Huff SJ and Nerbonne MA, "Comparison of the American Speech, Language and Hearing Association and Revised Tillman-Olsen Methods for Speech Threshold Determination," *Ear Hear*, 1982, 3:335-9.

References

Lloyd LL and Kaplan H, *Audiometric Interpretation: A Manual of Basic Audiometry*, Baltimore, MD: University Park Press, 1978, 89-149.

Lovrinic JH, "Pure Tone and Speech Audiometry," *Audiology for the Physician*, Keith RW, ed, Baltimore, MD: Williams & Wilkins, 1980, 13-31.

Schill HA, "Thresholds for Speech," *Handbook of Clinical Audiology*, 3rd ed, Katz J, ed, Baltimore, MD: Williams & Wilkins, 1985, 224-34.

Speech Discrimination Audiometry

CPT 92556

Related Information

Pure Tone Audiometry *on page 175*

Speech Audiometry, Threshold Only *on page 181*

Synonyms Speech Audiometry, Threshold and Discrimination

Abstract **PROCEDURE COMMONLY INCLUDES:** Testing speech comprehension at suprathreshold, conversational levels. A series of phonetically balanced words is presented to the listener at a specific sound intensity level. The listener repeats this list of words back to the examiner and the percentage of correct responses is determined at that intensity level. The procedure is repeated at different intensity levels with new word lists. Each time, the percentage of correct responses is recorded, the "discrimination score". Data accumulated in this manner is plotted as a performance-intensity function, the "articulation curve," with discrimination score on the vertical axis and sound pressure level (in dynes/cm^2) on the horizontal axis. From this curve several useful points may be read directly, including:

- optimal discrimination score, "PB_{max}," the highest point on the articulation curve
- speech reception threshold, the speech intensity corresponding to a 50% correct response rate
- the discrimination loss, the difference of PB_{max} from 100%

These parameters, along with the shape of the articulation curve, are compared with established norms. Both the degree and nature of hearing loss may be characterized. Speech discrimination testing is an integral part of the standard audiologic battery and plays an important role in evaluating conversation-level hearing.

INDICATIONS: Speech discrimination tests have been applied to a number of clinical situations, with variable degrees of success.[1] Among these are:

- evaluation of hearing skills necessary for day-to-day conversation and social adequacy
- determination of the site of an audiologic lesion (somewhat limited value; must be combined with other audiometric tests)
- selection of patients who might benefit from otologic surgery
- assessment of aural rehabilitation
- screening for central auditory disorders (procedure well-suited due to complexity of stimuli)
- selection of candidates eligible for hearing aids (important role)

CONTRAINDICATIONS: There are no absolute contraindications for this procedure.

Patient Care/Scheduling **PATIENT PREPARATION:** In most cases, patients should be examined by a physician prior to speech audiometry. Reversible or self-limited causes of hearing loss are ruled out (impacted cerumen, labyrinthitis, acute otitis media, etc). The procedure is explained to the patient in a step-by-step manner. No dietary or activity restrictions are necessary and the patient may take usual medications including nasal sprays, decongestants, etc. Hearing aid should be brought to test center (if applicable).

Method EQUIPMENT: Speech discrimination testing is performed using a standard audiometer, an electronic device capable of transmitting recorded speech to each ear independently via earphones. Instead of recorded speech, monitored live voice (MLV) may be alternatively employed for speech stimuli presentation. Speech discrimination tests have evolved over the past 40 years and may be classified by test format:[2]

- monosyllabic words with open response (repeat the words): Harvard Psychoacoustic Laboratory PB-50; Central Institute for the Deaf (CID) W-22; Northwestern University Tests 4 and 6
- monosyllabic words with closed response (multiple choice answers): Rhyme Test, California Consonant Test
- sentences with open response: CID "Everyday" Sentences; SPIN Test
- sentences with closed response: Synthetic Sentence Identification; Kent State University Speech Discrimination Test

TECHNIQUE: The patient is seated in a sound-dampened room with earphones on. The listener is instructed to simply repeat the words heard through the earphones with no "penalty" for an incorrect response. Each ear is tested separately (monoaurally) as well as binaurally. The audiologist selects a word list appropriate for the listener and presents the list using either a recording or MLV technique. Stimuli are presented at a sound level approximating conversational speech. On the average this would be 70 dB sound pressure level (dynes/cm^2 x 0.0002). For soft speech at 1 meter, intensity would be 60 dB SPL (sound pressure level), and for loud speech, 80 dB SPL. Usually the intensity levels selected reflect this 60-80 dB range (at least). The percentage of correct responses is determined at a specific frequency (eg, 50 dB). A new list of words is then presented at a different frequency (eg, 70 dB) and the discrimination score again noted. This procedure is continued at the discretion of the audiologist. If a wide range of sound intensity levels is assessed, an articulation curve may be plotted, that is, discrimination score on vertical axis and sound pressure level (re: 0.0002 dyne/cm^2) on the horizontal axis. This is a time-consuming process, but sometimes necessary in complicated cases. The maximum discrimination score, "PB_{max}," may be read directly from the curve (highest point), as well as the speech reception threshold (intensity at which discrimination score is 50%). During monaural testing, speech stimuli presented to the test ear may also be perceived in the nontest ear, primarily by bone conduction. Thus, as with other forms of audiometric testing, masking techniques are necessary to offset this problem. Filtered white noise is transmitted to the contralateral ear while the word list is being transmitted to the test ear. Speech discrimination testing may also be performed with competing noise in the test ear, "discrimination in noise". This technique is felt to better simulate day-to-day social communication. Various types of competing noise may be used: cafeteria noise, filtered white noise, competing voice, voice babble. Both the speech stimulus (the word list) and the competing noise are presented to the same ear simultaneously. This technique is particularly useful in hearing aid evaluation. DATA ACQUIRED:

- performance – intensity function for both right and left ears; if testing is extensive a complete articulation curve may be plotted
- PB_{max}
- speech reception threshold
- discrimination in noise (optional)

Interpretation NORMAL FINDINGS: Interpretation is done by a licensed audiologist or otologist on the same day. Normal values for the articulation curve have been derived from testing normal hearing young adults. However, depending on the particular speech discrimination test selected, normal curves may differ substantially. As one example, the configuration of the typical curve for a normal individual taking the PB W-22 test differs significantly from the same individual taking the Rush-Hughes test. Scores from different tests should not be compared directly. In the figure on the following page, a normal performance-intensity function is depicted. The normal value for PB_{max} is 100% for most tests, and this is generally achieved at 40-50 dB SPL. Once this maximum discrimination score is obtained, the normal listener will maintain the 100% score as sound intensity is in-

(Continued)

Speech Discrimination Audiometry *(Continued)*

creased. The normal value for the speech reception threshold (discrimination score of 50%) is around 30 dB SPL but varies considerably depending on the specific word list chosen. Speech reception threshold obtained directly from a formal articulation curve is the gold standard. The techniques described in the entry Speech Audiometry, Threshold Only are approximations of this value. It should be noted that the decibel scale on the performance-intensity graph represents actual SPL in units of dynes/cm^2. In contrast, the decibel scale used for pure tone audiometry and speech threshold audiometry is a relative value scale without physical units. This latter scale defines 0 dB hearing level (HL) as the average hearing acuity for a normal population, the so-called "audiometric zero". The value of 0 dB HL (audiometric zero) corresponds to 24.5 dB SPL at 250 Hertz. Another parameter is "discrimination loss," the difference between PB_{max} and 100%. The normal value is zero.

CRITICAL VALUES: The figure also depicts idealized curves seen with conductive loss, coch-

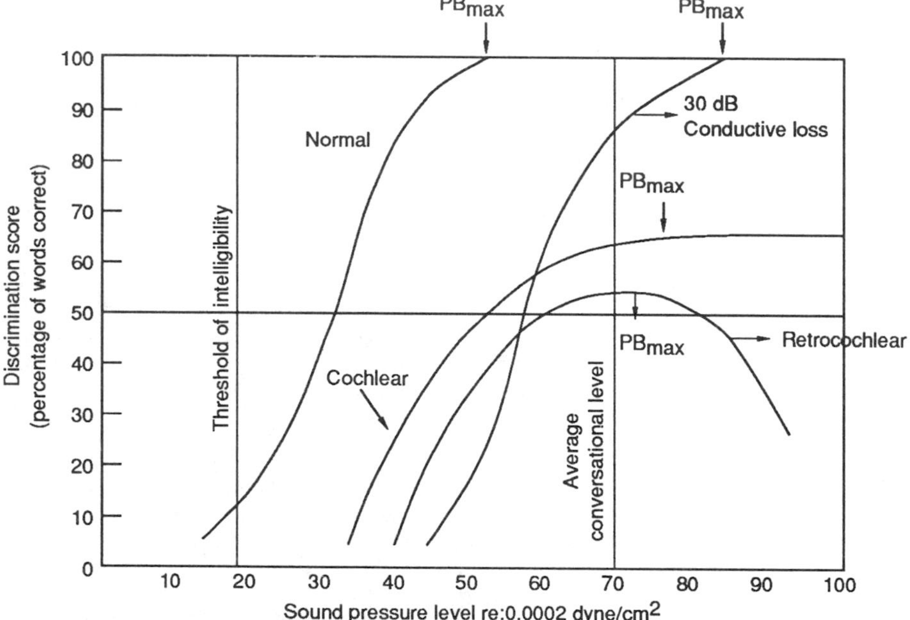

Idealized articulation curves for normal hearing, cochlear hearing loss, conductive loss, and retrocochlear loss. Reproduced with permission from Lloyd LL and Kaplan H, *Audiometric Interpretation: A Manual of Basic Audiometry*, Baltimore, MD: University Park Press, 1978, 93.

lear loss, or retrocochlear loss. General principles for interpretation are as follows.

- For pure conductive hearing loss, PB_{max} will eventually reach 100% but only at high intensity levels. Speech reception threshold is elevated. Clinically, an afflicted individual will display adequate speech discrimination if the stimulus is sufficiently loud.
- For sensorineural loss in the cochlea, PB_{max} is reduced (ie, best discrimination score much $<$100%) and this value is achieved only at high sound intensity levels. When sound intensity is increased even further, speech discrimination does not worsen (ie, the articulation curve plateaus).
- For retrocochlear, cranial nerve VIII loss, a characteristic "rollover phenomenon" is seen. After PB_{max} is reached, further increases in sound intensity actually cause a worsening of speech discrimination. "Rollover" refers to the shape of the curve. In the example shown, PB_{max} is 55% at 75 dB SPL. When word lists are presented at a higher sound intensity – 80 dB and above – more errors are made. Discrimination scores worsen to 20% correct at 90 dB.

- For central auditory dysfunction (lesion in brainstem or brain), the curve may resemble that of retrocochlear loss with rollover, but often the curve is not predictable.

These guidelines apply to the majority of cases, but many exceptions have been noted. Considerable overlap may exist between diagnostic groups, and this limits diagnostic utility. By itself, speech discrimination should not be relied upon for site-of-lesion determination. Other supporting tests are needed. Several classification schemes have been published to grade the loss in speech discrimination at any given intensity. These are based on the discrimination score. Categories include normal, slight discrimination difficulty, moderate difficulty, poor discrimination (50% to 60% correct response) and very poor discrimination (<50% correct).

Footnotes

1. Penrod JP, "Speech Discrimination Testing," *Handbook of Clinical Audiology*, 3rd ed, Katz J, ed, Baltimore, MD: Williams & Wilkins, 1985, 235-55.
2. Lovrinic JH, "Pure Tone and Speech Audiometry," *Audiology for the Physician*, Keith RW, ed, Baltimore, MD: Williams & Wilkins, 1980, 13-31.

References

Lloyd LL and Kaplan H, *Audiometric Interpretation: A Manual of Basic Audiometry*, Baltimore, MD: University Park Press, 1978, 89-149.

Speech Reception Threshold (SRT) *see* Speech Audiometry, Threshold Only *on page 181*

Speech Threshold *see* Speech Audiometry, Threshold Only *on page 181*

Spinal Tap *see* Lumbar Puncture *on page 165*

Spondee Threshold *see* Speech Audiometry, Threshold Only *on page 181*

Tympanometry *see* Pure Tone Audiometry *on page 175*

VERs *see* Visual Evoked Responses *on this page*

Vestibular Test *see* Electronystagmography *on page 164*

Visual Evoked Potentials *see* Visual Evoked Responses *on this page*

Visual Evoked Responses

CPT 92280

Related Information

Electroencephalography *on page 158*

Synonyms Pattern-Shift Visual Evoked Responses; VERs; Visual Evoked Potentials

Abstract PROCEDURE COMMONLY INCLUDES: Stimulation of the retina and optic nerve with a shifting checkerboard pattern. This external visual stimulus causes measurable electrical activity in neurons within the visual pathways. This is called the visual evoked response (VER) and is recorded by EEG electrodes located over the occiput. Using special computer techniques, the evoked responses measured over multiple trials are amplified and averaged. As with conventional EEG, a waveform may be plotted (electrical potential versus time). With pattern-shift VER, the waveform normally appears as a straight line with a single positive peak (100 msec after stimulus presentation). Abnormalities in this characteristic waveform may be seen in a variety of pathologic processes involving the optic nerve and its radiations. Pattern-shift VER is a highly sensitive means of documenting lesions in the visual system. It is especially useful when the disease process is subclinical (ie, ophthalmologic exam is normal and patient lacks visual symptoms). INDICATIONS: VER is used to confirm the diagnosis of multiple sclerosis, suspected on clinical grounds. VER testing can detect optic neuritis at an early, subclinical stage. In general, the diagnosis of "clinically definite" multiple sclerosis can be made by meeting the following criteria:

- past history of two or more episodes of a neurologic deficit
- an isolated white matter lesion demonstrable on clinical exam
- a second, independent lesion on laboratory testing (or again, on clinical exam); this last criterion may be fulfilled by documenting an abnormal VER (suggestive of optic neuritis). Thus, VER testing is indicated when multiple sclerosis is suspected, but clinical criteria are inconclusive.

(Continued)

Visual Evoked Responses *(Continued)*

- evaluate diseases of the optic nerve. VERs are abnormal in a number of diseases: glaucoma, ischemic optic neuropathy, pseudotumor cerebri, toxic amblyopias, nutritional amblyopias, and neoplasms compressing the anterior visual pathways. The VER may be abnormal in other conditions involving the central nervous system (primary or secondary) such as sarcoidosis, pernicious anemia, and Friedreich's ataxia. However, abnormalities are nonspecific and are not diagnostic of a specific disease entity.
- assess visual function in the infant or child; this procedure is reliable even in the neonate, since a verbal response is not required
- rule out hysterical blindness
- monitor the visual system during optic nerve (or related) surgery
- assess visual acuity in special circumstances (eg, amblyopia)

CONTRAINDICATIONS: VER can be reliably performed in patients with mild to moderate loss of visual acuity. In the severely myopic patient (visual acuity is worse than 20/200), the checkerboard pattern cannot be seen adequately and testing should not be performed. Also, the patient must be reasonably cooperative and attentive enough to watch the checkerboard for a several minute period. Muscular spasms involving the head and neck will compromise test results. Appropriate medications should be given or the procedure rescheduled.

Patient Care/Scheduling

PATIENT PREPARATION: The procedure is explained and verbal consent is obtained. Routine medications may be taken on the morning of the procedure, including prescription ophthalmics. Patient should wash hair the night beforehand (to facilitate electrode placement). Fasting prior to testing is not necessary; in fact, patient may eat shortly before the exam (to avoid relative hypoglycemia). Corrective lenses should be brought to the testing room. **AFTERCARE:** No specific restrictions are necessary postprocedure. Previous level of activity may be resumed. Since sedatives are not used during VER testing, outpatients may drive themselves home. **SPECIAL INSTRUCTIONS:** In most cases, this procedure is ordered directly by a neurologist. If ordered by a general physician, requisition should include brief clinical history, pertinent neurologic findings, and overall impression. When testing children and neonates, special techniques are necessary and the laboratory should be notified of this in advance. **COMPLICATIONS:** VER testing is a safe, pain-free procedure. In theory, there is a risk of inducing a seizure in a susceptible patient from the flashing checkerboard. However, this risk appears clinically negligible. The stimulus used for VER testing is quite different from the flashing strobe light used for seizure "activation" in EEG testing. The alternating checkerboard maintains a constant level of luminescence, unlike the strobe light.

Method

EQUIPMENT:

- surface (scalp) electrodes, the same used for conventional EEG
- pattern-shift stimulator, either a television screen or a projected image
- signal amplifier with filters
- computer system for signal averaging

TECHNIQUE: VER is performed in a specially-equipped electrodiagnostic procedure room. At the start, the patient is seated comfortably approximately 1 meter away from the pattern-shift screen. Surface electrodes are placed on the scalp overlying the occipital and parietal regions with reference electrodes in the frontal region and ear. The patient is asked to focus his gaze onto the center of the screen. Each eye is tested separately (monocular testing). A shifting checkerboard pattern is presented on the screen, with each square reversing color every 0.5-1 second. Usually, 100 or more pattern shifts are presented. Each pattern alteration is considered a separate stimulus. Electrical activity in the optic nerve and its radiations are detected by the scalp electrodes. Electrical potentials are recorded for a 500 msec interval following a stimulus. Characteristically, VERs are of low amplitude and require considerable amplification. Computer signal averaging must be used to diminish random, background electrical signals, and isolate the VER. Conventional EEG does not utilize this technology. It is unable to distinguish VERs (from strobe light stimuli) from background "noise". The results of the numerous consecutive trials are computer averaged. The composite signal appears as a waveform, with potential on the vertical axis and time on the horizontal. **DATA ACQUIRED:** A computer-averaged visual evoked response at each electrode.

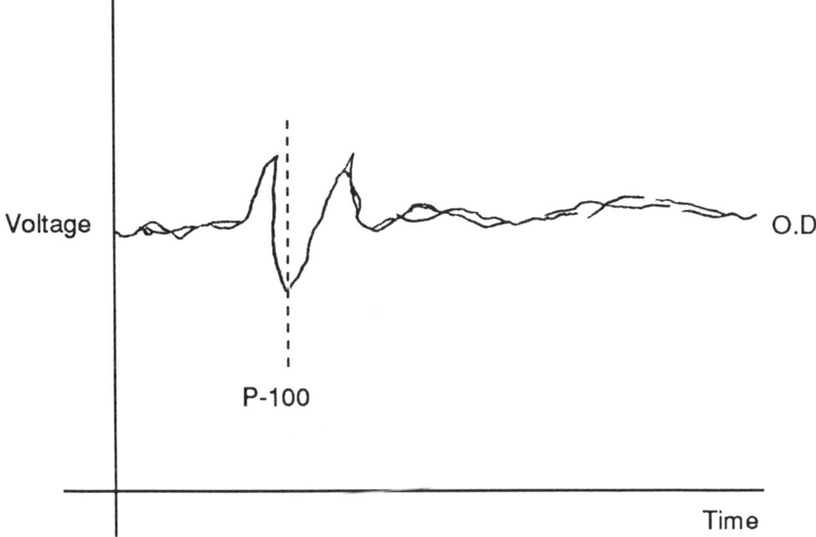

Visualized evoked response for one eye, depicting "P-100." Stimulus is presented at time 0.

Interpretation **NORMAL FINDINGS:** Data are interpreted by an experienced neurologist, usually on the same day. The normal visual evoked response is a single, triphasic wave. This is shown in the above figure. The peak of this wave occurs approximately 100 msec after stimulus presentation and is referred to as "P100". Several parameters of the evoked response are measured, including:

- absolute P100 latency – the time interval between the stimulus and the first large positive (downward) peak of P100. Normal range is 90-110 msec.
- interocular latency – the difference in P100 latency between the right and left eyes. Normally, the latency difference is <8-10 msec.
- amplitude of the VER (less important)
- duration of the triphasic wave (less important)

Normal values for these parameters are established for each laboratory and are age and gender dependent.

CRITICAL VALUES: Any disease which slows conduction of optic nerve fibers will prolong the absolute P100 latency. For example, in unilateral optic neuritis from multiple sclerosis, the P100 wave may be detected as late as 200 msec after the stimulus (instead of the normal 100 msec). Both the absolute P100 latency and the difference in latency between the two eyes would be abnormal. The advantage of VER testing, however, lies in its sensitivity, not specificity. Only limited information can be obtained regarding the nature of the visual lesion. P100 latencies may be prolonged in multiple sclerosis, ischemic optic neuropathy, tumors, etc. VER testing may be useful in localizing the site of the lesion. See table on the following page. Abnormalities of P100 duration or amplitude have more limited diagnostic utility, due to a lack of specificity. **ADDITIONAL INFORMATION:** Pattern shift VER is useful in the confirmatory diagnosis of multiple sclerosis. Well-designed studies have shown that PS-VER is abnormal in a significant number of multiple sclerosis patients whose formal ophthalmological examinations are normal. The rate of false negativity with pattern-shift VER is quite low. Some experts feel that a normal VER essentially rules out optic neuritis.

References

Asselman P, Chadwick DW, and Marsden CD, "Visual Evoked Responses in the Diagnosis and Management of Patients Suspected of Multiple Sclerosis," *Brain*, 1975, 98:261-82.

Chiappa KH, *Evoked Potentials in Clinical Neurology*, New York, NY: Raven Press, 1983.

(Continued)

Visual Evoked Responses *(Continued)*

Chiappa KH and Ropper AH, "Evoked Potentials in Clinical Medicine," *N Engl J Med*, 1982, 306:1140-50.

Shahroki F, Chiappa KH, and Young RR, "Pattern Shift Visual Evoked Responses: Two Hundred Patients With Optic Neuritis and/or Multiple Sclerosis," *Arch Neurol*, 1978, 35:65-71.

Visual Evoked Responses

VER Abnormality	Lesion Site
Prolonged latency, right eye only	Right optic nerve, anterior to the optic chiasm
Prolonged latency, left eye only	Left optic nerve, anterior to the optic chiasm
Prolonged latencies, right and left eye symmetrically	Localization not possible
Normal latency, midline electrodes	Either no lesions, or lesion is posterior to optic chiasm, or false-negative/technical error

OPHTHALMOLOGY

Lawrence E. Lohman, MD

Over the years, ophthalmology has been quick to embrace new technologies. This fact, along with terminologies which are confusing to other medical practitioners, often leads to difficulty in the understanding of various eye tests.

While many of the ophthalmic procedures in this handbook are well established, refinements continue to take place. Photography is more sophisticated as evidenced by our expanding knowledge of retinal diseases (fluorescein angiography) and the cornea (endothelial photography). Older procedures, such as visual field testing, have been modified by the application of computerized programming and analysis of results.

As more sophisticated testing and interpretive techniques are applied, even further information about the visual system will be obtained. Although test results are becoming more detailed and specific, they should actually seem more understandable, and therefore valuable, to the patient's general health care management team.

Aid for the Partially Sighted *see* Low Vision Center *on page 196*
Aid for the Visually Impaired *see* Low Vision Center *on page 196*
Angiogram *see* Fluorescein Angiography *on page 195*
Automated Perimetry *see* Perimetry *on page 197*

Axial Length, A-Scan

CPT 76511; 76516; 76519

Synonyms Ultrasound, A-Scan; IOL Measurement; Pseudophakos Measurement

Applies to Diagnostic Preoperative Cataract and Intraocular Lens Implant Surgical Assessment; Intraocular Lens Calculation

Abstract PROCEDURE COMMONLY INCLUDES: Keratometry readings, intraocular lens power calculation for various lens types INDICATIONS: Provide measurement of axial length of eye, identify abnormalities in globe length. Measurement is used in preoperative intraocular lens (IOL) power calculation. Helps in differential diagnosis of intraocular pathology (ie, tumors, membranes).

Patient Care/Scheduling PATIENT PREPARATION: Patient should bring spectacles to the testing area. If glaucoma patient, delete routine glaucoma drops one dose just prior to appointment, with ophthalmologist's approval. Pupils may be dilated. AFTERCARE: Patient will be cautioned not to rub or touch around eyes for 30 minutes after testing because of local anesthesia. May have eyes dilated, dark glasses are helpful. Patient should arrange for a ride home from testing site. SPECIAL INSTRUCTIONS: Type of intraocular lens to be implanted must be known for proper power calculation. Simultaneous B-scan ultrasound may be needed for proper orientation and interpretation of intraocular pathology.

Method EQUIPMENT: Changes in acoustic density of ocular tissue are displayed on an oscilloscope. TECHNIQUE: Digital biometric ruler uses A-scan ultrasound to accurately measure axial length of globe. Various calculation formulas (of either theoretical or regression types) are used to determine power of IOL to be implanted. Ultrasound probe is applied to the surface of anesthetized eye. Probe may be handheld or fixed in apparatus such as a mounted tonometer. Patient is usually in sitting position. DATA ACQUIRED: Axial length of the eye is the distance from the stationary transducer to the retinal echo spike.

Specimen TURNAROUND TIME: Immediately if indicated.

Interpretation LIMITATIONS: Results may be variable in patients with poor central visual fixation. Patient cooperation is required. ADDITIONAL INFORMATION: Axial length and keratometry measurements are used in various formulas for calculation of intraocular lens power. The acoustical density (height of echo spikes) helps to differentiate between intraocular tumor types or causes of intraocular membranes.

References

Duane TD, *Duane's Clinical Ophthalmology*, Philadelphia, PA: JB Lippincott Co, 1990.

Story PG and Wiesner PD, "Axial Length and the Average Ophthalmologist – Is Biometry Worthwhile?" *Ophthalmic Surg*, 1989, 20(5):327-31.

B-Scan *see* Ultrasound, B-Scan *on page 200*
Carotid Patency Evaluation *see* Oculoplethysmography *on page 196*
Central and Peripheral Field Testing *see* Perimetry *on page 197*
Coefficient of Outflow Facility *see* Tonography *on page 199*
Color Plates *see* Color Vision Testing *on this page*

Color Vision Testing

CPT 92283

Synonyms Color Plates

Applies to D-15 Test; Farnsworth-Munsell Test; FM-100 Test; H-R-R Plates; Ishihara Plates; Nagel Anomaloscope; Pseudoisochromatic Plates

Abstract INDICATIONS: Identification of hereditary color vision abnormalities, helpful in the diagnosis and management of optic nerve and retinal abnormalities.

Method EQUIPMENT: Pseudoisochromatic plates (H-R-R, Ishihara) consist of letter, number, or pattern arrangements of colored dots surrounded by complementary or gray dots. The

Nagel anomaloscope uses a prism to separate the colors of the visible spectrum which are then matched by the patient. The Farnsworth-Munsell test consists of a series of color chips mounted on a cap. **TECHNIQUE:** Under daylight, or simulated daylight conditions, the patient examines a series of pseudoisochromatic plates and indicates the figure seen. Incorrect responses are recorded by the examiner. With the Nagel anomaloscope, the patient matches the hue and saturation of yellow with mixtures of red and green. Color deficient individuals use inappropriate mixtures. The Farnsworth-Munsell tests are either the D-15 or FM-100. The patient arranges 15 buttons according to color with the D-15 exam. The patient is asked to arrange 85 chips in order or increasing hue in the FM-100 test. **DATA ACQUIRED:** The tests identify those patients with abnormal color vision and may help to identify different patterns of inherited color deficiency. The FM-100 test can identify persons with above average, average and deficient color discrimination along with identifying typical zones of color confusion.

Specimen **CAUSES FOR REJECTION:** Testing performed under incandescent lights may by inaccurate. **TURNAROUND TIME:** Immediate, but some interpretation may be necessary.

Interpretation **NORMAL FINDINGS:** The normal patient will sequence colors correctly or identify the correct patterns on color plate testing. **LIMITATIONS:** Some tests will not identify those with mild color deficits. In addition, some tests will not distinguish between different inherited color deficiencies. **ADDITIONAL INFORMATION:** Hereditary color deficiencies occur in approximately 7% of men and <1% of women. Acquired deficiencies occur secondary to optic nerve dysfunction or retinal disorders (especially those effecting the macular area where the cone receptors are concentrated).

References

Benson WE, "An Introduction to Color Vision," *Clinical Ophthalmology*, Duane TD and Jaeger EA, eds, Philadelphia, PA: Harper and Row, 1987.

D-15 Test *see* Color Vision Testing *on previous page*

Diagnostic Preoperative Cataract and Intraocular Lens Implant Surgical Assessment *see* Axial Length, A-Scan *on previous page*

Disc Photography *see* Fundus Photography *on page 196*

Electro-oculogram

CPT 92270

Synonyms Electrophysiologic Testing; EOG

Abstract **INDICATIONS:** When used in conjunction with the electroretinogram, this test supplies additional information concerning the retina and supporting tissues.

Patient Care/Scheduling **PATIENT PREPARATION:** The eyes may be dilated **AFTERCARE:** Patient should arranged for a ride home from the testing site.

Method **EQUIPMENT:** Electrodes are placed at the medial and lateral canthi of the eyelids. A ground electrode is placed on the forehead. **TECHNIQUE:** The average value of the resting potential of the eyes is measured as they move horizontally a standard distance by fixating alternately on two targets. The change in this resting potential across the retina is compared between the light and dark adapted states. **DATA ACQUIRED:** The ratio of the maximum amplitude in the light adapted state to the minimum amplitude in the dark adapted state is computed.

Specimen **TURNAROUND TIME:** Immediate, interpretation is required.

Interpretation **NORMAL FINDINGS:** The normal EOG ratio is >200. **ADDITIONAL INFORMATION:** The EOG reflects the health of the retinal pigment epithelium. It helps in differential diagnosis of retinal diseases, especially when used in conjunction with the electroretinogram.

Electrophysiologic Testing *see* Electro-oculogram *on this page*

Electrophysiologic Testing *see* Electroretinography *on this page*

Electroretinography

CPT 92275

Synonyms Electrophysiologic Testing; ERG

Abstract **INDICATIONS:** Helps in differential diagnosis of blindness in infancy, hereditary retinal diseases, toxic retinopathies, and degenerations. May help in the management of dia-

(Continued)

Electroretinography *(Continued)*

betic retinopathy, central retinal vein occlusion, blindness where retinal status is in doubt. **CONTRAINDICATIONS:** Sensitivity to topical anesthetics or dilating drops. The eye should not be dilated in the presence of narrow angle glaucoma.

Patient Care/Scheduling **PATIENT PREPARATION:** Pupils will be dilated and topical anesthetic instilled in the eyes. Testing may require dark adaptation. **AFTERCARE:** Dark glasses may be helpful. Patient should arrange for a ride home from the testing site.

Method **EQUIPMENT:** A contact lens electrode is applied to the eye surface. A reference electrode is applied to the forehead and a ground to an earlobe. The action potential produced by light stimulation is photographed from an oscilloscope record. **TECHNIQUE:** The retina is stimulated after either dark (scotopic) or light (photopic) adaptation. The light stimulus can be varied in intensity, color, and frequency. **DATA ACQUIRED:** The first negative deflection is termed the "a wave" and reflects outer retinal layer (photoreceptor) activity. The positive "b wave" follows and is generated by intermediate retinal layers. The "c wave" is generated by the pigment epithelium. Oscillatory potentials are identified on the ascending portion of the "b wave". The time from light stimulus to onset of "a wave" is the latency. The implicit time is measured from stimulus to peak of the "b wave".

Specimen **TURNAROUND TIME:** Immediate, interpretation is required.

Interpretation **NORMAL FINDINGS:** The response may be categorized as supernormal, normal, subnormal, or nonrecordable. **ADDITIONAL INFORMATION:** The light adapted response primarily reflects cone function. The dark adapted response is primarily from the rods. A flicker (rapid light stimulus) ERG is more specific for cone function.

References

Duane TD, *Duane's Clinical Ophthalmology*, Philadelphia, PA: JB Lippincott Co, 1990.

International Standardization Committee, "Standard for Clinical Electroretinography," *Arch Ophthalmol*, 1989, 107(6):816-9.

Endothelial Cell Count *see* Endothelial Photography *on this page*

Endothelial Photography

CPT 92286

Synonyms Endothelial Cell Count; Preoperative Corneal Evaluation; Specular Microscopy

Abstract **PROCEDURE COMMONLY INCLUDES:** Evaluation of corneal endothelium when diseased or prior to surgery. Microphotographs of corneal endothelium, determination of cellular density and morphology, pachymetry (measurement of corneal thickness). **INDICATIONS:** Helpful to screen patients with suspected inherited corneal endothelial disease (eg, Fuchs' dystrophy, posterior polymorphous dystrophy, iridocorneal endothelial syndrome); to evaluate endothelium prior to: fitting extended wear aphakic contact lenses, intraocular surgery when there is a history of previous intraocular surgery, cataract removal by the phacoemulsification technique, and cataract surgery in the presence of suspected endothelial abnormality.

Patient Care/Scheduling **PATIENT PREPARATION:** If done in conjunction with intraocular lens power measurement, pupils will be dilated **AFTERCARE:** Patient is advised not to rub eyes for 30 minutes after exam because of topical anesthesia. Patient should arrange for a ride home from the testing site.

Method **EQUIPMENT:** Light reflected at the endothelial layer of the cornea is microscopically studied and displayed on a video monitor or 35 mm film. The most accurate and commonly used microscopes contact the corneal surface. **TECHNIQUE:** After instillation of topical anesthesia, the objective lens of the microscope is gently applanated on the corneal surface. The observer focuses the instrument on the endothelial layer for photographic documentation. **DATA ACQUIRED:** Endothelial photographs evaluated for cell density ("cell count") and cellular morphology.

Specimen **TURNAROUND TIME:** Available immediately if indicated. Evaluation of 35 mm photographs require film developing time.

Interpretation **NORMAL FINDINGS:** Cell count variable **CRITICAL VALUES:** Cell count preferably >1500 cells/mm^2 prior to intraocular surgery, but varies by clinical situation **ADDITIONAL INFORMATION:** Preoperative evaluation helps predict the endothelial tolerance to surgical trauma and postoperative function. Simultaneous pachymetry (corneal thickness) measurements quantitate the endothelial role in the maintenance of corneal dehydration and clarity.

EOG *see* Electro-oculogram *on page 193*

ERG *see* Electroretinography *on page 193*

Facility of Aqueous Outflow *see* Tonography *on page 199*

Farnsworth-Munsell Test *see* Color Vision Testing *on page 192*

Field of Vision *see* Perimetry *on page 197*

Fluorescein Angiogram *see* Fluorescein Angiography *on this page*

Fluorescein Angiography

CPT 92235

Synonyms Angiogram; Fluorescein Angiogram; Fluorescein Angioscopy

Abstract PROCEDURE COMMONLY INCLUDES: Intravenous injection of fluorescein dye followed by multiframe photography (angiography) or ophthalmoscopic evaluation (angioscopy). Medical evaluation of photographic record. INDICATIONS: Helpful in evaluation of wide range of retinal and choroidal diseases. Less commonly used to evaluate abnormalities of the optic nerve and iris. Most frequently applied in diagnosis and management of macular and vascular (including diabetic) diseases. CONTRAINDICATIONS: Sensitivity to fluorescein dye, uncooperative patient.

Patient Care/Scheduling PATIENT PREPARATION: Pupils will be dilated AFTERCARE: Patient should arrange for a ride home from the testing sight. SPECIAL INSTRUCTIONS: Patient should expect temporary decrease in vision and red after image secondary to flash photography. Fluorescein dye will cause temporary skin and urine discoloration. COMPLICATIONS: Transient symptoms of nausea and possible vomiting occur in 2% to 4% of patients. Hives or asthmatic symptoms are treated with diphenhydramine hydrochloride or cortisone. Rare severe reactions such as anaphylactic reaction or respiratory and cardiac arrest have been reported.

Method EQUIPMENT: A fundus camera with motorized camera back is used to take serial photographs after fluorescein injection. Fluorescein absorbs light in the blue range and emits light in the yellow-green range. The fundus camera is fitted with appropriate filters to allow precise evaluation of the choroidal and retinal circulation. TECHNIQUE: Ten percent or 25% fluorescein dye is injected in a peripheral vein in a 2-second bolus. Serial photographs through a red-free filter document the dye transit through choroidal and retinal vessels. Routine processing of standard black and white film onto contact sheets and positive transparencies allow in-depth analysis. DATA ACQUIRED: Flow characteristics through the choroidal and retinal circulation along with assessment of integrity of retinal vessels are obtained. Fine details of retinal circulation and retinal pigment epithelium not obtainable by routine ophthalmoscopy can be discerned by this technique.

Specimen TURNAROUND TIME: Results can occasionally be obtained the same day in urgent cases. Time required for photographic developing and interpretation.

Interpretation LIMITATIONS: Poor pupillary dilation or media opacities (such as corneal scarring, cataract, vitreous hemorrhage) limit fundus view. ADDITIONAL INFORMATION: Test should be ordered in consultation with ophthalmologist.

References

Berkow JW, Kelley JS, and Orth DH, "Fluorescein Angiography: A Guide to the Interpretation of Fluorescein Angiograms," *American Academy Ophthalmology*, San Francisco, CA: 1984.

Fluorescein Angioscopy *see* Fluorescein Angiography *on this page*

FM-100 Test *see* Color Vision Testing *on page 192*

Formal Fields *see* Perimetry *on page 197*

Fundus Photography

CPT 92250

Synonyms Disc Photography; Optic Nerve Photography

Abstract **INDICATIONS:** Documentation of retinal and optic nerve disease. Follow glaucomatous optic nerve damage. **CONTRAINDICATIONS:** Poor patient cooperation.

Patient Care/Scheduling **PATIENT PREPARATION:** Pupils will be dilated **AFTERCARE:** Patient should arrange for a ride home from the testing site.

Method **EQUIPMENT:** Fundus camera **TECHNIQUE:** 35 mm or Polaroid record may be obtained with fundus photography. Optical filters and stereoscopic techniques may be employed. **DATA ACQUIRED:** Baseline photographic record of fundus pathology. Stereoscopic photography helps in documentation and follow-up of glaucomatous optic nerve "cupping".

Specimen **TURNAROUND TIME:** Polaroid records immediately. Standard 35 mm film requires processing into slides.

Interpretation **LIMITATIONS:** Poor pupillary dilation or opacities of ocular media (such as corneal scarring, cataract, vitreous hemorrhage) limit fundus view. **ADDITIONAL INFORMATION:** Stereoscopic viewer necessary for evaluation of stereo photographs.

Goldmann Perimetry *see* Perimetry *on next page*

H-R-R Plates *see* Color Vision Testing *on page 192*

Intraocular Lens Calculation *see* Axial Length, A-Scan *on page 192*

Intraocular Tension *see* Tonometry *on page 199*

IOL Measurement *see* Axial Length, A-Scan *on page 192*

IOP *see* Tonometry *on page 199*

Ishihara Plates *see* Color Vision Testing *on page 192*

Low Vision Aids *see* Low Vision Center *on this page*

Low Vision Center

CPT 92392

Synonyms Low Vision Aids; Aid for the Partially Sighted; Aid for the Visually Impaired

Abstract **PROCEDURE COMMONLY INCLUDES:** Thorough evaluation of degree of visual handicap, trial of appropriate optical and nonoptical low vision aids **INDICATIONS:** Evaluation of the low vision patient. Counseling and provision of low vision aids when appropriate.

Patient Care/Scheduling **PATIENT PREPARATION:** A recent ophthalmological examination with diagnosis and best refraction should be included in the referral note. Patient should bring current glasses and any low vision aids (eg, hand magnifiers) in current use. Pupils should **not** be dilated.

Specimen **TURNAROUND TIME:** Immediately if indicated.

Interpretation **ADDITIONAL INFORMATION:** Low vision aids for trial may be available for loan to the patient.

Nagel Anomaloscope *see* Color Vision Testing *on page 192*

Ocular Pressure *see* Tonometry *on page 199*

Ocular Ultrasound *see* Ultrasound, B-Scan *on page 200*

Oculoplethysmography

CPT 93850

Synonyms OPG; Plethysmography, Ocular; Carotid Patency Evaluation

Replaces Ophthalmodynamometry

Abstract **PROCEDURE COMMONLY INCLUDES:** Evaluation of carotid patency, evaluation scale with results **INDICATIONS:** Noninvasive evaluation for carotid blood flow in suspected carotid stenosis **CONTRAINDICATIONS:** Recent retinal detachment, eye infection, cataract surgery within 3 months, prosthesism, uncooperative or disoriented patient.

Patient Care/Scheduling **PATIENT PREPARATION:** Contact lens will be removed for test **AFTERCARE:** Must not rub eyes for 30 minutes following test because of local anesthesia. Contact lens should not be inserted for 30 minutes following test. Vision may be blurry for short time after test. **SPECIAL INSTRUCTIONS:** Patient must have two eyes (no prosthesis). Careful evaluation of patients with retinal detachment history.

Method **TECHNIQUE:** Zira oculoplethysmograph using corneal air sensors and earlobe pulse sensors.

Specimen **TURNAROUND TIME:** Test results called to physician's office immediately on outpatients.

Interpretation **NORMAL FINDINGS:** Printed on reverse side of reporting form **LIMITATIONS:** Must not have had ocular surgery in past 6 months **ADDITIONAL INFORMATION:** Other indirect tests also require a high grade stenosis of the carotid in the 80% range to document alteration in blood flow. Direct imaging tests (such as Doppler, B-scan ultrasound and duplex scanning) are more sensitive tests of extracranial carotid flow. Arteriography is required for definitive diagnosis.

ODM *see* Ophthalmodynamometry *on this page*

OPG *see* Oculoplethysmography *on previous page*

Ophthalmodynamometry *replaced by* Oculoplethysmography *on previous page*

Ophthalmodynamometry

CPT 92260

Synonyms ODM

Abstract **PROCEDURE COMMONLY INCLUDES:** Approximation of central retinal artery pressure (RAP) **INDICATIONS:** Screening test for reduction in carotid blood flow. **CONTRAINDICATIONS:** Recent intraocular surgery, prosthetic eye.

Patient Care/Scheduling **PATIENT PREPARATION:** Topical anesthetic is required. **AFTERCARE:** Patient advised not to rub eyes for 30 minutes after procedure.

Method **EQUIPMENT:** The ophthalmodynamometer is used to apply pressure in calibrated amounts to the globe. **TECHNIQUE:** Simultaneous ophthalmoscopy identifies pressure needed to cause onset of arterial pulsation and complete collapse of the central retinal artery. Comparison can be made to systemic blood pressure and to measured pressures in the opposite eye.

Specimen **TURNAROUND TIME:** Immediate.

Interpretation **CRITICAL VALUES:** A 70% to 90% stenosis of the carotid artery may cause a decrease in retinal artery pressure (RAP). **LIMITATIONS:** Embolic disease not associated with stenosis will not alter test results. High grade stenosis (70% to 90% range) is necessary for a decrease in RAP. **ADDITIONAL INFORMATION:** Other indirect tests (oculoplethysmography – OPG, oculopneumoplethysmography, and periorbital Doppler) also require a high grade stenosis of the carotid in the 80% range to document alteration in blood flow. Direct imaging tests (such as Doppler, B-scan ultrasound, and duplex scanning) are more sensitive tests of extracranial carotid flow. Arteriography is required for definitive diagnosis.

References

Strauss AL and Rieger H, "Variability of Doppler Ophthalmic Pressure Index With Occlusive Carotid Artery Disease," *J Vasc Surg*, 1990, 12(1):50-5.

Optic Nerve Photography *see* Fundus Photography *on previous page*

Orbital Ultrasound *see* Ultrasound, B-Scan *on page 200*

Perimetry

CPT 92082 (intermediate exam); 92083 (extended exam)

Synonyms Central and Peripheral Field Testing; Field of Vision; Formal Fields; Peripheral Vision Test; Topography Map of Visual Function; Visual Fields

Applies to Automated Perimetry; Goldmann Perimetry; Tangent Screen

Abstract **PROCEDURE COMMONLY INCLUDES:** Topography map of visual function by quantitative methods **INDICATIONS:** Useful in diagnosis and evaluation of optic nerve disease (including glaucoma), neuro-ophthalmic disease, neurologic disorders, some retinal diseases **CONTRAINDICATIONS:** Inability of patient to sit up; uncooperative, combative patient.

(Continued)

Perimetry *(Continued)*

Patient Care/Scheduling PATIENT PREPARATION: Pupils may be dilated AFTERCARE: If pupils are to be dilated, dark glasses may be helpful. Patient should arrange for a ride home from the testing site. SPECIAL INSTRUCTIONS: Patient should bring spectacles. Patient must be able to sit up for 60 minutes and be able to make cognitive judgments.

Method EQUIPMENT: The Goldmann bowl perimeter is the standard reference instrument. White and colored test objects of varying size and intensity are projected onto a background of standardized illumination. Automated perimeters eliminate some potential error introduced by inexperienced examiners. The tangent screen utilizes a plane target and a wand with varying test objects to be moved by the examiner. Amsler's grid is a handheld grid test pattern used to monitor central visual field defects. TECHNIQUE: Kinetic perimetry (moving test object) can be utilized to outline the points of peripheral vision where an object of designated intensity and size is first recognized by the patient. Defects within the visual field (scotoma) can be similarly outlined by going from nonseeing to seeing areas. Static perimetry utilizes a target of fixed size and position. The illumination intensity is increased until the target is recognized by the patient. Goldmann perimetry utilizes both kinetic and static testing. Automated and computer assisted perimeters most often utilize static testing. The later are very reproducible and are especially useful in following optic nerve disease due to glaucoma. DATA ACQUIRED: The peripheral isopter is the line connecting points at which a target is first recognized during kinetic perimetry. Alterations occur in various eye diseases and neurologic disorders affecting the visual pathways. Kinetic perimetry is frequently used to identify areas of reduced threshold of light sensitivity within the visual field. It is especially useful in following changes due to optic nerve disease including glaucoma.

Specimen CAUSES FOR REJECTION: An inexperienced examiner may induce error into the test results.

Interpretation NORMAL FINDINGS: Interpretations may be requested. A printed record of tested isopters may be provided. LIMITATIONS: Accurate test results depend on subjective patient responses. Individuals with short attention span, decreased awareness (ie, some neurologic disorders, very young children, extremely nervous, etc) have difficulty producing accurate tests. ADDITIONAL INFORMATION: Defects in the visual field can be categorized as peripheral, or central defects surrounded by seeing areas (scotomas). The pattern of central or peripheral defects helps to identify the underlying disease process.

References

Caprioli J, "Automated Perimetry in Glaucoma," *Am J Ophthalmol*, 1991, 111(2):235-9.

Lindenmuth KA, Skuta GL, Rabbani R, et al, "Effects of Pupillary Dilation on Automated Perimetry in Normal Patients," *Ophthalmology*, 1990, 97(3):367-70.

Werner EB, Krupin T, Adelson A, et al, "Effect of Patient Experience on the Results of Automated Perimetry in Glaucoma Suspect Patients," *Ophthalmology*, 1990, 97(1):44-8.

Periorbital Doppler

Abstract PROCEDURE COMMONLY INCLUDES: Placement of Doppler over the supraorbital or frontal artery with subsequent compression of branches of the external carotid artery to assess blood flow in the internal carotid artery INDICATIONS: Permits noninvasive detection of a hemodynamically significant stenosis or occlusion of the extracranial internal carotid artery.

Specimen TURNAROUND TIME: 24 hours.

Interpretation LIMITATIONS: Patients with facial fractures or reconstructive surgery on face ADDITIONAL INFORMATION: May be done in conjunction with the OPG or carotid ultrasound. The periorbital Doppler does not detect ulcerated plaques or nonobstructive disease.

Peripheral Vision Test *see* Perimetry *on previous page*

Plethysmography, Ocular *see* Oculoplethysmography *on page 196*

Preoperative Corneal Evaluation *see* Endothelial Photography *on page 194*

Pseudoisochromatic Plates *see* Color Vision Testing *on page 192*

Pseudophakos Measurement *see* Axial Length, A-Scan *on page 192*

Specular Microscopy *see* Endothelial Photography *on page 194*
Tangent Screen *see* Perimetry *on page 197*

Tonography

CPT 92130

Synonyms Coefficient of Outflow Facility; Facility of Aqueous Outflow

Abstract **PROCEDURE COMMONLY INCLUDES:** Measurement of flow of aqueous fluid from the eye as it relates to intraocular pressure. Electronic tracing of intraocular pressure over measured amount of time with known weight. Can include water provocative study. **INDICATIONS:** An adjunct in the diagnosis of open angle and angle closure glaucomas. Helps in determination of needed surgical procedure in angle closure glaucoma. Less commonly used to measure facility of outflow in ocular inflammation and myasthenia gravis. **CONTRAINDICATIONS:** Ocular infection.

Patient Care/Scheduling **PATIENT PREPARATION:** NPO 8-10 hours prior to testing . When water provocative study is requested, instruct patient to have nothing by mouth after midnight on the day before the test. **AFTERCARE:** Instruct patient not to rub eyes for 30 minutes following local anesthesia **SPECIAL INSTRUCTIONS:** When water provocative study is requested, please instruct patient to have nothing by mouth after midnight before test.

Method **EQUIPMENT:** Most commonly, an electronic indentation tonometer is utilized for continuous pressure measurements which are recorded on a paper strip. **TECHNIQUE:** Schiötz readings with Berkeley recorder. After instillation of topical anesthesia, the electronic tonometer is used to measure baseline intraocular pressure followed by a 4-minute uninterrupted tracing of pressure decline. **DATA ACQUIRED:** The declining slope of the tracing is converted to the "C value" (coefficient of outflow facility).

Specimen **TURNAROUND TIME:** Immediate.

Interpretation **CRITICAL VALUES:** C value >0.18 in 97.5% of normal patients.

References

Shields MB, *Textbook of Glaucoma*, Baltimore, MD: Williams & Wilkins, 1987.

Tonometry

CPT 92100

Synonyms Intraocular Tension; IOP; Ocular Pressure

Abstract **PROCEDURE COMMONLY INCLUDES:** Pressure within the eye, diagnosis of glaucoma **INDICATIONS:** Useful in diagnosis and management of glaucoma, ocular hypertension, routine eye examination, family history of glaucoma **CONTRAINDICATIONS:** Sensitivity to topical anesthesia.

Patient Care/Scheduling **AFTERCARE:** Instruct patient not to rub eyes for 30 minutes following topical anesthesia. **COMPLICATIONS:** Contact tonometers have potential for corneal abrasion or reaction to topical anesthetics. The potential for spread of infection is limited by proper disinfection techniques.

Method **EQUIPMENT:** Tonometers fall into three categories: indentation (Schiötz), applanation (Goldmann), and noncontact (air puff) **TECHNIQUE:** Schiötz (indentation) or Goldmann applanation tonometer. All tonometers except for the noncontact type are applied directly to the surface of the eye after topical anesthesia. **DATA ACQUIRED:** Intraocular pressure is measured in mm Hg.

Specimen **TURNAROUND TIME:** Immediate.

Interpretation **NORMAL FINDINGS:** Readings ≤20 mm Hg are considered normal screening values. Glaucoma can be present when readings fall in the "normal" range. High readings require clinical correlation and possible further testing to differentiate between "ocular hypertension" and glaucoma. Several measurements may be needed in borderline or questionable cases. **LIMITATIONS:** An irregular cornea interferes with pressure measurements. Several variations of applanation tonometers are accurate in these cases. **ADDITIONAL INFORMATION:** The Goldmann applanation tonometer is considered to be the standard against which other instruments are compared. Indentation tonometers are useful to identify wide variations in pressure. Noncontact tonometers are less accurate in increasing pressure ranges with abnormal corneas or with poor patient visual fixation.

References

Shields MB, *Textbook of Glaucoma*, Baltimore, MD: Williams & Wilkins, 1987.

Topography Map of Visual Function *see* Perimetry *on page 197*
Ultrasound, A-Scan *see* Axial Length, A-Scan *on page 192*

Ultrasound, B-Scan

CPT 76512; 76513; 76529

Synonyms B-Scan; Ocular Ultrasound; Orbital Ultrasound

Abstract **INDICATIONS:** Examination of the posterior portion of the eye when direct view is precluded by media opacities. Evaluation of intraocular or orbital masses.

Patient Care/Scheduling **AFTERCARE:** Patient will be cautioned not to rub or touch eyes for 30 minutes after testing because of topical anesthesia. Patient should arrange for a ride home from the testing site. **SPECIAL INSTRUCTIONS:** Special care must be exercised when performing test in the presence of a ruptured globe.

Method **TECHNIQUE:** Two-dimensional pictures of the eye are displayed on an oscilloscope as the ultrasound waves move in a linear fashion across the eye. A handheld transducer is covered with a coupling medium and applied over closed lids. As the probe is oriented in various directions, sectional views of the eye can be recorded with Polaroid photography. A water bath coupling mechanism may be needed for good images of the anterior portion of the eye. **DATA ACQUIRED:** Changes in acoustic impedance cause reflections building a picture of the eye, orbit, and any contained abnormalities.

Specimen **TURNAROUND TIME:** Immediately if indicated.

Interpretation **LIMITATIONS:** Moderate patient cooperation required **ADDITIONAL INFORMATION:** In many instances computed tomography or nuclear magnetic resonance imaging may yield a superior image of an abnormality. This is especially true for periocular or orbital lesions. A-scan ultrasonography and fluorescein angiography may help in differential diagnosis of intraocular masses.

Visual Fields *see* Perimetry *on page 197*

PULMONARY FUNCTION

Kevin McCarthy, RCPT and Joseph A. Golish, MD

The last 15 years have been a time for standardization of pulmonary function testing equipment and procedures. In that time, the American Thoracic Society (ATS) has published recommendations and guidelines on spirometry, bronchial provocation testing, single-breath diffusing capacity, and cardiopulmonary sleep studies, as well as guidelines for laboratory personnel and quality assurance programs. The National Board for Respiratory Care (NBRC) now administers certification and registry examinations for pulmonary function technologists.

It will take some time before these guidelines and recommendations are practiced on a widespread basis. All too often, pulmonary function testing is given a very small space in the training program of respiratory therapists. Many hospitals rotate poorly-trained respiratory therapists and pulmonary function technicians to staff a Pulmonary Function Laboratory. They are often given no feedback on the quality of the tests they perform; in fact, the quality of the work is seldom scrutinized.

Because most pulmonary function tests require full cooperation and understanding of the procedure on the part of the patient, and because the personnel administering the tests may lack a full understanding of the procedure themselves, it is quite common for results from tests that do meet current standards to be reported and accepted as valid.

It is imperative that the current recommendations for standardized procedures be well known to the medical director of Respiratory Therapy or the Pulmonary Function Laboratory. These procedures are best implemented by the supervisor or technical director of the laboratory. It is the responsibility of the testing personnel to apply these standards to every test performed and commit themselves to a statement on the test report that "all current ATS met" or specify which standards were not met and why. The interpreting physician must scrutinize the report for these comments which may alter the interpretation of the test result. Finally, an individual, either the lab supervisor or the medical director, should scrutinize **every** test report for adherence to standards and provide the feedback that will improve the performance of the testing personnel.

There are many good texts written on pulmonary function testing. Those wishing to know more about the technical aspects of the equipment and the tests will find *Pulmonary Function Testing: Guidelines and Controversies*, edited by Jack L. Clausen, MD, an invaluable reference tool. *Pulmonary Function Testing: Indications and Interpretations*, edited by Archie Wilson, MD provides an excellent discussion on the interpretation of the tests along with interesting case reports. Both books are necessary reference works for the Pulmonary Function Laboratory.

The following section presents a description of various common pulmonary function tests, how they are done, and notes on interpretation and test limitations. Readers are directed to references for more detailed reading about each test.

A-a Gradient *see* Alveolar to Arterial Oxygen Gradient *on page 204*

(A-a)O$_2$ *see* Alveolar to Arterial Oxygen Gradient *on page 204*

ABG *see* Arterial Blood Gases *on page 206*

Airway Resistance

CPT 93720 (plethysmography, total body, with interpretation and report)

Related Information

Thoracic Gas Volume *on page 252*

Applies to Conductance; Specific Airways Resistance; Specific Conductance

Abstract **PROCEDURE COMMONLY INCLUDES:** Airways resistance (R_{aw}) reported in cm H_2O pressure/L/second flow, specific airways resistance (SR_{aw}) reported in cm H_2O pressure/L/second flow/L FRC, airways conductance (G_{aw}) reported in L/second flow/cm H_2O pressure, and specific airways conductance (SG_{aw}) reported in L/second flow/cm H_2O/L FRC. **INDICATIONS:** Airway resistance is a measure of the resistance (measured in cm H_2O) to airflow (measured in L/second) afforded by all anatomical structures between the atmosphere and the lung alveoli, including the mouth, nasopharynx, and the central and peripheral airways. Evaluation of airway responsiveness, provocation testing, characterization of various types of obstructive lung disease, localization of the primary site of flow limitation, and evaluation of localized obstruction. **CONTRAINDICATIONS:** Patient must be willing and able to follow necessary instructions. Patient cooperation is very important for obtaining reliable results.

Patient Care/Scheduling **PATIENT PREPARATION:** Patient should avoid heavy meals 3 hours prior to testing. Patient should be conscious and able to follow simple instructions. Patient's height and weight should be measured without shoes. Loose comfortable clothing that does not restrict chest expansion should be worn. Smoking history, including last cigarette smoked, should be obtained. Current medications should be obtained with particular emphasis on bronchodilators and steroids. Indicate time period prior to testing that medication was last taken. **AFTERCARE:** Usually none. Patients complaining of lightheadedness and dizziness should be observed for 5 minutes after recovering and may benefit from rebreathing CO_2 from a paper bag. **SPECIAL INSTRUCTIONS:** Patients almost always have to be instructed to place palms flat against their cheeks during the closed shutter panting to avoid hysteresis of the mouth pressure signal from bulging cheeks when measuring TGV (thoracic gas volume). Thoracic gas volume value used in calculation of specific airways resistance and specific conductance must be measured just prior to measurement of airways resistance to ensure correct normalization of airway resistance and/or conductance to volume. Some body plethysmographs measure airways resistance during normal tidal breathing without requiring the patient to pant.

Method **EQUIPMENT:** Body plethysmograph **TECHNIQUE:** After proper instructions are given, the patient is seated in a calibrated body plethysmograph, noseclips and mouthpiece are adjusted, and the door is sealed. Allow box pressure to stabilize (temperature equilibration) then instruct the patient to pant lightly. Measurements are made in triplicate of the change in box pressure (delta P_{box}). versus flow. Mouthpiece shutter is closed at end tidal expiration and the patient is instructed to pant lightly against the closed shutter and triplicate measurements are made of delta P_{box} versus P_{mouth}. The mean of three angles of P_{mouth}/P_{box} are used in the calculation of TGV. The airway resistance should not be made from the mean angle of flow/P_{box}, but rather the mean of the values for R_{aw}. Measurements of box pressure are made at point of inspiratory and expiratory flow of 0.5 liter$_{BTPS}$/second. A shutter at the mouthpiece is closed and the subject is asked to pant against the closed shutter. Angle of change in mouth pressure [delta P_{mouth}] (Y axis) during closed shutter panting plotted against changes in box pressure [delta P_{box}] (X axis) is representative of thoracic gas volume at which measurement of airways resistance is made. This allows reporting of specific resistance.

Specimen **CAUSES FOR REJECTION:** Glottis closure during airways resistance measurement, cheeks bowing in or out during closed shutter panting, nonreproducible results. **TURNAROUND TIME:** Preliminary report usually ready in 1 day, interpreted report in 1 day.

Interpretation **NORMAL FINDINGS:** The normal range for airway resistance is 0.6-2.8 cm H_2O/L/second. The normal range for airway conductance is 0.36-1.7 L/second/cm H_2O. The normal range for specific conductance (conductance normalized to the lung volume at which it is measured) is 0.114-0.404 L/second/cm H_2O/L. **LIMITATIONS:** Lack of established criteria for measuring the angle of a resistance loop when there is significant hysteresis. An accepted practice is to measure the slope of a best fit line drawn through the curve at the more linear (low flow) portion of the curve. **ADDITIONAL INFORMATION:** Volume standardization of the airway resistance may be accomplished by dividing the conductance, SG_{aw} (the reciprocal of the resistance) by the TGV at which the resistance measurement was made. Changes in conductance values of >40% and resistance values >50% are considered significant when evaluating airway responsiveness to medication or challenge tests.

$$R_{aw} = \left(\frac{\tan \angle \dfrac{P_{mouth}}{P_{box}}}{\tan \angle \dfrac{\dot{V}}{P_{box}}} \times P_{mouth}\ \text{CAL factor} \times \dot{V}\ \text{CAL factor} \right) - R_{SYS}$$

Where:

R_{aw}	= airways resistance
$\tan < P_{mouth}/P_{box}$	= the tangent of the observed angle of mouth pressure plotted against box pressure
$\tan < \dot{V}/P_{box}$	= the tangent of the observed angle of flow plotted against box pressure
P_{mouth} CAL factor	= the calibration signal pressure (cm H_2O) divided by the calibration signal deflection (mm)
$\dot{V}$ CAL factor	= the calibration flow (L/sec) divided by the flow calibration signal deflection (mm)
R_{SYS}	= resistance of the testing system (cm H_2O/L/sec)

Airway Resistance and Conductance

	Normal Values
R_{aw}	0.6–2.8 cm H_2O/LPS_{BTPS}
G_{aw}	0.36–1.7 LPS_{BTPS}/cm H_2O
SG_{aw}	0.114–0.404 LPS_{BTPS}/cm H_2O/L_{BTPS}TGV

Categorization of Severity (FRC >2L)

Severity	R_{aw} (cm H_2O/LPS)
Mild	2.8–4.5
Moderate	4.5–8.0
Severe	>8.0

References

Aitken ML, Marini JJ, and Culver BH, "Humid Air Increases Airway Resistance in Asthmatic Subjects," *West J Med*, 1988, 149(3):289-93.

Desmond KJ, Demizio DL, Allen PD, et al, "An Alternate Method for the Determination of Functional Residual Capacity in a Plethysmograph," *Am Rev Respir Dis*, 1988, 137(2):273-6.

Littell NT, Carlisle CC, Millman RP, et al, "Changes in Airway Resistance Following Nasal Provocation," *Am Rev Respir Dis*, 1990, 141(3):580-3.

Alveolar to Arterial Oxygen Gradient

Related Information

Arterial Blood Gases *on page 206*

Synonyms A-a Gradient; $(A\text{-}a)O_2$; $P(A\text{-}a)O_2$

Abstract PROCEDURE COMMONLY INCLUDES: Results generally include the measured and calculated parameters of an arterial blood gas test plus the calculated gradient of the partial pressure of alveolar to arterial dissolved oxygen expressed in millimeters of mercury (mm Hg). INDICATIONS: The A-a gradient is used to assess oxygenation. It compares the arterial pO_2 (PaO_2) to the theoretical maximum alveolar pO_2 (PAO_2).

Patient Care/Scheduling PATIENT PREPARATION: Patient preparation includes assessment of peripheral circulation on both sides, the Allen test. Both the radial and ulnar arteries should be compressed at a level approximately 1 centimeter proximal to the wrist joint while the patient makes a tight fist for approximately 5 seconds. The patient is then instructed to open the fist in a relaxed fashion. The palmar surface of the hand should be blanched. Release compression on the ulnar artery. The palmar surface should flush within 5 seconds. Prolonged delay before flushing indicates decreased ulnar artery flow. Radial arteries lacking collateral ulnar circulation should be avoided as puncture sites if possible. The skin over the puncture site should be swabbed with a Betadine® solution followed by an alcohol swab. AFTERCARE: The puncture site should be compressed for a minimum of 5 minutes, longer if the patient is taking anticoagulant therapy, aspirin or has a prolonged prothrombin time. After 5 minutes, the puncture site should be inspected for several seconds to ensure that clotting has taken place. During this inspection, palpate the pulse proximal and distal to the puncture site to assess the presence of arterial spasm. A sterile bandage should be placed over the puncture site to keep the puncture site clean while healing. **Warning:** A bandage is **not** a substitute for compression of the puncture site.

Method TECHNIQUE: The calculated alveolar oxygen tension is generally obtained from the alveolar air equation :

$$PAO_2 = ((Pb - 47) \times FiO_2) - PaCO_2/0.8$$

where:

- PAO_2 = alveolar oxygen tension (mm Hg or torr)
- Pb = barometric pressure (mm Hg or torr)
- FiO_2 = fractional concentration of inspired oxygen
- $PaCO_2$ = partial pressure of dissolved CO_2 in arterial blood (mm Hg or torr)
- 0.8 = average, normal respiratory exchange ratio, the ratio of CO_2 output to O_2 intake.

The following parameters are needed for calculation of the A-a gradient:

- barometric pressure (Pb) in mm Hg
- arterial pCO_2 ($PaCO_2$) in mm Hg
- arterial pO_2 (PaO_2) in mm Hg
- fractional concentration of inspired oxygen (FiO_2)

$$\text{A-a gradient (mm Hg)} = (((Pb - 47) \times FiO_2) - pCO_2/0.8) - PaO_2$$

where:

- 47 = H_2O pressure at 37°C in mm Hg
- 0.8 = assumed normal respiratory exchange ratio

If the patient is breathing inspired oxygen concentrations >60%, the product ($PaCO_2/0.8$) can be eliminated from the alveolar air equation.

Specimen Heparinized arterial blood CONTAINER: Glass or plastic syringes (3-10 mL) may be used. Glass is preferred if sample measurement is delayed more than 1 hour. Glass capillary tubes are used for microsamples. It is impossible to maintain anaerobic integrity of a sample if evacuated glass tubes are used and their use is discouraged. COLLECTION: Personnel performing the arterial puncture should wear rubber gloves. Perform necessary tests to assess collateral circulation. After choosing the optimal puncture site, clean site with Betadine® solution followed by alcohol. Allow alcohol to air dry. Slight hyperextension of the brachial and radial puncture sites by placement of a rolled up towel under the elbow or wrist may facilitate palpation of the pulse. Draw up approximately 0.3 mL sodium heparin (1000 units/mL) into syringe. Replace needle with a sterile one. Needle sizes of 23- to 25-gauge x 5/8" to 1" in length are commonly used. Holding the syringe with the needle pointing upward, pull the syringe plunger back to the end of the syringe to allow the liquid heparin to come in contact with the internal surface of the syringe. Expel excess heparin into the needle cap, making sure that the dead space of the syringe and needle do not contain any air. Palpate the artery with the index finger and puncture the artery, holding the needle at an angle of approximately 25° to the surface of the skin. Allow the pressure of the artery to fill the syringe. Withdraw the needle and immediately apply pressure using a sterile gauze pad. Insert needle into rubber stopper. Hold pressure for a minimum of 5 minutes. Include collection procedures for capillary sampling and arterial mean line and catheter collection. **STORAGE INSTRUCTIONS:** Samples not analyzed within 10 minutes should be stored in an ice-slush mixture (approximately 2°C). Syringe barrel plunger assembly should be sufficiently tight to prevent sample dilution with the ice-slush mixture. **CAUSES FOR REJECTION:** Large air bubbles will cause all values to be erroneous. The magnitude of the error will be determined by the size of the air bubble, sample and sample air bubble interface, length of time bubble was in contact with sample before analysis and the gradient between sample gas tensions and room air gas tensions. Small bubbles, if immediately expelled will generally not cause any significant error. Samples with large (>0.2 mL) bubbles should be discarded and a new, anaerobic sample obtained. **TURNAROUND TIME:** Analysis of arterial blood gas typically takes less than 5 minutes, calculation of A-a gradient can be accomplished within 1 minute.

Interpretation **NORMAL FINDINGS:** <15 mm Hg in young adults, gradient increases with age. The following equations can be used to predict normal A-a gradients in the sitting and supine positions.

- $P(A\text{-}a)O_2$ sitting = 104.2 – (0.27 x age)
- $P(A\text{-}a)O_2$ supine = 103.5 – (0.42 x age)

LIMITATIONS: While the alveolar to arterial oxygen gradient should always yield a positive number, there are several assumptions made which, if deviated from, may cause the equation to yield a negative number. The major assumptions are listed.

- The FiO_2 is often not measured; the assumed FiO_2 may vary widely from that actually received by the patient.
- The barometric pressure is not measured or is not measured at the time the arterial blood gas is obtained (eg, the Pb is measured once at the beginning of the day and this value is used for the entire day).
- The increase in Pb when a patient is artificially ventilated is seldom taken into account.
- A value of 47 mm Hg is typically used to subtract water vapor pressure (PH_2O) from the barometric pressure (Pb). This assumes a constant body temperature of 37°C. Actual body temperature may vary from this and thus change the actual PH_2O.
- The alveolar air equation which solves for the PAO_2 assumes that arterial pCO_2 ($PaCO_2$) is equal to alveolar pCO_2 ($PACO_2$). Although the two may be nearly identical in normal lungs, in diseased lungs there can be a difference of several mm Hg.
- The alveolar air equation also assumes a normal respiratory exchange ratio (R) of 0.8. This is true only when the metabolic R value equals 0.8 and the patient is in a steady-state. Because of either changes in metabolism (largely diet dependent) or deviations from a steady-state (when the respiratory exchange ratio does **not** equal the metabolic exchange ratio, as in acute hyperventilation), the R used in the alveolar air equation can vary widely from 0.8.

Taken together, the assumptions inherent in the use of the alveolar gas equation can cause the calculated PaO_2 (and thus the (A-a) DO_2) to vary several mm Hg above or below the value that would be obtained if everything was precisely measured.

References

Overton DT and Bocka JJ, "The Alveolar-Arterial Oxygen Gradient in Patients With Documented Pulmonary Embolism," *Arch Intern Med*, 1988, 148(7):1617-9.

Arterial Blood Gases

CPT 36600 (arterial puncture, withdrawal of blood for diagnosis); 94700 (analysis of arterial blood gas [oxygen saturation, pO_2, pCO_2, pH] rest only); 94705 (analysis of arterial blood gas [oxygen saturation, pO_2, pCO_2, pH] rest and exercise including cannulization of artery); 94710 (analysis of arterial blood gas [oxygen saturation, pO_2, pCO_2, pH], 3 or more [O_2 administration, therapy, or exercise])

Related Information

Alveolar to Arterial Oxygen Gradient *on page 204*
Arterial Blood Oximetry *on page 210*
Arterial Cannulation *on page 60*
Pulse Oximetry *on page 241*
Shunt Determination *on page 243*

Synonyms ABG; Blood Gases, Arterial

Abstract PROCEDURE COMMONLY INCLUDES: Measured parameters include: pH, pCO_2, and pO_2; calculated parameters include: bicarbonate (HCO_3), base excess or deficit (BE), standard bicarbonate, standard base excess, alveolar to arterial oxygen gradient ($p[A\text{-}a]O_2$). INDICATIONS: Assessment of oxygenation of arterial blood and the blood's acid-base balance CONTRAINDICATIONS: Relative contraindications include peripheral artery spasm.

Patient Care/Scheduling PATIENT PREPARATION: Patient preparation includes assessment of peripheral circulation on both sides, the Allen test. Both the radial and ulnar arteries should be compressed at a level approximately 1 centimeter proximal to the wrist joint while the patient makes a tight fist for approximately 5 seconds. The patient is then instructed to open the fist in a relaxed fashion. The palmar surface of the hand should be blanched. Release compression on the ulnar artery. The palmar surface should flush within 5 seconds. Prolonged delay before flushing indicates decreased ulnar artery flow. Radial arteries lacking collateral ulnar circulation should be avoided as puncture sites if possible. If the radial artery is unsuitable as a puncture site, the brachial artery is the second choice, followed by the femoral artery. If the need for repeated measurements over several days exists, placement of an arterial catheter is indicated. The skin over the puncture site should be swabbed with a Betadine® solution followed by an alcohol swab. See the following illustration. AFTERCARE: The puncture site should be compressed for a minimum of 5 minutes, longer if the patient is taking anticoagulant therapy, aspirin or has a prolonged prothrombin time. After 5 minutes, the puncture site should be inspected for several seconds to ensure that clotting has taken place. During this inspection, palpate the pulse proximal and distal to the puncture site to assess the presence of arterial spasm. A sterile bandage should be placed over the puncture site to keep the puncture site clean while healing. **Warning:** A bandage is **not** a substitute for compression of the puncture site.

Specimen Adequately heparinized (sodium or lithium heparinate) arterial or "arterialized" capillary blood sample. Volume and/or concentration of heparin should be adjusted to yield a final blood concentration of 30-100 units/mL blood in a syringe sample or 50-250 units/mL blood in a capillary sample. CONTAINER: Glass or plastic syringes (3-10 mL) may be used. Glass is preferred if sample measurement is delayed more than 1 hour. Glass capillary tubes are used for microsamples. It is impossible to maintain anaerobic integrity of a sample if evacuated glass tubes are used and their use is discouraged. COLLECTION: Syringe sampling: Assemble the following equipment: syringe; needles (20- to 25-gauge (2)); anticoagulant, eg, sodium heparinate (1000 units/mL); sterile gauze sponges or cotton; skin antiseptic, eg, 70% alcohol and Betadine® swabs; rubber stopper or needle cap; tourniquet; adhesive bandage. Don disposable rubber gloves as an infection control measure. Preheparinized glass or plastic syringes are available in blood gas kits from several manufacturers. Syringes preheparinized with liquid heparin should be held vertically, needle up, and the liquid heparin should be pushed into the dead space of the syringe and needle, expelling all air out of the dead space. If preheparinized syringes are not used, the following procedure should be used. Fit a needle onto the syringe and draw 0.5-1.0 mL anticoagulant into it. Remove the original needle and replace with a sterile needle. Pull and push syringe plunger several times to coat syringe surface. Holding the syringe with the needle up, expel all liquid heparin into needle cap, taking care not to leave any air bubbles in the dead space of the needle. Perform the Allen test for collateral circulation to determine the best site for puncture. Sites listed in order of preference are as follows: radial, brachial, and femoral arteries. Palpate and visualize the artery. Apply antiseptic to the

ALLEN'S TEST FOR COLLATERAL CIRCULATION

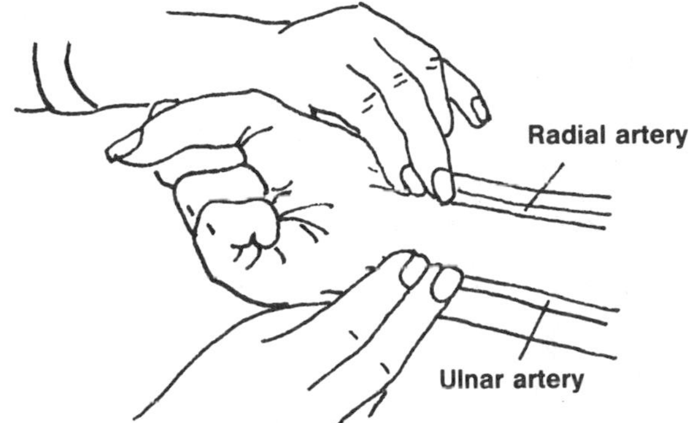

Fist clenched tightly, radial and ulnar arteries compressed

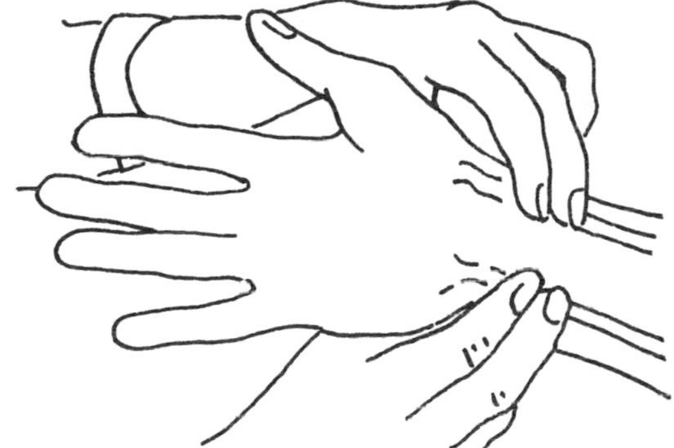

The hand is opened and relaxed; the palm and fingers are blanched

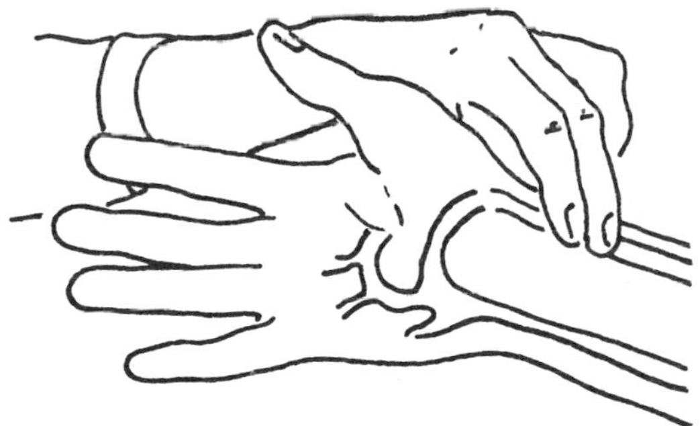

Pressure removed from ulnar artery, entire hand should flush within 15 seconds

Reproduced with permission from Shapiro BA, Harrison RA, and Walton JR, "Guidelines for Sampling and Quality Control," *Clinical Application of Blood Gases*, 2nd ed, Chapter 14, Chicago, IL: Year Book Medical Publishers, Inc, 1977, 148.

(Continued)

Arterial Blood Gases *(Continued)*

sampling site. Palpate the site once again, trying to stabilize the artery. Slight hyperextension of the wrist or elbow can be achieved by placing a rolled up towel under the joint; this can aid palpation and stabilization of the artery. Hold the syringe so the bevel of the needle faces upward, keeping the needle at a 25° to 30° angle to the artery. Insert the needle through the skin into the artery taking care not to puncture the posterior wall of the artery. Arterial pressure should cause the blood to flow into the syringe if the plunger fits properly and the barrel has been lubricated with anticoagulant. Withdraw the needle when an adequate sample has been obtained. Immediately place dry gauze or cotton over the puncture site. Maintain pressure over puncture site for a minimum of 5 minutes (longer if the patient has taken aspirin or anticoagulants). Expel any air bubbles from the sample. Insert needle into a rubber stopper or needle cap. Remove needle/cap assembly and replace with a syringe cap. Mix sample by rolling syringe for 20 seconds immediately prior to analysis. If not analyzed immediately, store the sample in iced water (2°C). Iced samples should be analyzed within 3 hours.

Capillary sampling: Assemble the following equipment: preheparinized capillary sample tubes; capillary tube end caps; mixing wire; magnet; water soluble jelly, if desired; sterile gauze sponges or cotton; skin antiseptic (eg, 70% alcohol). Select the puncture site (typically the heel on infants, fingertips on adults). Establish increased regional circulation by wrapping the extremity with a warm, moist towel for 5-10 minutes. Loosely mount a capillary tube cap on the end of the capillary tube and insert a mixing wire into the capillary, allowing the mixing wire to slide to the same end of the tube as the loosely mounted capillary cap. Apply antiseptic to the sampling site. Make a skin puncture that forms drops of blood rapidly and fill the capillary with blood from the **middle** of the drop without introducing air into the capillary. Firmly seat both capillary end caps. Mix blood and anticoagulant initially by moving the mixing wire along the full length of the capillary approximately 20 times with a magnet and repeat mixing immediately prior to analysis. If not analyzed immediately, store the sample in iced water.

STORAGE INSTRUCTIONS: Samples not analyzed within 10 minutes should be stored in an ice-slush mixture (approximately 2°C). Syringe barrel plunger assembly should be sufficiently tight to prevent sample dilution with the ice-slush mixture. **CAUSES FOR REJECTION:** Large air bubbles will cause all values to be erroneous; the magnitude of the error will be determined by the size of the air bubble, sample and sample air bubble interface, length of time bubble was in contact with sample before analysis and the gradient between sample gas tensions and room air gas tensions. Small bubbles, if immediately expelled, will generally not cause any significant error. Samples with large (>0.2 mL) bubbles should be discarded and a new, anaerobic sample obtained. **TURNAROUND TIME:** Results are available immediately after analysis. Stat results should be available 10 minutes after receipt of the sample.

Interpretation **NORMAL FINDINGS:** Normal values (arterial blood), pH: 7.35-7.45; pCO_2: 36-44. The normal partial pressure of oxygen in arterial blood at sea level is generally considered to be >80 mm Hg. Several factors confound interpretation of pO_2 by this simple means, notably altitude of residency, age, hypoventilation, and hyperventilation. Normal ranges of pO_2 are shown in the table on the following page. The arterial pO_2 should be evaluated according to the table of normal ranges shown. The most common causes of hypoxemia are:

- ventilation-perfusion (V/Q) abnormalities in the lungs
- physiologic shunting
- alveolar-capillary diffusion defects
- alveolar hypoventilation
- decreased inspired oxygen concentration

Interpretation of blood gases should start with the assessment of the ventilatory status by classification of the pCO_2. A low pCO_2 (<30 mm Hg) indicates alveolar hyperventilation. A high pCO_2 (>50 mm Hg) indicates ventilatory failure. A pCO_2 in the range of 30-50 mm Hg represents an acceptable level of alveolar ventilation. Because the lungs and the kidneys work together to achieve acid-base homeostasis, inspection of the arterial pH in conjunction with the pCO_2 will allow determination of the origin of the acid-base disturbance. Acid-base disturbances can be a primary ventilatory problem (respiratory acidosis, respiratory

Acceptable Arterial Oxygen Tensions at Sea Level Breathing Room Air (21% oxygen)

	mm Hg
Adult and Child	
Normal	97
Acceptable range	>80
Newborn	
Acceptable range	40–70
Aged	
Acceptable range	
60 y	>80
70 y	>70
80 y	>60
90 y	>50

alkalosis) or a primary metabolic problem (metabolic acidosis, metabolic alkalosis). Respiratory acid-base disturbances present for more than 24 hours will result in renal compensation by increasing or decreasing the plasma bicarbonate to normalize pH. Metabolic acid-base disturbances will result in partial or complete compensation by the respiratory system which increases or decreases alveolar ventilation (and thus the pCO_2). The following table lists the seven primary blood gas classifications based on inspection of the arterial pH and pCO_2.

Seven Primary Blood Gas Classifications*

Classification	$PaCO_2$	pH	$[HCO_3^-]p$	BE
Primary Ventilatory				
Acute ventilatory failure	↑	↓	N	N
Chronic ventilatory failure	↑	N	↑	↑
Acute alveolar hyperventilation	↓	↑	N	N
Chronic alveolar hyperventilation	↓	N	↓	↓
Primary Acid–Base				
Uncompensated acidosis	N	↓	↓	↓
Uncompensated alkalosis	N	↑	↑	↑
Partly compensated acidosis	↓	↓	↓	↓
Partly compensated alkalosis	↑	↑	↑	↑
Compensated alkalosis or acidosis	↑ or ↓	N	↑ or ↓	↑ or ↓

* Arrows indicate depressed or elevated values; N = normal; BE = base excess.
Reproduced with permission from Shapiro BA, Harrison RA, and Walton JR, *Clinical Application of Blood Gases,* 2nd ed, Chicago, IL: Year Book Medical Publishers, Inc, 1977, 137.

CRITICAL VALUES: pH values chronically outside of the normal range are a cause for concern. pCO_2 values >50 mm Hg may indicate ventilatory failure. pO_2 values <55 mm Hg while breathing room air may indicate the need for supplemental oxygen therapy. **LIMITATIONS:** Erroneous values can result from improper (aerobic) sample handling, excessive storage at room temperature (more than 10 minutes) before measurement, excessive storage at 2°C before measurement, improper calibration of the blood gas analyzer, and measurement errors. Potentially hazardous clinical judgments based solely on blood gas values without clinical correlation are discouraged. **ADDITIONAL INFORMATION:** Heparinized blood is required and may be obtained either from an artery or an "arterialized" capillary. Sodium heparin is generally used as an anticoagulant, it may be used as a powder or a liquid. Errors have been reported from the excessive dilution of the sample with liquid heparin. Disposable kits are available that supply needles with inner cannula that minimize syringe-needle combined dead space, making a minimum sample size of 0.5 mL sufficient. Blood

(Continued)

Arterial Blood Gases *(Continued)*

gas analyzers vary, but most can measure capillary samples of as little as 200 μL. Syringes and capillary tubes using powdered heparin obviate the need for concern regarding heparin dilution errors.

References

Emerman CL, Connors AF, Lukens TW, et al, "Relationship Between Arterial Blood Gases and Spirometry in Acute Exacerbations of Chronic Obstructive Pulmonary Disease," *Ann Emerg Med*, 1989, 18(5):523-7.

Hansen JE, "Arterial Blood Gases," *Clin Chest Med*, 1989, 10(2):227-37.

Preusser BA, Lash J, Stone, KS, et al, "Quantifying the Minimum Discard Sample Required for Accurate Arterial Blood Gases," *Nurs Res*, 1989, 38(5):276-9.

Arterial Blood Oximetry

CPT 82375 (carbon monoxide, carboxyhemoglobin, quantitative); 82793 (gases, blood, oxygen saturation, by spectrophotometry); 83050 (methemoglobin, quantitative); 85018 (hemoglobin, colorimetric)

Related Information

Arterial Blood Gases *on page 206*

Pulse Oximetry *on page 241*

Synonyms Co-oximetry; Hemoximetry

Applies to Carbon Monoxide Determination

Replaces Calculated Arterial or Venous Oxygen Saturation

Abstract **PROCEDURE COMMONLY INCLUDES:** Total hemoglobin (THb) in g/dL, oxygen saturation (HbO_2Sat) in percent or oxyhemoglobin (HbO_2) in percent, carboxyhemoglobin (HbCO) in percent, methemoglobin (metHb) in percent, and the calculated content of oxygen bound to hemoglobin (cO_2) in volumes percent **INDICATIONS:** Assessment of anemia or polycythemia, assessment of elevated levels of dysfunctional hemoglobins (carboxyhemoglobin, methemoglobin), assessment of oxygen content, correlation of pulse oximetry with blood oximetry (correction for dysfunctional hemoglobins).

Patient Care/Scheduling **PATIENT PREPARATION:** Patient preparation includes assessment of peripheral circulation on both arms, the Allen test. Both the radial and ulnar arteries should be compressed at a level approximately 1 centimeter proximal to the wrist joint while the patient makes a tight fist for approximately 5 seconds. The patient is then instructed to open the fist in a relaxed fashion. The palmar surface of the hand should be blanched. Release compression on the ulnar artery. The palmar surface should flush within 5 seconds. Prolonged delay before flushing indicates decreased ulnar artery flow. Radial arteries lacking collateral ulnar circulation should be avoided as puncture sites if possible. The skin over the puncture site should be swabbed with a Betadine® solution followed by an alcohol swab. **AFTERCARE:** The puncture site should be compressed for a minimum of 5 minutes, longer if the patient is taking anticoagulant therapy, aspirin or has a prolonged prothrombin time. After 5 minutes, the puncture site should be inspected for several seconds to ensure that clotting has taken place. During this inspection, palpate the pulse proximal and distal to the puncture site to assess the presence of arterial spasm. A sterile bandage should be placed over the puncture site to keep the puncture site clean while healing. **Warning:** A bandage is **not** a substitute for compression of the puncture site.

Method **TECHNIQUE:** Measurement systems use a calibrated system for measurement of the optical absorption and turbidity of blood samples. Absorbances measured are specific for reduced hemoglobin (RHb), HbO_2, HbCO, and metHb. The values for THb, HbO_2 sat, HbO_2, HbCO, metHb, and O_2 content are calculated from the data obtained from the measured absorbances.

Specimen Adequately heparinized (sodium or lithium heparinate) arterial or "arterialized" capillary blood sample. Volume and/or concentration of heparin should be adjusted to yield a final blood concentration of 30-100 units/mL blood in a syringe sample or 50-250 units/mL blood in a capillary sample. **CONTAINER:** Glass or plastic syringes, glass capillary tubes **SAMPLING TIME:** Samples should be analyzed within 15 minutes (see Storage Instructions). **COLLECTION:** Syringe sampling: Assemble the following equipment: syringe; needles (20- to 25-gauge (2)); anticoagulant, eg, sodium heparinate (1000 units/mL); sterile gauze sponges or cotton; skin antiseptic, eg, 70% alcohol and Betadine® swabs; rubber stopper or needle cap; tourniquet; adhesive bandage. Don disposable rubber gloves as an infection control measure. Preheparinized glass or plastic syringes are available in blood gas kits from several manufacturers. Syringes preheparinized with liquid heparin should be held vertically, needle up, and the liquid heparin should be pushed into the dead space of the syringe and needle, expelling all air out of the dead space. If preheparinized syringes are not used, the following procedure should be used. Fit a needle onto the syringe and draw 0.5-1.0 mL anticoagulant into it. Remove the original needle and replace with a sterile needle. Pull and push syringe plunger several times to coat syringe surface. Holding the syringe with the needle up, expel all liquid heparin into needle cap, taking care not to leave any air bubbles in the dead space of the needle. Perform the Allen test for collateral circulation to determine the best site for puncture (see Arterial Blood Gases). Sites listed in order of preference are as follows: radial, brachial, and femoral arteries. Palpate and visualize the artery. Apply antiseptic to the sampling site. Palpate the site once again, trying to stabilize the artery. Slight hyperextension of the wrist or elbow can be achieved by placing a rolled up towel under the joint; this can aid palpation and stabilization of the artery. Hold the syringe so the bevel of the needle faces upward, keeping the needle at a 25° to 30° angle to the artery. Insert the needle through the skin into the artery taking care not to puncture the posterior wall of the artery. Arterial pressure should cause the blood to flow into the syringe if the plunger fits properly and the barrel has been lubricated with anticoagulant. Withdraw the needle when an adequate sample has been obtained. Immediately place dry gauze or cotton over the puncture site. Maintain pressure over puncture site for a minimum of 5 minutes (longer if the patient has taken aspirin or anticoagulants). Expel any air bubbles from the sample. Insert needle into a rubber stopper or needle cap. Remove needle/cap assembly and replace with a syringe cap. Mix sample by rolling syringe for 20 seconds immediately prior to analysis. If not analyzed immediately, store the sample in iced water (2°C). Iced samples should be analyzed within 3 hours.

Capillary sampling: Assemble the following equipment: preheparinized capillary sample tubes; capillary tube end caps; mixing wire; magnet; water soluble jelly, if desired; sterile gauze sponges or cotton; skin antiseptic (eg, 70% alcohol). Select the puncture site (typically the heel on infants, fingertips on adults). Establish increased regional circulation by wrapping the extremity with a warm, moist towel for 5-10 minutes. Loosely mount a capillary tube cap on the end of the capillary tube and insert a mixing wire into the capillary, allowing the mixing wire to slide to the same end of the tube as the loosely mounted capillary cap. Apply antiseptic to the sampling site. Make a skin puncture that forms drops of blood rapidly and fill the capillary with blood from the **middle** of the drop without introducing air into the capillary. Firmly seat both capillary end caps. Mix blood and anticoagulant initially by moving the mixing wire along the full length of the capillary approximately 20 times with a magnet and repeat mixing immediately prior to analysis. If not analyzed immediately, store the sample in iced water.

STORAGE INSTRUCTIONS: If not analyzed immediately, samples should be chilled to 2°C in an ice/slush mixture to reduce erythrocyte metabolism. Iced samples should be analyzed within 3 hours after being drawn. **CAUSES FOR REJECTION:** Improperly stored samples **TURNAROUND TIME:** Measurement of sample takes 1-2 minutes. Report should be available at that time.

Interpretation

NORMAL FINDINGS: The table shows expected values. Elevated levels of HbCO can be secondary to exposure to cigarette, pipe and cigar smoke, faulty gas furnaces, automobile exhaust, or any site of incomplete combustion. Elevated methemoglobin may (Continued)

Arterial Blood Oximetry

Component	Whole Blood	Expected Values
tHb	Newborn	14.0–24.0 g/dL
	Adult male	13.5–18.0 g/dL
	Adult female	12.0–16.0 g/dL
HbO_2 saturation	Arterial	91.9%–98.5%
HbO_2	Arterial	94%–100%
HbCO	Nonsmokers	<1.5% of tHb
	Smokers	1.5%–5.0% of tHb
	Heavy smokers	5.0%–9.0% of tHb
MetHb		<3% of tHb or 0–0.24 g/dL
O_2 content	Arterial	15–23 vol %
SHb		0

Arterial Blood Oximetry *(Continued)*

be hereditary (hemoglobin M disease or enzyme [$NADH_2$-reductase] deficiency) or acquired through exposure to certain drugs or chemicals such as nitrites, nitrates, chlorates, quinones, aminobenzenes, nitrobenzenes, or nitrotoluenes. **CRITICAL VALUES:** Oxyhemoglobin values <85%. Sum of dysfunctional hemoglobins (COHb + MetHb) >15%. **LIMITATIONS:** Oxyhemoglobin or oxygen saturation values for samples that contain air bubbles should be questioned. Bubble size, length of time from obtaining sample, and analysis and gradient of partial pressure of oxygen between sample and atmosphere will determine the magnitude of the error introduced by the bubble. Other values should be unaffected by air contamination. Methylene blue in a concentration of approximately 60 mg/L blood interferes with the measurement of methemoglobin, total hemoglobin, and HbO_2 measurements yielding falsely low values of total hemoglobin and methemoglobin and falsely high values of HbO_2. Excessively high or low pH values will yield erroneously low and high values respectively of methemoglobin. Sulfhemoglobin levels ≥10% will increase $HbCO_2$ and decrease metHb values. Milking or squeezing the area of a capillary puncture will result in mixing of blood and tissue fluids with the liability of erroneous measurements. Inadequate mixing of either a syringe or capillary sample just prior to analysis will result in erroneous total hemoglobin measurements.

References

Goldhill DR, Hill AJ, Whitburn RH, et al, "Carboxyhemoglobin Concentrations, Pulse Oximetry and Arterial Blood-Gas Tensions During Jet Ventilation for Nd-YAG Laser Bronchoscopy," *Br J Anaesth*, 1990, 65(6):749-53.

Pierson DJ, "Pulse Oximetry Versus Arterial Blood Gas Specimens in Long-Term Oxygen Therapy," *Lung*, 1990, 168(suppl):782-8.

Assessment of Pulmonary Disability *see* Flow Volume Loop *on page 228*

Assessment of Pulmonary Disability *see* Spirometry *on page 245*

Bedside Spirometry

CPT 94160 (vital capacity screening tests: total capacity, with timed forced expiratory volume and peak flow rate)

Related Information

Bronchial Challenge Test *on page 215*
Flow Volume Loop *on page 228*
Spirometry *on page 245*
Spirometry, Sitting and Supine *on page 250*

Synonyms Portable Spirometry

Abstract **INDICATIONS:** Early monitoring of patient with high potential for respiratory problems, monitoring of the acutely ill patient, monitoring recuperating mechanically ventilated patient.

Patient Care/Scheduling **PATIENT PREPARATION:** Avoid heavy meals 3 hours prior to testing. Patient should be conscious and able to follow simple instructions. Patient's height and weight should be measured without shoes. Loose comfortable clothing that does not restrict chest expansion should be worn. Smoking history including last cigarette smoked should be obtained. Current medications should be obtained with particular emphasis on bronchodilators and steroids. **AFTERCARE:** Usually none, although patients that complain of lightheadedness and dizziness should not be allowed to walk unobserved until recovery. **SPECIAL INSTRUCTIONS:** Patients that have a tracheostomy stoma may be tested by attaching an infant anesthesia mask to the mouthpiece. Mouthpieces can be adapted directly to most tracheostomy tubes.

Method **EQUIPMENT:** Exhaled sample is collected or passed through a volume or flow measuring device known as a spirometer. Spirometers should meet certain minimum standards defined by the American Thoracic Society. Other equipment needed varies with the type of spirometer being used but should include a disposable mouthpiece and noseclips. Special circumstances may require adaptation of the mouthpiece to a mask, face seal, or tracheostomy adapters. **TECHNIQUE:** A spirometer is used to measure exhaled gas and to record the time of collection. Many such devices have recently been miniaturized and advertised as ideal for bedside spirometry. Regardless of whether measurements are made at bedside or in the Pulmonary Function Laboratory, equipment used to measure forced expiratory volumes or flows should meet or exceed equipment standards recommended by the American Thoracic Society (ATS). **DATA ACQUIRED:** Vital capacity (VC), forced vital capacity (FVC), timed forced expiratory volumes; $FEV_{0.5}$, FEV_1, FEV_3, midexpiratory flow rate ($FEF_{25\%-75\%}$), peak expiratory flow rate (PEFR or PF).

Specimen **COLLECTION:** Bedside spirometry is limited to patients on partial or complete bedrest for whom the seated position is contraindicated or for patients whose conditions make frequent serial measurements of pulmonary function desirable. The vital capacity and forced vital capacity maneuvers can be performed in virtually any position. Whenever possible, the patient should be tested in the upright position. Because of postural changes in lung function, it is imperative that the patient's position and angle of elevation of the bed, if any, be kept constant and recorded on the report so that valid comparisons can be made. After applying noseclips, the subject is instructed to take a full inspiration, hold it briefly, then exhale through a mouthpiece into the spirometer as forcefully and completely as possible, keeping the chin slightly elevated throughout the maneuver. Test is repeated a minimum of three times until two reproducible efforts have been obtained. See Causes for Rejection. A maximum number of eight attempts is recommended. **CAUSES FOR REJECTION:** **Cough,** when occurring in the early part of forced expiration, may render all data except total expired volume useless. **Hesitant start:** Peak effort must be applied as close to the start of exhalation as possible or timed forced expiratory volumes may be invalid. The volume exhaled before maximum effort is applied is known as back extrapolated volume and must not exceed 5% of total FVC. **Premature cessation of expiratory effort:** One of the three following conditions defines satisfactory end-of-test.

- Expiratory time is at least 6 seconds and no volume change for at least 2 seconds.
- If no plateau is seen, patient should sustain expiration for a reasonable length of time; "reasonable" in moderately severe obstruction is suggested to be 15 seconds.
- Patient **cannot** or **should** not continue the expiration for medical reasons.

Early termination of expiration will falsely increase the FEV_1/FVC% and the $FEF_{25\%-75\%}$. **Submaximal effort:** Indicated by a very low, often nonreproducible peak flow. Neuromuscular disease may produce the same pattern. **Nonreproducibility:** The two largest FVCs and the two largest FEV_1s should show <5% variability. Three acceptable tests should be obtained.

TURNAROUND TIME: Preliminary results should be available same day. Depending on the facility, an interpreted report may be available in 1-2 days.

Interpretation **NORMAL FINDINGS:** Spirometric values are dependent on patient's position during testing. Any position other than seated or standing will generally result in less than maximal values. This should be considered when comparing results with normal values generated by a study whose subjects were tested in an upright posture. Pain, especially thoracic or upper abdominal incisional pain, will further limit inspiratory efforts. One study cites a 40% reduction in vital capacity persisting several days after upper abdominal surgery. Normal range for spirometric indexes is typically ±20% of a reference value based on age, height, and gender. Abnormalities of pulmonary function can be separated into three broad descriptive categories: restrictive, obstructive, and mixed. See Patterns of Spirometric Abnormalities table. Restrictive ventilatory defects are characterized by proportional decreases in FVC and FEV_1, leaving the FEV_1/FVC% normal or even slightly elevated. Any lesion affecting the lung, chest wall, or respiratory muscles' ability to take in a normal amount of air yet does not affect the conducting airways' FVC can be classified as a restrictive lung disease. Obstructive diseases are characterized by their involvement of the airways and the resultant reduction in expiratory flow. Spirometric studies in the presence of obstructive lung disease generally show a reduced FEV_1, FEV_1/FVC% and flow rates with a relatively normal FVC. In severe obstructive lung disease, the FVC may also be reduced. Asthma, emphysema, and chronic bronchitis are the most common obstructive lung diseases. Mixed disorders generally present with a reduction in all parameters on spirometric examination. Some studies advocate the use of 95% confidence limit rather than percentage of predicted value.[1] While this is a more scientifically sound method, it has not yet gained widespread acceptance. Spirometric values expressed as % of predict-

(Continued)

Bedside Spirometry *(Continued)*

Patterns of Spirometric Abnormalities

	NML* (% of predicted)	Obstructive Diseases	Restrictive Diseases
FVC	≥80*	NML or ↓	↓ to ↓↓↓
FEV_1	≥80*	↓ to ↓↓↓	↓ to ↓↓↓
FEV_1/FVC %	≥75	↓ to ↓↓↓	NML or ↑
$FEF_{25\%-75\%}$	≥76*	↓↓ to ↓↓↓	↓ to ↓↓↓

*Expressed as actual ratio of FEV_1/FVC x 100.
↓ mildly reduced
↓↓ moderately reduced
↓↓↓ severely reduced

Quantification of Impairment by Spirometry (% of predicted)

	FVC	FEV_1	FEV_1/FVC%*†	$FEF_{25\%-75\%}$
Normal	≥80	≥80	75-85	>76
Minimal (slight)	70-79	70-79	65-74	60-75
Moderate	55-69	55-69	55-64	45-59
Severe	45-54	40-54	45-54	30-44
Very severe	<45	<45	<45	<30

*Expressed as actual ratio of FEV_1/FVC x 100.
†Female age >40 years.

ed can be used to grade the severity of abnormalities. See Quantification of Impairment by Spirometry table. **CRITICAL VALUES:** Severe or very severe reductions (see Quantification of Impairment by Spirometry table). **LIMITATIONS:** Spirometry requires a great deal of cooperation and a thorough understanding of expectations on the part of the patient. Poor understanding or lack of motivation will yield falsely low values that may be incorrectly interpreted. Reproducibility of the two best repeat FVCs and FEV_1s within 5% must be demonstrated before a meaningful interpretation can be made. Most portable (handheld) spirometers have severe limitations in their ability to present information necessary to evaluate the acceptability of spirometric efforts according to American Thoracic Society (ATS) standards. A recent evaluation of spirometers found many portable spirometers did **not** meet current ATS performance standards. Whenever possible, spirometry should be performed in the Pulmonary Function Laboratory rather than at the bedside. **ADDITIONAL INFORMATION:** Patients with asthma may show progressive decline in spirometric values with repeated efforts, yielding excessive variability between the two largest efforts. This may be distinguished from variable effort only by a trained pulmonary technologist noting maximal inspiration on each effort followed by an adequately forceful expiration (sharp peak of expiratory flow volume curve). In such cases, the largest and smallest acceptable efforts should be reported giving the physician a rough assessment of bronchial hyperreactivity. (See Bronchial Challenge Test.) Patients with neuromuscular disease (myasthenia gravis) may show progressive decline of values with repeated efforts but are seldom able to generate an adequate peak effort and may therefore mimic poor effort or understanding.

Footnotes

1. Morris JF, Koski A, and Johnson LC, "Spirometric Standards for Healthy Nonsmoking Adults," *Am Rev Respir Dis*, 1971, 103:57-67.

References

Bass H, "The Flow Volume Loop: Normal Standards and Abnormalities in Chronic Obstructive Pulmonary Disease," *Chest*, 1973, 63:171-6.

Cherniack RM and Raber MB, "Normal Standards for Ventilatory Function Using an Automated Wedge Spirometer," *Am Rev Respir Dis*, 1972, 106:38-46.

Gardner RM, Hankinson JL, Clausen JL, et al, "ATS Statement on Standardization of Spirometry – 1987 Update," *Am Rev Respir Dis*, 1987, 136:1285-98.

Ghio AJ, Crapo RO, and Elliott CG, "Reference Equations Used to Predict Pulmonary Function," *Chest*, 1990, 97(2):400-3.

Kass I, Bell WB, Epler GE, et al, "Evaluation of Impairment Disability Secondary to Respiratory Disease," *Am Rev Respir Dis*, 1982, 126:945-51.

Knudson RJ, Slatin RC, Lebowitz MD, et al, "The Maximal Expiratory Flow-Volume Curve: Normal Standards, Variability and Effects of Age," *Am Rev Respir Dis*, 1976, 113:587-600.

Morris JF, "Spirometry in the Evaluation of Pulmonary Function," *West J Med*, 1976, 125:110-8.

Nelson SB, Gardner RM, Crapo RO, et al, "Performance Evaluation of Contemporary Spirometers," *Chest*, 1990, 97(2):288-97.

Pattishall EN, "Pulmonary Function Testing Reference Values and Interpretations in Pediatric Training Programs," *Pediatrics*, 1990, 85(5):768-73.

Schoenberg JB, Beck GJ, and Bough SA, "Growth and Decay of Pulmonary Function in Healthy Blacks and Whites," *Respir Physiol*, 1978, 33:367-93.

Townsend MC, Duchene AG, and Fallat RJ, "The Effects of Underrecorded Forced Expirations on Spirometric Lung Function Indexes," *Am Rev Respir Dis*, 1982, 126:734-7.

Blood Gases, Arterial *see* Arterial Blood Gases *on page 206*

Bronchial Challenge Test

CPT 94070 (prolonged postexposure evaluation of bronchospasm with multiple spirometric determinations after test dose of bronchodilator or antigen); 95070 (inhalation bronchial challenge testing [not including necessary pulmonary function tests], with histamine, methacholine, or similar compounds)

Related Information

Bedside Spirometry *on page 212*
Flow Volume Loop *on page 228*
Ingestion Challenge Test *on page 20*
Spirometry *on page 245*
Spirometry Before and After Bronchodilators *on page 248*

Synonyms Bronchial Provocation Tests; Histamine Challenge Test; Mecholyl Challenge; Mecholyl Provocation Test; Methacholine Challenge; Methacholine Provocation Test; Provocholine® Challenge

Abstract **PROCEDURE COMMONLY INCLUDES:** $PD_{20}FEV_1$ (provocative dose necessary to cause a 20% reduction from baseline FEV_1). $PD_{35}SG_{aw}$, % change in FEV_1 or SG_{aw} at the end of study, % improvement in FEV_1 or SG_{aw} after administration of bronchodilators. **INDICATIONS:**

- identify and characterize severity of nonspecific bronchial hypersensitivity, especially helpful in the diagnosis of cough-variant asthma or asthma in remission
- evaluate the effectiveness of pharmacological agents in the prevention of provoked bronchospasm
- study the pathophysiology of bronchospasm

CONTRAINDICATIONS: Relatively contraindicated in the presence of severe restrictive or obstructive lung disease (FEV_1 <1 $liter_{BTPS}$).

Patient Care/Scheduling **PATIENT PREPARATION:** Patients should abstain from the use of: sympathomimetic drugs for 6 hours, metaproterenol for 8 hours, terbutaline or Salbutamol for 12 hours, methylxanthines for 12 hours, sustained release methylxanthines for 48 hours, cromolyn sodium for 48 hours, corticosteroids for 12 hours, smoking for 12 hours, coffee, tea, cola or chocolate for 6 hours, significant exercise for 2 hours, and exposure to cold air for 2 hours. Patient should be questioned as to these drugs and conditions prior to testing. Record time and nature of recent respiratory illnesses as viral respiratory infections have been shown to leave residual bronchial hyperreactivity that may linger for months. **AFTERCARE:** Administration of an aerosol bronchodilator and measurement of response to bronchodilator should be done on virtually every patient, even those that do not show a clearly positive response to methacholine. Spontaneous reversal of methacholine induced bronchospasm usually takes place within 90 minutes. Methacholine induced

(Continued)

Bronchial Challenge Test *(Continued)*

bronchospasm is usually readily reversible after inhaled bronchodilator therapy. **COMPLICATIONS:** Severe bronchospasm may occur, particularly if baseline airways obstruction is present.

Method **EQUIPMENT:** Standard equipment includes a spirometer which meets ATS equipment specifications, mouthpiece, noseclip, 10 compressed gas nebulizers, 20 psi compressed gas source, dosimeter (which delivers a 0.6 second burst of compressed gas to the nebulizer upon actuation) and various doses of methacholine chloride solution. See table. **TECHNIQUE:** Two protocols are widely in use, five breaths per challenge level or 2 minutes of tidal breathing per challenge level. In the 2 minute challenge, the test material is placed in a nebulizer cup attached to a constant output compressor. The patient is instructed to perform tidal breathing for 2 minutes. Measurement of response is done 3 minutes after each exposure. In the 5-breath challenge the patient inhales slowly from FRC to TLC through a dosimeter driven nebulizer cup containing the test material. The dosimeter delivers a 0.6 second nebulization (at 20 psig) of the test material. The breath is held for 3-5 seconds. Both protocols use the same schedules of test material concentrations. Forced expiratory maneuvers are performed before and 3 minutes after inhalation challenge with either a diluent solution or gradually increasing doses of a solution of methacholine. Testing consists of measurement of reproducible FVC and FEV_1 before and after administration of aerosolized diluent solution and aerosolized methacholine chloride/diluent solution. Measurement of spirometry should be done on calibrated spirometers that meet standards recommended by the American Thoracic Society (ATS). Duplicate FEV_1 at each challenge level should be reproducible within 5%. **DATA ACQUIRED:** For clinical use, the PD_{20} FEV_1 (the lowest concentration which produces a 20% reduction in FEV_1 from baseline) is generally reported. Researchers often plot the log of the cumulative dose of methacholine against the FEV_1 response reported as a percentage of the control FEV_1 (FEV_1 after inhalation of the diluent solution).

Standardized Methacholine Challenge Protocol

Methacholine Concentration (mg/mL)	Cumulative Number of Breaths	Units/ Breath	Cumulative Dose Units (CDU)
0.075	5	0.075	0.375
0.15	10	0.15	1.125
0.31	15	0.31	2.68
0.62	20	0.62	5.78
1.25	25	1.25	12.0
2.50	30	2.5	24.5
5.00	35	5	49.5
10.00	40	10	99.5
25.00	45	25	225.0

Specimen **CAUSES FOR REJECTION:** Nonreproducible forced expiratory maneuvers. FEV_1 should be reproducible to within 5% on any given level of challenge. Drop in FEV_1 should be sustained for 5 minutes to be considered valid. End expiratory coughing may result in nonreproducible FVC values. If the FEV_1 values show reproducibility, efforts that show end-expiratory coughing may be used only if the FEV_1/FVC% and $FEF_{25\%-75\%}$ are ignored. **TURNAROUND TIME:** Preliminary results are usually available on the day of testing. An interpreted report usually follows in 1-2 days.

Interpretation **NORMAL FINDINGS:** There is a certain amount of overlap between normal and asthmatic responses to methacholine chloride and histamine toward the end of the challenge procedure. Provocative doses are usually reported as either the concentration of methacholine in solution or the cumulative dose unit (CDU) necessary to provide a 20% reduction in the baseline FEV_1 or a 35% reduction in the specific conductance (SG_{aw}). A dose unit (DU) is defined as the number of breaths inhaled multiplied by the strength of solution in mg/mL being inhaled. Less than a 20% fall in FEV_1 or 35% fall in SG_{aw} by the end of a challenge, typically 200-225 cumulative dose units of methacholine, makes the diagnosis of asthma or nonspecific airway hyperreactivity unlikely. A positive methacholine challenge does not always indicate asthma. Recent viral infections and pre-existing obstructive lung disease in the absence of detectable asthma have been shown to cause false-positive reactions to challenge testing. **LIMITATIONS:** While methacholine challenge testing is a sensitive test for bronchial hyperreactivity, a positive test is not specific for the diagnosis of asthma. Other diseases associated with nonspecific bronchial hyperreactivity include COPD, bronchiolitis, viral upper respiratory infections, hay fever, cystic fibrosis, sarcoidosis, chemical irritant exposure, and recovery from adult respiratory distress syndromes. Appropriate preparation is imperative for proper interpretation of challenge response. Negative methacholine challenges in patients with positive specific bronchial challenges with chemical agents suspected of causing occupational asthma have been reported. **ADDITIONAL INFORMATION:** Methacholine chloride is available in ready to mix ampules from LaRoche Laboratories that are marketed under the name Provocholine®. The following dosage schedule is recommended when using Provocholine®:

- baseline spirometry
- diluent solution spirometry
- 0.025 mg/mL methacholine spirometry
- 0.25 mg/mL methacholine spirometry
- 2.5 mg/mL methacholine spirometry
- 10 mg/mL methacholine spirometry
- 25 mg/mL methacholine spirometry
- aerosolized bronchodilator spirometry

Bronchial Provocation Tests *see* Bronchial Challenge Test *on page 215*

Calculated Arterial or Venous Oxygen Saturation *replaced by* Arterial Blood Oximetry *on page 210*

Carbon Dioxide Challenge Test

CPT 94400

Synonyms CO_2 Response Test; Hypercapnic Challenge Test

Abstract **PROCEDURE COMMONLY INCLUDES:** Minute ventilation ($\mathring{V}_E$) in liter$_{BTPS}$/minute, respiratory rate (RR) and tidal volume ($\mathring{V}_E$) at the start and end of the hypercapnic challenge slope of ventilation ($\mathring{V}_E$) plotted against end-tidal carbon dioxide concentration ($P_{ET}CO_2$) or $\mathring{V}_E/P_{ET}CO_2$. **Optional:** Mouth occlusion pressure at 100 msec after occlusion (P_{100}), slope of PO_{100} plotted against $P_{ET}CO_2$. **INDICATIONS:** To quantify the effect of increasing levels of carbon dioxide on the respiratory center of patients suspected of decreased ventilatory drive to carbon dioxide. To quantify the effects of therapeutic agents on respiratory chemosensitivity to carbon dioxide.

Patient Care/Scheduling **PATIENT PREPARATION:** Respiratory stimulants such as caffeine containing beverages (coffee, tea, cola), theophylline preparations, medroxyprogesterone, and protriptyline should be discontinued for at least 12 hours before testing unless the effects of these substances on ventilatory response to CO_2 is desired. Patients should empty their bladder just before testing. **COMPLICATIONS:** Inhalation of high levels of carbon dioxide during this test can cause generalized vasodilatation which sometimes causes flushing, diaphoresis, and headaches.

Method **EQUIPMENT:** No commercially made devices are currently available for the performance of the rebreathing method for measurement of ventilatory response to CO_2. Rebuck describes the construction of a device using materials commonly available in hospitals[1]. The heart of this device is a bag in a box system used to allow the patient to rebreathe the test gas from the bag in the box while ventilation is measured at the other box opening. This unit is shown in the figure on the following page. **TECHNIQUE:** The 6-10 L anesthesia bag is filled with a volume equal to the patient's vital capacity plus 1 L of a gas mixture containing 7% CO_2 and 93% O_2. The 7% CO_2 is chosen to approximate average mixed venous concentrations of CO_2, and the 93% O_2 is chosen to eliminate concern for hypoxia during the test. After normal breathing followed by a full expiration, valves are turned that provide the anesthesia bag as a reservoir for ventilation during the test. Exhaled gases are returned to the bag. End-tidal CO_2 is monitored during the test. If occlusion pressures are desired, the inspiratory portion of the circuit is occluded by means of a Starling resistor at random intervals throughout the test. The output of a pressure transducer is then recorded on a high speed (at least 50 mm/second) recorder. The test continues until one of the following occurs:

- 4 minutes have elapsed or
- the patient's end-tidal CO_2 concentration equals 9% or

(Continued)

Carbon Dioxide Challenge Test *(Continued)*

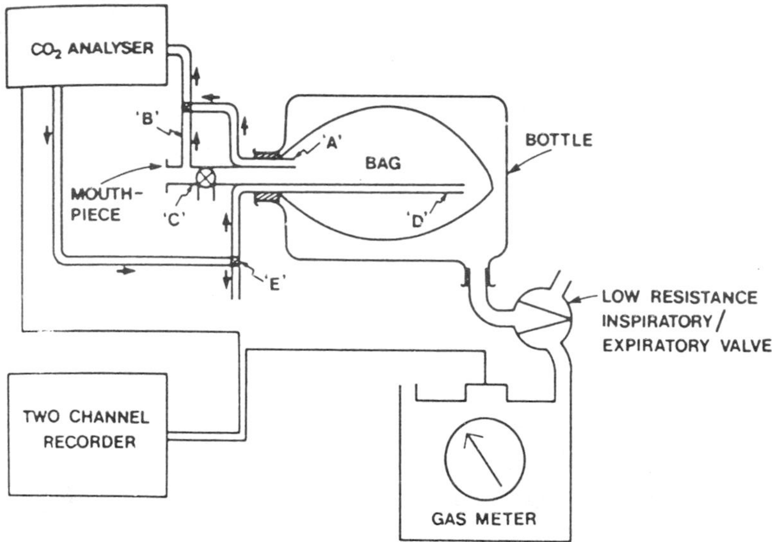

Circuit required for measuring the ventilatory response to CO_2 by rebreathing. The short thick arrows indicate the direction of gas flow to and from the CO_2 analyzer. Reprinted with permission from Rebuck AS, "Measurement of Ventilatory Response to CO_2 by Rebreathing," *Chest*, 1976, 70(suppl):118-21.

- when the patient complains of dyspnea
- the first 30 seconds of rebreathing are excluded from data analysis.

Specimen CAUSES FOR REJECTION: Hypercapnic patients that exhibit pCO_2 values >55 mm Hg at rest do not usually provide sufficient sample to plot ventilatory response by the end of the test (63 mm Hg). Voluntary erratic breathing caused by malingering will yield misleading data.

Interpretation NORMAL FINDINGS: In a study of 21 normals by Read, a mean slope of 2.65 ± 1.21 L/minute/mm Hg was found.[2] The range was quite large; 1.16-6.18 L/minute/mm Hg. Similar values were found in a larger study by Irsliger.[3] He studied 126 adults and found a mean slope of 2.6 ± 1.2 with a range of 0.47-6.22 L/minute/mm Hg. When interpreting ventilatory response tests, it is important to know if abnormal pulmonary mechanics (eg, emphysema) are present. This can help distinguish those who cannot breathe (limited by abnormalities in pulmonary mechanics) from those who will not breathe (abnormal sensitivity to carbon dioxide). The occlusion pressure measured at 100 msec is a relatively direct indicator of the output of the respiratory center to the diaphragm and is independent of airflow obstruction. Normal values for a normocapnic P_{100} is 2.6 cm H_2O (range 1.5-5). The occlusion pressure increased at a rate of approximately 0.5-6 cm H_2O for every mm increase in end-tidal CO_2. LIMITATIONS: A wide range of normal responses exists, making interpretation difficult.

Footnotes

1. Rebuck AS, "Measurement of Ventilatory Response to CO_2 by Rebreathing," *Chest*, 1976, 70(suppl):118-21.
2. Read DJC, "A Clinical Method For Assessing the Ventilatory Response to Carbon Dioxide," *Aust Ann Med*, 1967, 16:20-32.
3. Irsliger GB, "Carbon Dioxide Response Lines in Young Adults: The Limits of the Normal Response," *Am Rev Respir Dis*, 1976, 114:529-36.

Carbon Monoxide Determination *see* Arterial Blood Oximetry *on page 210*

Carbon Monoxide Diffusing Capacity, Single Breath

CPT 94720

Synonyms DLCO; SB DLCO; Transfer Factor

Abstract **PROCEDURE COMMONLY INCLUDES:** Diffusion capacity of the lung for carbon monoxide (DLCO) reported in mL CO_{STPD}/minute/mm Hg. Alveolar volume (VA), based on dilution of a vital capacity sized breath of test gas by the patient's residual volume, is reported in $liter_{BTPS}$. The "specific diffusing capacity" is the DLCO normalized to lung volume and is reported in mL CO_{STPD}/minute/mm Hg/$liter_{BTPS}$ VA. **INDICATIONS:**

- diagnose or following the course of interstitial lung disease, emphysema, sarcoidosis, pulmonary vascular disease, and intrapulmonary hemorrhage
- distinguish chronic bronchitis (normal DLCO) from emphysema (low DLCO) and interstitial from pleural fibrosis. The specific diffusing capacity (DL/VA) may be useful in separating patients with interstitial lung disease (low DLCO, low DL/VA) from patients with extrapulmonary restrictions such as obesity and diaphragm paralysis (low DLCO, normal or high DL/VA)
- elucidate operative cause of hypoxemia

Reduction of DLCO % of predicted value to <55% has been shown to be predictive of exercise arterial O_2 desaturation. A diffusing capacity ≤50% of predicted is considered to be a criterion for disability in interstitial lung disease.

Patient Care/Scheduling **PATIENT PREPARATION:** Patient should discontinue smoking for 24 hours pretest. Recent hemoglobin and carboxyhemoglobin are desired to allow for correction for high levels of carbon monoxide and high and low levels of hemoglobin. See also Spirometry. **AFTERCARE:** None usually needed.

Method **EQUIPMENT:** Test is performed on a device which contains a calibrated reservoir of test gas, a helium analyzer, a carbon monoxide analyzer, a timing circuit, an automatic or manually controlled five-way valve, a sample bag, and a sample pump. The testing unit should conform to standards put forth by the ATS.

Specimen Measurement of inspired volume, breath-holding time and inspired and expired concentrations of helium and carbon monoxide before and after respectively, approximately 10 seconds of breath-holding of a vital capacity sized breath of lung diffusion test gas (69% nitrogen, 21% oxygen, 10% helium and 0.3% carbon monoxide). **COLLECTION:** Test gas is held in reservoir (usually a spirometer). Patient should be sitting. Patient exhales until reaching a maximum end-expiration (residual volume – RV). Patient rapidly inspires from test gas reservoir until he reaches full inspiration (total lung capacity). Patient exhales rapidly after 10 seconds of breath-holding. A fraction of the exhaled air (usually 750 mL) is allowed to escape to the atmosphere before an exhaled sample (500 1000 mL) is collected to account for anatomical dead space. When testing patients with a VC <2 L, reduce the discard volume before sample collection from 750-500 mL and note this on the report. Exhaled sample is analyzed for helium and carbon monoxide. Test is repeated after a minimum wait of 4 minutes until reproducibility of 5% or 3 mL/minute/mm Hg is achieved. **CAUSES FOR REJECTION:** Inspiratory vital capacity <90% of the best previously measured vital capacity, breath-holding time <9 seconds or >11 seconds. Slow inspiration or expiration can affect results; inspiratory times should be <4 seconds in patients with obstructive lung disease or 2.5 seconds in the absence of airway obstruction. These represent conditions that fall below ATS standards for performance of a single breath diffusing capacity. They may represent the best performance obtained in spite of repeated efforts and should, therefore, **not** be discarded. They should be reported with a statement on the report which describes which specific standard was not met. **TURNAROUND TIME:** Depends on institution, results are usually available on the same day. Interpreted report is usually available the next day.

Interpretation **NORMAL FINDINGS:** Many prediction equations exist. No one set of prediction equations can be recommended for all labs and patient populations. Appropriate normal regression equations should be chosen by comparing a group of 10 nonsmoking normals free of pulmonary disease with the prediction equation which is being used. The measured DLCO should be corrected for abnormally low or high levels of hemoglobin and carboxyhemoglobin before comparison with predicted value. Values >80% of predicted or >95% confidence interval are considered normal. A **decreased** diffusing capacity is seen in emphysema, idiopathic pulmonary fibrosis, asbestosis, sarcoidosis, scleroderma lung disease, pneumonia, multiple pulmonary emboli, collagen vascular disease, histiocytosis-X,

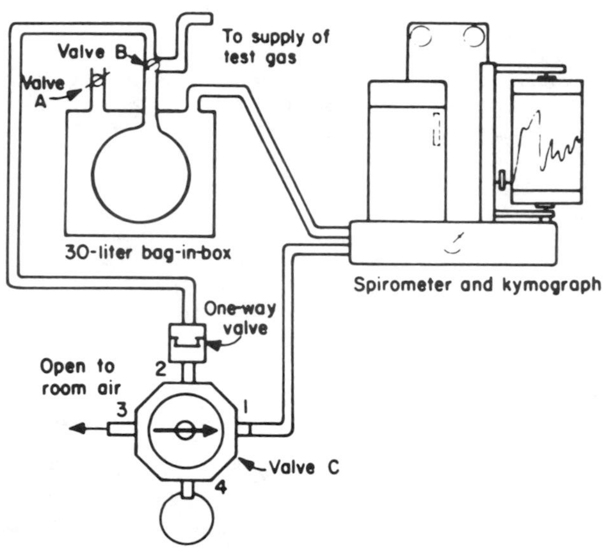

Suggested Instrument set-up for single-breath DLCO measurement. Reproduced with permission from Clausen JL, *Pulmonary Function Testing Guidelines and Controversies: Equipment, Methods, and Normal Values*, New York, NY: Academic Press, 1982, 176.

Pulmonary Diffusing Capacity for Carbon Monoxide

s

Washout volume

1/2 VC

t

Vital capacity

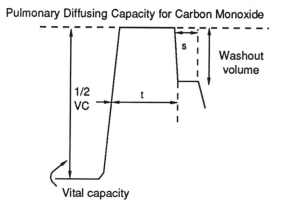

Determination of breath holding time (t) as recommended by Gaensler. The kymograph speed in this example is 160 mm/min or 32 mm/12 sec. The breath holding time is measured from the point of midinspiration (half of vital capacity) to the onset of alveolar gas collection. Washout and sample collection time is designated by s. Reproduced with permission from Clausen JL, *Pulmonary Function Testing Guidelines and Controversies: Equipment, Methods, and Normal Values*, New York, NY: Academic Press, 1982, 179.

extrathoracic restrictive lung disease, and anemia. The DLCO may be corrected to alveolar volume (DL/VA) to assess nonparenchymal reduction in DLCO, but this practice is controversial and may be inappropriate. Adjustment of the measured DLCO for abnormally high or low levels of hemoglobin may be made by the following equation:

corrected DLCO = actual DLCO x 10.2 + observed Hgb (g/dL) / 1.7 + observed Hgb (g/dL).

An **increased** diffusing capacity is seen in polycythemia, asthma, left-to-right shunts, exercise, supine position, intrapulmonary hemorrhage, and increased heart rates.

LIMITATIONS: Measured values must be corrected for known abnormal hemoglobin and carboxyhemoglobin or methemoglobin values. Overinterpretation of a normal DL/VA in the presence of an abnormal DLCO may decrease the sensitivity of the DLCO to detect early interstitial lung disease.

References

Crapo RO and Forster RE, "Carbon Monoxide Diffusing Capacity," *Clin Chest Med*, 1989, 10(2):187-98.

Ghio AJ, Crapo RO, and Elliott CG, "Reference Equations Used to Predict Pulmonary Function," *Chest*, 1990, 97(2):400-3.

Hathaway EH, Tashkin DP, and Simmons MS, "Intraindividual Variability in Serial Measurements of DLCO and Alveolar Volume Over One Year in Eight Healthy Subjects Using Three Independent Measuring Systems," *Am Rev Respir Dis*, 1989, 140(6):1818-22.

Kanengiser LC, Rapoport DM, Epstein H, et al, "Volume Adjustment of Mechanics and Diffusion in Interstitial Lung Disease: Lack of Clinical Relevance," *Chest*, 1989, 96(5):1036-42.

McKeage MJ, Evans BD, Atkinson C, et al, "Carbon Monoxide Diffusing Capacity is a Poor Predictor of Clinically Significant Bleomycin Lung," *J Clin Oncol*, 1990, 8(5):779-83.

Viegi G, Paoletti P, Prediletto R, et al, "Carbon Monoxide Diffusing Capacity, Other Indices of Lung Function, and Respiratory Symptoms in a General Population Sample," *Am Rev Respir Dis*, 1990, 141(4 Pt 1):1033-9.

Cardiopulmonary Exercise Testing

CPT 94620

Related Information

Maximum Voluntary Ventilation (MVV) *on page 237*
Pulse Oximetry *on page 241*
Spirometry *on page 245*

Synonyms Cardiopulmonary Stress Test; Incremental Exercise Testing

Applies to Disability Assessment; Disability Examination; Exercise Blood Gases; Exercise Oximetry

Abstract PROCEDURE COMMONLY INCLUDES: Maximum workload achieved (reported in watts, kilopond-meters (kpm), resting energy equivalents (METS), or maximum speed and grade achieved on treadmill), measured or calculated maximum oxygen uptake ($\dot{V}O_{2max}$), ventilation measured at maximum exercise ($\dot{V}_{E\ max}$), maximum carbon dioxide output ($\dot{V}CO_{2max}$), respiratory exchange ratio (R), maximum oxygen pulse, maximum heart rate achieved (HR_{max}), tidal volume (VT), respiratory rate (frequency of breathing or f_b), calculated dead space to tidal volume ratio (VD/VT), oxygen saturation measured by pulse oximetry (O_2 sat %). When necessary, arterial blood gas samples may be obtained during exercise for disability purposes; see Arterial Blood Gases. Some centers obtain noninvasive cardiac output measurements during exercise by CO_2 rebreathing technique. INDICATIONS:

- rule out significant cardiopulmonary disease in the presence of normal static pulmonary function (spirometry, lung volumes, diffusion capacity, arterial blood gases)
- detect cardiopulmonary abnormalities when symptoms (generally dyspnea) are out of proportion to findings on tests of static function
- assess cardiopulmonary fitness in disability evaluations
- detect the presence of exercise-induced bronchoconstriction
- assess the presence of peripheral vascular disease
- detect coronary artery disease

(Continued)

Cardiopulmonary Exercise Testing *(Continued)*

- assess the presence of some neuromuscular diseases such as McArdle's syndrome (muscle phosphorylase deficiency)

CONTRAINDICATIONS: Absolute contraindications include: acute febrile illness, acute ECG changes of myocardial ischemia, uncontrolled heart failure, pulmonary edema, unstable angina, acute myocarditis, uncontrolled hypertension (>250 mm Hg systolic, 120 mm Hg diastolic), uncontrolled asthma.

Relative contraindications include: recent (less than 4 weeks previous) myocardial infarction, aortic valve disease, resting tachycardia (heart rate >120 beats/minute), severe electrolyte disturbances, resting electrocardiographic abnormalities, poorly controlled diabetes, epilepsy, cerebrovascular disease, respiratory failure.

Patient Care/Scheduling **PATIENT PREPARATION:** Patient should be instructed to wear loose, comfortable clothing and tennis shoes or other comfortable shoes. Heavy meals should be avoided for 2 hours prior to testing. **AFTERCARE:** Patient should be allowed to "cool down" gradually rather than allowing abrupt, complete cessation of work. Blood pressures should be taken immediately after reduction in workload and at least once a minute until stabilization at or near baseline value has been reached.

Method **EQUIPMENT:** Volume measuring device, O_2 analyzer, CO_2 analyzer, mouthpiece and noseclips (or mask), ECG analyzer, ABG equipment (optional), pulse oximeter, sphygmomanometer, bicycle ergometer or treadmill. Ventilation exhaled or inhaled gas passes through a calibrated volume or flow measuring device (typically a pneumotach for exhaled flows or a dry gasometer for inhaled volumes). Heart rate is measured by electrocardiogram. Oxygen saturation is measured by electrocardiography. Exhaled concentrations of oxygen and carbon dioxide are measured by calibrated oxygen and carbon dioxide analyzers. Signals from these measuring devices are typically sent to a waveform analyzer or computer for subsequent calculation of reported values. Some systems sample on a breath by breath mode while others will take an average sample representative of conditions during a given workload. **TECHNIQUE:** Appropriate medical and medication history

Diagnostic Flow Chart for Stress Testing

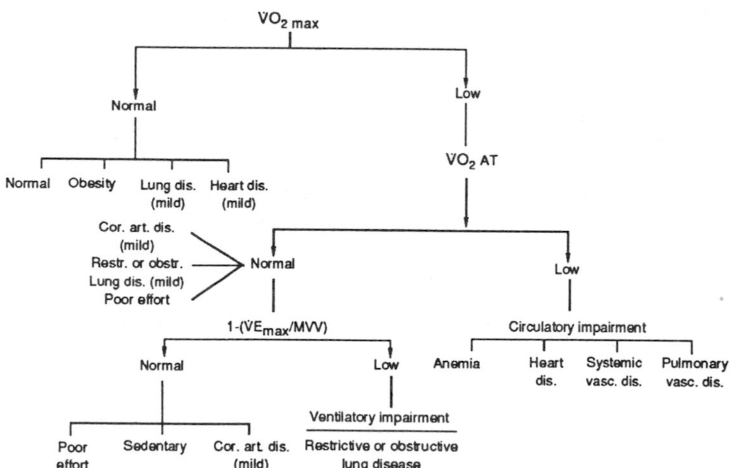

Wasserman's flow chart is especially helpful in the differential diagnosis of dyspnea. The vital relationship of the anaerobic threshold is clearly seen in this schema. The $\dot{V}_2$ AT is low if less than 40% of the subject's predicted $\dot{V}_{2max}$ and indicates circulatory impairment. The breathing reserve is low if 1-($\dot{V}E_{max}$/MVV) is less than 30%. Printed with permission from Wasserman K, *Principles of Exercise Testing and Interpretation*, Philadelphia, PA: Lea & Febiger, 1987.

must be obtained (see Contraindications). The patient's barefoot height and weight should be measured. Pre-exercise spirometry including MVV should be obtained (see Spirometry). Electrocardiograph leads should be carefully placed at the appropriate sites after adequate skin preparation. Skin preparation includes shaving, if necessary, and rubbing with acetone and a nylon abrader. It may be necessary to secure the electrodes in place with a surgical net vest to avoid excessive noise associated with movement. Baseline electrocardiogram should be obtained. Peripheral circulation should be evaluated and the best site (finger, ear, bridge of nose) for placement of a pulse oximetry probe should be determined. Sphygmomanometer cuff should be taped in place and a baseline blood pressure recorded. The patient should be instructed in the operation of the treadmill or cycle ergometer and appropriate workload incrementations based on the patient's history of physical activity, dyspnea on exertion, spirometry and physical findings. Workload incrementations are designed to achieve patient exhaustion between 8-12 minutes. The mouthpiece/noseclips or mask should be applied. Resting measurements are obtained for 2-3 minutes (until stable). Three minutes of unloaded cycling generally precede application of resistance to ergometer. Thereafter, the workload is increased by the constant, predetermined increment. Incrementation of workload is estimated to yield 8-12 minutes of exercise and is based on the patient's history of activities which cause breathlessness and/or fatigue. This continues until the patient cannot continue because of exhaustion, or should not continue because of medical reasons (eg, hypotensive response, ischemic changes on ECG, severe cardiac arrhythmia, etc).

Specimen CAUSES FOR REJECTION: Inadequate effort will cause erroneously low values to be reported as maximum. In such cases, no obvious limitation will be seen. Some patients will voluntarily hyperventilate throughout the test, again causing erroneously low values for $\mathring{V}O$ and workload. Because ventilation during exercise in this case is inappropriately high, it may appear that a ventilatory limitation is present, however, end-tidal CO_2 levels <35 mm Hg should indicate falsely high levels of ventilation. TURNAROUND TIME: Preliminary report is usually available on the same day, interpreted report is available in 1-2 days.

Interpretation NORMAL FINDINGS: Normal values for maximum oxygen uptake ($\mathring{V}O_2$) usually indicate a normal study. Prediction equations are available. Normally, the heart rate will approach the age-related predicted maximum heart rate (220 − age) at the end of the study. Typically, there will be a ventilatory reserve of 30% to 35% in normals. Predicted maximum ventilation can be calculated by multiplying the FEV_1 by 35 or 40. Normally there is no desaturation associated with exercise. Calculated V_D/V_T generally shows a decline with progressive levels of exercise. A calculated V_D/V_T that remains stable or increases is generally indicative of pulmonary vascular disease. CRITICAL VALUES: A maximum $\mathring{V}O_2$ <15 mL/kg (with good patient effort) is generally considered to indicate disability. LIMITATIONS: Proper evaluation of exercise performance requires that maximum patient effort be applied during the test. Malingering is possible and may be difficult to evaluate. ADDITIONAL INFORMATION: Postheart or heart-lung transplant patient should be allowed a minimum of 3 minutes between increments in workload to allow for the denervated heart to adjust stroke volume and rate. Measurement of spirometry up to 30 minutes postexercise can aid in detection of exercise induced asthma. A 20% drop in FEV_1 postexercise is indicative of exercise-induced asthma.

Cardiopulmonary Exercise Test

	Units
Measured Parameters	
Minute ventilation ($\mathring{V}E$)	LPM
Respiratory frequency (f_b)	breath/min
Tidal volume (V_T)	mL
Heart rate (HR)	beats/min
Blood pressure (SYS/DIAS)	mm Hg
Oxygen saturation	%
Calculated Parameters	
Oxygen uptake ($\mathring{V}O_2$)	mL/min
Oxygen pulse ($\mathring{V}O_2$/HR)	mL/beat
CO_2 production ($\mathring{V}CO_2$)	mL/min
Respiratory exchange ratio (R)	
Dead space to tidal volume ratio (V_D/V_T)	
Anaerobic threshold (AT)	mL $\mathring{V}O_2$/min

References

Eschenbacher WL and Mannina A, "An Algorithm for the Interpretation of Cardiopulmonary Exercise Tests," *Chest*, 1990, 97(2):263-7.

(Continued)

Cardiopulmonary Exercise Testing *(Continued)*

Savin WM, Schroeder JS, and Haskell WL, "Response of Cardiac Transplant Recipients to Static and Dynamic Exercise: A Review," *Heart Transplantation*, 1986, 1:72-9.
Wasserman K, "The Anaerobic Threshold Measurement in Exercise Testing," *Clin Chest Med*, 1984, 5(1):77-88.

Cardiopulmonary Sleep Study

CPT 95828 (polysomnography, recording, analysis and interpretation of the multiple simultaneous physiological measurements of sleep)

Related Information

Pulse Oximetry *on page 241*

Synonyms Polysomnography (PSG); Sleep Apnea Study; Sleep Oximetry; Sleep Study; Titration of Oxygen or Nasal CPAP During Sleep

Applies to Respiratory Inductive Plethysmography

Abstract **PROCEDURE COMMONLY INCLUDES:** Sleep studies for the evaluation of cardiopulmonary sleep-related disorders commonly include assessment of the stages of sleep, respiratory airflow, respiratory effort, arterial oxygen saturation by ear oximeter or pulse oximetry, monitoring of body position and periodic leg movements, monitoring of the electrocardiogram. **INDICATIONS:**

- Chronic obstructive pulmonary disease (COPD): patients with COPD whose PaO_2 is <55 mm Hg, patients with COPD whose PaO_2 is >55 mm Hg whose illness is complicated by pulmonary hypertension, right heart failure or polycythemia
- Restrictive ventilatory disorders: patients with restrictive ventilatory impairment secondary to chest wall and neuromuscular disturbances whose illness is complicated by chronic hypoventilation, polycythemia, pulmonary hypertension, disturbed sleep, morning headaches, daytime somnolence, and fatigue
- Disorders of respiratory control: patients with disturbances of respiratory control whose awake $PaCO_2$ is >45 mm Hg or whose illness is complicated by pulmonary hypertension, polycythemia, disturbed sleep, morning headaches, daytime somnolence, and fatigue
- Symptoms arising from sleep apnea: patients with excessive daytime sleepiness or sleep maintenance insomnia
- Cardiovascular manifestations of sleep apnea: patients with nocturnal cyclic bradyarrhythmias, nocturnal abnormalities of atrioventricular conduction, and ventricular ectopy during sleep that appears increased relative to wakefulness

CONTRAINDICATIONS: Although they do not represent contraindications, the following represent circumstances in which a cardiopulmonary sleep study is **not** indicated: patients with COPD whose awake PaO_2 is >55 mm Hg and are free of complications; patients with restrictive chest wall, neuromuscular or interstitial lung diseases who are not chronically hypoventilating and who are free of polycythemia, pulmonary hypertension, disturbed sleep, morning headaches or daytime somnolence and fatigue; patients that have the risk factors for sleep apnea of obesity and/or snoring but are free of any symptoms of sleep apnea; patients with systemic hypertension; patients with nocturnal nonspecific cardiac arrhythmias.[1]

Patient Care/Scheduling **PATIENT PREPARATION:** Patients scheduled for sleep studies should continue taking all medications as prescribed. Any medication which is scheduled to be taken before bedtime should be brought with them. Hair should be clean and free of hair care products such as mousse and hairspray.

Method **EQUIPMENT:** Equipment varies with the complexity of the study. Studies may be categorized as simplified (screening) or complete cardiopulmonary sleep study. A full cardiopulmonary sleep study is one in which a full polysomnogram with EEG is performed in which the focus of the study is on cardiac and respiratory parameters. A simplified cardiopulmonary sleep study is one in which only cardiac and respiratory parameters are measured. The role of the simplified study in the diagnosis of sleep apnea has not been definitively established. The following equipment is used to measure the various physiological markers used in a cardiopulmonary sleep study.

- Electroencephalogram (EEG): Electrodes are placed at the C3, C4, A1, and A2 positions (International 10-20 system).[2] Sleep staging is recorded using C3/A2; C4/A1 may be used as an alternative if technical difficulties are encountered.

- Electrooculogram (EOG): One electrode is placed on the outer canthus of each eye with the electrode on the right outer canthus being 1 cm above the horizontal and the electrode on the left being 1 cm below the horizontal.
- Electromyogram (EMG): **Chin muscles:** One electrode is applied at the center of the chin with two others beneath the chin (one of these is used as a back-up electrode). **Skeletal muscle EMG:** EMG of the anterior tibialis muscle will allow detection of periodic movements in sleep and assessment of body position.[3] **Respiration:** In a cardiopulmonary sleep study, it is important to measure both actual movement of airflow and the presence of respiratory effort in order to differentiate between obstructive and central sleep apneas. A large number of devices exist which generate either quantitative or semiquantitative assessment of respiratory activity. Semiquantitative techniques that will allow adequate differentiation of central and obstructive events may be used. To detect mouth or nasal airflow, various devices such as CO_2 analyzers, thermistors,[4] laryngeal and tracheal microphones[5,6,7] and impedance pneumography[8,9] have been used successfully. Quantitative techniques such as a pneumotachograph attached to a mask, magnetometers[10,11] and respiratory inductive plethysmography[12,13] have been used successfully. Respiratory inductive plethysmography systems may be used to qualitatively separate central from obstructive apneas. Esophageal balloon/catheter systems or pressure catheters have been used successfully to monitor respiratory effort.[14] **Oxygen saturation:** Ear oximeters and pulse oximeters have proved useful in documenting fluctuations of arterial oxygen saturation. Recent studies have shown that oximeters may underestimate or overestimate the oscillations in arterial oxygen saturation associated with apneic events.[15,16]

TECHNIQUE: The monitoring of the parameters listed may be done during a daytime nap or an overnight sleep study. A recent study concluded that afternoon nap studies may be inadequate for the evaluation of sleep-related breathing disorders.[17] Patients with severe daytime sleepiness and suspected obstructive sleep apnea are best suited for daytime studies because of the ease with which they fall asleep. A minimum of 2-4 hours of sleep should be obtained, including both REM and non-REM sleep and sleep in the supine position. If this is not done, the severity of sleep apnea may be underestimated. A therapeutic trial of nasal CPAP may be done in patients with severe, uncomplicated sleep apnea as a part of the diagnostic study night. **DATA ACQUIRED:** Sleep staging may be performed in fixed intervals (usually 30 seconds) using the criteria proposed by Rechtschaffen and Kales[18] or by other systems which modify the standard sleep scoring system for use in sleep apnea patients.[19] In addition to the scoring of the sleep state, the number of arousals during sleep and the frequency of occurrence of periodic movements in sleep should be tabulated. The total number of movements, the total number of movements associated with arousal or awakenings, and the movement index (number of movements/hour of sleep) should be calculated. Respiratory parameters reported include the number of apneic events and an apnea index (number of apneas/hour of sleep). Recent investigators suggest the reporting of a respiratory disturbance index (number of apneas plus the number of hypoapneas/hour of sleep). Various parameters have been reported using the oxygen saturation as measured by pulse or ear oximetry. Nadir values, mean oxygen saturation, mean oxygen saturation per sleep state, and the number of desaturations >4% have been used. Reporting the percentage of time spent below 90%, 80%, 70%, 60%, and 50% saturation are conveniently expressed by means of a cumulative oxygen saturation histogram plot.

Interpretation **NORMAL FINDINGS:** Most investigators agree that the standard definition of apnea is a cessation of airflow for more than 10 seconds. Less agreement is found for the definition of hypoapneas. Proposed definitions include reduction in airflow as measured by thermistors,[20,21] reduction in ventilation measured by a calibrated respiratory inductive plethysmograph,[22] or the combination of reduction in airflow and reduction of oxygen saturation >4%.[23] Such definitions are weakened by the relatively imprecise methods used to measure ventilation. An apnea index <5 apneas/hour of sleep is normal in young to middle-aged adults. An apnea index >5 apneas/hour of sleep is abnormal in this population and confirms the diagnosis of sleep apnea.[24] The older population has a considerably higher incidence of this disorder if an apnea index of 5 is used as the cutoff for normal and abnormal. Therefore, standards for the elderly population need to be established.[25] **CRITI-**

(Continued)

Cardiopulmonary Sleep Study *(Continued)*

CAL VALUES: Saturations measured by pulse oximetry <88% for prolonged periods may indicate the need for continuous and/or nocturnal oxygen therapy, nocturnal nasal continuous positive airway pressure (CPAP) or both. **LIMITATIONS:** Limitations of a cardiopulmonary sleep study are primarily associated with limitations of the methods used for measuring ventilation. Pneumotachography and a mask provide the most accurate method for measuring ventilation, but the use of this set-up is not tolerated well by most patients. Likewise, measurement of esophageal pressure is the best quantitative method for the assessment of respiratory efforts but this may also be poorly tolerated by many patients. Other methods for measuring ventilation (magnetometers, respiratory inductive plethysmography, etc) are at best semiquantitative. Measurements made by respiratory inductive plethysmography may be improved by the use of a body jerkin rather than separate thoracic and abdominal bands which have a tendency to move during sleep. Daytime nap studies may not adequately assess the severity of sleep apnea. If the results of a daytime study do not confirm a clinical suspicion of sleep apnea, an all night sleep study is indicated. A limited sleep study in which only cardiac and respiratory parameters are measured suffers the limitation of being unable to characterize the architecture of REM and non-REM sleep. **ADDITIONAL INFORMATION:** The Association of Sleep Disorders Centers and the American College of Chest Physicians[1] recommend that sleep study reports contain the following:

- variables measured and methods used to make measurements
- sleep staging – the percentage of each sleep stage and the relationship to age-matched normals; the total sleep time, sleep efficiency, and sleep latency should be noted
- type(s) of respiratory patterns, as well as the total number, number per hour of sleep time, and range and mean duration of patterns, and relationship to sleep stage; the patterns should be defined
- relationship of body position to disordered breathing, if pertinent
- oxygen saturation – the awake baseline level; arterial oxygenation should be described in quantitative terms, using either a continuous saturation versus time technique or discrete intervals
- cardiac rate and rhythm should be described and the relationship of any abnormalities to other cardiopulmonary events noted.
- technician's comments
- interpretation.

Footnotes

1. American Thoracic Society, "Indications and Standards for Cardiopulmonary Sleep Studies," *Am Rev Respir Dis*, 1989, 139(2):559-68.
2. Jasper HH, "The Ten Twenty Electrode System of the International Federation," *Electroencephalogr Clin Neurophysiol*, 1985, 10:371-5.
3. Coleman RM, "Periodic Movements in Sleep (Nocturnal Myoclonus) and Restless Legs Syndrome," *Sleeping and Waking Disorders: Indications and Techniques*, Guilleminault C, ed, Boston, MA: Butterworth's Publishers, 1982, 265-95.
4. Fisher JG, Garza G, Flickinger R, et al, "An Alternate Method of Recording Airflow During Sleep," *Sleep*, 1980, 21:461-3.
5. Krumpe PE and Cummiskey JM, "Use of Laryngeal Sound Recordings to Monitor Apnea," *Am Rev Respir Dis*, 1980, 122:797-801.
6. Cummiskey JM, Williams TC, Krumpe PE, et al, "The Detection and Quantification of Sleep Apnea by Tracheal Sound Recordings," *Am Rev Respir Dis*, 1982, 126:221-4.
7. Peirick J and Shepard JW Jr, "Automated Apnea Detection by Computer: Analysis of Tracheal Breath Sounds," *Med Biol Eng Comput*, 1983, 21:632-5.
8. Baker LE and Geddes LA, "The Measurement of Respiratory Volumes in Animals and Man With Use of Electrical Impedance," *Ann N Y Acad Sci*, 1970, 170:667-88.
9. Larsen VH, Christensen PH, Oxhojand, et al, "Impedance Pneumography for Long-Term Monitoring of Respiration During Sleep in Adult Males," *Clin Physiol*, 1984, 4:333-42.
10. Mead J, Peterson N, Grimby G, et al, "Pulmonary Ventilation Measured From Body Surface Movements," *Science*, 1967, 156:1383-4.
11. Sharp JT, Druz WS, Foster JR, et al, "Use of the Respiratory Magnetometer in Diagnosis and Classification of Sleep Apnea," *Chest*, 1980, 77:350-3.

12. Sackner MA, "Monitoring of Ventilation Without a Physical Connection to the Airway," *Diagnostic Techniques in Pulmonary Disease*, Sackner MA, ed, New York, NY: Marcel Dekker, 1980, 503-37.
13. Cohn MA, Roa ASV, Broudy M, et al, "The Respiratory Inductive Plethysmograph: A New Noninvasive Monitor of Respiration," *Bull Eur Physiopathol Respir*, 1982, 18:643-58.
14. Sampson MG, Walsleben JA, Gujavarty KS, et al, "Effect of Esophageal Balloon on Sleep Structure," *Sleep Res*, 1984, 13:211, (abstract).
15. West P, George CF, and Kryger MH, "Dynamic *in vivo* Response Characteristics of Three Oximeters: Hewlett-Packard 47201A, Biox III, and Nellcor N-100," *Sleep*, 1987, 10:263-71.
16. Naifeh KH and Severinghaus JW, "How Accurate Are Pulse Oximeters to Profound Brief Hypoxia?" *Sleep Res*, 1987, 161:569, (abstract).
17. Silvestri R, Guilleminault C, Coleman R, et al, "Nocturnal Sleep Versus Daytime Nap Findings in Patients With Breathing Abnormalities During Sleep," *Sleep Res*, 1982, 11:174, (abstract).
18. Rechtschaffen A and Kales A, *A Manual of Standardized Terminology, Techniques and Scoring Systems for Sleep Stages of Human Subjects*, No 204, Washington, DC: National Institute of Health, 1968, 204.
19. Schmidt-Nowara WW, Sano J, and Appel D, "Stage T: A Scoring Modification for Breathing Disturbed Sleep," *Sleep Res*, 1983, 12:356, (abstract).
20. Bliwise D, Bliwise NC, Kramer HC, et al, "Measurement Error in Visually Scored Electrophysiological Data; Respiration During Sleep," *J Neurosci Methods*, 1984, 12:49-56.
21. Catterall JR, Calverley PM, Shapiro CM, et al, "Breathing and Oxygenation During Sleep Are Similar in Normal Men and Normal Women," *Am Rev Respir Dis*, 1985, 132:86-8.
22. Bradley TD, Brown IG, Zamel N, et al, "Differences in Pharyngeal Properties Between Snorers With Predominantly Central Sleep Apnea and Those Without Sleep Apnea," *Am Rev Respir Dis*, 1987, 135:387-91.
23. Block AJ, Boysen PG, Wynne JW, et al, "Sleep Apnea, Hypoapnea and Oxygen Desaturation in Normal Subjects: A Strong Male Predominance," *N Engl J Med*, 1979, 300:513-7.
24. Guilleminault C, van den Hoed J, and Mitler MM, "Clinical Overview of the Sleep Apnea Syndromes," *Sleep Apnea Syndromes*, Guilleminault C and Dement WC, eds, New York, NY: Alan R Liss, 1978, 1-12.
25. Berry DTR, Webb WB, and Block AJ, "Sleep Apnea Syndrome: A Critical Review of the Apnea Index as a Diagnostic Criterion," *Chest*, 1984, 86:529-31.

Cardiopulmonary Stress Test *see* Cardiopulmonary Exercise Testing *on page 221*

Chord Compliance *see* Pulmonary Compliance (Dynamic) *on page 239*

Closing Capacity *see* Single Breath Nitrogen Elimination *on page 244*

Closing Volume *see* Single Breath Nitrogen Elimination *on page 244*

CO_2 Response Test *see* Carbon Dioxide Challenge Test *on page 217*

Conductance *see* Airway Resistance *on page 202*

Co-oximetry *see* Arterial Blood Oximetry *on page 210*

CPAP Titration *see* Pulse Oximetry *on page 241*

Density Dependent Spirometry *see* Volume of Isoflow (V iso $\mathring{V}$) *on page 254*

Desaturation Oximetry *see* Pulse Oximetry *on page 241*

Disability Assessment *see* Cardiopulmonary Exercise Testing *on page 221*

Disability Examination *see* Cardiopulmonary Exercise Testing *on page 221*

DLCO *see* Carbon Monoxide Diffusing Capacity, Single Breath *on page 219*

Ear Oximetry *see* Pulse Oximetry *on page 241*

Exercise ABG *replaced by* Pulse Oximetry *on page 241*

Exercise Blood Gases *see* Cardiopulmonary Exercise Testing *on page 221*

Exercise Oximetry *see* Cardiopulmonary Exercise Testing *on page 221*

Expiratory Reserve Volume *see* Lung Subdivisions *on page 235*

Finger Oximetry *see* Pulse Oximetry *on page 241*

Flow Volume Curves *see* Flow Volume Loop *on this page*

Flow Volume Loop

CPT 94375

Related Information

Bedside Spirometry *on page 212*
Bronchial Challenge Test *on page 215*
Spirometry *on page 245*
Spirometry Before and After Bronchodilators *on page 248*
Spirometry, Sitting and Supine *on page 250*

Synonyms Flow Volume Curves; Spirometry With Flow Volume Loop

Applies to Assessment of Pulmonary Disability; Preoperative Evaluation

Abstract **PROCEDURE COMMONLY INCLUDES:** Forced expiratory vital capacity (FVC), forced inspiratory vital capacity (FIVC), expiratory flow rates at specific percentage of expired vital capacity (eg, $FEF_{25\%}$, $FEF_{50\%}$, $FEF_{75\%}$), inspiratory flow rates at specific percentage of FVC vital ($FIF_{25\%}$, $FIF_{50\%}$, $FIF_{75\%}$), peak flow rates during expiration and inspiration (PEFR, PIFR). Ratio of expiratory and inspiratory flow rates at 50% of vital capacity ($FEF_{50\%}/FIF_{50\%}$) expressed as a percent, and a graphic presentation of the maneuver showing expiratory and inspiratory flow plotted against volume. **INDICATIONS:** To detect upper airway obstructions.

Patient Care/Scheduling **PATIENT PREPARATION:** Patient should avoid heavy meals 3 hours prior to testing. Patient should be conscious and able to follow simple instructions. Patient's height and weight should be measured without shoes. Loose comfortable clothing that does not restrict chest expansion should be worn. Smoking history including last cigarette smoked should be obtained. Current medications should be obtained with particular emphasis on bronchodilators and steroids. **AFTERCARE:** Usually none, although patients that complain of lightheadedness and dizziness should not be allowed to walk unobserved until recovery.

Method **EQUIPMENT:** Exhaled and inhaled air is collected or passed through a volume or flow measuring device known as a spirometer. Spirometers should meet certain minimum standards defined by the American Thoracic Society (ATS) **TECHNIQUE:** BA spirometer is used to measure inspiratory and expiratory volumes and flows and record the time of sample collection during a maximal forced exhalation from total lung capacity (TLC) to residual volume (RV) followed by a maximal forced inhalation from RV to TLC. Flow is plotted against volume and instantaneous flows are measured at 25%, 50%, and 75% of exhaled forced vital capacity on both the inspiratory and expiratory limbs. Peak inspiratory and expiratory flows are measured. Reproducibility of the expiratory limb is accomplished using the same criteria as spirometry. Reproducibility of the inspiratory limb is best accomplished by superimposing or visually comparing repeated efforts. (See following figures.) Test may be performed on adults in a seated or standing position. Children must be tested while seated. After applying a noseclip, the patient is instructed to take a full inspiration (TLC), hold it briefly, then exhale through a mouthpiece into a spirometer as forcefully and completely as possible. When exhalation has been judged to be complete (patient reaches obvious plateau at RV), the patient is coached to inhale as forcefully and completely as possible until reaching TLC. Allowing the patient to recover between efforts, the test is repeated a minimum of three times until two reproducible efforts have been recorded. When possible, superimposition of repeated flow volume loops can aid in assessment of reproducibility of data.

Specimen **CAUSES FOR REJECTION:** The flow volume loop test consists of a forced expiratory maneuver followed by a forced inspiratory maneuver. In addition to the same causes for rejection for spirometry (see Causes for Rejection under Spirometry) poorly performed forced inspiration can limit the usefulness of graphic or numeric data obtained. Many patients perform a low flow stridorous inspiration while attempting to inhale forcefully after a forced exhalation. Have the patient keep an upright posture with an elevated chin to maximize tracheal diameter. **TURNAROUND TIME:** Preliminary results should be available same day. Depending on the facility, an interpreted report may be available in 1-2 days.

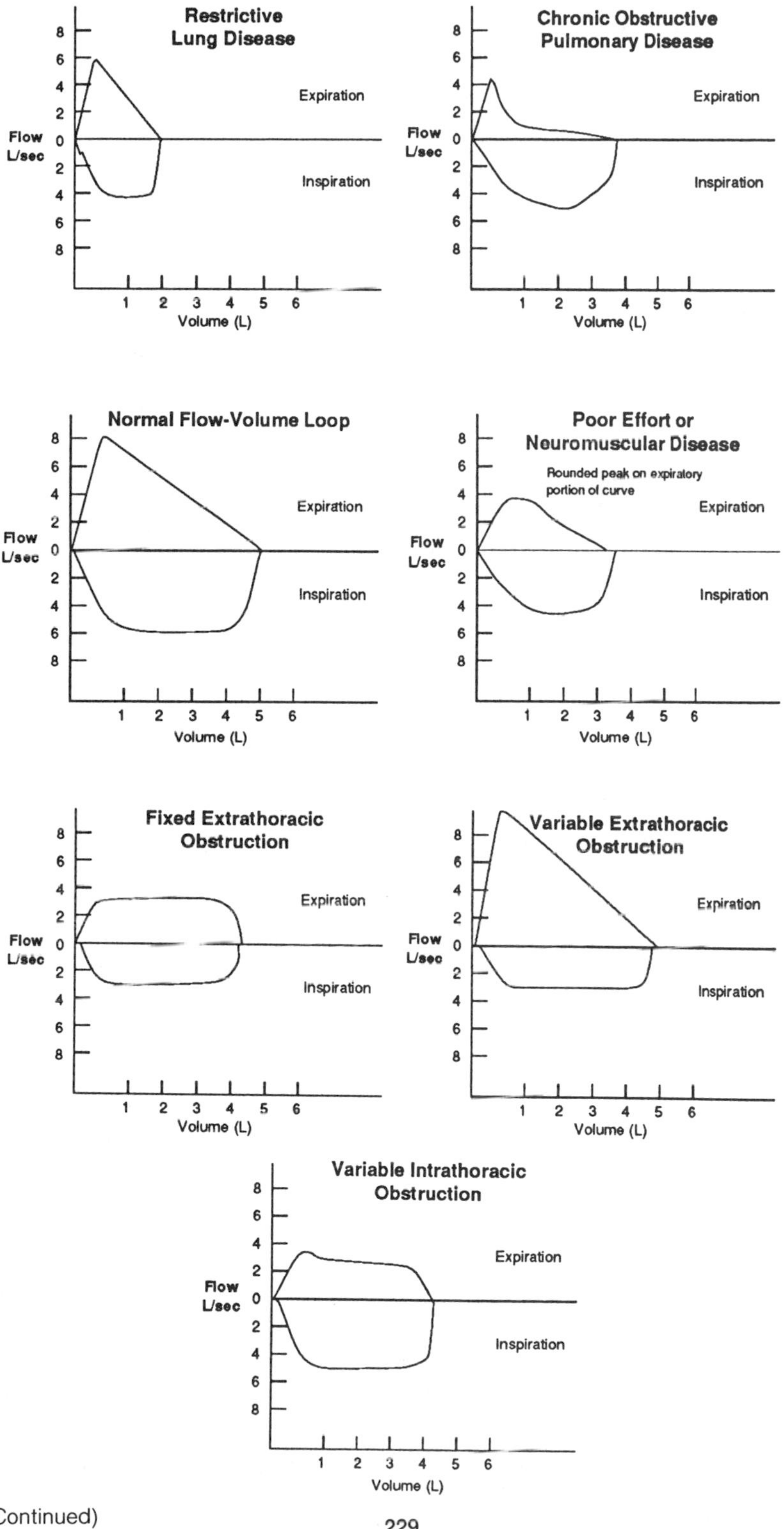
Restrictive
Lung Disease
Expiration
Inspiration
Flow
L/sec
Volume (L)
Chronic Obstructive
Pulmonary Disease
Expiration
Inspiration
Flow
L/sec
Volume (L)
Normal Flow-Volume Loop
Expiration
Inspiration
Flow
L/sec
Volume (L)
Poor Effort or
Neuromuscular Disease
Rounded peak on expiratory
portion of curve
Expiration
Inspiration
Flow
L/sec
Volume (L)
Fixed Extrathoracic
Obstruction
Expiration
Inspiration
Flow
L/sec
Volume (L)
Variable Extrathoracic
Obstruction
Expiration
Inspiration
Flow
L/sec
Volume (L)
Variable Intrathoracic
Obstruction
Expiration
Inspiration
Flow
L/sec
Volume (L)

(Continued)

Flow Volume Loop *(Continued)*

Interpretation **NORMAL FINDINGS:** Studies of normal instantaneous inspiratory and expiratory flow rates have been reported by several authors.[1,2,3,4,5] The graphic presentation of the flow volume loop allows for inspection of the shape of the curve and its comparison with a normal loop. Three general types of upper airway obstructions (UAO) which show characteristic configurations are: fixed, variable extrathoracic, variable intrathoracic. These are described as follows.

Fixed UAO refers to the fixed nature of the obstruction with respect to inspiratory and expiratory effort. The expiratory flow plateaus at a high lung volume and peak flow is severely diminished. Inspiratory and expiratory flows are diminished proportional to the degree of obstruction. The inspiratory and expiratory loops may resemble each other quite closely. Causes include goiters, endotracheal neoplasms, stenosis of both main bronchi, postintubation stenosis, and performance of the test through a tracheostomy tube or other fixed orifice device. Estimation of the diameter of a stenotic lesion may be made from ratio of midinspiratory and midexpiratory flows $FIF_{50\%}/FEF_{50\%}$.[6] See figure.

Variable extrathoracic lesions cause a reduction in flow rates seen during forced inspiration, the configuration of the expiratory limb of the flow volume loop remains normal (barring coexisting obstructive lung disease). Thus, the obstructive nature of the lesion varies with the phase of respiration. Inspiratory flows are decreased proportional to the degree of obstruction. Causes of variable extrathoracic UAO include unilateral and bilateral vocal cord paralysis, adhesions of the vocal cords, vocal cord constriction, laryngeal edema secondary to burns, and upper airway abnormalities associated with obstructive sleep apnea. See figure.

Variable intrathoracic lesions are characterized by an early plateau of expiratory flow followed by a normal inspiratory flow volume curve. Rarely a small peak is seen preceding the expiratory flow plateau, mimicking the picture seen in severe chronic lower airways obstruction. The main cause of variable intrathoracic obstruction is localized noncircumferential tumors of the lower trachea or a mainstem bronchus. Variable intrathoracic obstruction patterns have also been described in polychondritis and tracheomalacia. See figure.

The following illustrations explain the physiology of variable upper airway obstructions. Figures 1a and 1b show a variable intrathoracic upper airway obstruction. During inspiration (1a) tracheal pressure is negative but greater than pleural pressure. This gradient favors an outward displacement of the tracheal wall. During expiration (1b), however, the driving pressure of expiration falls from pleural pressure at the alveolus along the entire pathway to the mouth. At some point along this path, airway or tracheal pressure falls to a value less than pleural pressure. This pressure gradient favors an inward displacement of airway walls, leading to airway narrowing or collapse. Figures 2a and 2b show a variable extrathoracic (above the manubrium of the sternum) upper airway obstruction. During inspiration (2a), tracheal pressures are less than atmospheric, favoring airway collapse. During expiration (2b), tracheal pressures exceed atmospheric pressures which favors an open airway.

LIMITATIONS: Requires patient cooperation. Poor effort on inspiration or partial glottis closure may mimic variable extrathoracic obstruction but can usually be distinguished by its lack of reproducibility. Upper airway cross sectional diameter must be reduced to 8 mm or less before the shape of the flow volume loop is affected, making the flow volume loop an unreliable method for **ruling out** clinically suspected UAO. **ADDITIONAL INFORMATION:** Patients with obstructive sleep apnea may show a characteristic sawtoothing of either the expiratory limb, the inspiratory limb, or both.

Footnotes

1. Bass H, "The Flow Volume Loop: Normal Standards and Abnormalities in Chronic Obstructive Pulmonary Disease," *Chest*, 1973, 63:171-6.
2. Cherniack RM and Raber MB, "Normal Standards for Ventilatory Function Using an Automated Wedge Spirometer," *Am Rev Respir Dis*, 1972, 106:38-46.
3. Knudson RJ, Slatin RC, Lebowitz MD, et al, "The Maximal Expiratory Flow-Volume Curve: Normal Standards, Variability and Effects of Age," *Am Rev Respir Dis*, 1976, 113:587-600.
4. Schoenberg JB, Beck GJ, and Bouhuys A, "Growth and Decay of Pulmonary Function in Healthy Blacks and Whites," *Respir Physiol*, 1978, 33:367-93.

5. Jordanoglory J and Pride NB, "A Comparison of Maximum Inspiratory an Expiratory Flow in Health and in Lung Disease," *Thorax*, 1968, 23:38-45.
6. Gamsu G, Borson DB, Webb WR, et al, "Structure and Function in Tracheal Stenosis," *Am Rev Respir Dis*, 1980, 121:530.

References

Gardner RM, Crapo RO, and Nelson SB, et al, "Spirometry and Flow-Volume Curves," *Clin Chest Med*, 1989, 10(2):145-54.

Gardner RM, Hankinson JL, Clausen JL, et al, "ATS Statement on Standardization of Spirometry – 1987 Update," *Am Rev Respir Dis*, 1987, 136:1285-98.

Ghio AJ, Crapo RO, and Elliott CG, "Reference Equations Used to Predict Pulmonary Function," *Chest*, 1990, 97(2):400-3.

Nelson MS, Gardner RM, Crapo RO, et al, "Performance Evaluation of Contemporary Spirometers," *Chest*, 1990, 97(2):288-97.

Pattishall EN, "Pulmonary Function Testing Reference Values and Interpretations in Pediatric Training Programs," *Pediatrics*, 1990, 85(5):768-73.

Vollmer WM, McCamant LE, Johnson LR, et al, "Long-Term Reproducibility of Tests of Small Airways Function. Comparisons With Spirometry," *Chest*, 1990, 98(2):303-7.

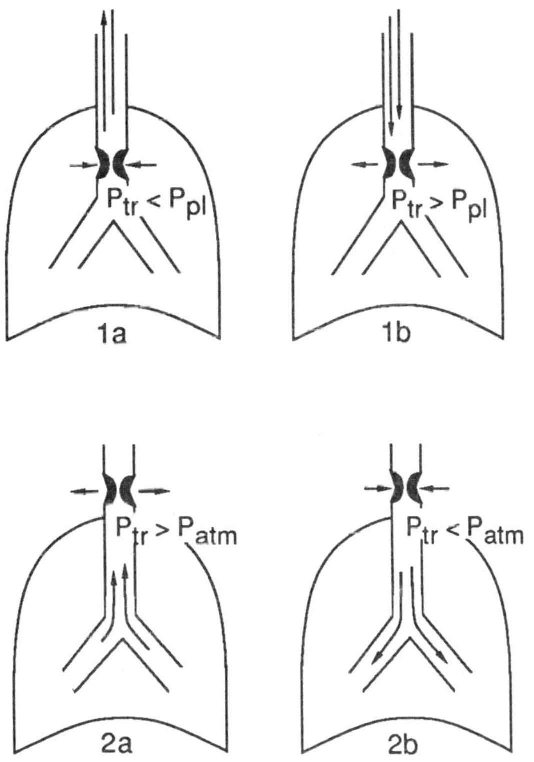

Forced Expirogram *see* Spirometry *on page 245*

FRC *see* Functional Residual Capacity *on next page*

Frequency Dependence of Compliance *see* Pulmonary Compliance (Static) *on page 240*

Functional Residual Capacity

CPT 94240 (functional residual capacity or residual volume: helium method, nitrogen open circuit method, or other method)

Related Information

Lung Subdivisions *on page 235*
Spirometry *on page 245*
Thoracic Gas Volume *on page 252*

Synonyms FRC; Helium Dilution; Nitrogen Washout; Static Lung Volumes

Applies to Residual Volume; Total Lung Capacity

Abstract **PROCEDURE COMMONLY INCLUDES:** Functional residual capacity (FRC), expiratory reserve volume (ERV), residual volume (RV), total lung capacity (TLC) are all reported in $liter_{BTPS}$, and residual volume to total lung capacity ratio (RV/TLC%). Report usually includes the actual measured values, the predicted values, and the percentage of the predicted value the actual value represents. **INDICATIONS:** Restrictive abnormalities seen on spirometry should be confirmed by measurement of lung volumes. Used to assess the severity of restrictive abnormalities and used to assess the degree of hyperinflation in obstructive abnormalities. **CONTRAINDICATIONS:** Patients known to have active pulmonary tuberculosis may be tested, but the common breathing circuit should be removed, cleaned, and gas or cold sterilized before testing other patients.

Patient Care/Scheduling **PATIENT PREPARATION:** See Spirometry test listing. Also, this test should not precede or follow a pulmonary function test that uses gas concentrations other than room air unless at least a 5-minute wait has been observed. **AFTERCARE:** Usually none needed. **SPECIAL INSTRUCTIONS:** Some patients may have a communicating channel to atmosphere secondary to a previously punctured tympanic membrane. To avoid a leak during testing and resultant artificially high values for FRC, cotton plegettes should be inserted in the ear to block the outer ear canal during testing.

Method **EQUIPMENT:** Test is usually performed on a full pulmonary function analyzer. This device should meet all standards set forth for spirometers by the American Thoracic Society (ATS). This device's gas analyzers as well as flow or volume system should be calibrated on the day of the test. Nitrogen needle valve should be properly peaked. **TECHNIQUE:** Patient is tested in the seated position at least 1 hour after eating a meal or smoking a cigarette. Patient should be allowed to breathe through the mouthpiece open to atmosphere with noseclip in place for several minutes to allow for relaxation and settling to a normal resting end-expiratory level. A minimum of 10 breaths should be allowed before the valve should be turned into the test gas at FRC. Test should continue until complete "washout" (end-expiratory N_2 <2% for nitrogen washout test) or complete "equilibration" (<0.05% change in helium concentration during 1 minute for the helium equilibration test).

Nitrogen washout test: Patient breathes through a one-way valve that is attached to but not yet connected to a reservoir filled with 100% O_2 or a demand valve connected to a pressurized O_2 source. At the end of a normal resting expiration the valve is opened, allowing the patient to breathe through the one-way valve. Expired nitrogen is measured at the mouth. Inspired or expired minute ventilations are measured continuously. Test continues until exhaled N_2 concentrations fall <2%, indicating a "washout" of communicating airways and alveoli. Total inhaled volume and final N_2 concentration can be used to calculate the FRC. Computerized systems calculate FRC with each breath and adjust calculated value after each subsequent breaths.

Helium dilution test: Patient breathes through a valve that is open to room air but connected to a reservoir (spirometer) containing 5% to 10% helium. At the end of a normal resting expiration (FRC) the valve is opened allowing the patient to breathe from the reservoir. Carbon dioxide is chemically scrubbed from the rebreathing circuit and oxygen is added to keep the end expiratory level constant. Test continues until concentration of helium in the system is constant (<0.02% change in helium concentration) for a minimum of 15 seconds. Initial and final helium concentrations, the volume of helium and air added to the system, and the system dead space can then be used to calculate the volume added to the system to achieve that dilution (FRC).

Both: Immediately after measurement of FRC measurement of lung subdivisions should be made. See Lung Subdivisions.

DATA ACQUIRED: Functional residual capacity (FRC) $liter_{BTPS}$, washout or equilibration time in minutes, average tidal volume (Vt) in mL, average respiratory rate (RR).

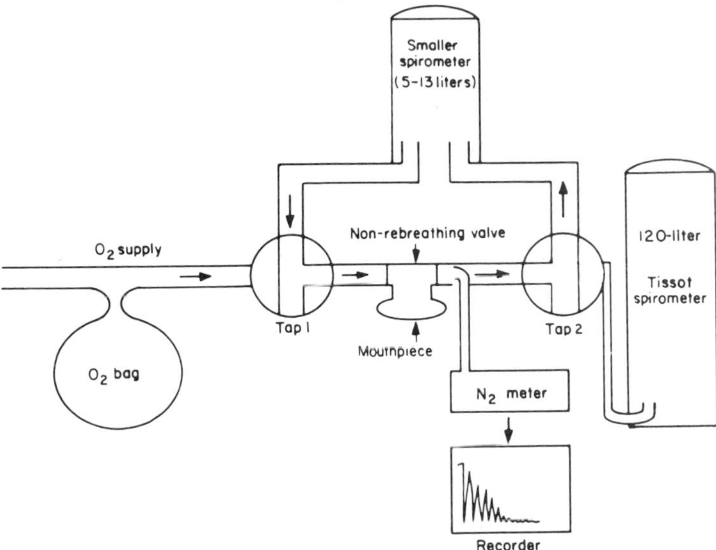

Apparatus for the measurement of FRC by nitrogen washout. Taps 1 and 2 are provided so that the subject may be switched between the small spirometer circuit and the N_2 washout circuit. When turned to the spirometer circuit, ERV and IC may be measured; also, observation of tidal breathing allows correct switching to the washout circuit at FRC. Reproduced with permission from Jalowayski AA and Dawson A, "Measurement of Lung Volume: The Multiple Breath Nitrogen Method," *Pulmonary Function Testing Guidelines and Controversies*, Clausen JL, ed, New York, NY: Academic Press, 1982, 117.

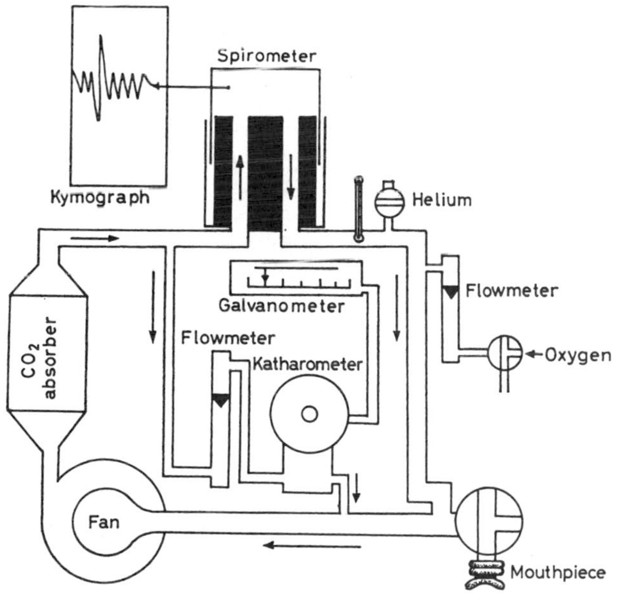

Apparatus for the measurement of FRC by helium dilution. The flowmeter, katharometer, and galvanometer together comprise the helium analyzer. The CO_2 absorber is usually combined with a dessicant as well. Reproduced with permission from Cotes JE, *Lung Function*, Oxford, England: Blackwell Scientific Publications, 1979, 112.

(Continued)

Functional Residual Capacity *(Continued)*

Specimen CAUSES FOR REJECTION: Variation on repeat studies of 500 mL or more, any obvious leaks during the procedure as evidenced (during a N_2 washout) by an increase in expired N_2 not related to a sigh, or (during a helium dilution) by a change in the end expiratory level and/or the amount of O_2 added to keep system volume constant. The total amount of O_2 added to the circuit during the helium dilution test should average the patient's resting O_2 consumption (3.5 mL/kg/minute ±1 mL). TURNAROUND TIME: Preliminary report is usually available on the same day, interpreted report is usually available the following day.

Interpretation NORMAL FINDINGS: Many equations for the prediction of normal lung volumes exist and the range of predictive values is considerable. No one equation can be recommended to apply to all labs and patient populations. Each laboratory should test at least 10 normal individuals and compare their results to the normal values predicted by the equations they wish to use. If more than one individual is shown to be abnormal, those prediction equations may be unsuitable for use in that laboratory and prediction equations more suitable to their population should be sought. Values may be presented as percentage of predicted value or compared with the 95% confidence intervals as has been recently advocated. Alveolar filling diseases, lung resection, and pleural disease result in a decrease in VC, FRC, TLC, and RV. Interstitial lung disease results in a decreased VC and TLC with slightly less reduction in FRC and RV. Inspiratory neuromuscular dysfunction results in a decreased VC and TLC and a normal FRC and RV. Expiratory neuromuscular dysfunction results in a normal FRC and TLC and a reduction in VC with a proportional increase in RV. Combined neuromuscular disease results in normal FRC with reduction of VC, RV, and TLC. Kyphoscoliosis results in reduction of FRC, VC, and TLC and slightly less reduction of the RV. Ankylosing spondylitis causes reduction in the VC and TLC and an increase in the RV and FRC (pseudohyperinflation). Chronic airway obstruction generally results in an increase in the RV, FRC, and TLC with an increased RV/TLC ratio. LIMITATIONS: FRC may be artificially high if the measurement is made at a higher lung volume secondary to pain or anxiety. Subject cooperation is necessary. Erroneous FRC can be made if patient has not established a stable end-expiratory level or if patient is switched into system at a point other than end-expiration.

References

Ghio AJ, Crapo RO, and Elliott CG, "Reference Equations Used to Predict Pulmonary Function," *Chest*, 1990, 97(2):400-3.

Hathaway EH, Tashkin DP, and Simmons MS, "Intraindividual Variability in Serial Measurements of DLCO and Alveolar Volume Over One Year in Eight Healthy Subjects Using Three Independent Measuring Systems," *Am Rev Respir Dis*, 1989, 140(6):1818-22.

Kanengiser LC, Rapoport DM, Epstein H, et al, "Volume Adjustment of Mechanics and Diffusion in Interstitial Lung Disease: Lack of Clinical Relevance," *Chest*, 1989, 96(5):1036-42.

Heliox Spirometry *see* Volume of Isoflow (V iso V̊) *on page 254*

Helium Dilution *see* Functional Residual Capacity *on page 232*

Hemoximetry *see* Arterial Blood Oximetry *on page 210*

Histamine Challenge Test *see* Bronchial Challenge Test *on page 215*

Hypercapnic Challenge Test *see* Carbon Dioxide Challenge Test *on page 217*

Incremental Exercise Testing *see* Cardiopulmonary Exercise Testing *on page 221*

Inspiratory Capacity *see* Lung Subdivisions *on next page*

Inspiratory Reserve Volume *see* Lung Subdivisions *on next page*

Low Density Gas Spirometry *see* Volume of Isoflow (V iso V̊) *on page 254*

Lung Compartments *see* Lung Subdivisions *on next page*

Lung Subdivisions

CPT 94240 (unlisted pulmonary procedure, usually done as part of functional residual capacity)

Related Information

Functional Residual Capacity *on page 232*

Spirometry *on page 245*

Synonyms Expiratory Reserve Volume; Inspiratory Capacity; Inspiratory Reserve Volume; Lung Compartments; Static Lung Volumes

Abstract **PROCEDURE COMMONLY INCLUDES:** Expiratory reserve volume (ERV), inspiratory capacity (IC), vital capacity (VC), or slow vital capacity (SVC) **INDICATIONS:** Assessment of severity of disease, diagnostic aid for classification of lung disease into restrictive, obstructive, and mixed disorders. Used with FRC measurement to calculate residual volume (RV), total lung capacity (TLC), and RV/TLC %. The effort which shows the largest vital capacity measurement following a **stable** end-expiratory level should be used for calculating expiratory reserve volume (ERV) and inspiratory capacity (IC). This ERV should be subtracted from the functional residual capacity (FRC) (see Functional Residual Capacity) to obtain a calculated residual volume (RV). The calculated RV is then added to the vital capacity (VC) to obtain a calculated total lung capacity (TLC). The RV is then divided by the TLC to obtain a calculated RV to TLC ratio. **CONTRAINDICATIONS:** Patients who are unable to sit upright, maintain an airtight seal, or perform vital capacity maneuvers.

Patient Care/Scheduling **PATIENT PREPARATION:** Patient should avoid heavy meals 3 hours prior to testing. Patient should be conscious and able to follow simple instructions. Patient's height and weight should be measured without shoes. Loose comfortable clothing that does not restrict chest expansion should be worn. Smoking history including last cigarette smoked should be obtained. Current medications should be obtained with particular emphasis on bronchodilators and steroids. **AFTERCARE:** Usually none.

Method **EQUIPMENT:** Exhaled sample is collected or passed through a volume or flow measuring device known as a spirometer. Spirometers should meet certain minimum standards defined by the American Thoracic Society. Other equipment needed varies with the type of spirometer being used but should include a disposable mouthpiece and noseclips. Special circumstances may require adaptation of the mouthpiece to a mask, face seal, or tracheostomy adapters. **TECHNIQUE:** Patient should be sitting erect, legs uncrossed, chin slightly elevated. Proper seal should be made with lips on mouthpiece. Noseclips should be applied. Patient should be instructed to relax and breathe in a normal relaxed fashion.

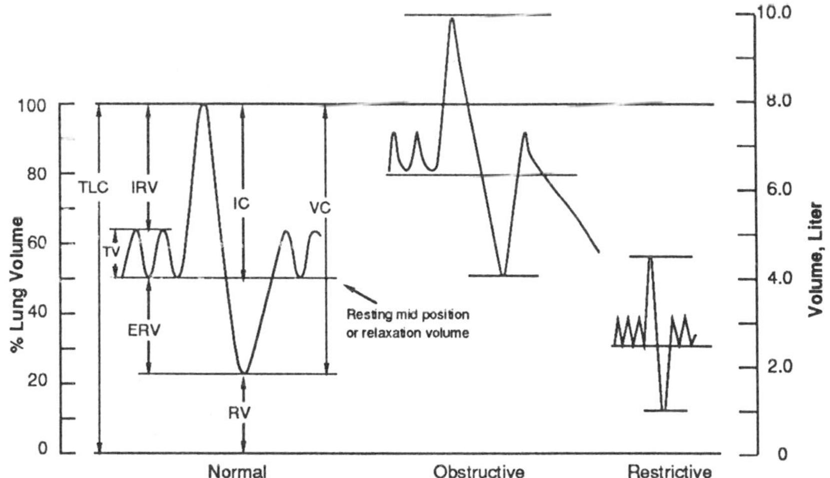

Schematic representation of the subdivisions of the lung in health and disease. Each of the basic subdivisions is termed a volume, and combinations of volumes are termed a capacity. FRC, not designated in the figure, is the sum of RV and ERV. Reproduced with permission from Miller WF, *Laboratory Evaluation of Pulmonary Function*, Philadelphia, PA: J.B. Lippincott Co, 1987, 106.

(Continued)

Lung Subdivisions *(Continued)*

An end-expiratory level that remains stable for approximately 10 seconds should be obtained before instructing the patient to inhale as deeply as possible and then exhale slowly and completely for as long as possible or until no volume increment is observed for at least 2 seconds. At this point, the patient should be instructed to return to normal breathing. This procedure is repeated at least in triplicate after visualizing a return to a stable end-expiratory level. Volume displacement spirometers should have a CO_2 absorbent canister, circulating fan, and supplemental O_2 source if repeat measurements without flushing the reservoir with room air are desired.

Specimen Inspired and expired volumes versus time are recorded during tidal breathing followed by a vital capacity maneuver. **CAUSES FOR REJECTION:** Insufficient tidal breathing sample to determine an average resting end-expiratory level, excessive variation from resting end-expiratory level (variable FRC), poor patient effort, nonreproducibility of SVC and ERV **TURNAROUND TIME:** Preliminary report is available on the day of the test, interpreted report is given in 1-2 days.

Interpretation **NORMAL FINDINGS:** Numerous reference equations are available and show considerable variability. The following table shows an arbitrary assignment of severity of lung disease based on percentage of predicted value for FRC, TLC, and RV. Values below predicted are suggestive of restrictive lung disease, values above predicted are suggestive of hyperinflation. Conditions associated with increased lung volumes include obstructive lung diseases (asthma, emphysema, chronic bronchitis, bullous lung disease), acromegaly, ankylosing spondylitis. Isolated elevated RV is associated with expiratory muscle weakness and is seen in amyotrophic lateral sclerosis and C_5 spinal cord injuries. Conditions associated with decreased lung volumes include, among others, interstitial fibrosis, pleural fibrosis, lung resection, alveolar filling processes, congestive heart failure, thoracoplasty, ALS, and myasthenia gravis. A reduced ERV is commonly seen in obesity. **LIMITA-**

Degrees of Severity of Lung Disease
Based on % of Predicted Lung Volume

Volume/Capacity	Mild (%)	Moderate (%)	Severe (%)
TLC	70–80 120–130	60–70 130–150	<60 >150
FRC	55-65 135–150	45-55 150-200	<45 >200
RV	55–65 135–150	45-55 150-250	<45 >250

Ries AL and Clausen JL, "Lung Volumes," *Pulmonary Function Testing, Indications and Interpretations,* New York, NY: Grune & Stratton, Inc, 1985, 69–85.

TIONS: The total picture of lung compartments can be obscured if the patient is breathing at a higher than normal end-expiratory level (secondary to incisional pain, chest wall pain, or anxiety) or breathing at a lower than normal end-expiratory level (active expiration secondary to anxiety during the measurement of FRC or ERV or both.) Full expiration must be made during the measurement of ERV or the RV will be artificially elevated. Vital capacity and expiratory reserve volume measurements should be duplicated to within 5% reproducibility.

References

Damia G, Mascheroni D, Croci M, et al, "Perioperative Changes in Functional Residual Capacity in Morbidly Obese Patients," *Br J Anaesth*, 1988, 60(5):574-8.

Thorsteinsson A, Jonmarker C, Larsson A, et al, "Functional Residual Capacity in Anesthetized Children: Normal Values and Values in Children With Cardiac Anomalies," *Anesthesiology*, 1990, 73(5):876-81.

Maximum Breathing Capacity (MBC) *see* Maximum Voluntary Ventilation (MVV) *on next page*

Maximum Expiratory Flow Rate *see* Peak Flow *on page 238*

Maximum Voluntary Ventilation (MVV)

CPT 94200

Related Information

Cardiopulmonary Exercise Testing *on page 221*
Spirometry *on page 245*

Synonyms Maximum Breathing Capacity (MBC)

Abstract **PROCEDURE COMMONLY INCLUDES:** Maximum voluntary ventilation (MVV) reported in $liter_{BTPS}$/minute, the mean respiratory rate used during the test and the total test time in seconds. **INDICATIONS:** As a nonspecific assessment of integrative function of the airways, lung parenchyma, thoracic cage, diaphragm and respiratory neuromuscular apparatus; preoperative pulmonary evaluation; prediction of maximum ventilatory reserve for exercise testing; respiratory disability evaluation **CONTRAINDICATIONS:** Patients that are unable to follow instructions or put forth a sustained maximal voluntary respiratory effort.

Patient Care/Scheduling **PATIENT PREPARATION:** Patient should avoid heavy meals 3 hours prior to testing. Patient should be conscious and able to follow simple instructions. Patient's height and weight should be measured without shoes. Loose comfortable clothing that does not restrict chest expansion should be worn. Smoking history including last cigarette smoked should be obtained. Current medications should be obtained with particular emphasis on bronchodilators and steroids. **AFTERCARE:** When done correctly, the MVV test produces an acute transient hypocapnia and resultant alkalemia. Patients often complain of dizziness and lightheadedness. Adequate rest, up to 5 minutes, should follow each effort. **COMPLICATIONS:** Lightheadedness or dizziness secondary to acute hyperventilation is common. Patients may also complain of numbness and/or tingling of the lips and fingers. Adequate rest (up to 5 minutes) between each effort will minimize this.

Method **EQUIPMENT:** Sample may be measured on any properly calibrated spirometer that meets the standards recommended by the American Thoracic Society. **TECHNIQUE:** Measurement of exhaled volumes (or inhaled and exhaled volumes) is made over a 10-15 second time increment and a count of the number of respirations during this time period is made. Patients are coached to breathe in and out with maximum respiratory effort with the goal of moving as much air in and out of their lungs during the 10- to 15-second collection time. Respiratory rates of 90-120 breaths/minute generally result in optimal performance. At least three measurements should be made until the two largest calculated MVVs are within 5% of each other. Generally a real time tracing of inspiratory and expiratory volume or accumulated expiratory volume alone is plotted against time.

Maximum Voluntary Ventilators (MVV)

Severity of Impairment	% of Predicted
Mild	65–80
Moderate	50–64
Severe	35–49
Very severe	<35

Specimen **CAUSES FOR REJECTION:** Nonreproducibility of best two efforts (>5% variability). Respiratory rates <90 or >120 breaths/minute may result in less than optimal performance. **TURNAROUND TIME:** Preliminary results are usually available on the day of testing, interpreted results usually follow in 1-2 days.

Interpretation **NORMAL FINDINGS:** Several authors present reference equations for the prediction of a normal MVV. The MVV expressed as a percentage of predicted value may be used along with the standard spirometric measurements VC, FVC, and FEV_1 to grade functional impairment according to the table. **LIMITATIONS:** The MVV is an extremely effort dependent test. Low values may merely reflect a lack of understanding or effort. Low values do not identify which component of the respiratory apparatus has a deficit. Many laboratories have abandoned the routine use of this test because of this limitation. Some find value in using the MVV to predict potential maximum ventilation during an incremental exercise test. Ventilatory reserve is calculated by subtracting the maximum minute ventilation measured during exercise from the MVV. **ADDITIONAL INFORMATION:** In the absence of upper airway obstruction, the MVV may be predicted by multiplying the FEV_1 by 35 or 40 (the so-called "indirect MVV.").

Mecholyl Challenge *see* Bronchial Challenge Test *on page 215*

Mecholyl Provocation Test *see* Bronchial Challenge Test *on page 215*
Methacholine Challenge *see* Bronchial Challenge Test *on page 215*
Methacholine Provocation Test *see* Bronchial Challenge Test *on page 215*
Nitrogen Washout *see* Functional Residual Capacity *on page 232*
Oxygen Titration Test *see* Pulse Oximetry *on page 241*
$P(A\text{-}a)O_2$ *see* Alveolar to Arterial Oxygen Gradient *on page 204*
Peak Expiratory Flow *see* Peak Flow *on this page*

Peak Flow

CPT 94799 (unlisted pulmonary procedure)

Related Information

Spirometry *on page 245*

Synonyms Maximum Expiratory Flow Rate; Peak Expiratory Flow

Abstract **PROCEDURE COMMONLY INCLUDES:** Peak expiratory flow rate is reported in either $liter_{BTPS}$/second or $liters_{BTPS}$/minute. **INDICATIONS:** The peak flow measurement is widely used epidemiologically and clinically to follow diurnal variations in airway tone. Peak flow diaries which plot measured peak flow against time of day have been used to investigate occupational asthma and to detect the onset of exacerbations of asthma before clinical symptoms appear. The extreme effort of dependence of this measurement diminish its usefulness in these situations. The peak expiratory flow rate has been shown to be one of the most sensitive spirometric indices to decreasing tracheal diameter.

Patient Care/Scheduling **PATIENT PREPARATION:** Patient should avoid heavy meals 3 hours prior to testing. Patient should be conscious and able to follow simple instructions. Patient's height and weight should be measured without shoes. Loose comfortable clothing that does not restrict chest expansion should be worn. Smoking history including last cigarette smoked should be obtained. Current medications history should be obtained with particular emphasis on bronchodilators and steroids. **AFTERCARE:** Usually none **SPECIAL INSTRUCTIONS:** Because of the portability and ease of use of the peak flow meter, peak expiratory flow is being used in epidemiology studies and the study of occupational asthma. Because of the effort dependence of this test, interpretation of unsupervised peak flow measurements recorded in a "patient diary" must be looked at with some degree of suspicion.

Method **TECHNIQUE:** The patient is asked to inhale to total lung capacity (TLC) and then the mouthpiece of the flow meter or spirometer is inserted in his mouth. Some devices allow mouthpiece to be in place before maximum inhalation. Mouthpiece should be inserted between the teeth or dentures and an airtight seal should be achieved with the lips. A strong, sharp burst of exhalation using maximum available force should be exhaled. Full exhalation is not necessary or desired unless other spirometric indices are being measured. The test is very effort dependent and active coaching is necessary. Peak flow measurements should be repeated until 10% reproducibility is achieved. Careful attention should be placed on orientation of peak meter during measurement. Most peak flow meters should be held horizontally level to measure accurately.

Specimen The maximum flow rate during a forced expiration is measured by a spirometer or handheld peak flow meter (Wright peak flow meter). **CAUSES FOR REJECTION:** Submaximal effort, submaximal inhalation before exhalation, lack of seal around mouthpiece, improper mouthpiece placement. **TURNAROUND TIME:** Same day.

Interpretation **NORMAL FINDINGS:** Numerous prediction equations are available. **LIMITATIONS:** The sensitivity of the peak flow is somewhat tempered by its extreme dependence on effort and lung volume. Malingering should always be considered when peak flow diaries are being used to document occupational asthma. Peak flow studies should be used as an adjunct to, not a replacement for, laboratory spirometry evaluations of airway function.

References

Janson-Bjerklie S and Shnell S, "Effect of Peak Flow Information on Patterns of Self-Care in Adult Asthma," *Heart Lung*, 1988, 17(5):543-9.

Jones KP and Mullee MA, "Measuring Peak Expiratory Flow in General Practice: Comparison of Mini Wright Peak Flow Meter and Turbine Spirometer," *BMJ*, 1990, 300(6740):1629-31.

Klaustermeyer WB, Kurohara M, and Guerra GA, "Predictive Value of Monitoring Expiratory Peak Flow Rates in Hospitalized Adult Asthma Patients," *Ann Allergy*, 1990, 64(3):281-4.

Polysomnography (PSG) *see* Cardiopulmonary Sleep Study *on page 224*

Portable Spirometry *see* Bedside Spirometry *on page 212*

Postbronchodilator Spirometry *see* Spirometry Before and After Bronchodilators *on page 248*

Preoperative Evaluation *see* Flow Volume Loop *on page 228*

Preoperative Evaluation *see* Spirometry *on page 245*

Provocholine® Challenge *see* Bronchial Challenge Test *on page 215*

Pulmonary Compliance (Dynamic)

CPT 94750

Related Information

Pulmonary Compliance (Static) *on next page*

Applies to Chord Compliance

Abstract **PROCEDURE COMMONLY INCLUDES:** Pulmonary compliance reported in units of $liter_{BTPS}$/cm H_2O, maximum static elastic recoil pressure reported in units of cm H_2O, dynamic compliance at 60 breaths/minute reported as a percentage of the static compliance measurement ($Cdyn_{60}$). **INDICATIONS:** To assess small airways dysfunction **CONTRAINDICATIONS:** Patients that are unable to follow instructions and relax, patients in whom placement of an esophageal balloon is contraindicated.

Patient Care/Scheduling **PATIENT PREPARATION:** Patient should not take anything by mouth for 2-3 hours prior to testing. Nasal passage should be treated with a topical Xylocaine®/epinephrine solution to widen nasal passage and minimize discomfort. Patient should take small sips of ice water (if not contraindicated) before and during passage of a nasogastric balloon. **AFTERCARE:** Usually none, occasionally patient will experience vagal stimulation during passage of the nasogastric balloon. Placement in a feet up supine position may aid in the treatment of hypotension, dizziness and nausea. **SPECIAL INSTRUCTIONS:** Balloon should be coated with a topical anesthetic treated lubricant to aid in minimizing the gag reflex. Balloon should contain a small amount (usually 0.5 mL) of air. If excessive amounts of air are used esophageal pressures will be overstated resulting in an erroneously low pulmonary compliance.

Method **TECHNIQUE:** With the patient in a seated position, an uninflated, 10 cm x 1 cm, thin walled, latex balloon-catheter set-up attached to a pressure transducer is inserted transnasally after topical anesthesia and positioned in the lower one-third of the esophagus. Sips of water will aid in the passage of the balloon. The patient is instructed to perform a Valsalva maneuver with the end of the balloon catheter open to a loose fitting glass syringe. The balloon is then inflated with approximately 0.2-0.5 mL air. Several volume histories are obtained (inhalation to TLC) prior to making any measurement. Measurement of maximal static recoil pressure may be made while holding breath at TLC for several seconds. Peak pressure should be ignored and stable pressure recorded. After several static recoil measurements are made, relaxed shutter interrupted exhalations from TLC to FRC (or RV if the entire pressure volume curve is desired) are made while plotting transpulmonary pressure (pleural pressure minus mouth pressure) against exhaled volume. Compliance measurements (so-called "chord compliance") are made along the exhalation pressure volume curve from points corresponding to FRC and FRC plus 0.5 $liter/_{BTPS}$. Patients are then asked to increase their breathing rate 10 breaths/minute to a maximum rate of 100 breaths/minute. Measurement of transpulmonary pressure and volume are plotted on an X-Y plotter. Dynamic compliance is measured by dividing volume change by pressure change at points of zero flow. Dynamic compliance is typically reported as a percentage of the static compliance or $Cdyn_{60}$ = dynamic compliance measured during 60 breaths/minute panting/static compliance x 100.

Specimen Transpulmonary pressures (mouth pressure minus esophageal (**pleural**) pressures) are plotted against volumes obtained from an interrupted, passive, expiratory volume history from TLC to RV. Compliance measurements are made along the recorded

(Continued)

Pulmonary Compliance (Dynamic) *(Continued)*

pressure lines at points corresponding to FRC and FRC + 1 $liter_{BTPS}$. **COLLECTION:** Measurement is made by recording mouth pressure and pressures recorded from an esophageal balloon inserted transnasally into the lower one-third of the thorax of an upright seated patient. Volume should be measured from a device that meets standards recommended by the American Thoracic Society (ATS). **CAUSES FOR REJECTION:** Wide variations in baseline level of FRC. Active expiratory efforts made against the shutter during interrupted passive exhalation. **TURNAROUND TIME:** Preliminary report usually available same day, interpreted reports available in 1-2 days.

Interpretation **NORMAL FINDINGS:** Normal value for pulmonary compliance can be derived from the following equation:

C_{st} in $liter_{BTPS}$ = (0.00343 x height in cm) – 0.425

LIMITATIONS: Technically difficult secondary to correct placement of the balloon and the need for the patient to relax against an obstruction while maintaining an open glottis. Patients often find transnasal passage of the esophageal balloon unpleasant.

References

Vollmer WM, McCamant LE, Johnson LR, et al, "Long-Term Reproducibility of Tests of Small Airways Function. Comparisons With Spirometry," *Chest*, 1990, 98(2):303-7.

Pulmonary Compliance (Static)

CPT 94750

Related Information

Pulmonary Compliance (Dynamic) *on previous page*

Applies to Frequency Dependence of Compliance

Abstract **PROCEDURE COMMONLY INCLUDES:** Pulmonary compliance reported in units of $liter_{BTPS}$/cm H_2O **INDICATIONS:** Characterize the pressure-volume curve of the lung to aid in the diagnosis of emphysema, pulmonary vascular congestion, interstitial lung disease, and pulmonary fibrosis **CONTRAINDICATIONS:** Patients that are unable to follow instructions and relax, patients in whom placement of an esophageal balloon is contraindicated.

Patient Care/Scheduling **PATIENT PREPARATION:** Patient should not take anything by mouth for 2-3 hours prior to testing. Patient should take small sips of ice water (if not contraindicated) before and during passage of a nasogastric balloon. **AFTERCARE:** Usually none, occasionally patient will experience vagal stimulation during passage of the nasogastric balloon. Placement in a feet up supine position may aid in the treatment of hypotension, dizziness, and nausea. **SPECIAL INSTRUCTIONS:** Balloon should be coated with a topical anesthetic treated lubricant to aid in minimizing the gag reflex. Balloon should contain a small amount (usually 0.5 mL) of air. If excessive amounts of air are used esophageal pressures will be overstated resulting in an erroneously low pulmonary compliance.

Method **TECHNIQUE:** With the patient in a seated position, an uninflated, 10 cm x 1 cm, thin walled, latex balloon-catheter set-up attached to a pressure transducer is inserted transnasally after topical anesthesia and positioned in the lower one-third of the esophagus. Sips of water will aid in the passage of the balloon. The patient is instructed to perform a Valsalva maneuver with the end of the balloon catheter open to a loose fitting glass syringe. The balloon is then inflated with approximately 0.2-0.5 mL air. Several volume histories are obtained (inhalation to TLC) prior to making any measurement. Measurement of maximal static recoil pressure may be made while holding breath at TLC for several seconds. Peak pressure should be ignored and stable pressure recorded. After several static recoil measurements are made, relaxed shutter interrupted exhalations from TLC to FRC (or RV if the entire pressure volume curve is desired) are made while plotting transpulmonary pressure (pleural pressure minus mouth pressure) against exhaled volume. Compliance measurements (so-called "chord compliance") are made along the exhalation pressure volume curve from points corresponding to FRC and FRC plus 0.5 $liter_{BTPS}$.

Specimen Transpulmonary pressures (mouth pressure minus esophageal (**pleural**) pressures) are plotted against volumes obtained from an interrupted, passive, expiratory volume history from TLC to RV. Compliance measurements are made along the recorded pressure lines at points corresponding to FRC and FRC + 1 $liter_{BTPS}$. **COLLECTION:** Measurement is made by recording mouth pressure and pressures recorded from an esophageal balloon inserted transnasally into the lower one-third of the thorax of an upright seated patient. Volume should be measured from a device that meets standards recommended by the American Thoracic Society (ATS). **CAUSES FOR REJECTION:** Wide variations in baseline level of FRC. Active expiratory efforts made against the shutter during interrupted passive exhalation. **TURNAROUND TIME:** Preliminary report usually available same day, interpreted reports available in 1-2 days.

Interpretation **NORMAL FINDINGS:** Normal value for pulmonary compliance can be derived from the following equation:

C_{st} in $liter_{BTPS}$ = (0.00343 x height in cm) – 0.425

LIMITATIONS: Technically difficult secondary to correct placement of the balloon and the need for the patient to relax against an obstruction while maintaining an open glottis. Patients often find transnasal passage of the esophageal balloon unpleasant.

Pulse Oximetry

CPT 94760 (noninvasive ear or pulse oximetry for oxygen saturation, single determination); 94761 (multiple determinations, eg, during exercise); 94762 (by continuous overnight monitoring, separate procedure)

Related Information

Arterial Blood Gases *on page 206*
Arterial Blood Oximetry *on page 210*
Arterial Cannulation *on page 60*
Cardiopulmonary Exercise Testing *on page 221*
Cardiopulmonary Sleep Study *on page 224*

Synonyms CPAP Titration; Desaturation Oximetry; Oxygen Titration Test

Applies to Ear Oximetry; Finger Oximetry

Replaces Exercise ABG

Abstract **PROCEDURE COMMONLY INCLUDES:** Report generally includes baseline heart rate and functional O_2 saturation, heart rate and lowest functional O_2 saturation during whatever event may be taking place: exercise, sleep or therapeutic intervention such as nasal CPAP or oxygen therapy. **INDICATIONS:** To determine an estimate of the level of arterial oxygenation at rest and in the presence of positive and negative intervention. These include exercise, sleep, and during procedures such as surgery, bronchoscopy, ventilator assist/support therapy, etc. **CONTRAINDICATIONS:** Not to be used in the presence of flammable anesthetics. Contraindications for exercise may be found in the section on cardiopulmonary exercise testing.

Patient Care/Scheduling **PATIENT PREPARATION:** Fingernail polish should be removed with acetone. Permanent or disposable sensors should be applied according to the manufacturer's instructions. When finger probes are used, the patient should be instructed not to grip treadmill rail or handlebars tightly to avoid reduction of circulation to the digits. Preparation depends on the type of test being performed. Exercise patients should wear loose comfortable clothing. Patients should refrain from smoking 24 hours prior to test to avoid functional versus fractional O_2 saturation discrepancy that occurs with elevated carboxyhemoglobin levels. If possible, an arterial blood gas should be drawn and pH, pCO_2, pO_2, Hb, oxyhemoglobin ($O_2Hb\%$), carboxyhemoglobin (COHb%) and methemoglobin (metHb%) should be measured. Draw the heparinized arterial blood sample while the pulse oximetry sensor is in place and is stable. (See Arterial Blood Oximetry and Arterial Blood Gases.) Correlation of oxyhemoglobin ($O_2Hb\%$) (measured by blood oximetry) and $SpO_2\%$ (measured by pulse oximetry) should be made. The discrepancy between the $O_2Hb\%$ – $SpO_2\%$ should be used to determine the endpoint of the maneuver inducing arterial desaturation. For example, if the pulse oximeter displays a SpO_2 reading of 93% and a simultaneously obtained arterial blood sample shows an $O_2Hb\%$ of 91%, 2% should be subtracted from subsequent SpO_2 measurements during exercise for a more valid estimate of arterial oxygen saturation. This adjustment should also be made to determine the therapeutic endpoint when titrating supplemental oxygen therapy at rest, during sleep, or exercise. **AFTERCARE:** After exercise, allow patient to walk slowly on level treadmill or pedal bicycle ergometer at zero load slowly to allow gradual cooldown period. Monitor ECG, blood pressure, and patient status frequently during the first 5 minutes after a maximum exercise test. **SPECIAL INSTRUCTIONS:** Poor collateral circulation may be compensated for by warming the hands with warm towels. Fluctuation $\pm 1\%$ is acceptable. Range of fluctuation should be noted.

(Continued)

Pulse Oximetry *(Continued)*

Method TECHNIQUE: Methodology may differ widely depending on the type of challenge or intervention planned. Basic methodology should include correlation with blood oximetry as outlined in Patient Preparation. External ECG should correlate within 5 beats/minute of the pulse oximeter's pulse display. Record baseline functional saturation, external ECG rate and pulse oximeter heart rate along with patient status, workload, and supplemental oxygen given at each stage of the test.

Specimen Spectrophotometric measurement is made by passing light at two specific wavelengths through a pulsing capillary bed (finger, toe, bridge of nose, and ear are the most common sites for sensor placement). Light collection on the other side of the site is proportional to the amount of oxyhemoglobin present in the arterial capillary bed relative to the amount of hemoglobin available for binding with oxygen (exclusive of the dyshemoglobins: carboxyhemoglobin and methemoglobin). CAUSES FOR REJECTION: Unstable readings secondary to any cause: external light, poor peripheral circulation, or skin pigmentation are common causes. TURNAROUND TIME: Preliminary report should be available same day, interpreted report should follow in 1-2 days.

Interpretation NORMAL FINDINGS: Normal adult oxyhemoglobin saturation is >95%. Drops in oxyhemoglobin are usually the result of cardiac, pulmonary, or combined cardiopulmonary disease. Significant declines (>5%) during exercise or sleep are abnormal. LIMITATIONS: Test does not measure or take into consideration total hemoglobin or the dyshemoglobins, carboxyhemoglobin, and methemoglobin. May overestimate total oxygen delivery (oxygen content) if not correlated with blood oximetry. Not accurate in the presence of poor peripheral circulation. Accuracy at most units is ±2%, standard deviation is usually 1%. ADDITIONAL INFORMATION: Guidelines for reimbursement of home oxygen therapy state that a resting arterial pO_2 <55 torr or a resting oxygen saturation (SpO_2%) <88% with evidence of improvement with oxygen therapy qualify a patient for continuous oxygen therapy reimbursement. Guidelines for reimbursement for nocturnal and exercise oxygen therapy state that O_2 saturations during exercise or sleep that fall to <88% that improve with oxygen therapy will be reimbursed. Because of the limitations of pulse oximetry, decisions regarding discontinuing oxygen therapy should **not** be made on the basis of pulse oximetry alone. Assessment of the PaO_2 by arterial blood gas and/or O_2Hb% by arterial blood oximetry should be done before such decisions are made. Carlin et al has shown that patients with PaO_2 ≤55 torr may be denied oxygen therapy if the decision was based on pulse oximetry measurements alone (a significant number of these patients had SpO_2% measurements >88%).

References

Carlin BW, Clausen JL, and Ries AL, "The Use of Cutaneous Oximetry in the Prescription of Long-Term Oxygen Therapy," *Chest*, 1988, 94(2):239-41.

Escourrou PJ, Delaperche MF, and Visseaux A, "Reliability of Pulse Oximetry During Exercise in Pulmonary Patients," *Chest*, 1990, 97(3):635-8.

Joyce WP, Walsh K, Gough DB, et al, "Pulse Oximetry: A New Noninvasive Assessment of Peripheral Arterial Occlusive Disease," *Br J Surg*, 1990, 77(10):1115-7.

Jubran A and Tobin MJ, "Reliability of Pulse Oximetry in Titrating Supplemental Oxygen Therapy in Ventilator-Dependent Patients," *Chest*, 1990, 97(6):1420-5.

Kumar A, Chawla R, Ahuja S, et al, "Nitrobenzene Poisoning and Spurious Pulse Oximetry," *Anaesthesia*, 1990, 45(11):949-51.

Pierson DJ, "Pulse Oximetry Versus Arterial Blood Gas Specimens in Long-Term Oxygen Therapy," *Lung*, 1990, 168(suppl):782-8.

Residual Volume *see* Functional Residual Capacity *on page 232*

Respiratory Inductive Plethysmography *see* Cardiopulmonary Sleep Study *on page 224*

Right to Left Shunt Determination *see* Shunt Determination *on next page*

SB DLCO *see* Carbon Monoxide Diffusing Capacity, Single Breath *on page 219*

Shunt Determination

CPT 36600 (single arterial puncture); 94700 (analysis of arterial blood gas); 94799 (unlisted pulmonary procedure)

Related Information

Arterial Blood Gases *on page 206*

Synonyms Right to Left Shunt Determination; Shunt Study, 100% O_2

Abstract PROCEDURE COMMONLY INCLUDES: Alveolar to arterial gradient of partial pressure of dissolved oxygen while breathing 100% O_2 for a minimum of 20 minutes, reported in mm Hg and the shunt fraction ($Q_s/Q_t\%$) expressed as a percentage of the cardiac output. INDICATIONS: Determine the nature of hypoxemia and the nature of a right to left shunt.

Patient Care/Scheduling PATIENT PREPARATION: As with all arterial puncture procedures, a prothrombin time, if available, can alert one to the need to spend extra time applying direct pressure to the puncture site to allow for coagulation to occur. Test for collateral circulation (Allen test) should be negative before the radial puncture site is used. (See Arterial Blood Gases.) AFTERCARE: Apply direct pressure to the puncture site until bleeding has stopped and then apply a sterile bandage. Bandaging the puncture site does **not** substitute for the application of direct pressure to the puncture site for at least 5 minutes. Palpate pulse distal to the puncture site to evaluate arterial spasm. SPECIAL INSTRUCTIONS: Patient should be instructed to remain in the same position (upright seated posture is standard) throughout the O_2 breathing and obtaining of the ABG. The importance of maintaining an airtight seal on the mouthpiece and the use of noseclips should be stressed.

Method TECHNIQUE: Provide the patient with a 100% oxygen breathing supply. Typical setup uses a 100 L Douglas bag (that has been flushed three times to wash the dead space of bag, tubing, and valve dead space) attached to a bidirectional low resistance valve by a 3-way valve and a length of tubing. After flushing the reservoir and measuring the inspired oxygen concentration in the bag, begin the 20-minute oxygen breathing period. The patient is encouraged to take slow, deep breaths during the O_2 breathing. The patient's lips should maintain an airtight seal and noseclips should prevent nasal inspiration. After a minimum of 20 minutes a heparinized, arterial blood gas sample is obtained. If possible, sample end-tidal nitrogen from the breathing valve to ensure an expired N_2 of $<1\%$ before obtaining arterial blood sample. Calculate the percentage of right-to-left shunt according to the following equation:

$$Q_s/Q_t\% = \frac{0.0031 \times p(A\text{-}a)O_2}{0.0031 \times p(A\text{-}a)O_2 + 5} \times 100$$

Where:

$Q_s/Q_t\%$ – the fraction of the cardiac output that passes through a right-to-left shunt

$p(A\text{-}a)O_2$ = gradient of alveolar minus arterial oxygen partial pressure after breathing 100% O_2 for a minimum of twenty minutes

Specimen A heparinized arterial blood sample is obtained from the patient after a minimum of 20 minutes of breathing 100% oxygen. Sample can be obtained with patient in any position to evaluate the shunt status of the gravity-dependent portion of lung or lungs. Standard arterial blood gas parameters are measured (pH, pCO_2, and pO_2). CONTAINER: Although not studied, it is felt that heparinized glass syringes are preferred over plastic to minimize diffusion of high levels of dissolved oxygen across the walls of the syringe. Sample should be labeled with the patient's name and ID number, position during the 20-minute O_2 breathing and blood draw, and the number of minutes of oxygen breathing. CAUSES FOR REJECTION: Large air bubbles in sample, excessive (more than 15 minutes) interval between obtaining sample and sample analysis, inspiring room air during 100% O_2 breathing. TURNAROUND TIME: Same day.

Interpretation NORMAL FINDINGS: Two percent to 5% of the cardiac output passes through a right to left shunt at rest in the normal individual. LIMITATIONS: Erroneous results can be obtained if sample is not analyzed immediately, if the patient does not maintain an airtight seal with the O_2 supply, if insufficient (less than 20 minutes) time is allowed for wash-in of oxygen, or if oxygen electrode on the blood gas analyzer is alinear during measurement of high pO_2. Correct sample handling and observation during O_2 breathing can minimize errors. The shunt fraction calculation assumes an arterial to mixed venous oxygen content difference of 5 volume %. Significant variation from this value may occur in some patients.

Shunt Study, 100% O_2 *see* Shunt Determination *on previous page*

Single Breath Nitrogen Elimination

CPT 94370

Synonyms Closing Capacity; Closing Volume

Abstract PROCEDURE COMMONLY INCLUDES: Closing volume to vital capacity ratio (CV/VC%), closing capacity to total lung capacity ratio (CC/TLC%), slope of phase III (delta $N_{2(750\text{-}1250)}$ mL). INDICATIONS: To assess distribution of ventilation and presence of small airway dysfunction CONTRAINDICATIONS: Patients that are unable to limit inspiratory and expiratory flow rates to <0.5 $liter_{BTPS}$/second, patients with demonstrable airways obstruction.

Patient Care/Scheduling PATIENT PREPARATION: Patient should avoid heavy meals 3 hours prior to testing. Patient should be conscious and able to follow simple instructions. Patient's height and weight should be measured without shoes. Loose comfortable clothing that does not restrict chest expansion should be worn. Smoking history including last cigarette smoked should be obtained. Current medications should be obtained with particular emphasis on bronchodilators and steroids. SPECIAL INSTRUCTIONS: Generally, some sort of feedback circuit that monitors inspiratory and expiratory flow is needed to keep flows ≤0.5 L/second.

Method TECHNIQUE: The patient is attached to either a spirometer mouthpiece or a mouthpiece attached to a bag-in-box system. The spirometer used should conform to ATS recommended standards. The nitrogen analyzer should have a recent two-point calibration. The O_2 reservoir, either the bag in the box or the spirometer, should be flushed with oxygen until the N_2 measured at the mouthpiece is <0.1%. Initially, the patient valve should be turned to room air and the patient should breathe normally. Instruct the patient to take two deep breaths and then exhale to residual volume (RV). When the patient reaches RV, turn the patient valve so that the next inspiration to total lung capacity (TLC) comes from the 100% O_2 reservoir. Instruct the patient to inhale slowly (<0.5 L/second) to TLC, followed immediately by a slow (<0.5 L/second) exhalation to RV. Flow feedback devices are recommended. Flow, volume and expired nitrogen are continuously measured and recorded during the procedure. They should be repeated two more times. Repeat studies should be delayed until the inspiratory to expiratory nitrogen difference is <5% during room air breathing. Flow must not exceed 0.7 L/second for more than 300 mL expirate. Vital capacity measurements must show ≤10% variation on repeat maneuvers. Inspiratory and expiratory vital capacities must agree within 5%. Three acceptable tracings should be obtained. Mean values obtained from all valid efforts should be reported.

Specimen Measurement of expired nitrogen after one vital capacity breath of 100% O_2. CAUSES FOR REJECTION: Excessively high inspiratory or expiratory flow rates (>0.5 L/second), breath-holding at TLC. TURNAROUND TIME: Preliminary report is available the same day, interpreted report is usually available in 1-2 days.

Interpretation NORMAL FINDINGS: The onset of phase IV is not always seen. The normal values for closing volume (CV) are reported in units of [(VC – CV)/VC] x 100. The normal values for closing capacity (CC) are reported as [(VC – CV) + RV/VC] x 100. Closing volumes are age dependent and do not seem to vary with the size of the patient. Normal values range from around 10% at age 20 to around 20% to 25% at age 60. The slope of phase III (delta $N_{2(750\text{-}1250)}$) is reported as % nitrogen change/L volume expired and varies from around 1%/$liter_{BTPS}$ at age 20 to around 1.5%/$liter_{BTPS}$ at age 60. LIMITATIONS: Although seemingly simple, the test is actually difficult to perform correctly, with emphasis on the need to limit inspiratory and expiratory flows to <0.5 $liter_{BTPS}$/second. Large intraindividual coefficient of variation is noted even when careful attention to flow rates and absence of breath-holding during the procedure. Phase IV may not be evident in healthy young individuals and in patients with a high phase III slope. Poor correlation has been shown between phase IV and an abnormal flow rate $FEF_{25\%\text{-}75\%}$ measured on spirometry. A 1973 workshop at the National Heart and Lung Institute stated that the CV and CC are sensitive tests but are probably of low specificity and moderate precision and their validity as a diagnostic test is unknown.

References

Vollmer WM, McCamant LE, Johnson LR, et al, "Long-Term Reproducibility of Tests of Small Airways Function. Comparisons With Spirometry," *Chest*, 1990, 98(2):303-7.

Sleep Apnea Study *see* Cardiopulmonary Sleep Study *on page 224*

Sleep Oximetry *see* Cardiopulmonary Sleep Study *on page 224*

Sleep Study *see* Cardiopulmonary Sleep Study *on page 224*

Specific Airways Resistance *see* Airway Resistance *on page 202*

Specific Conductance *see* Airway Resistance *on page 202*

Spirogram *see* Spirometry *on this page*

Spirometry

CPT 94010

Related Information

Bedside Spirometry *on page 212*
Bronchial Challenge Test *on page 215*
Cardiopulmonary Exercise Testing *on page 221*
Flow Volume Loop *on page 228*
Functional Residual Capacity *on page 232*
Lung Subdivisions *on page 235*
Maximum Voluntary Ventilation (MVV) *on page 237*
Peak Flow *on page 238*
Spirometry Before and After Bronchodilators *on page 248*
Spirometry, Sitting and Supine *on page 250*
Volume of Isoflow (V iso $\mathring{V}$) *on page 254*

Synonyms Forced Expirogram; Spirogram

Applies to Assessment of Pulmonary Disability; Preoperative Evaluation

Abstract PROCEDURE COMMONLY INCLUDES: Vital capacity (VC); forced vital capacity (FVC); timed forced expiratory volumes, $FEV_{0.5}$, FEV_1, FEV_3; forced expiratory flow between 25% and 75% of the FEV ($FEF_{25\%-75\%}$); peak expiratory flow rate (PEFR or PF); total expiratory time in seconds INDICATIONS:

- establish baseline lung function
- detect disease
- follow the course of disease to monitor treatment
- evaluation of impairment
- preoperative evaluation
- identify high risk smokers
- occupational surveys

Patient Care/Scheduling PATIENT PREPARATION: Patient should avoid heavy meals 3 hours prior to testing. Patient should be conscious and able to follow simple instructions. Patient's height and weight should be measured without shoes. Loose comfortable clothing that does not restrict chest expansion should be worn. Smoking history including last cigarette smoked should be obtained. Current medications should be obtained with particular emphasis on bronchodilators and steroids. AFTERCARE: Usually none, although patients that complain of lightheadedness and dizziness should not be allowed to walk unobserved until recovery.

Method TECHNIQUE: A spirometer is used to measure exhaled gas and to record the time of collection. Two major categories of spirometers exist. Volume displacement spirometers such as the water seal, dry rolling seal, or bellows spirometers record volume change as vertical deflection on a kymograph or a moving stylus on a sheet of paper. The second category of spirometers integrates the measurement of expired flow over time to yield exhaled volume. Pneumotachograms, turbinometers, and hot wire mass flow meters are examples of flow integrating spirometers. Turbinometer type of spirometers have failed to meet current ATS standards of performance. Computer assisted flow integrating spirometers generate a CRT image of volume versus time or flow versus volume which can be inspected during testing and later printed. Graphic representation of spirometric data should be inspected along with numeric data to assess reliability of data (see Causes for Rejection).

Specimen Measurement of exhaled volumes and flow rates during a maximal forced expiratory maneuver from total lung capacity to residual volume. COLLECTION: Exhaled sample is collected or passed through a volume or flow measuring device known as a spirometer.

(Continued)

Spirometry *(Continued)*

Spirometers should meet certain minimum standards defined by the American Thoracic Society. Test may be performed on adults in a seated or standing position and children in a seated position. After applying noseclips, the subject is instructed to take a full inspiration, hold it briefly, then exhale through a mouthpiece into the spirometer as forcefully and completely as possible. Test is repeated a minimum of three times until two reproducible efforts have been obtained. See following figures. **CAUSES FOR REJECTION: Cough**, espe-

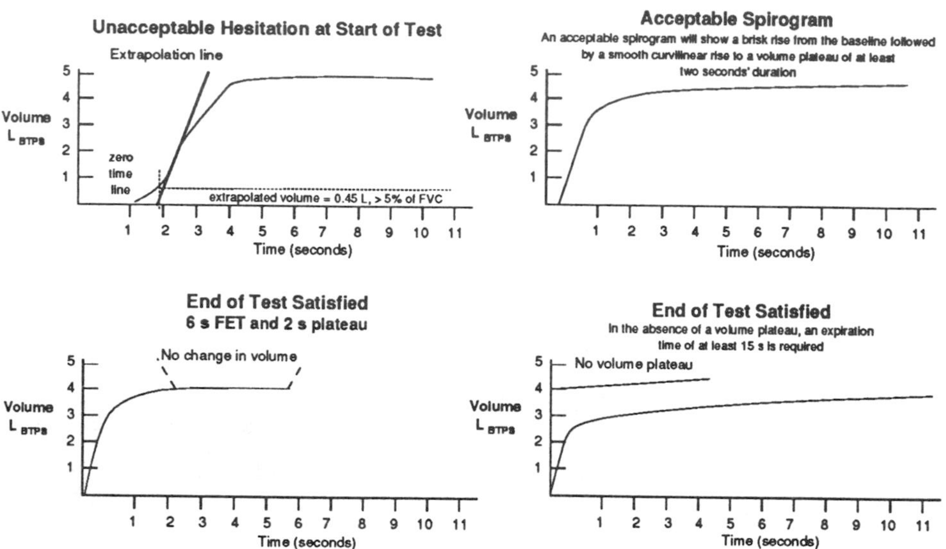

cially when it occurs in the early part of forced expiration, may render all data except expired volume useless. **Hesitant start:** Peak effort must be applied before 50% of total volume is exhaled, otherwise measurement of timed forced expiratory volume may be invalid. (Back extrapolated volume.) **Premature cessation of expiratory effort:** Expiratory effort must be maintained until a valid end-of-test has been observed. ATS has defined a valid end-of-test to be:

- when forced exhalation has continued for at least **6** seconds and a volume plateau (**no** volume change) of at least **2** seconds duration is seen
- in the absence of a volume plateau, a reasonable exhalation time of at least 15 seconds is observed
- when the patient cannot or should not sustain forced exhalation for valid medical reasons

Although difficult to achieve, the first two conditions for a valid end-of-test should be the goal of each testing session.

Early termination falsely increases $FEV_1FVC\%$ and increased mean and instantaneous flow rates at middle or low lung volumes. **Submaximal effort:** Indicated by a very low, often nonreproducible peak flow. Neuromuscular disease may produce the same pattern. **Nonreproducibility:** The two largest FVCs and FEV_1s should show <5% variability.

TURNAROUND TIME: Preliminary results should be available same day. Depending on the facility, an interpreted report may be available in 1-2 days.

Interpretation **NORMAL FINDINGS:** Typically ±20% of a reference value based on age, height and gender. Some studies advocate the use of 95% confidence limit. Spirometric values expressed as % of predicted can be used to grade the severity of abnormalities. **LIMITATIONS:** Requires patient cooperation. Transient obstruction secondary to cigarette smoking just prior to testing may be observed. **ADDITIONAL INFORMATION:** Patients with asthma may show progressive decline in spirometric values with repeated efforts yielding excessive variability between two largest efforts. This may be distinguished from variable effort only by a trained pulmonary technologist noting maximal inspiration on each effort followed by an adequately forceful expiration (sharp peak of expiratory flow volume curve). In such cases the largest and smallest acceptable efforts should be reported giving the physician a rough assessment of bronchial hyperreactivity. (See Bronchial Challenge Test.) Patients with neuromuscular disease (myasthenia gravis) may show progressive decline of values with repeated efforts but are seldom able to generate an adequate peak effort and may therefore mimic poor effort. See following tables. Good understanding of the

Patterns of Spirometric Abnormalities

	NML* (% of predicted)	Obstructive Diseases	Restrictive Diseases
FVC	≥80*	NML or ↓	↓ to ↓↓↓
FEV_1	≥80*	↓ to ↓↓↓	↓ to ↓↓↓
FEV_1/FVC %	≥75	↓ to ↓↓↓	NML or ↑
$FEF_{25\%-75\%}$	≥76*	↓↓ to ↓↓↓	↓ to ↓↓↓

*Expressed as actual ratio of FEV_1/FVC x 100.
↓ mildly reduced
↓↓ moderately reduced
↓↓↓ severely reduced

Quantification of Impairment by Spirometry (% of predicted)

	FVC	FEV_1	FEV_1/FVC%*†	$FEF_{25\%-75\%}$
Normal	≥80	≥80	75–85	>76
Minimal (slight)	70–79	70–79	65–74	60–75
Moderate	55–69	55–69	55–64	45–59
Severe	45–54	40–54	45–54	30–44
Very severe	<45	<45	<45	<30

*Expressed as actual ratio of FEV_1/FVC x 100.
†Female age >40 years.

expectations for maximum performance is the key for obtaining reproducible results. It is often helpful to include a demonstration of a proper forced expiratory maneuver as part of the initial instructions. Subsequent instructions should focus on correcting specific deficits in performance. The three most common deficits are:

- failure to inspire to TLC
- failure to begin exhalation with a prompt, forceful blow
- failure to sustain exhalation until valid end-of-test criteria is met.

References

Bass H, "The Flow Volume Loop: Normal Standards and Abnormalities in Chronic Obstructive Pulmonary Disease," *Chest*, 1973, 63:171-6.

Cherniack RM and Raber MB, "Normal Standards for Ventilatory Function Using an Automated Wedge Spirometer," *Am Rev Respir Dis*, 1972, 106:38-46.

Gardner RM, Baker CD, Broennle AM Jr, et al, "ATS Statement – Snowbird Workshop on Standardization of Spirometry." *Am Rev Respir Dis*, 1978, 118:1-120.

Gardner RM, Hankinson JL, Clausen JL, et al, "ATS Statement on Standardization of Spirometry – 1987 Update," *Am Rev Respir Dis*, 1987, 136:1285-98.

Ghio AJ, Crapo RO, and Elliott CG, "Reference Equations Used to Predict Pulmonary Function," *Chest*, 1990, 97(2):400-3.

Kass I, Bell WB, Epler GE, et al, "Evaluation of Impairment Disability Secondary to Respiratory Disease," *Am Rev Respir Dis*, 1982, 126:945-51.

Knudson RJ, Slatin RC, Lebowitz MD, et al, "The Maximal Expiratory Flow-Volume Curve: Normal Standards, Variability and the Effects of Age," *Am Rev Respir Dis*, 1976, 113:587-600.

(Continued)

Spirometry *(Continued)*

Morris JF, "Spirometry in the Evaluation of Pulmonary Function," *West J Med*, 1976, 125:110-8.
Nelson MS, Gardner RM, Crapo RO, et al, "Performance Evaluation of Contemporary Spirometers," *Chest*, 1990, 97(2):288-97.
Otulana BA, Higenbottam T, Ferrari L, et al, "The Use of Home Spirometry in Detecting Acute Lung Rejection and Infection Following Heart-Lung Transplantation," *Chest*, 1990, 97(2):353-7.
Pattishall EN, "Pulmonary Function Testing Reference Values and Interpretations in Pediatric Training Programs," *Pediatrics*, 1990, 85(5):768-73.
Schoenberg JB, Beck GJ, and Bough SA, "Growth and Decay of Pulmonary Function in Healthy Blacks and Whites," *Respir Physiol*, 1978, 33:367-93.
Townsend MC, Duchene AG, and Fallat RJ, "The Effects of Underrecorded Forced Expirations on Spirometric Lung Function Indexes," *Am Rev Respir Dis*, 1982, 126:734-7.
Vollmer WM, McCamant LE, Johnson LR, et al, "Long-Term Reproducibility of Tests of Small Airways Function. Comparisons With Spirometry," *Chest*, 1990, 98(2):303-7.

Spirometry Before and After Bronchodilators

CPT 94060

Related Information

Bronchial Challenge Test *on page 215*
Flow Volume Loop *on page 228*
Spirometry *on page 245*
Volume of Isoflow (V iso $\mathring{V}$) *on page 254*

Synonyms Postbronchodilator Spirometry

Abstract PROCEDURE COMMONLY INCLUDES: Vital capacity; forced vital capacity; timed forced expiratory volumes, $FEV_{0.5}$, FEV_1, FEV_3; forced expiratory flows; $FEF_{25\%-75\%}$; peak flow; $FEF_{25\%}$, $FEF_{50\%}$, $FEF_{75\%}$, $\mathring{V}_{E\ max\ 25\%}$; $\mathring{V}_{E\ max\ 50\%}$; $\mathring{V}_{E\ max\ 75\%}$ INDICATIONS: Assessment of physiologic response to bronchodilator, evaluate the need for additional medication, diagnosis of asthma.

Patient Care/Scheduling PATIENT PREPARATION: Patient should avoid heavy meals 3 hours prior to testing. Cigarettes should be avoided for 2 hours prior to testing. Patient should be conscious and able to follow simple instructions. Patient's height and weight should be measured without shoes. Loose comfortable clothing that does not restrict chest expansion should be worn. Smoking history including last cigarette smoked should be obtained. Current medication history should be obtained with particular emphasis on bronchodilators and steroids. If assessment of physiologic response to bronchodilator is desired, regularly prescribed bronchodilators should be withheld for 6 hours for inhaled sympathomimetics, 12 hours for short-acting theophylline preparations, and 24 hours for long-acting theophylline preparation. If assessment of the need for additional medication is desired, prebronchodilator and postbronchodilator testing may be performed while patient continues current bronchodilator therapy without interruption. Resting pulse should be recorded before bronchodilator is given, as administration of a bronchodilator in the presence of resting tachycardia is a relative contraindication. AFTERCARE: Usually none, although patients that complain of lightheadedness and dizziness should not be allowed to walk unassisted. Some patients, especially those that have not withheld bronchodilators prior to testing may develop tachycardia. Resting pulse rates should be monitored periodically until <100 beats/minute. SPECIAL INSTRUCTIONS: Patients that have a tracheostomy stoma may be tested by attaching an infant anesthesia mask to the mouthpiece. Mouthpieces can be adapted directly to most tracheostomy tubes. Effective administration of metered dose bronchodilators may be facilitated by use of a spacing device, especially one that limits inspiratory flow rates. Slow inhalation of the bronchodilator from FRC to RV should be followed by a 5- to 10-second breath-holding period before exhalation.

Method TECHNIQUE: A spirometer is used to measure exhaled gas and to record the time of collection. Two major categories of spirometers exist. Volume displacement spirometers such as the water seal, dry rolling seal, or bellows spirometers record volume change as vertical deflection on a kymograph or a moving stylus on a sheet of paper. The second category of spirometers integrates the measurement of expired flow over time to yield exhaled volume. Pneumotachograms, turbinometers, and hot wire mass flow meters are examples of flow integrating spirometers. Computer assisted flow integrating spirometers generate a CRT image of volume time or flow volume which can be inspected during testing and later printed. Graphic representation of spirometric data should be inspected along with numeric data to assess reliability of data (see Causes for Rejection). Inhalation of bronchodilator from a metered dose inhaler should occur from FRC to TLC followed by breath-holding for 5-10 seconds. Following a 1-minute waiting period, a second inhalation should be repeated in the same fashion. Repeat testing should be performed when at least 75% of the peak response to the drug is expected (see manufacturer's instructions).

Specimen Measurement of exhaled volumes and flow rates during a maximal forced expiratory maneuver from total lung capacity (TLC) to residual volume (RV) done before and after administration of an (aerosolized) bronchodilator and an appropriate waiting period suitable for that bronchodilating agent. **COLLECTION:** Exhaled sample is collected or passed through a volume or flow measuring device known as a spirometer. Spirometers should meet certain minimum standards defined by the American Thoracic Society (ATS). Test may be performed on adults in a seated or standing position and children in a seated position. After applying noseclips the subject is instructed to take a full inspiration, hold it briefly, then exhale through a mouthpiece into the spirometer as forcefully and completely as possible, keeping the chin slightly elevated throughout the maneuver. The test is repeated a minimum of three times until two reproducible efforts have been obtained. Several minutes after baseline spirometry has been obtained and resting pulse shows no tachycardia, an aerosolized bronchodilator is administered via metered dose inhaler, metered dose inhaler and a spacing device, ultrasonic nebulizer, inhaled powder, rubber bulb-type nebulizers, or compressed air-powered nebulizers. Although any bronchodilator may be used, inhaled sympathomimetic amines such as isoproterenol or metaproterenol are usually used. Selective beta-2 agonists should be considered in patients with known cardiac arrhythmias. The timing of postbronchodilator should coincide with the peak response time of the drug being used (5-30 minutes postinhalation with isoproterenol and 10-45 minutes with metaproterenol). The standards for data quality and reproducibility and cause for rejection used for prebronchodilator testing apply to postbronchodilator testing as well. The amount of drug administered and time before performance of postbronchodilator test should be reported. **CAUSES FOR REJECTION:** **Cough**, especially when it occurs in the early part of forced expiration, may render all data except expired volume useless. **Hesitant start:** Peak effort must be applied before 50% of total volume is exhaled, otherwise measurement of timed forced expiratory volume may be invalid. (Back extrapolated volume.) **Premature cessation of expiratory effort:** Expiratory effort must be maintained until a valid end-of-test has been observed. ATS has defined a valid end-of-test to be:

- when forced exhalation has continued for at least **6** seconds and a volume plateau (**no** volume change) of at least **2** seconds duration is seen
- in the absence of a volume plateau, a reasonable exhalation time of at least 15 seconds is observed
- when the patient cannot or should not sustain forced exhalation for valid medical reasons

Although difficult to achieve, the first two conditions for a valid end-of-test should be the goal of each testing session.

Early termination falsely increases FEV_1/FVC% and increased mean and instantaneous flow rates at middle or low lung volumes (LV). **Submaximal effort:** Indicated by a very low, often nonreproducible peak flow. Neuromuscular disease may produce the same pattern. **Nonreproducibility:** The two largest FVCs and FEV_1s should show <5% variability.

TURNAROUND TIME: Preliminary results should be available same day. Depending on the facility, an interpreted report may be available in 1-2 days.

Interpretation **NORMAL FINDINGS:** Various criteria have been suggested for definition of a significant response to bronchodilators. The FVC, FEV_1, and $FEF_{25\%-75\%}$ have been the most widely used single parameters for assessment of reversibility. Use of the $FEF_{25\%-75\%}$ alone should be made cautiously as it shows the greatest intrasubject variability (9.3% in patients) of the three. It is also dependent upon the FVC and pre- and postbronchodilator comparisons should be made volumetrically. The table shows recommendations for definition of degree of reversibility made by the Committee on Emphysema, American College of Chest Physicians. Perhaps the most universally agreed upon criterion for significant re-

(Continued)

Spirometry Before and After Bronchodilators *(Continued)*

sponse to bronchodilator is 15% to 20% improvement in the FEV_1. **LIMITATIONS:** Requires patient cooperation. Poor effort will cause most values reported to be unreliable for evaluative purposes. Transient obstruction secondary to cigarette smoking just prior to testing. If the forced vital capacity (FVC) increases following bronchodilator administration the $FEF_{25\%-75\%}$ will not be calculated at the same absolute lung volumes as the prebronchodilator determination and will, therefore, be underestimated. Postbronchodilator comparison of the $FEF_{25\%-75\%}$ should be made isovolumetrically (see Volume of Isoflow (V iso $\dot{V}$)). Postbronchodilator changes in lung volume may also influence the ratio $FEV_1/FVC\%$. If the FEV_1 and FVC increase equally, or the FVC increases more than FEV_1, the $FEV_1/FVC\%$ will show no change or a decline respectively. See figure. **ADDITIONAL INFORMATION:** Paradoxical decline in spirometric indices have been seen. These may be related to airway sensitivity to metabisulfites used as preservatives in some bronchodilator preparations. Patients with asthma may show progressive decline in spirometric values with repeated efforts yielding excessive variability between two largest efforts. This may be distinguished from variable effort only by a trained pulmonary technologist noting maximal inspiration on each effort followed by an adequately forceful expiration (sharp peak of expiratory flow volume curve). In such cases, the largest and smallest acceptable efforts should be reported giving the physician a rough assessment of bronchial hyperreactivity. (See Bronchial Challenge Test.) Patients with neuromuscular disease (myasthenia gravis) may show progressive decline of values with repeated efforts but are seldom able to generate an adequate peak effort and may therefore mimic poor effort. Good understanding of the expectations for maximum performance is the key for obtaining reproducible results. It is often helpful to include a demonstration of a proper forced expiratory maneuver as part of the initial instructions. Subsequent instructions should focus on correcting specific deficits in performance. The three most common deficits are:

Spirometry Before and After Bronchodilator

Degree of Reversibility	% Improvement in FVC, FEV_1, or $FEF_{25\%-75\%}$
Mild	15–25
Moderate	25–50
Marked	>50

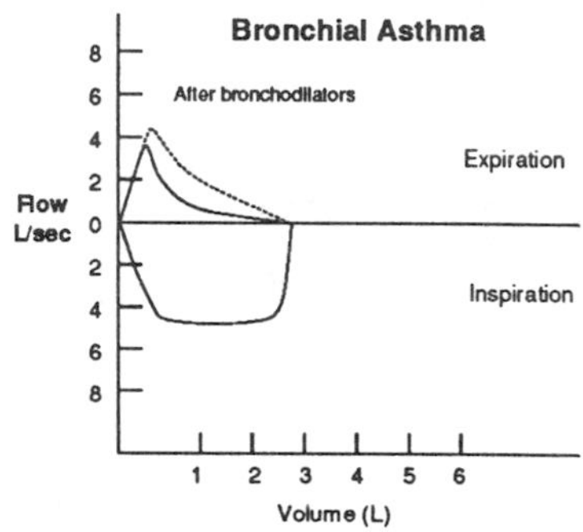

- failure to inspire to TLC
- failure to begin exhalation with a prompt, forceful blow
- failure to sustain exhalation until valid end-of-test criteria is met.

References

Gardner RM, Hankinson JL, Clausen JL, et al, "ATS Statement on Standardization of Spirometry – 1987 Update," *Am Rev Respir Dis*, 1987, 136:1285-98.

Ghio AJ, Crapo RO, and Elliott CG, "Reference Equations Used to Predict Pulmonary Function," *Chest*, 1990, 97(2):400-3.

Nelson MS, Gardner RM, Crapo RO, et al, "Performance Evaluation of Contemporary Spirometers," *Chest*, 1990, 97(2):288-97.

Pattishall EN, "Pulmonary Function Testing Reference Values and Interpretations in Pediatric Training Programs," *Pediatrics*, 1990, 85(5):768-73.

Spirometry, Sitting and Supine

CPT 94010

Related Information

Bedside Spirometry *on page 212*
Flow Volume Loop *on page 228*
Spirometry *on page 245*

Abstract **INDICATIONS:**

- detect abnormalities in diaphragm function
- assess the efficacy of Mestinon® in treatment of myasthenia gravis
- assess the need for night-time ventilatory support

Patient Care/Scheduling **PATIENT PREPARATION:** Patient should avoid heavy meals 3 hours prior to testing. Patient should be conscious and able to follow simple instructions. Patient's height and weight should be measured without shoes. Loose comfortable clothing that does not restrict chest expansion should be worn. Smoking history including last cigarette smoked should be obtained. Current medications should be obtained with particular emphasis on bronchodilators and steroids. **AFTERCARE:** Usually none, although patients that complain of lightheadedness and dizziness should not be allowed to walk unobserved until recovery. **SPECIAL INSTRUCTIONS:** Patients that have a tracheostomy stoma may be tested by attaching an infant anesthesia mask to the mouthpiece. Mouthpieces can be adapted directly to most tracheostomy tubes. Patients with diaphragm dysfunction may find the supine position uncomfortable or intolerable. Every effort should be made to minimize time spent by the patient in the supine position for each effort. Adequate rest in an upright position between efforts is essential. Spirometers that allow patients to inhale from and exhale into the spirometer may require a length of tubing be added to allow testing in the supine position. Only one or two tidal breaths should pass before commencing the vital capacity maneuver, as prolonged breathing of dead space air will increase the patient's sense of panic.

Method **TECHNIQUE:** Patient should be treated in the same fashion as a regular spirometry, measuring a vital capacity in the seated position. Repeat testing until two acceptable efforts show <5% variability. (Largest VC – second largest VC/largest VC) x 100 <5%. Allow patient to rest for at least 5 minutes in the seated position. After recovery, have patient lie flat on back and repeat the vital capacity maneuver using the same standards for reproducibility. Allow patient to rest in an upright position after each effort until recovered. Report sitting and supine vital capacity and calculate absolute (mL) and percent decline with change of position. Flow volume loop in sitting and supine position may be done instead of or in addition to vital capacity to obtain additional information.

Specimen Measurement of exhaled volumes and flow rates during a maximal forced expiratory maneuver from total lung capacity to residual volume made while in an upright, seated position and in a supine position. **COLLECTION:** Exhaled sample is collected or passed through a volume or flow measuring device known as a spirometer while the patient is in a seated position. Spirometers should meet certain minimum standards defined by the American Thoracic Society. After applying noseclips the subject is instructed to take a full inspiration, hold it briefly, then exhale through a mouthpiece into the spirometer as forcefully and completely as possible. Test is repeated a minimum of three times until two reproducible efforts have been obtained. After good results have been obtained in a seated position, the test is repeated with the patient in a supine position. The expiratory maneuver is repeated a minimum of three times until two reproducible efforts have been obtained. **CAUSES FOR REJECTION:** Nonreproducibility of test results data is a relative cause for rejection of data. As this test evaluates diaphragm's ability to contract during inspiration, the vital capacity is the most important parameter; the expiratory flow rates (FEV_1, $FEF_{25\%-75\%}$, $\dot{V}_{E\ max\ 25\%-50\%,\ and\ 75\%}$) are relatively unimportant. Progressive decline of FVCs or VCs on repeated efforts are often seen in myasthenia gravis and other neuromuscular disorders. Particular attention should be made to ensure that full inspiration to supine TLC is made, adequate seal is made around mouthpiece without air leakage, full expiration (to RV) is made, and adequate time for the patient's recovery is given between repeat efforts. **TURNAROUND TIME:** Preliminary results should be available same day. Depending on the facility, an interpreted report may be available in 1-2 days.

Interpretation **NORMAL FINDINGS:** Normals show either no decline or very slight decline in vital capacity when tested in a supine position. Although no good studies have been done, a 500 mL decline in VC or FVC is considered evidence of diaphragm dysfunction. **LIMITATIONS:** Requires patient cooperation. Insufficient or inconsistent effort will render sitting vs supine changes in VC unreliable for evaluative purposes. **ADDITIONAL INFORMATION:** If flow volume loop is done in seated and supine positions, forced expiratory volume in 1 second (FEV_1) in the supine position can be used to predict night-time hypoventilation. If the su-

(Continued)

Spirometry, Sitting and Supine *(Continued)*

pine FEV_1 is <800-1000 mL, night-time supine hypoventilation is likely. Supine arterial blood gas test during sleep should be done to verify and quantitate degree of alveolar hypoventilation.

References

Bass H, "The Flow Volume Loop: Normal Standards and Abnormalities in Chronic Obstructive Pulmonary Disease," *Chest*, 1973, 63:171-6.

Cherniack RM and Raber MB, "Normal Standards for Ventilatory Function Using an Automated Wedge Spirometer," *Am Rev Respir Dis*, 1972, 106:38-46.

Gardner RM, Baker CD, Broennle AM Jr, et al, "ATS Statement – Snowbird Workshop on Standardization of Spirometry," *Am Rev Respir Dis*, 1978, 118:1-120.

Kass I, Bell WB, Epler GE, et al, "Evaluation of Impairment Disability Secondary to Respiratory Disease," *Am Rev Respir Dis*, 1982, 126:945-51.

Knudson RJ, Slatin RC, Lebowitz MD, et al, "The Maximal Expiratory Flow-Volume Curve: Normal Standards, Variability, and Effects of Age," *Am Rev Respir Dis*, 1976, 113:587-600.

Morris JF, Koski A, and Johnson LC, "Spirometric Standards for Healthy Nonsmoking Adults," *Am Rev Respir Dis*, 1971, 103:57-67.

Schoenberg JB, Beck GJ, and Bough SA, "Growth and Decay of Pulmonary Function in Healthy Blacks and Whites," *Respir Physiol*, 1978, 33:367-93.

Townsend MC, Duchene AG, and Fallat RJ, "The Effects of Underrecorded Forced Expirations on Spirometric Lung Function Indexes," *Am Rev Respir Dis*, 1982, 126:734-7.

Spirometry With Flow Volume Loop *see* Flow Volume Loop *on page 228*

Static Lung Volumes *see* Functional Residual Capacity *on page 232*

Static Lung Volumes *see* Lung Subdivisions *on page 235*

Thoracic Gas Volume

CPT 94260

Related Information

Airway Resistance *on page 202*

Functional Residual Capacity *on page 232*

Abstract **PROCEDURE COMMONLY INCLUDES:** Thoracic gas volume (TGV) reported in $liter_{BTPS}$ **INDICATIONS:** Used in the calculation of **static lung volumes** in the same fashion as the functional residual capacity. Static lung volumes are used to categorize lung function into obstructive, restrictive, and combined abnormalities. May be used to assess the severity of lung disease. May be compared with FRC measured by helium dilution or nitrogen washout techniques to assess the volume of noncommunicating air spaces within the lungs (cysts or bullae). **Caution**: See Additional Information. Usually measured in conjunction with measurements of airway resistance, which must be standardized to the lung volume at which it is measured to calculate specific airway resistance. **CONTRAINDICATIONS:** Severe claustrophobia may contraindicate this measurement. Patients that cannot follow simple instructions should be excluded.

Patient Care/Scheduling **PATIENT PREPARATION:** Patient should avoid heavy meals 3 hours prior to testing. Patient should be conscious and able to follow simple instructions. Patient's height and weight should be measured without shoes. Loose comfortable clothing that does not restrict chest expansion should be worn. Smoking history including last cigarette smoked should be obtained. Current medications should be obtained with particular emphasis on bronchodilators and steroids. **AFTERCARE:** Usually none needed **SPECIAL INSTRUCTIONS:** Patients must often be instructed to press the palms of the hands against their cheeks during occluded airway panting to avoid bowing out of the cheeks. Patients should be instructed to apply gentle effort against the closed shutter, effort should be equal on inspiration and expiration.

Method **TECHNIQUE:** Thoracic gas volume is the measurement of all air in the thorax at end expiration (FRC) by plethysmographic technique as opposed to gas dilution technique. (See Functional Residual Capacity.) The patient is placed in a closed chamber which can monitor chamber pressure, mouth pressure (just distal to the mouthpiece), and flow. The

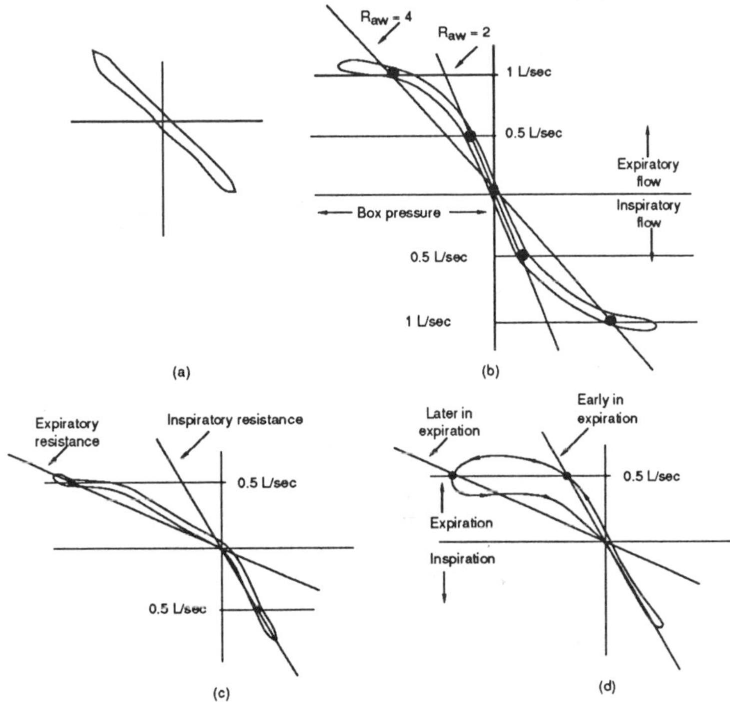

Plethysimographic loops for (a) TGV and (b, c, d) R_{aw}

Reproduced with permission from Clausen JL, *Pulmonary Function Testing Guidelines and Controversies*, London, England: Grund & Stratton, Inc, 1984, 148.

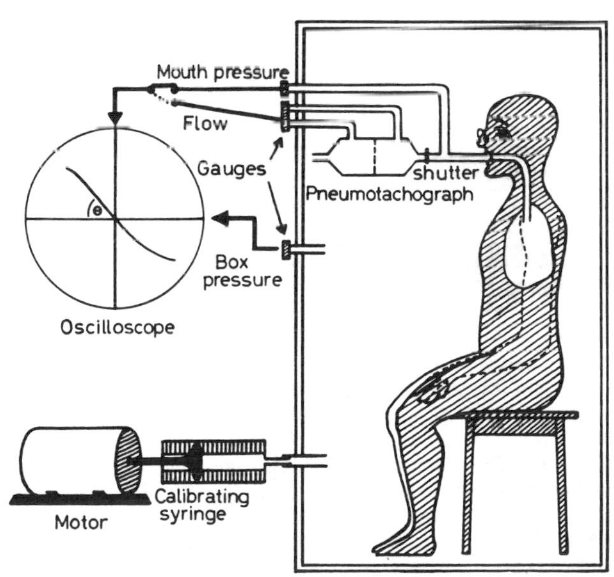

Configuration of a pressure (constant volume) body plethysmograph. Not shown are the large and small ports for pressure relief within the box. Reproduced with permission from Cotes JE, *Lung Function*, Oxford, England: Blackwell, 1979, 116.

(Continued)

Thoracic Gas Volume *(Continued)*

patient breathes through a special manifold which contains a shutter for occlusion of the airway. This shutter is closed at end expiration and the subject is asked to pant lightly against the closed shutter, alternately compressing and expanding the volume of air in the lungs and the chamber. During conditions of zero flow (closed shutter) mouth pressure changes reflect alveolar pressure changes. Changes in box pressure secondary to thoracic volume changes are proportional to alveolar gas pressure changes. Because the inverse relationship between mouth (alveolar) and box pressure is linear, Boyle's law, $P_1V_1=P_2V_2$, can be used to solve for the volume of gas being compressed, the thoracic gas volume.

Specimen Measurement of mouth pressure versus box pressure during end-tidal occluded airway panting in a body plethysmograph. **CAUSES FOR REJECTION:** Loops that do not close are usually secondary to compression of gas in the cheeks or varying inspiratory and expiratory effort. **TURNAROUND TIME:** Preliminary result usually available same day, interpreted report to follow in 1-2 days.

Interpretation **NORMAL FINDINGS:** Regression equations derived from studies that used helium dilution technique or nitrogen washout technique for measurement of FRC may be used. No studies used plethysmographic technique to develop normal values for TGV. **LIMITATIONS:** Some patients find being enclosed in a body box uncomfortable, even unacceptable. Some patients find it difficult to pant against a closed shutter. **ADDITIONAL INFORMATION:** Plethysmographically thoracic gas volume is felt by many to be the "gold standard" for lung volume determination because it measures all gas within the thorax, even gas trapped in pockets that do not communicate with the central airways. Mouth pressures may underestimate alveolar pressures in patients with severe airways obstruction leading to overestimation of thoracic gas volume. Panting with the accessory muscles may compress intra-abdominal gas and lead to erroneously high TGV. This error is insignificant with normal panting technique.

References Peslin R, Hannhart B, Duvivier C, et al, "Thoracic Gas Volume Measurements in Chronic Obstructive Pulmonary Disease by Low Frequency Ambient Pressure Changes," *Am Rev Respir Dis*, 1988, 137(2):277-80.

Titration of Oxygen or Nasal CPAP During Sleep *see* Cardiopulmonary Sleep Study *on page 224*

Total Lung Capacity *see* Functional Residual Capacity *on page 232*

Transfer Factor *see* Carbon Monoxide Diffusing Capacity, Single Breath *on page 219*

Volume of Isoflow (V iso $\mathring{V}$)

CPT 94799 (unlisted pulmonary procedure)

Related Information

Spirometry *on page 245*
Spirometry Before and After Bronchodilators *on page 248*

Synonyms Density Dependent Spirometry; Heliox Spirometry; Low Density Gas Spirometry

Abstract **PROCEDURE COMMONLY INCLUDES:** Volume of isoflow (V iso $\mathring{V}$), percent increase in maximum flow measured at 50% of the vital capacity (change $FEF_{50\%}$ or change $\mathring{V}_{max\ 50\%}$) and percent increase in maximum flow measured at 25% of the vital capacity measured from residual volumes (change $FEF_{75\%}$ or change $\mathring{V}_{max\ 75\%}$).

Patient Care/Scheduling **PATIENT PREPARATION:** Patient should avoid heavy meals 3 hours prior to testing. Patient should be conscious and able to follow simple instructions. Patient's height and weight should be measured without shoes. Loose comfortable clothing that does not restrict chest expansion should be worn. Smoking history including last cigarette smoked should be obtained. Current medications should be obtained with particular emphasis on bronchodilators and steroids. See also Spirometry. **AFTERCARE:** Usually none, although patients that complain of lightheadedness and dizziness should not be allowed to walk unobserved until recovery. **SPECIAL INSTRUCTIONS:** Patients that have a tracheostomy stoma may be tested by attaching an infant anesthesia mask to the mouthpiece. Mouthpieces can be adapted directly to most tracheostomy tubes.

Method **TECHNIQUE:** Forced vital capacity maneuvers are performed at least in triplicate breathing room air and during heliox breathing. The change $\mathring{V}_{E\ max\ 50\%}$ value is calculated as follows: Change $\dot{V}_{E\ max\ 50\%}$ = $\dot{V}_{E\ max\ 50\%}$ (HeO_2) – $\dot{V}_{E\ max\ 50\%}$ (AIR) x 100 / $\dot{V}_{E\ max\ 50\%}$. The change $\dot{V}_{E\ max\ 75\%}$ value is calculated in an identical fashion, measuring flows at 25% of the VC (from RV).

Specimen Measurement of exhaled volumes and flow rates during a maximal forced expiratory maneuver from total lung capacity (TLC) to residual volume (RV). Test is performed during air breathing and low density gas breathing (typically 80% helium, 20% oxygen – heliox). A bag in the box system is interposed between the patient and the spirometer, that is the spirometer measures the room air that is displaced as the patient inhales and exhales from a reservoir (bag) contained in a rigid "box" that is open only to the spirometer. Flow volume curves that represent best $\dot{V}_{E\ max\ 50\%}$ and $\dot{V}_{E\ max\ 75\%}$ are chosen. **CAUSES FOR REJECTION:** **Cough**, especially when it occurs in the early part of forced expiration, may render all data except expired volume useless. **Hesitant start:** Peak effort must be applied before 10% of total volume is exhaled, otherwise measurement of timed forced expiratory volume may be invalid. Back extrapolated volume. **Premature cessation of expiratory effort:** Expiratory effort must be maintained for a minimum of 6 seconds or until the volume-time tracing shows <25 mL volume increment for 1/2 a second. **Early termination** falsely increased FEV_1/FVC% and increased mean and instantaneous flow rates at middle or low lung volume (LV). **Submaximal effort:** Indicated by a very low, often nonreproducible peak flow. Neuromuscular disease may produce the same pattern. **Nonreproducibility:** The second largest FVCs should show 15% variability, the two largest FEV_1 should show <10% variability. **TURNAROUND TIME:** Preliminary results should be available same day. Depending on the facility, an interpreted report may be available in 1-2 days.

Interpretation **NORMAL FINDINGS:** Normal values for the change $\dot{V}_{E\ max\ 50\%}$ and $\dot{V}_{E\ max\ 75\%}$ of 47.3 and 13.7% (mean ±SD) and 29.12 ±23.4% respectively for nonsmokers have been reported. Volume of isoflow is generally reported as a percentage of the vital capacity and shows a significant rise with increasing age. The regression equation, V iso $\dot{V}$ = 0.291 x age + 4.917 ±6.88 SD describes the relationship of V iso $\dot{V}$ and changes in $\dot{V}_{E\ max\ 50\%}$ and V iso $\dot{V}$ following bronchodilators can be interpreted as follows. **LIMITATIONS:** Requires pa-

Interpretation of Changes in $\dot{V}_{E\ max}$ and Delta $\dot{V}_{E\ max\ 50\%}$ After Bronchodilators

$\dot{V}_{E\ max}$	Delta $\dot{V}_{E\ max\ 50\%}$	Interpretation
Increased	Increased	Predominant peripheral airways bronchodilation
Increased	Decreased	Predominant central airways bronchodilation
Increased	Unchanged	Proportionally equal peripheral and central airways bronchodilation

tient cooperation. Transient obstruction secondary to cigarette smoking just prior to testing. FVC of the forced expirations used for comparison of air and heliox flow measurements must be within 25% of each others. Flow rates must be compared isovolumetrically, that is at the same absolute lung volume. **ADDITIONAL INFORMATION:** A great deal of controversy exists regarding the clinical usefulness of V of iso $\dot{V}$. Lam and Berend suggest that the test is not very useful for detection of early airways obstruction secondary to its high coefficients of variation. A study by Mink et al has shown that airway geometry differs during air and heliox breathing. Flow comparisons have been made under the assumption that airway geometry was constant.

References

Bass H, "The Flow Volume Loop: Normal Standards and Abnormalities in Chronic Obstructive Pulmonary Disease," *Chest*, 1973, 63:171-6.

Cherniack RM and Raber MB, "Normal Standards for Ventilatory Function Using an Automated Wedge Spirometer," *Am Rev Respir Dis*, 1972, 106:38-46.

Gardner RM, Baker CD, Broennle AM Jr, et al, "ATS Statement – Snowbird Workshop on Standardization of Spirometry," *Am Rev Respir Dis*, 1978, 118:1-120.

Kass I, Bell WB, Epler GE, et al, "Evaluation of Impairment Disability Secondary to Respiratory Disease," *Am Rev Respir Dis*, 1982, 126:945-51.

(Continued)

Volume of Isoflow (V iso V̊) *(Continued)*

Knudson RJ, Slatin RC, Lebowitz MD, et al, "The Maximal Expiratory Flow-Volume Curve: Normal Standards, Variability, and Effects of Age," *Am Rev Respir Dis*, 1976, 113:587-600.

Morris JF, Koski A, and Johnson LC, "Spirometric Standards for Healthy Nonsmoking Adults," *Am Rev Respir Dis*, 1971, 103:57-67.

Schoenberg JB, Beck GJ, and Bough SA, "Growth and Decay of Pulmonary Function in Healthy Blacks and Whites," *Respir Physiol*, 1978, 33:367-93.

Townsend MC, Duchene AG, and Fallat RJ, "The Effects of Underrecorded Forced Expirations on Spirometric Lung Function Indexes," *Am Rev Respir Dis*, 1982, 126:734-7.

Vollmer WM, McCamant LE, Johnson LR, et al, "Long-Term Reproducibility of Tests of Small Airways Function. Comparisons With Spirometry," *Chest*, 1990, 98(2):303-7.

PULMONARY MEDICINE

Joseph A. Golish, MD and Carlos M. Isada, MD

The respiratory system is the site of many important ailments that afflict patients. The most common ones include pneumonia, asthma, emphysema, AIDS, and lung cancer. Lung cancer has become the number one cancer killer in our hemisphere. In addition, many nonpulmonary diseases involve the respiratory system. The lungs are one of the most common sites of metastases of a variety of malignancies. Adult respiratory distress syndrome (ARDS) may occur secondary to a large variety of medical and surgical disorders. Infections originating elsewhere often involve the lungs. Autoimmune disease frequency manifests in the chest. The cardinal manifestations of cardiac disease may appear to be pulmonary in origin.

Evolving technology has added greatly to our armamentarium for the diagnosis of respiratory illness. Pulmonary function can be readily assessed by accurate, efficient, and inexpensive devices. Whole new batteries of such tests are now available, as evidenced by an entire section dedicated to the topic. The advent of the Swan-Ganz catheter allows in-depth monitoring of the critical care patient that was heretofore impossible.

Fiberoptic technology has led to the development of flexible endoscopes which can allow visualization of the inner reaches of the body. The hollow channels of such scopes permit the passage of a variety of instruments for obtaining diagnostic specimens. With the availability of laser technology, some surgical procedures can be performed utilizing endoscopic techniques without the need for an incision.

The fiberoptic bronchoscope has become the central medical instrument in pulmonary medicine. A multitude of diagnostic procedures have been developed which center around this device. This section reviews the currently available techniques. Along with the Pulmonary Function and Critical Care sections, this represents a comprehensive review of the multitude of diagnostic tests available in pulmonary disease.

Bronchial Brushings

CPT 31717

Related Information

Bronchoscopy, Fiberoptic *on page 260*

Synonyms Brush Biopsy

Abstract **PROCEDURE COMMONLY INCLUDES:** Cytologic examination for the diagnosis of malignancy. Can also be used to collect cytologic material for culture (protected brush). **INDICATIONS:** The main utility is the diagnosis of malignancy and cell type. It may also be used to obtain material for Gram staining and culture but in the past frequent contamination by upper airway flora limited its usefulness. Newer protected brush catheters (PBC) have become available to avoid contamination by upper airway flora. Such sampling now makes this a useful diagnostic technique in pneumonia. **CONTRAINDICATIONS:** Bleeding diathesis.

Patient Care/Scheduling **PATIENT PREPARATION:** NPO after midnight for a morning bronchoscopy and NPO after liquid breakfast for afternoon procedures. Routine medications (especially antiasthmatic drugs) may be taken at any time with a small amount of water. Routine lab work including clotting times, BUN, CBC, and platelet count are essential to exclude a coagulopathy – especially if a biopsy is to be performed. Some measure of pulmonary function is useful (spirometry, blood gases) to assess pulmonary reserve and document bronchospasm. Premedication with a narcotic (meperidine 25-75 mg) or minor tranquilizer (diazepam 10 mg) is given parenterally 15-30 minutes before the procedure. Atropine 0.4 mg I.M. is given as a vagolytic agent at the same time unless contraindicated by the presence of arrhythmia, narrow angle glaucoma, or urinary retention. **AFTERCARE:** NPO for 2 hours or longer after the procedure until the gag reflex is fully recovered. Because of the premedication, outpatients are not allowed to drive until the following day. Transient fever and mild hemoptysis may be noted for the next 24 hours. **COMPLICATIONS:** Occasionally, endobronchial bleeding may occur. It is usually quite mild and self-limited; suctioning and local instillation of epinephrine is normally all that is required for treatment.

Method **EQUIPMENT:** Both disposable and reusable brushes are available, most made of nylon. Large and small size bristles are also available. For diagnosis of bacterial pneumonia, a specially-designed protected brush catheter is utilized. It consists of a brush within a catheter, within a second catheter, with a wax plug at its top. This configuration prevents contamination by upper airway flora. **TECHNIQUE:** The brush is passed through the channel of the bronchoscope and advanced to the lesion either under direct visualization or for peripheral lesions under fluoroscopic guidance. The lesion is gently brushed and then the brush is withdrawn through the channel. Alternatively, the brush may be left in the channel and the entire bronchoscope may be withdrawn (facilitated by the use of an end-tracheal tube) although the diagnostic yield is no greater. The material is then transferred onto glass slides by pressing the brush onto the slide using either a circular or back and forth motion. Generally, 1-2 slides can be made per brush depending on the abundance of material. It is imperative that the slides be immersed immediately in 95% ethyl alcohol for proper fixation as any drying will distort cellular morphology. Another method for processing brush specimens involves agitating the brush in a tube of isotonic solution (normal saline). This fluid can then be spun down and examined as smears and cell block. The PBC requires sequential advancing of the inner catheter followed by the brush into an area of suspected pneumonia. The gentle brushing motion is followed by reversal of the above sequence. The brush tip is then sent in total for culture by the Bacteriology Laboratory. **DATA ACQUIRED:** Prior to microscopic examination all smears are stained with Papanicolaou's stain.

Specimen Cellular material is obtained by brushing the area in question. **CONTAINER:** Both disposable and reusable brushes are available, most made of nylon. Large and small size bristles are also available. **CAUSES FOR REJECTION:** Inadequate cellular material; excessive drying of specimen, thus distorting cellular morphology **TURNAROUND TIME:** Depends on the institution but may be processed and read the same day.

Interpretation **NORMAL FINDINGS:** No malignant cells, or, no growth on bacterial culture **LIMITATIONS:** The diagnostic yield from endobronchially visible lesions in a group of 106 patients was 92% for brushing and 93% for biopsy.

References

Kvale PA, "Collection and Preparation of Bronchoscopic Specimens," *Chest*, 1978, 73(suppl):707-12.

Mak VH, Johnston ID, Hetzel MR, et al, "Value of Washings and Brushings at Fiberoptic Bronchoscopy in the Diagnosis of Lung Cancer," *Thorax*, 1990, 45(5):373-6.

Örtqvist Å, Kalin M, Lejdeborn L, et al, "Diagnostic Fiberoptic Bronchoscopy and Protected Brush Culture in Patients With Community-Acquired Pneumonia," *Chest*, 1990, 97(3):576-82.

Stokes DC, Shenep JL, Parham D, et al, "Role of Flexible Bronchoscopy in the Diagnosis of Pulmonary Infiltrates in Pediatric Patients With Cancer," *J Pediatr*, 1989, 115(4):561-7.

Bronchial Washings

CPT 31622

Related Information

Bronchoscopy, Fiberoptic *on next page*

Abstract **PROCEDURE COMMONLY INCLUDES:** Bronchial washings for cytology, fungi, and acid-fast bacilli **INDICATIONS:** For bronchoscopically visible tumors, the diagnostic yield is 76%. For peripheral nonvisible tumors, the yield is 52%. Cytologic cell typing in one study was 92% for squamous cell carcinoma, 87% for small cell carcinoma, 83% for adenocarcinoma, and only 38% for large cell carcinoma.[1] Bronchial washings when used along with bronchial brushing and biopsy allow for a diagnosis in >90% of cases of neoplasm. **CONTRAINDICATIONS:** Bleeding diathesis.

Patient Care/Scheduling **PATIENT PREPARATION:** NPO after midnight for a morning bronchoscopy and NPO after liquid breakfast for afternoon procedures. Routine medications (especially antiasthmatic drugs) may be taken at any time with a small amount of water. Routine lab work including clotting times, BUN, CBC, and platelet count are essential to exclude a coagulopathy – especially if a biopsy is to be performed. Some measure of pulmonary function is useful (spirometry, blood gases) to assess pulmonary reserve and document bronchospasm. Premedication with a narcotic (meperidine 25-75 mg) or minor tranquilizer (diazepam 10 mg) is given parenterally 15-30 minutes before the procedure. Atropine 0.4 mg I.M. is given as a vagolytic agent at the same time unless contraindicated by the presence of arrhythmia, narrow angle glaucoma, or urinary retention. **AFTERCARE:** NPO for 2 hours or longer after the procedure until the gag reflex is fully recovered. Because of the premedication, outpatients are not allowed to drive until the following day. Transient fever and mild hemoptysis may be noted for the next 24 hours.

Method **EQUIPMENT:** Fiberoptic bronchoscope **TECHNIQUE:** The bronchoscope is passed in the usual manner. Isotonic saline is instilled through the inner channel of the bronchoscope. Fluid is aspirated into a trap connected in-line to the suction tubing. Usually 2-5 ml aliquots of fluid are instilled with each washing and approximately one-fourth to one-half of this volume is recovered. For endoscopically visible lesions, the fluid is washed directly over the area in question. For lesions which are not visible, the bronchoscope is wedged in the respective segment and washings are aspirated. For tumors which are diagnosed on sputum cytology, but remain radiographically and endobronchially invisible, washings of each segment can be performed for localization of the tumor.

Specimen 5-30 mL aspirated 0.9% normal saline along with bronchial secretions **CONTAINER:** Suction trap **CAUSES FOR REJECTION:** Inadequate volume of aspirated fluid **TURNAROUND TIME:** 24-48 hours for cytology; several weeks for mycobacterial or fungal cultures.

Interpretation **NORMAL FINDINGS:** No evidence of malignancy, mycobacterium, or fungi **LIMITATIONS:** Cultures for *Mycobacterium tuberculosis* may be inhibited by the topical anesthetics. Because of the invariable contamination which occurs by introducing the bronchoscope through the upper airway, there is no indication for the routine culturing of bronchial washings. It is a useful technique, however, for the recovery of fungi, cultures for fungi, and *Mycobacterium* species. Nonbacteriostatic topical anesthesia may increase the culture yield.

Footnotes

1. Jay SJ, Wehr K, Nicholson DP, et al, "Diagnostic Sensitivity and Specificity of Pulmonary Cytology: Comparison of Techniques Used in Conjunction With Flexible Fiberoptic Bronchoscopy," *Acta Cytol*, 1980, 24:304-12.

References

Kvale PA, "Collection and Preparation of Bronchoscopic Specimens," *Chest*, 1978, 73(suppl):707-12.

(Continued)

Bronchial Washings *(Continued)*

Yoss EB, Berd D, Cohn JR, et al, "Flow Cytometric Evaluation of Bronchoscopic Washings and Lavage Fluid for DNA Aneuploidy as an Adjunct in the Diagnosis of Lung Cancer and Tumors Metastatic to the Lung," *Chest*, 1989, 96(1):54-9.

Bronchoalveolar Lavage (BAL)

CPT 31622

Related Information

Bronchoscopy, Fiberoptic *on this page*

Abstract PROCEDURE COMMONLY INCLUDES: An irrigation of peripheral lung followed by collection of the aspirate INDICATIONS: This procedure was originally utilized to assess the activity of alveolitis in chronic interstitial lung disease, such as sarcoid or idiopathic pulmonary fibrosis (IPF). More recently, it has been useful in uncovering the etiology of opportunistic pneumonia, especially in AIDS.[1] CONTRAINDICATIONS: Bleeding diathesis.

Method EQUIPMENT: Fiberoptic bronchoscope, suction trap TECHNIQUE: The bronchoscope is passed in the usual manner. 100 mL isotonic saline is instilled through the inner channel of the scope into a lung segment isolated by "wedging" the scope's tip. Aspiration generally provides 30-60 mL fluid. This fluid is then sent for cytologic and microbiologic analysis along with differential cell count.

Specimen 30-60 mL aspirated fluid CONTAINER: Suction trap CAUSES FOR REJECTION: <30 mL fluid return TURNAROUND TIME: 24-48 hours for cell differential, cytology, special stains for pneumocysts/AFB/fungus, and bacterial culture. Several weeks for AFB and fungal cultures.

Interpretation NORMAL FINDINGS: No evidence of malignancy or pathologic organisms. Normal differential cell count includes 92% alveolar macrophages, 7% lymphocytes, and 1% neutrophils. CRITICAL VALUES: Differential cell count showing >28% lymphocytes suggests sarcoid activity[2] while >10% neutrophils suggests active IPF.[3] LIMITATIONS: Neutrophils in lavage fluid have little meaning in the face of smoking, chronic bronchitis, and active respiratory infection.

Footnotes

1. Miles PR, Baughman RP, and Linnemann CC Jr, "Cytomegalovirus in the Bronchoalveolar Lavage Fluid of Patients With AIDS," *Chest*, 1990, 97(5):1072-6.
2. Keogh BA, Hunninghake GW, Line B, et al, "The Alveolitis of Pulmonary Sarcoidosis," *Ann Rev Respir Dis*, 1983, 128:256-65.
3. Keogh B, Line B, Rust M, et al, "Clinical Staying of Patients With Idiopathic Pulmonary Fibrosis," *Ann Rev Respir Dis*, 1981, 123:89A.

Bronchoscopy, Fiberoptic

CPT 31622

Related Information

Bronchoalveolar Lavage (BAL) *on this page*
Bronchial Brushings *on page 258*
Bronchial Washings *on previous page*

Synonyms Flexible Bronchoscopy

Abstract PROCEDURE COMMONLY INCLUDES: Direct visual examination of upper airway, vocal cords, and tracheobronchial tree out to the fourth to sixth division bronchi. Other procedures such as washings, brush biopsy bronchoalveolar lavage, endobronchial and transbronchial biopsy are also included depending on the clinical indications. INDICATIONS: The major utility is in the assessment of malignant disease, early diagnosis of carcinoma, assessment of operability, transbronchial or endobronchial lung biopsy, hemoptysis (not massive), persistent chronic cough, removal of foreign bodies (minor role), and diagnosis of lung infections especially in immunocompromised hosts. Other uses include difficult endotracheal intubation. CONTRAINDICATIONS: Asthma, severe hypoxemia, serious arrhythmia unstable angina pectoris, recent myocardial infarction, and poor patient cooperation. All of these are only relative contraindications and vary depending on the clinical situation and experience of the bronchoscopist. When bronchoscopy involves biopsy procedures, coagulopathies or bleeding tendencies are contraindications.

Patient Care/Scheduling PATIENT PREPARATION: NPO after midnight for a morning bronchoscopy and NPO after light breakfast for afternoon procedures. Routine medications (especially antiasthmatic drugs) may be taken at any time with a small amount of water. Routine lab work including clotting times, BUN, CBC, and platelet count is essential to exclude a coagulopathy – especially if a biopsy is to be performed. Some measure of pulmonary function is useful (spirometry, blood gases) to assess pulmonary reserve and document bronchospasm. Premedication with a narcotic (meperidine 25-75 mg) or minor tranquilizer (diazepam 10 mg) is given parenterally 15-30 minutes before the procedure. Atropine 0.4 mg I.M. is given as a vagolytic agent at the same time unless contraindicated by the presence of arrhythmia, narrow angle glaucoma, or urinary retention. **AFTERCARE:** NPO for 2 hours or longer after the procedure until the gag reflex is fully recovered. Because of the premedication, outpatients are not allowed to drive until the following day. Transient fever and mild hemoptysis may be noted for the next 24 hours.

Method **EQUIPMENT:** A fiberoptic bronchoscope and halogen or xenon light source are necessary for this airway exam. The bronchoscope is equipped with a thumb lever which allows angulation of the distal end of the instrument. A 2-2.6 mm hollow channel runs the length of the scope and allows injection of medication and aspiration of secretions for airway clearance and obtaining bronchial washings and lavage. It is also utilized for the passage of instruments, such as bronchial brushes and forceps. **TECHNIQUE:** Procedure may be performed with the patient in supine or sitting position. Patient gargles with 2% lidocaine solution or alternatively tetracaine 2% aerosolized spray (Cetacaine®) is used to anesthetize the pharynx. The bronchoscope tip is lubricated with Xylocaine® jelly and introduced transnasally or transorally with the use of a bite block. Lidocaine 2% solution is then injected through the bronchoscopic channel in 2 mL aliquots for anesthesia of the vocal cords and entire tracheobronchial tree. Lidocaine has definite toxicity (seizures and respiratory arrest) and the total dosage should generally not exceed 400 mg. The duration of action generally lasts 20-30 minutes.[1] Once adequate anesthesia has been obtained, a detailed visual examination is performed. Subsequently other procedures such as biopsies, washings, and brushings can be carried out. **DATA ACQUIRED:** This examination provides information regarding the patency and normality of the central airways. It is used as a vehicle for sampling the airways and lung parenchyma itself via brushing and biopsy techniques.

Specimen Bronchial washings, brushings, biopsy, or lavage **CONTAINER:** Formalin jars, mucous specimen containers, slides in 95% alcohol **TURNAROUND TIME:** Reports: Written in chart at time of procedure.

Interpretation **NORMAL FINDINGS:** Normal endobronchial examination. **LIMITATIONS:** Limited usefulness in retrieving foreign bodies and the management of massive hemoptysis. **ADDITIONAL INFORMATION:** The procedure is markedly safe. Large reviews have shown that approximately 50% of the life-threatening complications are associated with premedication or topical anesthesia. The risk seems highest in patients with underlying cardiac disease and the elderly. Patients with underlying bronchospastic disease are particularly prone to bronchospasm and laryngospasm and thus should be under optimal treatment before undertaking bronchoscopy. A drop in pO_2 of approximately 20 mm Hg occurs, and therefore supplemental oxygen administration is indicated. Transient fever and pneumonia occur in a small number of patients. Bleeding can occur from the nose or tracheobronchial tree although this complication is mainly associated with transbronchial biopsy.[2]

Footnotes

1. Perry LB, "Topical Anesthesia for Bronchoscopy," *Chest*, 1978, 73(5):691-3.
2. Lukomsky GI, Ovchinnikov AA, and Bilal A, "Complications of Bronchoscopy: Comparison of Rigid Bronchoscopy Under General Anesthesia in Flexible Bronchoscopy Under Topical Anesthesia," *Chest*, 1981, 79:316-21.

References

Ackart RS, Foreman DR, and Klayton RJ, "Fiberoptic Bronchoscopy in Outpatient Facilities," *Arch Intern Med*, 1983, 143:30.

Fulkerson WJ, "Fiberoptic Bronchoscopy: Current Concepts," *N Engl J Med*, 1984, 311(8):511-15.

Ikeda S, *Atlas of Flexible Bronchofiberoscopy*, Baltimore, MD: University Park Press, 1974.

Marini JJ, Pierson DJ, and Hudson LD, "Acute Lobar Atelectasis: A Prospective Comparison of Fiberoptic Bronchoscopy and Respiratory Therapy," *Am Rev Respir Dis*, 1979, 119:971-8.

Mitchell DM, Emerson CJ, and Collyer J, "Fiberoptic Bronchoscopy: Ten Years On," *Br Med J [Clin Res]*, 1980, 281:360-3.

(Continued)

Bronchoscopy, Fiberoptic *(Continued)*

Pereira W, Kovnat DM, Khan MA, et al, "Fever and Pneumonia After Flexible Fiberoptic Bronchoscopy," *Am Rev Respir Dis*, 1975, 112:59-64.

Perry LB, "Topical Anesthesia for Bronchoscopy," *Chest*, 1978, 73(5):691-3.

Sackner MA, "Bronchofiberoscopy: State of the Art," *Am Rev Respir Dis*, 1975, 111:62-88.

Schnapf BM, "Oxygen Desaturation During Fiberoptic Bronchoscopy in Pediatric Patients," *Chest*, 1991, 99(3):591-4.

Sen RP and Walsh TE, "Fiberoptic Bronchoscopy for Refractory Cough," *Chest*, 1991, 99(1):33-5.

Trouillet JL, Guiguet M, Gilbert C, et al, "Fiberoptic Bronchoscopy in Ventilated Patients," *Chest*, 1990, 97(4):927-38.

Bronchoscopy, Transbronchial Biopsy

CPT 31628

Synonyms Forceps Biopsy; Transbronchoscopic Biopsy

Replaces Trephine Drill Biopsy

Abstract **PROCEDURE COMMONLY INCLUDES:** Histologic examination of tissue. Depending on the clinical situation, the tissue can be cultured directly. **INDICATIONS:** Useful in the diagnosis of both malignant and nonmalignant lung disease. In diffuse lung disease, transbronchial biopsy is especially helpful in demonstrating lung parenchymal infiltration by noncaseating granulomas. Regardless of the stage of the disease, transbronchial biopsy is now the procedure of choice to confirm sarcoidosis with diagnostic yields ranging from 60% to 90%.[1,2] The diagnostic yield in other diffuse lung diseases, most commonly idiopathic pulmonary fibrosis, is much more variable, given the patchy nature of lung involvement and the investigator's willingness to correlate the histologic findings with the clinical picture. With the exception of malignancy, demonstration of acid-fast or fungal elements, or noncaseating granulomas, transbronchial biopsy is often inadequate to make a specific diagnosis in diffuse lung disease.[3] In malignant disease, the diagnostic yield for endobronchially visible tumors is approximately 90%.[4] For endobronchially occult tumors, the yield is considerably lower (50%) even utilizing fluoroscopic guidance. The yield may be increased slightly by the addition of cytologic brushing.[5] **CONTRAINDICATIONS:** Uncorrected bleeding diathesis, severe pulmonary hypertension, unstable cardiorespiratory status (relative), active bronchospasm.

Patient Care/Scheduling **PATIENT PREPARATION:** The same preparations as for Bronchoscopy, Fiberoptic with special attention to factors which may predispose the patient to complications. Specifically, a normal PT, PTT, bleeding time, and platelet count >50,000 should be documented. Uremia and pulmonary hypertension are also risk factors for bleeding. The incidence of pneumothorax is increased in fibrotic lung disease and also patients who are being ventilated with positive pressure.[6] In general, the procedure can be safely done in the outpatient setting.[7] **AFTERCARE:** Generally, the patient may be discharged 1 hour after the procedure with instructions to return if any unusual chest pain, shortness of breath, or hemoptysis occurs. **COMPLICATIONS:** The same precautions that apply to fiberoptic bronchoscopy apply to transbronchial biopsy, with a higher risk of bleeding (1.3%) and pneumothorax (5.5%).[6] The pneumothorax may be delayed.[7] Mild hypoxemia, with an average drop in pO_2 of 20 torr, may occur during bronchoscopy but gradually resolves.

Method **EQUIPMENT:** Several types of forceps are available including small and large "alligator" forceps, cup forceps, and curette. The small "alligator" forceps are preferred because of the generally larger pieces of tissue obtained with a minimum of bleeding or crush artifact.[8] **TECHNIQUE:** Procedure is the same as for fiberoptic bronchoscopy. The bronchoscope is directed toward the segment or subsegment where the biopsy is to be taken. The biopsy forceps are inserted into the channel of the bronchoscope and advanced into the respective segment. Although the forceps can be advanced blindly until resistance is met and the biopsy is taken, it is generally felt that the incidence of pneumothorax is higher, and therefore fluoroscopic guidance is advisable. The forceps are advanced until the lesion or specific area of the lung is encountered. The scope is wedged in the respective bronchial segment to tamponade any bleeding as the biopsy forceps with the specimen are withdrawn. Patient cooperation is necessary at the time of biopsy. The patient is instructed to take in a deep breath after the forceps are advanced to target area. The forceps' jaws are opened, and the patient is instructed to exhale. As this is occurring, the "open jawed" forceps are advanced slightly and closed, thus obtaining a piece of tissue. Although the optimal number of biopsies is not clearly known, multiple pieces (3-6) should be obtained.[4] Bleeding can be controlled by tamponading the involved segment. Topical epinephrine 1:1000 in 10% solution can be useful as well. At the end of the procedure, either fluoroscopy or an expiratory chest x-ray can be used to check for pneumothorax. **DATA ACQUIRED:** Tissue specimens are embedded in paraffin and sectioned for staining and histologic examination. Direct staining of flesh or frozen tissue can be done as well. Tissue can also be cultured.

Specimen Bronchial or lung parenchymal tissue. **CONTAINER:** Tissues are placed in jar of formalin for histologic studies and sterile saline for culture. **CAUSES FOR REJECTION:** Inadequate tissue sample. **TURNAROUND TIME:** 24-48 hours; 3-4 days if special stains are performed.

Interpretation **NORMAL FINDINGS:** Normal pulmonary parenchyma **LIMITATIONS:** Due to sampling error, the tissue obtained via biopsy may not reflect the entire pulmonary pathogenic process. Clinical correlation is required to assess the significance of the pathogenic findings.

Footnotes

1. Koontz CH, Joyner LR, and Nelson RA, "Transbronchial Lung Biopsy via the Fiberoptic Bronchoscope in Sarcoidosis," *Ann Intern Med*, 1976, 85:64-6.
2. Khan MA, Corona F, Masson RG, et al, "Transbronchial Lung Biopsy for Sarcoidosis," *N Engl J Med*, 1976, 295:225.
3. Wall CP, Gaensler EA, Carrington CB, et al, "Comparison of Transbronchial and Open Biopsies in Chronic Infiltrative Lung Diseases," *Am Rev Respir Dis*, 1981, 123:280-5.
4. Popovich J, Kvale PA, Eichenhorn MS, et al, "Diagnostic Accuracy of Multiple Biopsies From Flexible Fiberoptic Bronchoscopy: A Comparison of Central Versus Peripheral Carcinoma," *Am Rev Respir Dis*, 1982, 125:521-3.
5. Cortese DA and McDougall JC, "Biopsy and Brushing of Peripheral Lung Cancer With Fluoroscopic Guidance," *Chest*, 1979, 75:141-5.
6. Herf SM and Suratt PM, "Complications of Transbronchial Lung Biopsies," *Chest*, 1978, 73(suppl):759-60.
7. Ahmad M, Livingston DR, Golish JA, et al, "The Safety of Outpatient Transbronchial Biopsy," *Chest*, 1986, 90:403-5.
8. Zavala DC, "Transbronchial Biopsy in Diffuse Lung Disease," *Chest*, 1978, 73:727-33.

References

Kovalski R, Hansen-Flaschen J, Lodato RF, et al, "Localized Leukemic Infiltrates. Diagnosis by Bronchoscopy and Resolution With Therapy," *Chest*, 1990, 97(3):674-8.

Brush Biopsy *see* Bronchial Brushings *on page 258*

Conventional Bilateral Bronchography Via a Nasotracheal Catheter *replaced by* Localized Bronchogram *on next page*

Endobronchial Biopsy

CPT 31625

Abstract **INDICATIONS:** Diagnostic yield for malignant neoplasm is slightly greater than that for brushings, however, this is dependent on each particular institution. It can also be useful in the diagnosis of endobronchial sarcoid granulomatous infection, polyps, and benign tumor. **CONTRAINDICATIONS:** Similar indications that apply to bronchoscopy as well as any uncorrected bleeding diatheses, uremia, pulmonary hypertension, mechanical ventilation, or severe anemia.

Patient Care/Scheduling **PATIENT PREPARATION:** NPO after midnight for a morning bronchoscopy and NPO after light breakfast for afternoon procedures. Routine medications (especially antiasthmatic drugs) may be taken at any time with a small amount of water. Routine lab work including clotting times, BUN, CBC, and platelet count is essential to exclude a coagulopathy – especially if a biopsy is to be performed. Some measure of pulmonary function is useful (spirometry, blood gases) to assess pulmonary reserve and docu-

(Continued)

Endobronchial Biopsy *(Continued)*

ment bronchospasm. Premedication with a narcotic (meperidine 25-75 mg) or minor tranquilizer (diazepam 10 mg) is given parenterally 15-30 minutes before the procedure. Atropine 0.4 mg I.M. is given as a vagolytic agent at the same time unless contraindicated by the presence of arrhythmia, narrow angle glaucoma or urinary retention. **AFTERCARE:** NPO for 2 hours or longer after the procedure until the gag reflex is fully recovered. Because of the premedication, outpatients are not allowed to drive until the following day. Transient fever and mild hemoptysis may be noted for the next 24 hours. **COMPLICATIONS:** Occasionally, endobronchial bleeding may occur. It is usually quite mild and self-limited; suctioning and local instillation of epinephrine is normally all that is required for treatment.

Method **EQUIPMENT:** Several types of forceps are available including small and large "alligator" forceps, cup forceps, and curette. The small "alligator" forceps are preferred because of the generally larger pieces of tissue obtained with a minimum of bleeding or crush artifact. **TECHNIQUE:** The bronchoscope is passed transorally or transnasally in the usual manner. Biopsy forceps are passed down the bronchoscope channel. The forceps are then positioned next to the lesion in question, the jaws are opened and closed upon the tissue. The tissue is then removed. The biopsy forceps are removed through the channel of the bronchoscope or the entire bronchoscope is pulled out through an endotracheal tube without passing the forceps through the bronchoscope channel. The tissue is then gently eased out of the forceps and transferred into a container with formalin for fixation. For large pieces of tissue which cannot be passed through the bronchoscopic channel, continuous suction can be applied and the entire bronchoscope can be withdrawn so the specimen can be retrieved. **DATA ACQUIRED:** Tissue specimens are embedded in paraffin and sectioned for staining and histologic examination. Furthermore, tissue can be directly plated and cultured.

Specimen Endobronchial tissue **COLLECTION:** Tissues are placed in a jar of formalin for histologic studies and in sterile saline for culture. **CAUSES FOR REJECTION:** Inadequate tissue **TURNAROUND TIME:** 48 hours.

Interpretation **NORMAL FINDINGS:** Normal bronchial mucosa **LIMITATIONS:** Sampling error can occasionally lead to faulty interpretation of malignancy as a benign lesion. **ADDITIONAL INFORMATION:** Specimens can also be retrieved and processed for cultures and for touch prep to rule out opportunistic organisms such as *Pneumocystis carinii* or to look for viral inclusions.

References

Fulkerson WJ, "Fiberoptic Bronchoscopy: Current Concepts," *N Engl J Med*, 1984, 311(8):511-50.

Tanaka M, Kohda E, Satoh M, et al, "Diagnosis of Peripheral Lung Cancer Using a New Type of Endoscope," *Chest*, 1990, 97(5):1231-4.

Flexible Bronchoscopy *see* Bronchoscopy, Fiberoptic *on page 260*

Forceps Biopsy *see* Bronchoscopy, Transbronchial Biopsy *on page 262*

Localized Bronchogram

CPT 31656

Related Information

Bronchogram *on page 291*

Synonyms Localized Bronchography

Replaces Conventional Bilateral Bronchography Via a Nasotracheal Catheter

Abstract **INDICATIONS:** To document radiographically localized bronchiectasis in patients with recurrent pneumonias or chronic purulent sputum production **CONTRAINDICATIONS:** Same as with bronchoscopy with addition of hypersensitivity to iodine-based dye.

Patient Care/Scheduling **PATIENT PREPARATION:** NPO after midnight for a morning bronchoscopy and NPO after light breakfast for afternoon procedures. Routine medications (especially antiasthmatic drugs) may be taken at any time with a small amount of water. Routine lab work including clotting times, BUN, CBC, and platelet count is essential to exclude a coagulopathy – especially if a biopsy is to be performed. Some measure of pulmonary function is useful (spirometry, blood gases) to assess pulmonary reserve and document bronchospasm. Premedication with a narcotic (meperidine 25-75 mg) or minor tranquilizer (diazepam 10 mg) is given parenterally 15-30 minutes before the procedure. Atropine 0.4 mg I.M. is given as a vagolytic agent at the same time unless contraindicated by the presence of arrhythmia, narrow angle glaucoma, or urinary retention. **AFTERCARE:** Same as for Bronchoscopy, Fiberoptic. Patients typically experience more coughing after a bronchogram. Patient is returned to floor or clinic for observation. Encourage cough and postural drainage for 1 hour. Nothing by mouth until gag reflex returns; to be determined by physician. Outpatient, NPO for 3 hours. **SPECIAL INSTRUCTIONS:** Procedure is done in fluoroscopy suite. **COMPLICATIONS:** Hypoxemia may be greater with bronchography than with other bronchoscopic procedures. Therefore, pulse oximetry should be monitored during the procedure, and the oxygen dose should be titrated accordingly.

Method **EQUIPMENT:** 20 mL Dionisol iodine-based dye, bronchoscope **TECHNIQUE:** The bronchoscope is inserted in the usual manner. The area of suspected bronchiectasis is either identified on chest x-ray or endobronchially. The bronchoscope is wedged in a lobar or segmental bronchus, or utilizing the bronchoscope, a separate catheter is placed. Dionisol (10-20 mL prewarmed) is rapidly injected through the bronchoscope channel or other tube and monitored fluoroscopically. Still pictures are taken as well. **DATA ACQUIRED:** Radiographs of contrast-filled bronchi in the area of suspected bronchiectasis.

Interpretation **NORMAL FINDINGS:** Normal endobronchial anatomy. **LIMITATIONS:** Unlike complete bronchography, localized bronchoscopy does not show bronchial anatomy throughout the entire tracheobronchial tree, and therefore, if surgical resection is contemplated, an assessment of both lungs is recommended. **ADDITIONAL INFORMATION:** Although uncommon today due to widespread use of antibiotics, bronchiectasis still occurs. Frequently the bronchiectasis results from endobronchial obstruction (right middle lobe syndrome). Bronchography can help document this disorder and thereby ensure proper treatment. Localized bronchography is tolerated better by the patient than the complete study.

References

Fennessy JJ, "Selective Catheterization of Segmental Bronchi With the Aid of a Flexible Fiberoptic Bronchoscope," *Radiology*, 1970, 95:689-91.

Flower CDR and Shnurson JM, "Bronchography via the Fiberoptic Bronchoscope," *Thorax*, 1984, 39:260-3.

Jenkins P, Dick R, and Clarke SW, "Selective Bronchography Using the Fiberoptic Bronchoscope," *Br J Dis Chest*, 1982, 76:88-90.

Saha SP, Mayo P, Long GA, et al, "Middle Lobe Syndrome: Diagnosis and Management," *Ann Thorac Surg*, 1982, 33:28-31.

Taber RE, "Bronchography After Bronchoscopy," *Ann Thorac Surg*, 1984, 37:264.

Localized Bronchography *see* Localized Bronchogram *on previous page*

Open Tube Bronchoscope *see* Rigid Bronchoscopy *on this page*

Pleural Fluid "Tap" *see* Thoracentesis *on page 267*

Rigid Bronchoscopy

CPT 31622

Synonyms Open Tube Bronchoscope

Abstract **PROCEDURE COMMONLY INCLUDES:** Visual examination of trachea and bronchi under general anesthesia. **INDICATIONS:** The indications for rigid bronchoscopy are generally therapeutic: removal of foreign bodies, control of massive hemoptysis, and endobronchial laser photoresection. The large channel and wide field of vision make this instrument ideal for removing foreign bodies or debulking endobronchial tumors. Some have advocated the use of the flexible scope for removal of foreign bodies however.[1] It has also been utilized when endobronchial lesions have evaded fiberoptic bronchogenic diagnosis. Larger biopsies are feasible. **CONTRAINDICATIONS:** All contraindications are relative if this procedure is being done for life-threatening reasons. Otherwise, the typical contraindications to any general surgical procedure apply.

Patient Care/Scheduling **PATIENT PREPARATION:** Rigid bronchoscopy is a surgical procedure done under general anesthesia. **AFTERCARE:** Routine postoperative care. **COMPLICATIONS:** Hemorrhage and ventilatory insufficiency.

(Continued)

Rigid Bronchoscopy *(Continued)*

Method EQUIPMENT: Rigid bronchoscope, fiberoptic telescope, directable optical forceps for upper lobe biopsy TECHNIQUE: Procedure is done under general anesthesia with ventilation carried out using side arm or high frequency jet ventilator. The neck is hyperextended and the scope is introduced into the trachea. Bleeding sites can be visualized; foreign bodies may be removed. Biopsies of suspicious lesions may be obtained. A large array of instruments are available for use with the rigid scope. It is particularly well-suited for laser photoresection of large central endobronchial tumors. DATA ACQUIRED: Visual examination of the central airways.

Specimen If diagnosis of malignancy is sought bronchial washings and endobronchial biopsies may be obtained.

Interpretation NORMAL FINDINGS: Potency and normality of the central airways LIMITATIONS: Ineffective in evaluating or retrieving objects from lower lobe distal airways. Visualization of upper lobes may be limited due to inability to angulate the rigid bronchoscope.

Footnotes

1. Cunanan OS, "The Flexible Fiberoptic Bronchoscope in Foreign Body Removal: Experience in 300 Cases," *Chest*, 1978, 73(suppl):725-6.

References

Holinger PH and Holinger LD, "Use of the Open Tube Bronchoscope in the Extraction of Foreign Bodies," *Chest*, 1978, 73:721-4.

Núñez H, Perez-Rodriquez E, Alvarado C, et al, "Foreign Body Aspirate Extraction," *Chest*, 1989, 96(3):698.

Simpson GT, "Rigid vs Flexible Bronchoscopy for Foreign Body Aspiration," *N Engl J Med*, 1984, 310:1190-1.

Sputum Collection *see* Sputum Induction *on this page*

Sputum Induction

CPT 89350

Synonyms Sputum Collection

Abstract PROCEDURE COMMONLY INCLUDES: Induction of sputum expectoration by inhaling nebulized pyrogen-free or 3% saline INDICATIONS: To collect noninvasive sputum specimen for microbiology or cytology in patients with suspected malignancy or respiratory infections, but unable to expectorate sputum. This technique has been shown to be 94% sensitive in the diagnosis of *Pneumocystis* pneumonia associated with AIDS. More invasive procedures, such as bronchoscopy, may be avoided.[1] CONTRAINDICATIONS: Asthma, respiratory distress, bronchospasm.

Patient Care/Scheduling PATIENT PREPARATION: The teeth should be brushed and mouth rinsed and gargled to remove debris and other contaminating materials. SPECIAL INSTRUCTIONS: Patient must be able to cough deeply and vigorously. COMPLICATIONS: Although rib fractures due to vigorous coughing are possible they have not been reported.

Method EQUIPMENT: Ultrasonic nebulizer TECHNIQUE: Pyrogen-free or 3% saline is administered to the patient by ultrasonic nebulizer for 5-15 minutes. This saturates the airways, liquifies thick sputum, and leads to a productive cough. The expectorated sputum is then collected in a specimen container.

Specimen Sputum CONTAINER: Sterile, leakproof, screw capped jars STORAGE INSTRUCTIONS: Place the specimen in a plastic, sterile, airtight container to prevent dehydration. It should be immediately stained and plated for culture. CAUSES FOR REJECTION: >25 squamous epithelial cells/lpf is indicative of oropharyngeal contamination. A preponderance of neutrophils, ciliated epithelial cells, or alveolar macrophages with <10 squamous epithelial cells/lpf indicates lower respiratory secretions warranting culture.[2] TURNAROUND TIME: Specimen immediately transferred to laboratory. Test results determine turnaround time.

Interpretation NORMAL FINDINGS: No malignant cells and no pathogenic organisms found LIMITATIONS: Weak cough, sputum tenacious and difficult to expectorate, patient not alert enough to cough ADDITIONAL INFORMATION: If patient unable to cough, may use orotracheal or nasotracheal suction catheter to aspirate specimen.

Footnotes

1. Kovacs JA, Ng VL, Masur H, et al, "Diagnosis of *Pneumocystis carinii* Pneumonia: Improved Detection in Sputum With Use of Monoclonal Antibodies," *N Engl J Med*, 1988, 318(10):589-93.
2. Geckler DW, Gremillion DH, McAllister CK, et al, "Microscopic and Bacteriological Comparison of Paired Sputa and Transtracheal Aspirate," *J Clin Microbiol*, 1977, 6:396-9.

References

Leigh TR, Parsons P, Hume C, et al, "Sputum Induction for Diagnosis of *Pneumocystis carinii* Pneumonia," *Lancet*, 1989, 2(8656):205-6.

Thoracentesis

CPT 32000

Related Information

Pleural Biopsy *on page 68*
Ultrasound, Thoracentesis *on page 412*

Synonyms Pleural Fluid "Tap"

Abstract **PROCEDURE COMMONLY INCLUDES:** At the bedside, a physician utilizes a needle and catheter system to withdraw fluid from a patient with radiographically demonstrable pleural effusion for diagnostic or therapeutic purposes. **INDICATIONS:** The major diagnostic indication is the presence of pleural fluid of unclear etiology. In those instances where the etiology of a pleural effusion is clinically apparent, thoracentesis may be deferred at physician's discretion. For example, the patient with recurrent congestive heart failure who presents with typical left ventricular failure and pleural effusion may appropriately undergo a trial of diuresis prior to thoracentesis.[1] The major therapeutic indication for thoracentesis is respiratory compromise secondary to a large pleural effusion. Less commonly, the procedure may be used to evacuate trapped air in the pleural space (rather than fluid) as with a tension pneumothorax. **CONTRAINDICATIONS:** Platelet count $<50,000/mm^3$; severe, uncorrectable coagulopathy; effusions <10 mm thick on decubitus radiograph[2] (or effusions not freely movable on decubitus radiograph); inability to define rib landmarks (necessary for proper needle placement); an uncooperative patient, unable to sit immobile. Other high-risk situations, not necessarily representing contraindications, include: mechanical ventilation with positive end expiratory pressure (PEEP); severe emphysema with blebs; patients who have undergone pneumonectomy with pleural effusion located on the side of the remaining lung. In these instances, ultrasound or CT guided aspiration of pleural fluid may be more prudent; a common complication such as pneumothorax could have profound consequences.

Patient Care/Scheduling **PATIENT PREPARATION:** Technique and risks of procedure are explained and consent is obtained. Chest x-ray is routinely performed prior to procedure, including a PA, lateral, and lateral decubitus view, and should be available for physician review. Recent prothrombin, partial thromboplastin time, and platelet count on the chart. Laboratory requisitions completed in advance. Premedication for pain (such as parenteral meperidine) is rarely required and local anesthesia during the procedure is usually sufficient. **AFTERCARE:** Immediately postprocedure, a "stat" chest x-ray is performed, usually at end-expiration. Vital signs must be monitored closely, especially if >1 L fluid is removed. Hypoxemia is a known complication of thoracentesis and some patients may require temporary supplemented oxygen.[3] If dyspnea or hypotension develops, physician must be contacted promptly. Otherwise, if vital signs and postprocedure chest x-ray are satisfactory, patient activity may be ad lib. **COMPLICATIONS:** Although numerous complications have been reported, diagnostic thoracentesis is generally at low risk.[1] Complications may be classified as traumatic or nontraumatic. Nontraumatic complications are related to predictable physiologic responses and include:

- syncope
- cough
- hypotension, either immediate (vasovagal reaction) or delayed (fluid shifts)
- noncardiogenic pulmonary edema (following rapid expansion of a collapsed lung, especially on removal of large volumes of a chronic effusion)
- hypoxemia; PaO_2 may drop by 10 mm Hg within minutes and not return to baseline until the following day. Some authorities recommend supplemental oxygen routinely.[4]

(Continued)

Thoracentesis *(Continued)*

Traumatic complications are iatrogenic and include:

- pneumothorax, simple or tension (requiring chest tube); lateral decubitus radiograph demonstrating a pleural effusion <10 mm thick substantially increases the risk of pneumothorax
- hemothorax
- laceration of intercostal artery, potentially lethal
- puncture of liver or spleen
- miscellaneous, subcutaneous emphysema, air embolism, infection

Of note, the recovery of a grossly bloody pleural effusion (RBC >100,000/mm^3) does not automatically imply needle trauma since blood may be seen in several pleural diseases as well. To differentiate this, traumatic effusions tend to clot rapidly and become more clear as serial samples are withdrawn; bloody effusions from pleural disease generally are slow to clot due to defibrination over time.[5] In doubtful cases, a hematocrit should be obtained on the bloody effusion and compared with plasma hematocrit.

Method **EQUIPMENT:** Several complete thoracentesis kits are available commercially. Alternatively, individual components commonly found in most clinics and hospitals may be assembled separately. Common items include sterile drapes, iodine, alcohol pads, gauze, local anesthesia (1% lidocaine), at least four sterile tubes, syringes, and anaerobic culture media. Two red top tubes and two lavender top (EDTA containing) tubes may be used in place of the four sterile tubes. If cytologic studies are planned, heparin (1:1000) is needed as an additive. If pleural fluid pH is planned, a heparinized syringe and ice bag are needed. Several needle and catheter assemblies are available. For diagnostic thoracentesis (only 50-100 mL fluid removed), a 2" angiocatheter is convenient (18- or 20-gauge needle within catheter). For therapeutic thoracentesis with >1 L removed, a catheter within needle arrangement is effective. A 12" long plastic catheter (16-gauge) within a 14-gauge needle allows more complete pleural space drainage. Also required are liter-sized vacuum bottles and connecting tubing for collection of large volumes of fluid. Commercial thoracentesis kits represent variations of the above and are most useful when >1 L fluid is to be removed. **TECHNIQUE:** Ideally, patient is positioned so that he is seated and leaning forward slightly, arms crossed in front and resting comfortably on a bedside table. The highest level of pleural effusion is determined on physical examination and a mark is placed one intercostal space below. The area is prepped and draped, and the skin and subcutaneous tissues are infiltrated with local anesthetic. Generally, the site is located 5-10 cm lateral to the spine, near the posterior axillary line. At this point technique varies with equipment used. If a catheter within needle is used, the needle (14-gauge) is passed bevel down over the superior aspect of the rib in the anesthetized intercostal space (avoiding the neurovascular bundle). Once the needle has penetrated the parietal pleura and fluid easily aspirated, the smaller plastic catheter (16-gauge) can be advanced its entire length into the pleural space. The needle is then completely withdrawn through the skin. Pleural fluid can be aspirated through the plastic catheter into a 50 mL syringe. Multiple samples of 50 mL may be obtained in this fashion. Alternatively, the catheter may be attached to sterile connecting tubing and fluid collected with liter-sized vacuum bottles. Once the desired amount is obtained, the catheter is pulled out completely and pressure held over the puncture site. If an angiocatheter is used (needle within catheter), the technique is similar. Immediately after collection, serum is drawn for LDH, protein, and further additional studies depending on the clinical situation (see interpretation).

Specimen For diagnostic thoracentesis, 50-100 mL is adequate for routine studies. If cytology desired, larger volumes have been recommended (100-250 mL), although occasionally as little as 5 mL have been sufficient.[6] For therapeutic thoracentesis, removal of 1000-1500 mL is generally well tolerated. **CONTAINER:** Lavender top tube for cell count, red top tube for chemistries, sterile syringe adequate for transport to Microbiology Laboratory. For cytology samples add 5000-10,000 units of heparin into syringe or vacuum bottle and label. For pleural fluid pH send specimen in anaerobic syringe (air bubbles removed) on ice immediately to acute care (blood gas) laboratory. **COLLECTION:** Samples should be hand carried to respective laboratories immediately. **CAUSES FOR REJECTION:** Lack of heparin additive to cytology (or cell count, if plain glass tube used in place of lavender top tube), improper collection technique for pH (not on ice).

Interpretation **NORMAL FINDINGS:** Pleural effusions are traditionally classified as either "transudates" or "exudates" based on the underlying mechanism of pleural fluid formation. This is the first and most crucial step in pleural fluid analysis. Transudates are ultrafiltrates of plasma which result from alterations in the osmotic or hydrostatic focus across pleural membranes. The pleural surface itself is usually disease-free. Examples include congestive heart failure (elevated hydrostatic pressure), nephrotic syndrome, and other hypoproteinemic states (decreased oncotic pressure), cirrhosis, myxedema, sarcoidosis, and Meig's syndrome. Exudates occur when the pleural membrane is involved in a disease process which increases pleural capillary permeability or obstructs lymphatics. Causes of exudates include pulmonary infections (pneumonia, empyema, abscess), malignancy (mesothelioma or metastases), collagen vascular diseases, pulmonary embolism, gastrointestinal diseases (pancreatitis, esophageal rupture), hemothorax, chylothorax, and miscellaneous causes such as postmyocardial infarction syndrome, uremia, and postradiation. In general, discovering a transudate allows therapy to be focused on the underlying systemic disease causing the effusion (eg, cirrhosis). Further studies of the pleural space are not necessary. Discovering an exudate, however, is more ominous and mandates additional, thorough diagnostic testing to rule out entities such as occult malignancy and pleural space infection. **CRITICAL VALUES:** The following biochemical criteria were found by Light to accurately predict an exudate:[7]

- pleural fluid protein to serum protein ratio >0.5
- pleural fluid LDH to serum LDH ratio >0.6
- pleural fluid LDH >200 units/mL (or >2/3 the upper limit of normal of serum LDH)

Exudates satisfy one or more of these three criteria. Effusions are classified as transudates only if none of the these criteria are met. Misclassification rate is <1%, based on several prospective studies.[7,8] In the past, specific gravity (SG) was used as the sole criteria for separating transudates (SG <1.016) from exudates (SG >1.016). Despite its appeal as a simple and inexpensive test, it is no longer recommended due to its high misclassification rate (≤30%). Similarly, older criteria using pleural fluid protein alone to differentiate transudates (protein <3 mg/dL) from exudates (>3 mg/dL) carries a misclassification rate near 15% and should no longer be used.

ADDITIONAL INFORMATION: Supplemental tests are available for more specific evaluation of the exudate. To minimize expense, test selection should be based on the differential diagnosis of an individual case. Malignant effusions are often grossly bloody with RBCs from 5000-100,000/mm^3. Cytologic exam is initially positive for malignancy in approximately 60% of cases of later documented pleural malignancy; if three separate samples are sent, yield improves to 90%.[5] Pleural fluid pH is often <7.3 and glucose is low (<60 mg/dL) in 15% of cases.[6] In patients with empyema, enormous numbers of polymorphonuclear cells are present in pleural fluid. Parapneumonic effusions are sterile effusions secondary to pneumonia and require pleural pH measurement for optimal management. A pH <7.2, in the absence of systemic acidosis, indicates that the effusion will behave clinically like an empyema and will require chest tube drainage for resolution.[9,10] Note that pleural fluid pH <7.2 may occur in other conditions (malignancy, TB, rheumatoid arthritis) which do not necessarily require tube thoracotomy. Tuberculosis effusions are characterized by WBC count >10,000/mm^3 with >50% small lymphocytes. This latter finding is highly suggestive of either TB or malignancy and may warrant pleural biopsy. Mesothelial cells are absent in tuberculous effusions; some authors feel that the presence >1% mesothelial cells effectively rules out TB. AFB stains alone are initially positive in only 25% of proven cases. Rheumatoid effusions characteristically have low glucose levels and a value >30 mg/dL makes the diagnosis doubtful. Pleural pH levels are quite low (often <7). Rheumatoid factor testing on pleural fluid is nonspecific and not clinically useful. In suspected lupus effusions, the finding of lupus erythematosus (LE) cells in pleural fluid is pathognomonic for systemic lupus erythematosus. Effusions associated with both pancreatitis and esophageal rupture have similar laboratory profiles. Amylase levels are elevated >160 units/L with both esophageal rupture (salivary amylase) and pancreatitis (pancreatic amylase). Pleural fluid pH is low in both cases, and may be <7 with esophageal rupture.

Footnotes

1. Health and Public Policy Committee, American College of Physicians, "Diagnostic Thoracentesis and Pleural Biopsy in Pleural Effusions," *Ann Intern Med*, 1985, 103:799-802.
2. Light RW, *Pleural Diseases*, Philadelphia, PA: Lea & Febiger, 1983.
3. Brandstetter RD and Cohen BP, "Hypoxemia After Thoracentesis: A Predictable and Treatable Condition," 1979, 242(10):1060-1.

(Continued)

Thoracentesis *(Continued)*

4. Jay SJ, "Pleural Effusions: Preliminary Evaluation – Recognition of the Transudate," *Postgrad Med*, 1986, 80:165-77.
5. Light RW, "Pleural Effusions," *Med Clin North Am*, 1977, 61:1339-52.
6. Prakash UB, "Malignant Pleural Effusions," *Postgrad Med*, 1986, 80:201-9.
7. Light RW, MacGregor MI, and Luchsinger PC, "Pleural Effusions: The Diagnostic Separation of Transudates and Exudates," *Ann Intern Med*, 1972, 77:507-13.
8. Paradis IL and Caldwell EJ, "Diagnostic Approach to Pleural Effusion," *J Main Med Assoc*, 1977, 68:378-82.
9. Light RW, "Management of Parapneumonic Effusions," *Arch Intern Med*, 1981, 141:1339-41.
10. Light RW, Girard WM, Jenkinson SG, et al, "Parapneumonic Effusions," *Am J Med*, 1980, 69:507-12.

References

Corwin RW and Irwin RS, "Thoracentesis," *Intensive Care Med*, 3rd ed, Rippe JM, Irwin RS, Alpert JS, et al, eds, Boston, MA: Little, Brown and Co, 1985, 121-7.

Hausheer FH and Yarbro JW, "Diagnosis and Treatment of Malignant Pleural Effusion," *Semin Oncol*, 1985, 12:54-75.

Grogan DR, Irwin RS, Channick R, et al, "Complications Associated With Thoracentesis. A Prospective, Randomized Study Comparing Three Different Methods," *Arch Intern Med*, 1990, 150(4):873-7.

McVay PA and Toy PT, "Lack of Increased Bleeding After Paracentesis and Thoracentesis in Patients With Mild Coagulation Abnormalities," *Transfusion*, 1991, 31(2):164-71.

Sahn SA, "The Differential Diagnosis of Pleural Effusions," *West J Med*, 1982, 137:99-108.

Transbronchial Needle Aspiration

CPT 31629

Synonyms Wang Needle Aspiration

Abstract **PROCEDURE COMMONLY INCLUDES:** Bronchoscopic examination with washings, brushings, and biopsies if indicated. The transbronchial needle is used to sample nodal or tissue areas immediately adjacent to the central airways. **INDICATIONS:** Originally developed as a method to histologically stage bronchogenic carcinoma, this method has gained widespread acceptance as an adjunct in the diagnosis of suspected peribronchial carcinoma.[1] Several studies have shown an increased diagnostic yield utilizing the transbronchial needle in lesions which present as extrinsic compression of the central airways.[2,3] Also, in selected patients who have radiographic evidence of subcarinal or paratracheal nodal enlargement in the setting of known bronchogenic carcinoma, a positive diagnosis on transbronchial needle aspiration obviates the need for mediastinoscopy or thoracotomy. In several case reports, a large 18-gauge needle has been utilized to obtain histologic specimens for diagnosis of sarcoid mediastinal adenopathy. **CONTRAINDICATIONS:** Uncorrected bleeding diathesis, severe pulmonary hypertension, unstable cardiorespiratory status (relative), active bronchospasm.

Patient Care/Scheduling **PATIENT PREPARATION:** Exactly the same as for Bronchoscopy, Fiberoptic and Transbronchial Biopsy. **AFTERCARE:** Similar to Bronchoscopy, Fiberoptic. The major complication of transbronchial needle aspiration is bleeding. **SPECIAL INSTRUCTIONS:** Various needles are available including 20- and 18-gauge. **COMPLICATIONS:** Detailed knowledge of normal endobronchial and vascular anatomy is essential to minimize bleeding complications. However, even if a vascular structure is entered, the bleeding usually spontaneously resolves upon withdrawal of the needle.

Method **EQUIPMENT:** 22- and 18-gauge Wang transbronchial needle **TECHNIQUE:** Procedure is carried out during fiberoptic bronchoscopy. A catheter with a 22-gauge, 13 mm hollow needle is inserted through the channel of the bronchoscope. Once the tip of the catheter clears the distal end of the bronchoscope, the needle is advanced into the airway lumen and locked in place. The needle is then directed perpendicular to the tracheobronchial wall adjacent to the area to be sampled. The needle punctures the wall and is advanced completely to the hub. The guide wire is removed and negative pressure is applied using a 50 mL syringe primed with a small amount (5 mL) of normal saline. The needle and catheter are completely withdrawn from the channel of the scope and the first drop of the specimen is directly placed onto a dry slide and immersed in fixative. The remaining material is sent for cell block. Generally the procedure is repeated again.[4]

Specimen Aspirated cellular material or biopsy specimen **CONTAINER:** Material directly placed on slide and also flushed into dry container; biopsies are transported in formalin **CAUSES FOR REJECTION:** Insufficient cellular material **TURNAROUND TIME:** A wet reading can be given immediately. Final cytologic or histologic diagnosis generally takes 24-48 hours.

Interpretation **NORMAL FINDINGS:** Nonmalignant cytology does not rule out carcinoma adjacent to the central airways. **LIMITATIONS:** Caution is advised in interpreting a malignant transbronchial needle aspirate in the face of positive bronchial washings, especially when nodal enlargement is lacking, as false-positives have been reported.[5,6]

Footnotes

1. Wang KP, Marsh BR, Summer WR, et al, "Transbronchial Needle Aspiration for the Diagnosis of Lung Carcinoma," *Chest*, 1981, 80:48-50.
2. Shure D and Fedullo PF, "Transbronchial Needle Aspiration in the Diagnosis of Submucosal and Peribronchial Bronchogenic Carcinoma," *Chest*, 1985, 88:49-51.
3. Tita JA, Livingston DR, Mehta AC, et al, "Diagnostic Utility of Transbronchial Needle Aspiration in Bronchogenic Carcinoma Presenting as Extrinsic Compression," *Chest*, 1986, 89:449S, (abstract).
4. Wang KP and Terry PB, "Transbronchial Needle Aspiration in the Diagnosis and Staging of Bronchogenic Carcinoma," *Am Rev Respir Dis*, 1983, 127:344-7.
5. Sehenk DA, Chasen MH, McCarthy MF, et al, "Potential False-Positive Mediastinal Transbronchial Needle Aspiration in Bronchogenic Carcinoma," *Chest*, 1986, 4:649-50.
6. Cropp AJ, Dimaro AF, and Laukeroni M, "False-Positive Transbronchial Needle Aspiration in Bronchogenic Carcinoma," *Chest*, 1985, 5:696-7.

References

Mehta AC, Kavuru MS, Meeker DP, et al, "Transbronchial Needle Aspiration for Histology Specimens," *Chest*, 1989, 96(6):1228-32.

Shure D and Fedullo PF, "The Role of Transcarinal Needle Aspiration in the Staging of Bronchogenic Carcinoma," *Chest*, 1986, 5:693-6.

Wang KP, "Flexible Transbronchial Needle Aspiration Biopsy for Histologic Specimens," *Chest*, 1985, 88:860-3.

Transbronchoscopic Biopsy *see* Bronchoscopy, Transbronchial Biopsy *on page 262*

Trephine Drill Biopsy *replaced by* Bronchoscopy, Transbronchial Biopsy *on page 262*

Wang Needle Aspiration *see* Transbronchial Needle Aspiration *on previous page*

IMAGING PROCEDURES

COMPUTED TOMOGRAPHY

Peter B. O'Donovan, MD

In 1917, an Austrian mathematician named Radon, showed that a three-dimensional likeness of an object could be reconstructed from an infinite number of two-dimensional projections of that object. At the time, Radon was working with equations, describing gravitational fields. It was from this work that the principle of computed tomography evolved.[1]

Work done independently by Houndsfield in Nottinghamshire, England and Cormack at Tufts University in Boston, culminated in the application of this principle to clinical imaging and resulted in them sharing the Nobel prize for medicine and physiology in 1979. The first commercially produced scanners were made by EMI Limited of England and designed for brain scanning. These were placed in hospitals in England and the United States in the summer of 1973 and required 4½ minutes to produce two axial images of the brain. Today, less than 20 years later, scan times of 2 seconds or less are routinely available. Computed tomographic imaging is available in most community hospitals and has made a significant contribution to medical diagnosis and has aided in the physician's understanding of the natural history of disease.

[1] Hendee WR, PhD, "Cross-Sectional Medical Imaging: A History," *Radiographics*, 1989, 9(6):1155.

Abdomen, CT *see* Computed Transaxial Tomography, Abdomen Studies *on this page*

Arthrography, CT *see* Computed Transaxial Tomography, Arthrography *on next page*

Bone Densitometry, CT *see* Computed Transaxial Tomography, Bone Densitometry *on next page*

Brain, CT *see* Computed Transaxial Tomography, Head Studies *on page 277*

Cervical Spine, CT *see* Computed Transaxial Tomography, Spine *on page 282*

Computed Transaxial Tomography, Abdomen Studies

CPT 74150 (without contrast); 74160 (with contrast); 74170 (with and without contrast)

Related Information

Computed Transaxial Tomography, Pelvis *on page 281*

Synonyms Abdomen, CT; CT, Lower Abdomen; CT, Total Abdomen; CT, Upper Abdomen

Abstract PROCEDURE COMMONLY INCLUDES: CT scan of liver, spleen, kidneys, pancreas, aorta, retroperitoneum, gastrointestinal tract, pelvis. **Note:** In some departments, a request for a CT study of the abdomen will yield a study extending inferiorly to the pubic symphysis. In others, the study will extend only to the pelvic brim. See Computed Transaxial Tomography, Pelvis. INDICATIONS: Diagnosis and/or evaluation of cysts, tumors, masses, aneurysm, metastases, abscesses, and trauma. The modality is also often used for staging of known tumors. CONTRAINDICATIONS: Patient cooperation is of the utmost importance as the examination requires the patient to remain motionless for the duration of the study. The time of the study will vary from 20-40 minutes depending on the equipment being used. Children and uncooperative adults may require sedation.

Patient Care/Scheduling PATIENT PREPARATION: Patient's oral intake restricted to fluid only for 4 hours prior to the examination. Medication schedule should not be interrupted. Should the patient have recently undergone a barium examination of the gastrointestinal tract, a digital radiograph obtained with the scanner prior to commencement of the procedure may be helpful in excluding the presence of barium within the bowel. The latter may produce significant artifact and thus render the study nondiagnostic. Where possible, all CT scan studies of the abdomen should be performed prior to normal GI barium studies. A recent serum creatinine is requested on all patients 60 years of age and older, patients with known significant atherosclerotic disease, diabetes mellitus, or with pre-existing renal disease. Intravenous contrast material is routinely administered for this examination. Physician may opt to omit intravenous contrast. Patients undergoing a CT study of the abdomen are requested to drink approximately 450 mL of a dilute barium solution (approximately 1% barium) commencing 1 hour prior to the examination. Inclusion of the pelvis in this examination requires further patient preparation. See Computed Transaxial Tomography, Pelvis. SPECIAL INSTRUCTIONS: CT scan of the abdomen may be requested by a practicing physician. The abdominal area of interest should be specified along with pertinent clinical history. This will allow the diagnostic radiologist to tailor the examination for maximum diagnostic yield. For example, studies being performed for detection of renal calculi should be performed without contrast material, as the contrast, when excreted from the kidney, will mask the presence of small calculi within the collecting system. Adequate evaluation of small structures within the abdomen may require modification of technique such as thin slices or overlapping slices. A further example would be in the evaluation of the liver for primary or metastatic tumor. Maximum yield in the demonstration of such abnormalities requires examination both with and without contrast material.

Method EQUIPMENT: This examination may be performed on any one of many commercially available computerized tomography scanners. TECHNIQUE: Standard examination of the abdomen consists of 1 cm contiguous slices obtained from the dome of the diaphragm to the pelvic brim or pubic symphysis depending upon whether one groups the pelvis with the abdomen or treats it separately.

Specimen CAUSES FOR REJECTION: Patients with residual barium within the GI tract from a prior conventional barium study – this nondilute barium produces considerable artifact rendering the examination suboptimal and often nondiagnostic, uncooperative patients who are not candidates for sedation/anesthesia TURNAROUND TIME: A verbal telephone report of the scan will be given to the referring physician if specified. A written report will be available.

Interpretation ADDITIONAL INFORMATION: Patients should be informed that the examination may take 45 minutes to 1 hour and that oral contrast and intravenous contrast are commonly required. If the pelvis is included with the abdominal CT study, rectal contrast material and placement of a vaginal tampon in the case of females may also be required. The patient's medical record should accompany the patient. This will furnish the radiologist with sufficient information to tailor the examination as he/she deems appropriate. For example, patients suspected of an adrenal adenoma may require thin (2 mm) slices through the adrenal glands for the detection of such an abnormality.

References

Halvorsen RA and Thompson WM, "Computed Tomographic Staging of Gastrointestinal Tract Malignancies, Part I. Esophagus and Stomach," *Invest Radiol*, 1987, 22:2-16.

Thompson WM and Halvorsen RA, "Computed Tomographic Staging of Gastrointestinal Tract Malignancies, Part II," *Invest Radiol*, 1987, 22:96.

Computed Transaxial Tomography, Arthrography

CPT 73040 (shoulder); 73085 (elbow); 73115 (wrist); 73200 (upper extremity CT without contrast); 73201 (upper extremity CT with contrast); 73525 (hip); 73580 (knee); 73615 (ankle); 73700 (lower extremity CT without contrast); 73701 (lower extremity CT with contrast) (Note: There are no CPT codes for CT Arthrography at this time. One may choose to combine the CPT code for an extremity CT with that for a radiographic exam of the joint being examined.)

Synonyms Arthrography, CT

Abstract PROCEDURE COMMONLY INCLUDES: CT scanning of any joint subsequent to instillation of air and/or contrast material under fluoroscopic guidance to obtain thin, overlapping slices through the joint in question are obtained. INDICATIONS: CT arthrography of the shoulder is often undertaken to evaluate the unstable shoulder for an abnormality involving the glenoid labrum or in search of an abnormal joint capsule. When performed in the ankle, elbow, and knee joints, it is more frequently done for osteochondritis dissecans and confirmation/localization of a loose body. CONTRAINDICATIONS: Uncooperative patient.

Patient Care/Scheduling PATIENT PREPARATION: No intravenous contrast material is administered for this procedure, therefore no preliminary laboratory work is required. No dietary restrictions. AFTERCARE: Physical exertion should be restricted until the air and contrast material have been reabsorbed through the joint capsule. This is usually complete within 24-36 hours.

Method EQUIPMENT: This examination can be performed on any of the commercially available CT scanners. TECHNIQUE: In the case of the shoulder examinations, a slice thickness of 4 mm with the table incrementing at 3 mm prior to each slice is generally satisfactory. A 2 mm slice with equal or slightly greater table increments may be required in the elbow.

Interpretation ADDITIONAL INFORMATION: The improved spatial resolution afforded by magnetic resonance imaging coupled with the natural contrast that this modality provides may soon supersede CT arthrography in the knee and should advances continue in MR, the CT procedure may be totally replaced.

References

Hall FM, "Arthrography: Past, Present and Future," *AJR*, 1987, 149:561-2.

Sartoris DJ and Resnick D, "MR Imaging of the Musculoskeletal System: Current and Future Status," *AJR*, 1987, 149:457-67.

Computed Transaxial Tomography, Bone Densitometry

CPT 76070

Synonyms Bone Densitometry, CT; Single and Dual Energy Quantitative Computed Tomography

Abstract PROCEDURE COMMONLY INCLUDES: A noninvasive, quantitative bone mineral determination. The technique's usefulness lies in its ability to give a quantitative image. It can be used to measure trabecular, cortical, or integral bone, centrally or peripherally. INDICATIONS: The quantitative CT technique for vertebral mineral determination has been used to study skeletal changes in osteoporosis and other metabolic bone diseases. CONTRAINDICATIONS: Patient cooperation is of the utmost importance as the examination requires the patient to remain motionless for the duration of the study. The time of the study will vary from 10-20 minutes depending on the equipment being used.

(Continued)

Computed Transaxial Tomography, Bone Densitometry *(Continued)*

Patient Care/Scheduling PATIENT PREPARATION: This examination does not require the use of intravenous contrast material. Because of this, there are no dietary restrictions prior to the examination. Medication schedules should not be interrupted. SPECIAL INSTRUCTIONS: The use of computed tomographic scanners for quantitative purposes requires great attention to detail to ensure accurate and precise measurements. The use of a calibration phantom measured simultaneously with the patient is helpful in assuring quality and accuracy.

Method EQUIPMENT: This examination may be performed on most commercially available computed tomography scanners. TECHNIQUE: Generally, a total of four vertebral bodies between T-12 and L-4 are measured. Vertebral bodies with compression deformities are to be avoided. T-12 should also be avoided if the lungs are hyperinflated and the vertebral body remains in the lung field. An 8 or 10 mm thick slice is obtained through the center of each vertebral body. The slice should be obtained with the gantry tilted so that it lies parallel to the end plates of the vertebral body. Baseline and final measurement are to be performed in dual energy mode. Thus, two scans must be obtained through each vertebral body. One of these with a low kilo voltage per (kVp) setting and the second with a high kVp setting. It is important that these two scans are obtained back to back with a minimal time lapse between the acquisitions.

Specimen CAUSES FOR REJECTION: Residual barium in the gastrointestinal tract may produce beam hardening artifact thus negating the value of the study. TURNAROUND TIME: A verbal telephone report of the scan will be given to the referring physician if specified. A written report will be available.

Interpretation ADDITIONAL INFORMATION: It should be noted that table height influences the results. The standard table height should be selected for each commercially available CT scanner. Care should be taken not to include portions of the end plates within the thickness of the scan.

References

Genant HK, "Osteoporosis: Assessment by Quantitative Computer Tomography," *Orthop Clin North Am*, 1985, 16(3):557-68.

Computed Transaxial Tomography, Dynamic Study

CPT Note: This entry describes a technique, rather than a specific examination. Thus it is applicable to many anatomic areas and the appropriate CPT code should be selected.

Synonyms Dynamic Study, CT

Abstract PROCEDURE COMMONLY INCLUDES: Dynamic CT refers to rapid sequential imaging of an anatomic area of interest subsequent to delivery (usually intravenously, rarely intra-arterially) of a bolus of contrast material. While it is possible to extract some physiologic information utilizing this technique, this is not a major indication. INDICATIONS: The examination is most commonly utilized to highlight vasculature thus improving ability to demonstrate thrombosis, aneurysmal dilatation, or differential rate of flow in the case of aortic dissection. The technique may be used for evaluation of vascularity of abnormal masses. The latter may be helpful in the characterization of hepatic lesions such as hemangiomas which commonly demonstrate initial peripheral enhancement with later central enhancement and eventual equalization with the surrounding hepatic parenchyma. CONTRAINDICATIONS: Patient cooperation is of the utmost importance.

Patient Care/Scheduling PATIENT PREPARATION: The reader is referred to Patient Preparation for the area of anatomic interest (eg, for liver, see Computed Transaxial Tomography, Abdomen Studies). SPECIAL INSTRUCTIONS: The reader is referred to the special instructions for the anatomic area of interest (eg, dynamic CT of the chest, see Computed Transaxial Tomography, Thorax).

Method EQUIPMENT: Standard commercially available CT scanners TECHNIQUE: The volume of the bolus of contrast material, the slice thickness, and the delay between administration of the bolus and commencement of scanning will vary depending upon the anatomic area of interest and the information required. Most commercially available CT scanners include software that permits a rapid scanning technique to facilitate a dynamic examination.

References

Foley WD, "Dynamic Hepatic CT," *Radiology*, 1989, 170(3 Pt 1):617-22.

Computed Transaxial Tomography, Extremities

CPT 73200 (upper extremities without contrast); 73201 (upper extremities with contrast); 73202 (upper extremities with and without contrast); 73700 (lower extremities without contrast); 73701 (lower extremities with contrast); 73702 (lower extremities with and without contrast)

Synonyms Extremities, CT

Abstract PROCEDURE COMMONLY INCLUDES: Intravenous administration of contrast material with subsequent CT scans of the portion of the extremity in question. Both extremities are usually included in the field of view. In the majority of cases, this provides a normal side for comparative purposes. INDICATIONS: The modality has been employed primarily to evaluate bone and soft tissue neoplasms. Occasionally, the modality may be used in inflammatory conditions for localization of an abscess or evaluation of the extent of the abnormality. The cross-sectional display afforded by this modality is useful in localizing abnormalities of the extremities and in determining the intramedullary and extraosseous extent of such abnormalities. The modality is used infrequently for the evaluation of trauma involving the extremities; however, it has been found most useful in evaluating trauma involving the hip joints and shoulder joints. CONTRAINDICATIONS: Uncooperative patient. Patients with extremities in traction are not good candidates for this examination. The presence of a cast on the extremity will produce some significant artifact thus degrading the image somewhat.

Patient Care/Scheduling PATIENT PREPARATION: Diet should be restricted to liquids only for 4 hours prior to the examination. Medication schedule should not be interrupted. Intravenous contrast material may be administered at the discretion of the radiologist. Because of this, a recent serum creatinine is also requested on patients 60 years of age or older, those with significant atherosclerotic disease, those with a known diagnosis of diabetes mellitus, or with pre-existing renal disease.

Method EQUIPMENT: Examination may be performed on any of the commercially available CT scanners. TECHNIQUE: Examination usually consists of 1 cm contiguous slices obtained throughout the area of interest subsequent to the intravenous administration of contrast material. The size and location of the lesion may require modification of the examination technique by the radiologist.

Specimen TURNAROUND TIME: Written report available.

Interpretation LIMITATIONS: Patient's weight should be <300 lb. This is the table limitation on most commercially available CT scanners. ADDITIONAL INFORMATION: This method of imaging the extremities has, to a large degree, been superseded by magnetic resonance imaging in the recent past. Unfortunately, computed tomography lacks both the spatial resolution and the soft tissue contrast necessary for the evaluation of many different pathologic conditions involving bone. The inherent contrast of MRI is a major advantage when imaging the appendicular skeleton. The ever increasing array of surface coils now available coupled with the excellent spatial resolution provided by magnetic resonance has superseded computed tomography for the evaluation of the extremities.

References

Berger PE, Offstein RA, Jackson DW, et al, "MRI Demonstration of Radiographically Occult Fractures: What Have We Been Missing?" *Radiographics*, 1989, 9(3):407-36.

Binkovitz LA, Cahill DR, Ehman RL, et al, "Magnetic Resonance Imaging of the Wrist: Normal Cross Sectional Anatomy and Selected Abnormal Cases," *Radiographics*, 1988, 8:1171.

Demas BE, Heelan RT, Lane J, et al, "Soft-Tissue Sarcomas of the Extremities: Comparison of MR and CT in Determining the Extent of Disease," *AJR*, 1988, 150(3):615-20.

Computed Transaxial Tomography, Head Studies

CPT 70450 (CT head without contrast); 70460 (CT head with contrast); 70470 (CT head with and without contrast)

Synonyms Brain, CT; Head Studies, CT

Abstract PROCEDURE COMMONLY INCLUDES: CT scan of the brain INDICATIONS: Evaluation of known/suspected primary or secondary neoplasm, cystic lesions, hydrocephalus, head trauma, seizure disorder, multiple sclerosis, atrophy, Alzheimer's disease, normal pressure hydrocephalus, Parkinson's disease, dementia, depression, organic brain syndrome, etc.

(Continued)

Computed Transaxial Tomography, Head Studies *(Continued)*

CONTRAINDICATIONS: Assuming a cooperative or quiescent patient, there are no absolute contraindications to a CT scan of the head. A decision must be taken, however, as to whether the study is to be done with or without intravenous contrast material. While each case must be assessed individually, the following broad guidelines may be helpful. Those studies indicated by virtue of a recent infarct, cerebrovascular accident or stroke, or those being done for assessment of atrophy, Alzheimer's disease, normal pressure hydrocephalus, Parkinson's disease, hydrocephalus, evaluation of an intraventricular shunt, assessment of ventricular size, subdural hematoma, or suspected dementia are examined without contrast material. Patients for whom the indication is headache, psychiatric condition (such as anorexia or bulimia), tumor follow-up, rule out tumor, rule out metastasis, multiple sclerosis, seizure disorders, depression, and organic brain syndrome are generally studied with contrast material. Patients in whom the indication is one of infection, abscess, meningitis, transient ischemic attack, arteriovenous malformation, remote subdural hematoma, or who have recently undergone a craniotomy and are being studied for postoperative evaluation are best studied with and without contrast material. Patients with a known diagnosis of plasmacytoma or multiple myeloma should not receive intravenous contrast material. Patients with compromised renal function may or may not benefit from intravenous contrast material. A recent serum creatinine and BUN will be helpful in deciding whether or not the latter group of patients receive contrast material.

Patient Care/Scheduling **PATIENT PREPARATION:** The examination should be ordered and a requisition with information pertaining to the reason for the request and the clinical history should be completed by the referring physician. If there is the slightest possibility that intravenous contrast material will be administered, the patient's oral intake should be limited to liquids for at least 4 hours prior to the examination. Care must be taken to ensure the patient does not become dehydrated and medications should not be interrupted. A recent serum creatinine is requested on patients with pre-existing renal disease, diabetes mellitus, significant atherosclerotic disease, and advancing age (60 years and older). Agitated patients and children may require sedation prior to the examination. In these cases, an order for the appropriate sedative and dose should be recently recorded within the patient's chart. Sedatives should be administered by a physician within the Radiology Department.

Method **EQUIPMENT:** Any commercially available computed tomographic scanner **TECHNIQUE:** CT scans of the head are usually obtained at 15° angulation to the orbitomeatal line, a line connecting the lateral canthus of the eye with the external auditory canal. Contiguous slices 8 or 10 mm in thickness are obtained from the vertex of the skull to the foramen magnum. The orbital roof should be included. The patient is positioned supine for the examination. The head is placed securely in a head holder. The chin is flexed comfortably towards the chest. The appropriate 15° angulation can be obtained by angulation of the gantry if necessary.

Computed Transaxial Tomography, Larynx

CPT 70490 (CT of the neck without contrast material); 70491 (CT of the neck with contrast material); 70492 (CT of the neck with and without contrast material)

Synonyms Larynx, CT; Neck, CT

Replaces Laryngogram

Abstract **PROCEDURE COMMONLY INCLUDES:** 5 mL sequential sections through the neck extending from the base of the tongue to the lung apices **INDICATIONS:** For evaluation of laryngeal tumors, evaluation of anterior and posterior triangle for lymphadenopathy **CONTRAINDICATIONS:** Uncooperative patient.

Patient Care/Scheduling **PATIENT PREPARATION:** Intravenous contrast agent will occasionally be used to identify the relationship of tumor mass to vessels or to differentiate small lymph nodes from vessels. The patient should be limited to a liquid diet for at least 4 hours prior to the CT examination. A medication schedule should be maintained. The use of intravenous contrast material will be at the discretion of the diagnostic radiologist. Because of this, a recent serum creatine is requested in all patients 60 years of age or older and those patients with known significant atherosclerotic disease, diabetes mellitus, or pre-existing renal disease. **SPECIAL INSTRUCTIONS:** When interest is primarily focused on the larynx, the examination can be tailored to extend from the inferior aspect of the tongue or the superior aspect of the epiglottis inferiorly to just below the cricoid cartilage or upper trachea. Patients who have a metal tracheostomy tube should have this replaced with a plastic tube prior to the examination as the metallic tube will produce significant artifact. Phonation may be used to determine vocal cord mobility as well as distend the piriform sinuses. Phonation may also be valuable in evaluating the extent of supraglottic tumors around the piriform sinuses and aryepiglottic folds. Computer tomography of the larynx is an ideal method for evaluating carcinoma of the larynx and staging this tumor. It is also helpful in evaluation of the larynx in cases of laryngeal trauma.

Method EQUIPMENT: This examination may be performed on any one of many commercially available computerized tomographic scanners. TECHNIQUE: As mentioned, examinations of the neck and larynx are generally comprised of 5 mL consecutive slices through the area of anatomic interest.

Specimen TURNAROUND TIME: A verbal telephone report of the scan will be given to the referring physician if specified. A written report will be available.

References

Curtin HD, "Imaging of Larynx: Current Concepts," *Radiology*, 1989, 173(1):1-11.
Som PM, "Lymph Nodes of the Neck," *Radiology*, 1987, 165:593-600.

Computed Transaxial Tomography, Multiplanner Reconstruction and Display

CPT 76375

Synonyms Multiplanner Reconstruction and Display, CT; Sagittal and Coronal Reconstruction. CT

Abstract PROCEDURE COMMONLY INCLUDES: A standard CT examination of particular body part, eg, lumbar spine. These images are obtained in the axial projection. Subsequent to this, computer software may be programmed to reformat the acquired data into the sagittal and coronal projections. INDICATIONS: Helpful in the evaluation of pituitary tumor, spinal canal size, disc configuration. Also helpful in the evaluation of comminuted fractures of the spine, pelvis, and face.

Patient Care/Scheduling PATIENT PREPARATION: The reader is referred to Patient Preparation listed under the specific anatomic area to be studied. SPECIAL INSTRUCTIONS: The reader is referred to Special Instructions listed under specific anatomic areas to be studied.

Method EQUIPMENT: This examination may be performed on most commercially available computerized homographic scanners. TECHNIQUE: Generally speaking, thin contiguous or overlapping slices produce the best results.

Specimen CAUSES FOR REJECTION: Scan slices not in sequence, scan slices not all in same plane TURNAROUND TIME: A verbal telephone report of the scan will be given to the referring physician if specified. A written report will be available.

Interpretation ADDITIONAL INFORMATION: Computed tomographic multiplanner reconstructions have been demonstrated to have several applications. Software packages are also available to allow 3-D reformatting.

References

Herman GT, "Three-Dimensional Imaging on a CT or MR Scanner," *J Comput Assist Tomogr*, 1988, 12(3):450-8.
Magid D, Fishman EK, Sponseller PD, et al, "2-D and 3-D Computed Tomography of Pediatric Hip," *Radiographics*, 1988, 8:901.

Computed Transaxial Tomography, Orbits

CPT 70480 (computed axial tomography orbit without contrast material); 70481 (computed transaxial tomography orbit with contrast material); 70482 (computed axial tomography orbit with and without contrast)

Synonyms Orbits, CT

Abstract PROCEDURE COMMONLY INCLUDES: CT study of orbits INDICATIONS: Tumor, foreign body, trauma, ophthalmologic conditions that threaten vision CONTRAINDICATIONS: Assuming a cooperative or quiescent patient, there are no absolute contraindications to a CT study of the orbits. Administration of intravenous contrast material is variable depending

(Continued)

Computed Transaxial Tomography, Orbits *(Continued)*

upon the patient's suspected diagnosis. Intravenous contrast material is generally indicated in suspected tumor, pseudotumor, arteriovenous malformation, or vascular abnormality. The search for a foreign body is not an indication for contrast material.

Patient Care/Scheduling PATIENT PREPARATION: The examination should be ordered and a requisition with pertinent information pertaining to the reason for the request and the clinical history should be completed by the referring physician. If there is the slightest possibility that intravenous contrast material will be administered, the patient's oral intake should be limited to liquids for at least 4 hours prior to the examination. Care must be taken to ensure the patient does not become dehydrated and medications should not be interrupted. A recent serum creatinine is requested on patients with pre-existing renal disease, diabetes mellitus, significant atherosclerotic disease, and advancing age (60 years of age and older). Agitated patients and children may require sedation prior to the examination. In these cases, an order for the appropriate sedative and dose should be recently recorded within the patient's chart. Sedatives, when necessary, should be administered by a physician within the Radiology Department.

Method EQUIPMENT: Commercially available CT scanners TECHNIQUE: Contiguous 2 mm slices extending from the infraorbital margin to slightly above the supraorbital rim. The study may be extended if pathology indicates. 2 mm slices will facilitate sagittal/coronal reconstruction for optimal visualization of the optic nerve, superior ophthalmic vein, etc. A negative angulation of -20° to the orbitomeatal baseline while the eyes are maintained in the upward gaze position will facilitate optimum visualization of the optic nerve. If a blowout fracture of the orbit is suspected, the study should be continued inferiorly for visualization of the maxillary sinuses and nasal cavity.

References

Mafee MF, Miller MT, Tan W, et al, "Dynamic Computed Tomography and Its Application to Ophthalmology," *Radiol Clin North Am*, 1987, 25:715-31.

Computed Transaxial Tomography, Paranasal Sinuses

CPT 70486 (with contrast); 70487 (with contrast); 70488 (with and without contrast)

Related Information

Paranasal Sinuses *on page 301*

Synonyms Paranasal Sinuses, CT; Sinuses, CT

Abstract PROCEDURE COMMONLY INCLUDES: The examination is composed of contiguous 3-5 mm slices obtained from the inferior portion of the maxillary sinuses, cephalad to the superior extent of the frontal sinuses. INDICATIONS: For the diagnosis and/or evaluation of tumors, masses, metastases, inflammatory conditions, and traumatic involvement. The modality is commonly used for staging of tumors. CONTRAINDICATIONS: Patients who are not candidates for sedation/anesthesia, uncooperative patient; patient cooperation is of the utmost importance as the examination requires the patient to remain motionless for the duration of the study.

Patient Care/Scheduling PATIENT PREPARATION: Patients oral intake should be restricted to fluid for 4 hours prior to the examination. Medication schedule should not be interrupted. Administration of intravenous contrast material is at the discretion of the diagnostic radiologist. If a patient is being evaluated for trauma or inflammatory disease of the paranasal sinuses, no intravenous contrast material is usually administered. If a mass is identified in the course of the examination, or if a patient is known to have a tumor, then intravenous contrast material is usually given. Because of this, a recent serum creatinine is requested in all patients 60 years of age and older and those patients with known significant atherosclerotic disease, diabetes mellitus, or pre-existing renal disease. Children and uncooperative adults may require sedation. SPECIAL INSTRUCTIONS: If the nasopharynx is to be included in the examination, the study should be extended inferiorly to the hard palate or slightly below. The oral pharynx may be included by continuing to the base of the tongue. If there is a question of tumor invasion of the orbit from a sinus then coronal sections are very helpful.

Method TECHNIQUE: This examination may be performed in any one of many commercially available computerized tomographic scanners. Standard examination of the paranasal sinuses consist of 3-5 mm contiguous slices as previously described.

Specimen TURNAROUND TIME: Verbal telephone report of the scan will be given to the referring physician if specified. A written report will be available.

Interpretation ADDITIONAL INFORMATION: Some departments offer a limited CT study of the paranasal sinuses which is competitive with plain film radiographs of the sinus in terms of pricing. This consists of 5 or 6 transaxial images through the sinus obtained parallel to Reid's baseline. The examination is achieved by obtaining a lateral digital image of the skull. From this the distance between the hard palate and the superior aspect of the frontal sinuses is measured. The distance is then divided by 5 or 6 to get the interslice distance. The slice thickness is 3-5 mm.

References

Harnsberger HR, Osborn AG, and Smoker RK, "CT in the Evaluation of the Normal and Diseased Paranasal Sinuses," *Seminars in the Ultrasound, CT and MR*, 1986, 7:68-90.

Computed Transaxial Tomography, Pelvis

CPT 72192 (CT examination of pelvis without contrast); 72193 (CT examination of pelvis with contrast); 72194 (CT examination of pelvis with and without contrast)

Related Information

Computed Transaxial Tomography, Abdomen Studies *on page 274*

Synonyms Lower Abdomen, CT; Pelvis, CT

Abstract PROCEDURE COMMONLY INCLUDES: CT scan pelvic area includes bladder, prostate, ovaries, uterus, lower retroperitoneum, and iliac lymph node chains INDICATIONS: Evaluation of cysts, tumors, masses, metastasis, inflammatory processes, and lymphadenopathy CONTRAINDICATIONS: Uncooperative patient.

Patient Care/Scheduling PATIENT PREPARATION: Dietary restrictions include fluids only for 4 hours prior to the examination. Medication schedule should not be interrupted. Intravenous contrast material may be administered. This is at the discretion of the radiologist. A recent serum creatinine is requested in all patients 60 years of age and older and those patients with known significant atherosclerotic disease, diabetes mellitus, or pre-existing renal disease, in case intravenous contrast administration is necessary. 450 mL dilute barium (1%) is administrated orally commencing at least 1 hour prior to the examination. This facilitates good opacification of the small bowel. A small volume (4-8 oz) of dilute contrast material is given per rectum to facilitate opacification of the distal large bowel. In the case of females, placement of a vaginal tampon may be helpful in further defining the anatomy. SPECIAL INSTRUCTIONS: A CT study of the pelvis may be requested by a practicing physician. The patient's medical record should accompany them to furnish the radiologist with adequate clinical information thus facilitating tailoring of the examination to ensure maximum diagnostic benefit.

Method TECHNIQUE: Study may be performed on any one of the many commercially available computed tomographic scanners. Sequential 1 cm slices are obtained from the pelvic brim through the pubic symphysis. Intravenous administration of contrast material facilitates opacification of the major vascular structures in addition to the ureters and urinary bladder. Oral contrast, rectal contrast, and a vaginal tampon aid in defining the anatomy within the pelvis.

Specimen CAUSES FOR REJECTION: The presence of residual concentrated barium deposits within the large bowel secondary to a prior gastrointestinal exam, creates artifacts which usually detracts from diagnostic usefulness of the study. Where possible, CT studies of the abdomen and pelvis should be completed before conventional gastrointestinal barium examinations. Should these studies be performed in the reverse order, laxative use or cleansing enema may aid in elimination of the concentrated barium. TURNAROUND TIME: A verbal telephone report of the scan will be given to the referring physician if specified. A written report will be available.

Interpretation ADDITIONAL INFORMATION: The patient should be informed the examination may take 30-45 minutes and that oral, rectal, and intravenous contrast media may be necessary for the examination.

References

Thoeni RF, "Computed Tomography of the Pelvis," *Computed Tomography of the Body*, Moss AA, Gamsu G, Genant HK, eds, Philadelphia, PA: WB Saunders Co, 1983.

Computed Transaxial Tomography, Sella Turcica

CPT 70480 (CT sella without contrast); 70481 (CT sella with contrast); 70482 (CT sella with and without contrast)

Synonyms Sella Turcica, CT

Abstract **PROCEDURE COMMONLY INCLUDES:** Thin slices through the anatomic area of sella turcica for evaluation of suspected pathology **INDICATIONS:** Evaluation of patients suspected of having intrasella or extrasella abnormalities including those that present with amenorrhea, galactorrhea, or increased prolactin levels. **CONTRAINDICATIONS:** In the absence of a history of allergy to iodine, intravenous contrast material is administered in almost all cases. The exceptions include patients with known compromised renal function, patients with plasmacytoma, and multiple myeloma.

Patient Care/Scheduling **PATIENT PREPARATION:** The examination should be ordered and a requisition stating pertinent information pertaining to the reason for the request and the clinical history should be completed by the referring physician. If there is the slightest possibility that intravenous contrast material will be administered, the patient's oral intake should be limited to liquids for at least 4 hours prior to the examination. Care must be taken to ensure the patient does not become dehydrated and medications should not be interrupted. A recent serum creatinine is requested on patients with pre-existing renal disease, diabetes mellitus, significant atherosclerotic disease and advancing age (60 years of age and older). Agitated patients and children may require sedation prior to the examination. In these cases, an order for the appropriate sedative and dose should be recently recorded within the patient's chart. Sedatives should be administered by a physician within the Radiology Department.

Method **EQUIPMENT:** This examination can be performed on any commercially available CT scanner. **TECHNIQUE:** A slice thickness of 2-3 mm is suggested. Slices should be contiguous.

Interpretation **ADDITIONAL INFORMATION:** Instant oblique reconstruction or sagittal/coronal reconstruction can be utilized for additional evaluation. A slight overlapping of slices optimizes the sagittal/coronal reconstruction if the slice thickness is >2 mm. Optimum visualization of the sella turcica is best achieved with coronal sections. Axial sections are usually reserved for those patients in which it is difficult or impossible to achieve coronal scans. For coronal positioning the patient is positioned supine. The optimal position for coronal scanning is 90° from Reid's baseline. To achieve this position the patient is supine with the upper torso elevated by supports 10" to 12" above the table. Hyperextend the head and neck and secure the head holder. Alternatively, the patient may be scanned in the prone position. Here a vertical submental position is utilized. The head and neck are extended and secured in the head holder to provide a scanning plain at 90° to Reid's baseline. If the coronal position is impossible, then obtain axial images and reformat these in the sagittal and coronal projections utilizing instant oblique reconstruction. The coronal position is difficult to maintain and when utilized, rapid sequence scanning may be implemented to facilitate rapid completion of the study.

References

Daniels DL, Williams AL, Thornton RS, et al, "Differential Diagnosis of Intracellular Tumors by Computed Tomography," *Radiology*, 1981, 141:697-701.

Kucharczyk W, Davis DO, Kelly WM, et al, "Pituitary Adenomas: High Resolution MR Imaging at 1.5 Tesla," *Radiology*, 1986, 161:761-5.

Computed Transaxial Tomography, Spine

CPT 62284 (intrathecal contrast material); 72125 (CT cervical spine without contrast material); 72126 (CT cervical spine with contrast material); 72127 (CT cervical spine with and without contrast material); 72128 (CT thoracic spine without contrast material); 72129 (CT thoracic spine with contrast material); 72130 (CT thoracic spine with and without contrast material); 72131 (CT lumbar spine without contrast material); 72132 (CT lumbar spine with contrast material); 72133 (CT lumbar spine with and without contrast material)

Synonyms Cervical Spine, CT; Dorsal Spine, CT; Lumbar Spine, CT; Spine, CT

Replaces Discogram

Abstract **PROCEDURE COMMONLY INCLUDES:** CT scan of cervical, dorsal, lumbar, and/or sacral spine **INDICATIONS:**

- diagnosis of disc herniation

- evaluation of spinal canal stenosis
- evaluation of facet disease
- evaluation of spondylolysis
- evaluation of infectious disease involving an intervertebral disc or a vertebral body.

Patient Care/Scheduling PATIENT PREPARATION: No preparation by nursing personnel is required. Intravenous contrast material is generally not indicated. Intrathecal contrast material may be administered at the discretion of the radiologist depending upon the reason for the examination. There should be no barium present within the gastrointestinal tract as this will produce considerable artifacts when the lower thoracic, lumbar, or lumbosacral spine is being evaluated. Examination of the cervical spine is best performed when the patient suspends respiration and swallowing during the exposures. Slice thickness utilized may be 2-5 mm. Slight overlap is recommended if sagittal and coronal reconstructions are to be performed. When the primary area of interest is the upper cervical spine, the chin should be extended to eliminate artifacts created from dental hardware. When scanning patients with a history of cervical trauma, movement of the patient should be done with extreme care. When the thoracic spine is to be examined, the examination is usually tailored to a specific portion of the thoracic spine depending on the patient's symptomatology. Again, slice thickness of 2-5 mm may be employed at the discretion of the radiologist. Evaluation of the lumbar spine is not infrequently performed subsequent to myelography. In these cases, the thecal sac is opacified by water soluble contrast material. A slice thickness of 4-5 mm is utilized and the table moves in increments of 3-5 mm at the discretion of the radiologist. SPECIAL INSTRUCTIONS: The exam may be requested by a practicing physician. The area of interest must be specified along with pertinent clinical history and reason for the CT scan. To achieve optimal postscanning reconstruction, complete immobilization and patient cooperation is imperative. Coronal, sagittal, or instant oblique reconstruction is of definite value in assessing the neural canal and foramina. Isodensity and gray scale reversal may also be of value in visualizing herniated disc material.

Method EQUIPMENT: Examinations may be performed on all commercially available CT scanners. TECHNIQUE: Slice thickness and table incrementation are at the discretion of the radiologist. The parameters mentioned serve only as rough guidelines.

Specimen CAUSES FOR REJECTION: Inability of the patient to remain motionless, presence of barium within the bowel when lower thoracic, lumbar, and sacral spines are to be examined TURNAROUND TIME: A verbal telephone report of the scan will be given to the referring physician if specified. A written report will be available.

Interpretation ADDITIONAL INFORMATION: High resolution computed tomography has had a major impact on the neuroradiologic diagnosis of lumbar disc herniation. The modality facilitates noninvasive diagnoses with an accuracy approaching 93%. The modality is more accurate than myelography alone as it facilitates a diagnosis of lateral disc herniation. Magnetic resonance however has certain advantages over computed tomography of the spine. This modality allows direct multiplanner imaging, utilizes nonionizing radiation, and facilitates imaging of the entire lumbar spine and conus medullaris.

References

Chambers AA, "Thoracic Disc Herniation," *Semin Roentgenol*, 1988, 23:111-7.

Heiss JD and Tew JM Jr, "Discogenic Diseases of the Spine: Clinical Aspects," *Semin Roentgenol*, 1988, 23:93-9.

Lukin RR, Gaskill MF, and Wiot JG, "Lumbar Herniated Disc and Related Topics," *Semin Roentgenol*, 1988, 23:100-5.

Simon JE and Lukin RR, "Discogenic Disease of the Cervical Spine," *Semin Roentgenol*, 1988, 23:118-24.

Computed Transaxial Tomography, Temporal Bone

CPT 70480 (CT temporal bone without intravenous contrast); 70481 (CT temporal bone with contrast); 70482 (CT temporal bone with and without contrast)

Synonyms Middle and Inner Ear, CT; Temporal Bone, CT

Replaces Polytomography of the Temporal Bone

Abstract PROCEDURE COMMONLY INCLUDES: Thin sections through the temporal bone for evaluation of the middle and inner ear and the jugular fossa; contiguous thin slices through the

(Continued)

Computed Transaxial Tomography, Temporal Bone *(Continued)*

temporal bone for evaluation of suspected pathology **INDICATIONS:** CT is most valuable is assessing the temporal bone in cases of trauma, tumors, inflammatory processes, genetic or other abnormalities. **CONTRAINDICATIONS:** Patient cooperation is most important. The examination requires the patient to remain motionless for the duration of the study. The time of the study will vary from 10-20 minutes depending on the equipment being used. Children and uncooperative adults may require sedation.

Patient Care/Scheduling **PATIENT PREPARATION:** The patient should be limited to a liquid diet for at least 4 hours prior to the CT examination. Medication schedules should be maintained. The use of intravenous contrast material is at the discretion of the diagnostic radiologist. Generally speaking, no intravenous contrast material is administered unless the presence of tumor is suspected. In all patients 60 years of age and older and those patients with known significant atherosclerotic disease, diabetes mellitus, or pre-existing renal disease, a recent serum creatinine is required prior to administration of contrast material.

Method **EQUIPMENT:** The examination may be performed on all commercially available CT scanners. **TECHNIQUE:** The examination should extend from the petrous ridges superiorly to slightly below the external auditory meatus. The tilt line should be parallel with the orbitomeatal line. Consecutive 2 mm slices are suggested for evaluation of the temporal bone and ideally these should overlap slightly.

Specimen **TURNAROUND TIME:** A verbal telephone report of the scan will be given to the referring physician if specified. A written report will be available.

Interpretation **ADDITIONAL INFORMATION:** In cases of trauma where cerebrospinal fluid leak is to be excluded, intrathecal contrast material is helpful. An adequate study is dependent upon knowledge of pertinent, specific clinical information.

References

Swartz JD, "Current Imaging Approach to the Temporal Bone," *Radiology*, 1989, 171(2):309-17.

Computed Transaxial Tomography, Thorax

CPT 71250 (CT of the chest without intravenous contrast); 71260 (CT of the chest with intravenous contrast); 71270 (CT study of the chest with and without intravenous contrast)

Abstract **PROCEDURE COMMONLY INCLUDES:** CT study of the chest extending from the lung apices to the posterior costophrenic sulci. The study may extend inferiorly to image the adrenal glands because they are a relatively frequent site of metastasis from primary lung carcinoma. **INDICATIONS:** The examination facilitates evaluation of abnormalities of the lungs, mediastinum, pleura, and chest wall. Conventional PA and lateral views of the chest represent the basic screening tool in the identification of abnormalities involving the thorax. The axial anatomic display and superior density discrimination of computed tomography provides information pertaining to the extent of disease and more precise characterization of abnormalities initially noted on physical examination, chest films or on the barium swallow. **CONTRAINDICATIONS:** Patient cooperation is of utmost importance as the examination requires the patient to remain motionless for the duration of the study. The time of the study will vary from 10-30 minutes depending on the equipment being used. Children and uncooperative adults may require sedation.

Patient Care/Scheduling **PATIENT PREPARATION:** The patients should be limited to a liquid diet for at least 4 hours prior to the CT examination. Medication schedules should be maintained. The use of intravenous contrast material may be required at the discretion of the diagnostic radiologist. Because of this, a recent serum creatinine is requested in all patients 60 years of age and older, and those patients with known significant atherosclerotic disease, diabetes mellitus, or pre-existing renal disease. In the case of children who need sedation, a recent (within 30 days) recording of the child's weight and a written order by the child's physician must be in the patient's medical record. All children should be accompanied by a responsible adult. Opacification of the esophagus with thick barium paste may be of value in some cases and administration should be at the discretion of the diagnostic radiologist. **SPECIAL INSTRUCTIONS:** The exam may be requested by a practicing physician. The area of interest must be specified along with pertinent clinical history and reason for the CT scan. The test should be complete in 10-30 minutes. Intravenous contrast material may be administered.

Method EQUIPMENT: The examination may be performed on any number of commercially available CT scanners. TECHNIQUE: A routine CT study of the chest consists of sequential 1 cm slices obtained from the apices through the posterior costophrenic sulci. The study may be extended to include the adrenal glands if a diagnosis of primary bronchogenic carcinoma is known or suspected. The technique may vary depending upon the indications for the study. The examination may be tailored by the diagnostic radiologist to answer specific questions. For example, the questionably abnormal pulmonary hilum on conventional films may require 5 mm contiguous sections subsequent to the intravenous administration of contrast material. The latter will facilitate enhancement of major vascular structures thus highlighting normal and abnormal anatomy. Similarly, densitometric evaluation of a solitary pulmonary nodule will require contiguous 2 mm slices throughout the nodule without intravenous contrast material. This maneuver will facilitate evaluation of the nodule for the presence and distribution of calcium within it. All modifications of the conventional contiguous 1 cm slice protocol throughout the chest are made at the discretion of the radiologist. The patient's medical record should accompany the patient to the department in order to ensure that the radiologist is furnished with sufficient information to tailor the examination appropriately.

Specimen CAUSES FOR REJECTION: Inability of the patient to cooperate is the major problem. Should the uncooperative patient not be a candidate for sedation and/or anesthesia, the study cannot be performed. TURNAROUND TIME: A verbal telephone report of the scan will be given to the referring physician if specified. A written report will be available.

References

Naidich DP, Zerhouni EA, Hutchins GM, et al, "Computed Tomography of the Pulmonary Parenchyma, Part 1: Distal Air-space Disease," *J Thorac Imaging*, 1985, 1:39-53.

Zerhouni EA, Naidich DP, Stitik FP, et al, "Computed Tomography of the Pulmonary Parenchyma, Part 2: Interstitial Disease," *J Thorac Imaging*, 1985, 1:54-64.

Computed Transaxial Tomography, Treatment Planning

CPT 76370

Synonyms Radiotherapy Treatment Planning; Treatment Planning, CT

Abstract PROCEDURE COMMONLY INCLUDES: The area of the tumor is scanned while the patient reclines on a flat table top during quiet respiration. Care must be taken to ensure that the patient is in the treatment position. The CT study will allow accurate localization of tumor. Single transaxial imaging method provides multilevel accurate body contours. The modality provides accurate density detail formerly not available. Three dimensional treatment planning can now be performed with the accurate anatomical data available from computed tomographic scans. In addition to this, computed tomography can be utilized to monitor the response of a tumor to treatment. Scans through the proximal portion of the field, the central axis of the radiation field, and the distal portion of the field should be obtained. Should there be a marked distortion of anatomy, further scans between these landmarks may be required. The use of contrast material is at the discretion of the radiologist and radiotherapist and will be influenced by location and characteristics of tumor. INDICATIONS: Procedure indicated in those patients with a known tumor that is to be treated with radiotherapy. The purpose of the examination is to ensure that the radiotherapy administered is appropriately distributed throughout tumor volume and to minimize radiation to normal structures. CONTRAINDICATIONS: Patient cooperation is of utmost importance. The patient must be able to assume the treatment position and to remain motionless but without suspending respiration during the course of the study which generally can be completed in less than 15 minutes.

Patient Care/Scheduling PATIENT PREPARATION: Limitation to a liquid diet for a 4-hour period prior to the CT examination is not required unless the intravenous administration of contrast material is necessary. Medication schedules should be maintained. In patients 60 years of age and older, or those with known significant atherosclerotic disease, diabetes mellitus, or pre-existing renal disease, a recent serum creatinine will be required if the patient is to receive intravenous contrast material. SPECIAL INSTRUCTIONS: Scan may be requested by a radiation therapy physician who is in the process of planning therapy or assessing therapeutic results.

Method EQUIPMENT: The examination may be performed on any number of commercially available CT scanners. TECHNIQUE: The patient is scanned on a flat table top during quiet

(Continued)

Computed Transaxial Tomography, Treatment Planning *(Continued)*

respiration while in the treatment position. Scans are obtained through the central axis of the tumor and through the upper and lower extent of tumor. Further images between these scans may be required depending on anatomical considerations. The use of intravenous contrast material is at the discretion of the radiologist and radiation therapist.

Specimen TURNAROUND TIME: A verbal telephone report of the scan will be given to the referring physician if specified. A written report will be available.

Interpretation ADDITIONAL INFORMATION: Scan passes will be marked on the patient with radiopaque material by the Radiation Therapy Department personnel who will position the patient within the scanner.

References

Tremewan RN, "Computed Tomography in Radiotherapy Treatment Planning," *Australas Radiol*, 1988, 32:50-6.

CT, Lower Abdomen *see* Computed Transaxial Tomography, Abdomen Studies *on page 274*

CT, Total Abdomen *see* Computed Transaxial Tomography, Abdomen Studies *on page 274*

CT, Upper Abdomen *see* Computed Transaxial Tomography, Abdomen Studies *on page 274*

Discogram *replaced by* Computed Transaxial Tomography, Spine *on page 282*

Dorsal Spine, CT *see* Computed Transaxial Tomography, Spine *on page 282*

Dynamic Study, CT *see* Computed Transaxial Tomography, Dynamic Study *on page 276*

Extremities, CT *see* Computed Transaxial Tomography, Extremities *on page 277*

Head Studies, CT *see* Computed Transaxial Tomography, Head Studies *on page 277*

Laryngogram *replaced by* Computed Transaxial Tomography, Larynx *on page 278*

Larynx, CT *see* Computed Transaxial Tomography, Larynx *on page 278*

Lower Abdomen, CT *see* Computed Transaxial Tomography, Pelvis *on page 281*

Lumbar Spine, CT *see* Computed Transaxial Tomography, Spine *on page 282*

Middle and Inner Ear, CT *see* Computed Transaxial Tomography, Temporal Bone *on page 283*

Multiplanner Reconstruction and Display, CT *see* Computed Transaxial Tomography, Multiplanner Reconstruction and Display *on page 279*

Neck, CT *see* Computed Transaxial Tomography, Larynx *on page 278*

Orbits, CT *see* Computed Transaxial Tomography, Orbits *on page 279*

Paranasal Sinuses, CT *see* Computed Transaxial Tomography, Paranasal Sinuses *on page 280*

Pelvis, CT *see* Computed Transaxial Tomography, Pelvis *on page 281*

Polytomography of the Temporal Bone *replaced by* Computed Transaxial Tomography, Temporal Bone *on page 283*

Radiotherapy Treatment Planning *see* Computed Transaxial Tomography, Treatment Planning *on previous page*

Sagittal and Coronal Reconstruction. CT *see* Computed Transaxial Tomography, Multiplanner Reconstruction and Display *on page 279*

Sella Turcica, CT *see* Computed Transaxial Tomography, Sella Turcica *on page 282*

DIAGNOSTIC RADIOLOGY

Peter B. O'Donovan, MD

Almost immediately following the discovery of x-rays by WK Roentgen, on November 8, 1895, application of radiography to the identification and diagnosis of disease was pursued with vigor by the medical profession. As the centennial of the discovery of x-rays approaches, a glance back reveals a history studded with major developments, such as the development of the antiscatter grid (Buckey, 1911), the development of the phototimer (Morgan, 1942), the image intensifier (Langnuir, 1937) and its refinement (Coltman, 1948), the development of cineradiography (1954) and digital subtraction radiography (1970s). Landmark developments are interspersed with periods of consolidation. Conventional film screen radiography and fluoroscopy have continued to improve over the past 95 years. While some conventional radiographic examinations have been displaced by newer diagnostic techniques (endoscopy, bronchoscopy, computed tomography, etc) the vast majority of radiographic procedures are of the conventional kind and will be for the foreseeable future.

Abdomen for Fetal Age *see* Abdomen X-ray *on this page*

Abdomen X-ray

CPT 74000 (single AP view); 74010 (AP and additional oblique and cone down views); 74020 (complete, including decubitus and/or erect views)

Synonyms KUB

Applies to Abdomen for Fetal Age; Decubitus Abdomen

Abstract PROCEDURE COMMONLY INCLUDES: Abdomen series includes AP and upright abdomen and PA chest on patients who are able to stand. Lateral decubitus abdomen and supine chest on patients who cannot stand. Abdomen for kidney stones involves an AP abdomen and a coned-down view over the bladder area. Abdomen for gallstones involves the abdomen series and one coned-down view of the right upper quadrant. Abdomen for aneurysm or aortic calcification includes an AP and lateral. Abdomen for IUD placement includes an AP and lateral abdomen. Abdomen for multiple pregnancy, breech presentation, fetal age, position or death, or to rule out pregnancy includes AP abdomen only. Please see Ultrasound Section. INDICATIONS: Location of foreign bodies, tubes, free peritoneal or retroperitoneal air, displacement of the gastric air bubble, elevation of the diaphragm, displacement of the lateral and pelvic fat lines, disturbances of normal bowel patterns and renal shadow. Fetal age in late pregnancy. Detection and localization of calcifications. CONTRAINDICATIONS: Plain films of the abdomen are contraindicated in early pregnancy and ultrasound is the method of choice for evaluation of the abdomen under these circumstances.

Patient Care/Scheduling PATIENT PREPARATION: Consult physician in charge before giving any medication. Physician should write orders in cases of bleeding or obstruction. For a usual adult routine, some radiologists prefer not to use any cathartics prior to this examination. Cathartics are used in many cases when a plain film of the abdomen is obtained prior to excretory urography. In these cases, on the evening before the examination, the patient should have 2 oz of castor oil. The patient should omit breakfast for morning appointments and omit lunch for afternoon appointments. Since preparation of abdomen in pediatric patients is so dependent on age and clinical problem, it is left to judgment of referring physician. In special cases, consult Pediatric Radiologist. SPECIAL INSTRUCTIONS: Requisition **must** state type of pills patient is receiving and if patient can stand.

Method TECHNIQUE: AP film of the abdomen. This film is obtained in the recumbent position and is often referred to as a KUB as it is commonly employed in examinations of the urinary tract. The letters stand for kidneys, ureters, and bladder. The AP film of the abdomen obtained in the erect position will allow demonstration of gas fluid levels within the intestine. In the small intestine, the presence of such fluid levels frequently indicates intestinal obstruction. Free intraperitoneal air is readily identifiable in this projection, because, unless trapped by intestinal adhesions, it will rise to reside beneath the domes of the hemidiaphragms. A rapid exposure technique is recommended to ensure the absence of diaphragmatic motion on the film. For the lateral decubitus film, the patient is recumbent lying on one side. A horizontal x-ray beam is directed at the abdomen from the anterior aspect. This film again will allow demonstration of fluid levels in patients who are unable to assume the upright position. If employed for identification of free intraperitoneal air, the patient's left side should be dependent. The patient should be placed in this position for at least 5 minutes prior to exposure of the film to ensure any free gas present within the peritoneal space will migrate to the highest point along the right lateral abdominal wall.

Specimen CAUSES FOR REJECTION: Barium in colon in cases to rule out kidney stone.

Interpretation ADDITIONAL INFORMATION: A PA view of the chest is sometimes included in this examination. This is because patients presenting with abdominal pain sometimes have pulmonary pathology such as lower lobe pneumonia. The presence of retroperitoneal air will not be appreciated as readily as free intraperitoneal air. This is because it will not migrate freely to a subphrenic location due to the configuration and confines of the retroperitoneal space. It will usually be recognized by its tendency to outline those organs which lie in the retroperitoneum such as the kidneys, ascending and descending colons, pancreas, and duodenum.

References

Federle MP, "The Acute Abdomen: Computed Tomography," *Radiographics*, 1985, 5(2):307-22.

(Continued)

Abdomen X-ray *(Continued)*

Freeman LM, Lutzker LG, and Weissmann HS, "The Acute Abdomen: Radionuclide Imaging," *Radiographics*, 1985, 5(2):285-306.
Johnson CD and Rice RP, "The Acute Abdomen: Plain Radiographic Evaluation," *Radiographics*, 1985, 5(2):259-72.
Leopold GR, "The Acute Abdomen: Ultrasonography," *Radiographics*, 1985, 5(2):273-83.
McCort J, "The Acute Abdomen: Introduction," *Radiographics*, 1985, 5(2):257-8.

Air Contrast Study of Colon *see* Colon Films *on page 293*
Barium Meal *see* Gastrointestinal Series *on page 298*
Barium Swallow *see* Esophagram *on page 296*

Bone Age

CPT 76020

Abstract PROCEDURE COMMONLY INCLUDES: Single AP view of the hand and wrist used to assess the physical development status of children INDICATIONS: Precocious puberty, marked hypogonadism, or eunuchoidism; evaluation of skeletal status and general body maturity.

Method EQUIPMENT: Standard radiography room TECHNIQUE: Single AP view of the left hand.

Interpretation ADDITIONAL INFORMATION: There are a number of radiographic atlases of skeletal development of the hand and wrist. The patient's film is to be matched with a standard radiograph of the appropriate gender. The report should include information pertaining to skeletal age and chronological age. The standard deviation from the normal is included in the atlas. Comment can also be made on bone mineralization and any scars of interrupted growth that may provide a record of past illness or other misadventure.

References

Cole AJ, Webb L, and Cole TJ, "Bone Age Estimation: A Comparison of Methods," *Br J Radiol*, 1988, 61(728):683-6.
Greulich WW and Pyle SI, *Radiographic Atlas of Skeletal Development of the Hand and Wrist*, London, England: Oxford University Press, 1959.

Bone Biopsy

CPT 76003 (under fluoroscopic guidance); 76361 (under CT guidance)

Applies to Percutaneous Biopsy of Musculoskeletal Lesions and Synovial Membranes

Abstract PROCEDURE COMMONLY INCLUDES: This procedure involves the passage of a needle, either under fluoroscopic or computed tomographic guidance, into an area of bony abnormality to facilitate precise histologic and/or bacteriologic diagnosis. In many clinical situations, this procedure can establish definitive diagnosis without the disadvantages of surgery making it a useful alternative to open biopsy. In selected cases of arthritis, examination of the synovium may provide precise diagnostic clues or useful information about the nature of the arthritic process. A biopsy of the synovium can be performed through an open arthrotomy, percutaneous biopsy, or as part of an arthroscopic procedure during which the synovium can be visualized. INDICATIONS: The need for a tissue or bacteriologic diagnosis in situations where it is desirable to forego open biopsy.

Patient Care/Scheduling PATIENT PREPARATION: Biopsies are performed in the Radiology Department. Skeletal biopsies are usually done under local anesthesia, with the exception of children and restless patients who are placed under general anesthesia or heavy sedation. Local anesthesia facilitates communication between the patient and the physician performing the procedure. Should the patient complain of radiating pain, the needle can be repositioned. Spinal biopsies necessitate a 24-hour hospitalization. Other anatomic areas may be biopsied on an outpatient basis. The patient should not eat on the morning of the examination. An intravenous catheter is generally placed for I.V. access and the patient is usually administered both a sedative and a medication for pain.

Specimen There are a wide variety of commercially available needles for these procedures. A needle aspiration biopsy consists of aspiration of fluid for cytologic and/or bacteriologic analysis. A core biopsy, however, requires a larger needle and allows retrieval of a core of tissue for histopathologic interpretation.

References

Bard M and Laredo JD, *Interventional Radiology in Bone and Joint*, New York, NY: Springer-Verlag Wien, 1988.

Breast, X-ray *see* Mammogram *on page 300*

Bronchogram

CPT 71041 (complete unilateral); 71061 (complete bilateral)

Related Information

Localized Bronchogram *on page 264*

Applies to Bronchogram Bilateral; Bronchogram Unilateral

Abstract INDICATIONS: Indications for bronchography today are extremely limited. The major airways can be well evaluated by bronchoscopy. The smaller more peripheral airways can be very accurately assessed for the presence of bronchiectasis by thin section computed tomography. Formerly the indications for bronchography included:

- assessment of the severity and extent of bronchiectasis
- establishment of the diagnosis of neoplasm, particularly in patients with malignant cells in the sputum but a normal chest film
- evaluation of patients with hemoptysis and a normal chest film
- evaluation of patients with recurrent pneumonia localized to the same segment or lobe

CONTRAINDICATIONS: Marked diminished pulmonary function, an acute illness (pneumonia, asthmatic attack, etc).

Patient Care/Scheduling PATIENT PREPARATION: If the appointment is in the AM, nothing should be taken by mouth after midnight. If the appointment is in the afternoon, the patient may have breakfast consisting of clear liquids. The patient is usually premedicated 30-45 minutes prior to the procedure. Premedication would include atropine (0.4-0.8 mg) intramuscularly. This is usually given in conjunction with a mild sedative such as Valium®. AFTERCARE: The patient should be encouraged to cough and aid postural drainage for 1-2 hours subsequent to the procedure. The patient should receive nothing by mouth until the gag reflex returns. A postprocedural fever is not uncommonly encountered. The procedure is usually associated with a mild transient respiratory obstructive component which will clear usually within 24-48 hours. COMPLICATIONS: These include subcutaneous emphysema and intratracheal bleeding when a transtracheal approach is used. A postprocedural fever and laryngeal edema may be encountered when a nasolaryngeal approach is utilized.

Method EQUIPMENT: Fluoroscopy table with a standard overhead radiography tube TECHNIQUE: This consists of exposing radiographs in standard AP, oblique, and lateral projections subsequent to the instillation of radiopaque material (Dionosil®) into selected bronchi.

Interpretation LIMITATIONS: Outpatient studies are discouraged except in unusual conditions because of the nature of the examination. The study should not be performed within 3 months of an episode of pneumonia. The reversible bronchiectasis associated with pneumonia may be misdiagnosed should the study be performed soon after an episode of pneumonia. The procedure should also be avoided in patients with severe obstructive or restrictive lung disease.

References

Grenier P, Frantz M, Mussett D, et al, "Bronchiectasis: Assessment by Thin Section CT," *Radiology*, 1986, 161:95-9.

Bronchogram Bilateral *see* Bronchogram *on this page*

Bronchogram Unilateral *see* Bronchogram *on this page*

Cardiac Series *see* Esophagram *on page 296*

Cervical Spine

CPT 72040 (AP and lateral); 72050 (minimum 4 views); 72052 (complete, including oblique and flexion and/or extension views)

Abstract PROCEDURE COMMONLY INCLUDES: AP view of the cervical spine which is obtained with the patient in the supine position. Vertebral bodies below the level of C3 are well visualized in this view. An AP view of the upper cervical spine is obtained through the open mouth with the patient in the supine position. This allows good identification and evaluation of the odontoid process. Lateral view of the cervical spine may be performed in the upright or supine position. If the film is obtained to rule out fracture subsequent to trauma, the supine position should be maintained and the patient should not be moved until the films have been evaluated by the radiologist. The radiologist will decide if further views are necessary. In the nontraumatized patient, a lateral view of the cervical spine may be obtained with the patient in the upright position dropping the shoulders as much as possible to enhance visualization of C7. Traction on the arms by means of heavy weights held in the hands will aid in lowering the shoulders. Oblique views of the cervical spine are exposed in the supine position with the entire body rotated through 45° so that the head, neck, and torso are in straight alignment. Routine examination usually includes only the AP and lateral film. If oblique views are required, for example for evaluation of the neural foramina, then this should be written on the requisition. INDICATIONS: Evaluate cervical spine for presence of metastatic and primary neoplasm, trauma, infectious disease, degenerative and reactive processes.

Patient Care/Scheduling SPECIAL INSTRUCTIONS: Specify if patient can be removed from the stretcher in cases of injury.

Method EQUIPMENT: Standard radiography equipment.

References

Freemyer B, Knopp R, Piche J, et al, "Comparison of Five-View and Three-View Cervical Spine Series in the Evaluation of Patients With Cervical Trauma," *Ann Emerg Med*, 1989, 18(8): 818-21.

Vandemark RM, "Radiology of the Cervical Spine in Trauma Patients: Practice Pitfalls and Recommendations for Improving Efficiency and Communication," *AJR*, 1990, 155(3):465-72.

Chest Films

CPT 71010 (single view); 71020 (PA and lateral chest); 71030 (4 views of the chest)

Synonyms CXR; PA; PA and Lateral CXR

Abstract PROCEDURE COMMONLY INCLUDES: PA and lateral exposures of the chest. Sagel and his colleagues published an article in 1974 questioning the efficacy of screening examinations of the chest and whether or not lateral views should be obtained. Both medical and economic factors were considered. The study was based on a review of PA and lateral views of the chest in 10,597 examinations and reached the following conclusions.

- Routine screening for hospital admission or for surgery was not warranted for patients younger than 20 years of age.
- Lateral projection could be eliminated in routine screening of patients 20-39 years of age.
- Lateral projection should be obtained at any age when disease of the chest is suspected.
- Lateral projection should be obtained in screening examinations of patients older than 40 years of age.

INDICATIONS: Evaluate lungs and thoracic bones for presence of metastatic and primary neoplasm, infectious disease, degenerative and reactive processes, trauma, and surgical change. The chest film is also used to evaluate the heart and great vessels.

Patient Care/Scheduling PATIENT PREPARATION: Remove medals, lockets, and other jewelry from neck. Arrange hair, when long, high on head so that no locks hang over chest or shoulders. SPECIAL INSTRUCTIONS: The chest x-ray can be modified in various ways to answer specific questions. For example, while the standard PA view of the chest is obtained in full inspiration, a pneumothorax will be more readily appreciated when the film is exposed in expiration. Decubitus films are helpful in differentiating mobile fluid in the pleural space from fluid loculations or pleural thickening. A lordotic view of the chest may be helpful in evaluating the apices. Oblique views of the chest done with 45° angulation in the right anterior oblique projection and 60° angulation in the left anterior oblique projection with barium opacifying the esophagus at the time of exposure are helpful in evaluating the size of the various cardiac chambers. A standard radiographic examination of the chest in addition to the modifications mentioned may be scheduled by calling the Radiology Department.

References

Sagel SS, Evans RG, Forrest JV, et al, "Efficacy of Routine Screening and Lateral Chest Radiographs in a Hospital-Based Population," *N Engl J Med*, 1974, 291:1001-4.

Cholangiogram, Operative

CPT 74300

Synonyms Intraoperative Cholangiogram; Surgical Cholangiogram

Abstract PROCEDURE COMMONLY INCLUDES: Visualization of the bile ducts by means of contrast agent injection through an indwelling T-tube at the time of surgery to assess for calculi within the biliary system. Radiographs are exposed in the operating room during the procedure in the AP and/or oblique projections. INDICATIONS: Evaluate patency of biliary system, evaluate filling defects in bile ducts CONTRAINDICATIONS: History of allergic reaction to contrast media, barium in the bowel.

Patient Care/Scheduling PATIENT PREPARATION: Procedure is performed in the operating room after cholecystectomy before closure of abdominal incision.

Interpretation LIMITATIONS: Biliary duct system may not be optimally visualized due to respiratory motion or size of patient or barium in bowel.

Cholangiography, Postoperative, T-Tube

CPT 74305

Synonyms T-Tube

Applies to Postoperative Cholangiography

Abstract PROCEDURE COMMONLY INCLUDES: Injection of contrast material through indwelling T-tube for visualization of bile ducts in the postoperative period in those patients who have had cholecystectomy and/or common bile duct exploration with placement of T-tube at the time of surgery. INDICATIONS: Evaluate the patency of the biliary system prior to removal of the T-tube CONTRAINDICATIONS: Cholangitis, sepsis without antibiotic cover.

Patient Care/Scheduling AFTERCARE: Routine observation. Examination may be scheduled by calling the Radiology Department. Assuming the patient is not on dietary restriction, a light breakfast may be consumed the day of the procedure. SPECIAL INSTRUCTIONS: By appointment only. A completed and signed Radiology consult must be sent to Radiology before an appointment can be made.

Specimen CAUSES FOR REJECTION: Inadequate clinical information on the Radiology consult TURNAROUND TIME: Written report available within 24 hours of completed exam. Verbal report will be supplied immediately postprocedure if requested.

Interpretation ADDITIONAL INFORMATION: If sepsis is present the examination may be done in special circumstances following antibiotic care.

Cholecystography *see* Oral Cholecystogram, Gallbladder Series *on page 301*

Colon Films

CPT 74270 (barium enema); 74280 (air contrast barium with specific high density barium, with or without glucagon)

Applies to Air Contrast Study of Colon

Abstract INDICATIONS: Evaluate the colon for presence of embolism, aneurysm, neoplasms, hemorrhage, or atherosclerosis CONTRAINDICATIONS: Known perforation of the colon.

Patient Care/Scheduling PATIENT PREPARATION: Adequate bowel preparation is the key to the performance of a diagnostic barium enema. For appropriate preparation of the bowel we use a polyethylene glycol electrolyte gastrointestinal lavage solution. This product is contraindicated in patients with gastrointestinal obstruction, gastric retention, bowel perforation, toxic colitis, or megacolon. On the day prior to the examination, a clear liquid diet

(Continued)

Colon Films *(Continued)*

should start at lunchtime. Clear liquids include black tea or coffee, broth or bouillon, plain jello, strained fruit juice, popsicles, water, carbonated beverages or sherbet. The patient should not drink milk or cream. At 3 PM on the day before the examination, the patient should start drinking the product GoLYTELY® at a rate of 8 oz (240 mL) every 10 minutes until a total of 4 L has been consumed. Rapid drinking of each portion should be encouraged (as opposed to drinking sips continuously). It is important that each patient drink the entire volume of GoLYTELY® for an adequate GI examination. An alternative method of bowel cleansing may be required in patients with fluid restrictions, with renal failure, with congestive cardiac failure, or in patients younger than 18 years of age. The patient's primary physician should be consulted with regard to this. Orally administered GoLYTELY® induces a diarrhea which rapidly cleanses the bowel, usually within 4 hours. The material is available in a powdered form for oral administration as a solution following reconstitution. **AFTERCARE:** Correct aftercare of the barium enema patient is essential if examination is to be followed by a GI series. If colon is not cleansed of residual barium following barium enema, patient will not be accepted for GI series on the following morning. The following is advised. All patients on return from barium enema examination should be given 10 oz of magnesium citrate at 4 PM. On the following morning, patient should have a Fleet® enema before being sent for GI series. **SPECIAL INSTRUCTIONS:** By appointment only. When a series of gastrointestinal examinations are desired, the procedures should be scheduled as follows.

- First day: Gallbladder series: If it is known that the patient is to have a barium enema following the gallbladder series, then preparation for the barium enema should begin on the same day as preparation for the gallbladder series. Please see listing for Oral Cholecystogram, Gallbladder Series.
- Second day: Barium enema followed by adequate aftercare, consisting of 10 oz of magnesium citrate at 4 PM and a Fleet® enema on the following morning, if there is to be a GI series on the following morning. If this is not done, residual barium may remain in the colon so that a GI series is not possible on the following morning.
- Third day: Gastrointestinal series and small bowel series. Barium enema will be supplemented by an air contrast study at the discretion of the radiologist. There is no need for the requisition to state "air contrast study". The decision whether to do an air contrast study will reside with the radiologist. An air contrast study may also be done after routine barium enema by consultation with the radiologist. Pyelograms should be scheduled before barium studies of the GI tract.

Specimen **CAUSES FOR REJECTION:** Barium in colon or inadequate preparation.

Interpretation **LIMITATIONS:** If a rectal biopsy has been done, barium enema should not be ordered for 10 days. Exceptions to this will be permitted only after consultation with the surgeon involved. Hypotonic colon examination using glucagon will be ordered at the discretion of the radiologist or by consultation with the radiologist. If the patient is to have ultrasonography or computerized tomography, then barium enema should be delayed until these exams are completed. Barium in the abdomen will interfere with these exams. Air contrast examination is not optimally performed following sigmoidoscopy.

Contrast Study of the Esophagus and Pharynx *see* Esophagram *on page 296*

CXR *see* Chest Films *on page 292*

Cystogram *see* Cystourethrogram *on this page*

Cystourethrogram

CPT 74456

Synonyms Cystogram; Voiding Cystourethrogram

Abstract **PROCEDURE COMMONLY INCLUDES:** Catheterization of the urinary bladder which is then distended with contrast material until the patient feels the urge to micturate. Micturition is then recorded on videotape with appropriate views for confirmation or exclusion of ureteric reflux and appropriate evaluation of the urethra. **INDICATIONS:** Evaluation of the morphology of the urinary bladder, evaluation of the urethra for exclusion of obstructive processes such as posterior urethral valves or urethral strictures, evaluation for the presence and extent of ureteric reflux **CONTRAINDICATIONS:** Allergy to iodine.

Patient Care/Scheduling **PATIENT PREPARATION:** Obtain a signed procedure permit for cystourethrogram. Catheterization of the urinary bladder is performed. **SPECIAL INSTRUCTIONS:** Schedule this procedure before gastrointestinal barium studies.

Method **EQUIPMENT:** The ability to videotape the fluoroscopic record of this procedure will be most beneficial in assuring documentation of the appropriate diagnostic information.

Specimen **CAUSES FOR REJECTION:** Barium in pelvic region.

Interpretation **LIMITATIONS:** Previous barium studies within 24 hours.

Decubitus Abdomen *see* Abdomen X-ray *on page 289*

Dorsal Spine

CPT 72070 (AP and lateral); 72072 (AP, lateral and swimmer's); 72074 (complete including obliques, minimum of 4 views)

Synonyms Thoracic Spine

Abstract **PROCEDURE COMMONLY INCLUDES:** AP view of the thoracic spine obtained with the patient in the supine position. A lateral view of the thoracic spine obtained with the patient in the supine position. A lateral (slightly oblique) view of the upper two thoracic segments known as a Twining's or swimmer's view is obtained for evaluation of the lower cervical and upper thoracic spine. **INDICATIONS:** Evaluate thoracic spine for presence of metastasis and primary neoplasm, trauma, infectious disease, degenerative and reactive process.

Patient Care/Scheduling **PATIENT PREPARATION:** No preparation required for the examination. To schedule a study, call X-ray Department.

Enteroclysis

CPT 74356

Synonyms Small Bowel Enema

Abstract **PROCEDURE COMMONLY INCLUDES:** Intubation of the small bowel with a 12- or 14-gauge French catheter under fluoroscopic guidance. The catheter should be long enough to reach the first loop of jejunum. It should be the smallest possible diameter to minimize nasopharyngeal or oropharyngeal irritation. The catheter should possess an adaptation, such as a distensible balloon, to prevent reflux of contrast material thus preventing decompression of the small bowel during the examination. A barium mixture is then introduced into the small bowel. The examination may be performed in a single contrast or double contrast fashion. Where a double contrast examination is performed, methyl cellulose is introduced subsequent to infusion of high density contrast material. **INDICATIONS:** Enteroclysis is indicated after all radiologic and endoscopic tests have been unrevealing in the evaluation of gastrointestinal tract blood loss of unknown origin. Enteroclysis is the method of choice in the evaluation of malabsorptive states. While Crohn's disease involving the distal ileum can be well demonstrated on a conventional small bowel study, enteroclysis excels in the demonstration of the proximal and distal extent of disease and the presence of skip lesions or fistulas in patients with Crohn's disease. While contraindicated in patients with the clinical and radiographic findings of high grade obstruction, enteroclysis may be useful in determining the site, severity, and nature of the obstruction once the bowel has been satisfactorily decompressed. This method of examination may also be helpful in patients with periumbilical or right lower quadrant pain associated with abdominal distention, nausea, or vomiting, especially if the patient has had prior abdominal surgery. **CONTRAINDICATIONS:** Clinical and radiographic findings of high grade obstruction, extensive prior gastric surgery where the anatomy is ill-defined, lack of patient compliance.

Patient Care/Scheduling **PATIENT PREPARATION:** Patient should be fasting from midnight prior to the examination. A laxative or mild colon cleansing enema should be performed the day prior to the examination to ensure that not much fecal material is present in the ascending colon. **SPECIAL INSTRUCTIONS:** It is recommended that requests for enteroclysis be discussed with the attending radiologist prior to completion of the radiology consult. The importance of adequate bowel preparation is stressed. Metoclopramide administration

(Continued)

Enteroclysis *(Continued)*

prior to the study has been found useful as it eases transpyloric intubation and facilitates a faster infusion rate of contrast material. Intravenous diazepam in small doses (3-5 mg) may be helpful in particularly apprehensive patients.

Specimen TURNAROUND TIME: A written report available within 24 hours of the completed examination. Consultation with the radiologist prior to this upon request.

Interpretation ADDITIONAL INFORMATION: This is a specialized examination of the small bowel. Routine enteroclysis in the absence of prior investigations or an attempt at small bowel examination is not usually performed.

References

Barloon TJ, Lu CC, Franken EA Jr, et al, "Small Bowel Enteroclysis Survey," *Gastrointest Radiol*, 1988, 13(3):203-6.

Maglinte DD, Lappas JC, Kelvin FM, et al, "Small Bowel Radiography: How, When and Why?" *Radiology*, 1987, 163:297-305.

Epidural Venogram

CPT 75873

Synonyms Lumbar Venogram

Abstract PROCEDURE COMMONLY INCLUDES: This examination was developed to facilitate the diagnosis of lateral prolapse of intervertebral discs in the lumbar spine. The advent of computed tomography and nuclear magnetic resonance, both of which facilitate direct visualization of lateral herniation, has removed the need for this invasive procedure.

Esophagram

CPT 74210 (radiologic examination); 74220 (esophagus); 74230 (swallowing function, pharynx and/or esophagus, with cineradiography and/or video)

Synonyms Barium Swallow; Contrast Study of the Esophagus and Pharynx; Esophagus, X-ray

Applies to Cardiac Series; Heart Size; Positive Contrast Examinations of the Pharynx and Esophagus

Abstract PROCEDURE COMMONLY INCLUDES: Fluoroscopy, spot films, and survey radiographs. Videotaping may be helpful in the further detailed analysis of the swallowing mechanism. Spot films are at the discretion of the radiologist and may be obtained in any projection to more clearly delineate pathology. Survey films obtained include an anteroposterior film of the barium distended esophagus extending from the neck to the diaphragm and right anterior oblique projection of the barium distended esophagus to include the neck and thorax. The left anterior oblique projection including the same anatomic area is occasionally included in the examination. INDICATIONS:

- establish the presence of intrinsic abnormalities of the pharynx and esophagus including neoplasms, webs, tracheoesophageal fistulas, gastroesophageal reflux, Barrett's esophagus, and esophagitis
- demonstrate the type and location of foreign bodies within the pharynx and esophagus
- demonstrate narrowing or displacement of the barium-filled esophagus due to extrinsic pathology such as vascular rings, mediastinal masses, etc
- evaluate caliber and motility of the esophagus
- confirm the integrity of esophageal anastomoses in the postoperative patient

CONTRAINDICATIONS: While no definite contraindications to this examination are recognized, the study requires considerable modification under certain circumstances. Because of this, the type, location, and extent of suspected pathology should be clearly stated on the requisition.

Patient Care/Scheduling PATIENT PREPARATION: This examination is commonly performed in association with an upper GI series. Under these circumstances, the patient should have nothing to eat or drink after midnight before the examination. On the morning of the examination, the patient may wash the mouth with water but should not swallow the water. If a foreign body is suspected, this should be clearly stated on the requisition, thus allowing the examination to be tailored accordingly. AFTERCARE: None or mild laxative

SPECIAL INSTRUCTIONS: By appointment only. Where problem is complex, preliminary consultation with an attending radiologist is desirable. Such cases may require rapid serial spot filming or other modalities.

Method **TECHNIQUE:** A comprehensive discussion of the methodology employed in the evaluation of the pharynx and esophagus is beyond the scope of this text. A reference for this information is supplied.

Interpretation **ADDITIONAL INFORMATION:** The correct application of the full column technique, mucosal relief films, double contrast studies and motion recording is critical in obtaining maximum information from the examination. An article by Maglinte and his colleagues examines what constitutes a minimal esophageal survey in a patient referred for an upper GI series with nonspecific and/or vague upper abdominal complaints.[1] The author evaluated approximately 500 patients with nonspecific and/or vague upper GI complaints to examine what constituted a minimal esophageal survey and the extent of esophageal disease visible on radiography in these patients.

Footnotes

1. Maglinte DDT, Schultheis TE, Krol KL, et al, "A Survey of the Esophagus During the Upper Gastrointestinal Examination in 500 Patients," *Radiology*, 1983, 147:65-70.

References

Gelfand DW and Ott DJ, "Anatomy and Technique in Evaluating the Esophagus," *Semin Roentgenol*, 1981, 16(3):168.

Esophagus, X-ray *see* Esophagram *on previous page*

Facet Joint Arthrography/Injection

Abstract **PROCEDURE COMMONLY INCLUDES:** Arthrographic evaluation of facet joints or placement of needle within facet joints for injection of anti-inflammatory agents or a long lasting anesthesia. **INDICATIONS:**

- facet syndrome
- nerve root compression by a facet joint synovial cyst
- narrowing of the lumbar canal caused primarily by degeneration of the facet joint
- prerhizolysis survey
- spondylolysis with nodule protruding from the bony defect which may be producing nerve root compression
- inflammatory spondyloarthropathy
- septic facet joint arthritis

Patient Care/Scheduling **PATIENT PREPARATION:** No alteration of the patient's diet is required for this procedure. Scheduling is accomplished by contacting the Radiology Department. **SPECIAL INSTRUCTIONS:** Examination will be performed by appointment following consultation with the neurosurgeon or neurologist.

References

McCormick CC, Taylor JR, and Twomey LT, "Facet Joint Arthrography in Lumbar Spondylolysis: Anatomic Basis for Spread of Contrast Medium," *Radiology*, 1989, 171(1):193-6.

Wybire M and Laredo JD, "Facet Joint Arthropathy and Steroid Injection," *Interventional Radiology in Bone and Joint*, New York, NY: Springer-Verlag Wien, 1988.

Facial Bones

CPT 70140 (facial bones, less then 3 views); 70150 (complete, minimum of 3 views)

Related Information

Skull, X-ray *on page 305*

Applies to Zygomatic Arch, Left and Right

Abstract **PROCEDURE COMMONLY INCLUDES:** Radiographic evaluation of the facial bones including three views of the bones of the face. The first is a posterior-anterior view obtained with the patient in the prone position. This projection provides a good view of the maxilla, the zygomatic arches, the orbits, and the nasal cavity. The second view is known as the submentovertical view of the skull. It is obtained with the patient in the supine position and the x-ray tube angled in a caudocephalad direction. This projection facilitates visualization

(Continued)

Facial Bones *(Continued)*

of the foramina at the base of the skull, the petrous ridges, and the ethmoid and sphenoid bones. It also provides a tangential perspective on the zygomata, the zygomatic arches, and the maxillary bones. The third film in the facial bone series is a lateral view of the face. If a fracture of the zygomatic arch is suspected, a further view, entitled the verticosubmental projection, may be helpful. **INDICATIONS:** Facial trauma, specifically to exclude fracture of the facial bones.

Patient Care/Scheduling **PATIENT PREPARATION:** No specific preparation required. The examination may be scheduled by contacting the Radiology Department.

Fistulogram *see* Fistulous Tracts, X-ray *on this page*

Fistulous Tracts, X-ray

CPT 76081

Synonyms Fistulogram

Abstract **PROCEDURE COMMONLY INCLUDES:** Opacification under fluoroscopic guidance of abnormal communications between two epithelial surfaces. Example: Between the skin and the bowel (enterocutaneous fistula), between the stomach and the colon (gastrocolic fistula), etc. **INDICATIONS:** To determine the extent and organs involved in the fistula's tract to plan surgical therapeutic approach or to monitor the healing progress **CONTRAINDICATIONS:** Barium within the bowel may constitute a relative contraindication, depending upon whether it interferes with visualization of the opacified fistulous tract.

Patient Care/Scheduling **SPECIAL INSTRUCTIONS:** By appointment only.

Interpretation **ADDITIONAL INFORMATION:** In the case of enterocutaneous fistulas, opacification will require placement of an appropriate size catheter and injection of contrast material through the catheter to opacify the fistulous tract. This will generally be performed within the gastrointestinal radiology suite in the Radiology Department.

Gallbladder Series *see* Oral Cholecystogram, Gallbladder Series *on page 301*

Gallbladder X-ray *see* Oral Cholecystogram, Gallbladder Series *on page 301*

Gastrointestinal Series

CPT 74240 (radiologic examination, gastrointestinal tract, upper, with or without delayed films, without KUB); 74241 (with or without delayed films, with KUB); 74245 (with small bowel, included multiple serial films); 74246 (radiologic exam, gastrointestinal tract, upper, air contrast, with specific high density barium, effervescent agent, with or without glucagon, with or without delayed films, without KUB); 74247 (with or without delayed films, with KUB); 74249 (with small bowel follow-through); 74250 (radiologic examination small bowel, includes multiple serial films); 74260 (duodenography, hypotonic)

Synonyms Barium Meal; GI Series; Upper GI Examination

Abstract **PROCEDURE COMMONLY INCLUDES:** Radiographic and fluoroscopic evaluation of the esophagus, stomach, and duodenum while the patient is drinking a barium solution. Spot films will be obtained in various projections during the dynamic portion of the study. Subsequent to this, routine overhead films will also be obtained. The examination may be coupled with a study of the small bowel or may be done separately. **INDICATIONS:** Evaluation of the gastrointestinal tract for the presence of neoplasms, inflammatory diseases, ulcers, diverticula, obstruction, foreign body, hiatal hernia, and gastroesophageal reflux **CONTRAINDICATIONS:** Presence of barium within the colon, presence of food within the stomach.

Patient Care/Scheduling **PATIENT PREPARATION:** Adult patients should have a light, liquid supper the evening prior to the examination and should have nothing to eat or drink after midnight. Pediatric patients should refrain from eating or drinking for 4 hours prior to the examination. (The latter is at the discretion of the radiologist and depends on the age of the patient.) Some radiologists recommend a mild cathartic subsequent to the examination particularly in the case of older, chronically constipated patients. **SPECIAL INSTRUCTIONS:** Examination may be scheduled by calling the Radiology Department.

Interpretation **LIMITATIONS:** Pyelograms should be scheduled before barium studies of the GI tract. Hypotonic duodenography may be performed at the discretion of the radiologist.

If the patient is scheduled to have sonographic examination of the abdomen or a CT examination, the gastrointestinal series should be delayed until these exams have been completed. High concentration of barium within the gastrointestinal tract will produce artifacts on CT scan. When the patient is scheduled for both an upper gastrointestinal series and a barium enema, the barium enema should be performed first and the patient given a cathartic such as magnesium citrate to facilitate evacuation prior to the gastrointestinal series. **ADDITIONAL INFORMATION:** A number of different techniques are described for mucosal relief studies, double contrast examinations. There are also several different commercially available barium sulfate suspensions. In addition to this, pharmacological agents such as glucagon may be helpful in suppressing motility and facilitating hypotonic evaluation. A standard dose of 0.1 mg of glucagon diluted to 0.25 mL with sterile water is utilized routinely in some double contrast examinations.

References

Levine MS, Rubesin SE, Herlinger H, et al, "Double-Contrast Upper Gastrointestinal Examination: Technique and Interpretation," *Radiology*, 1988, 168(3):593-602.

GI Series *see* Gastrointestinal Series *on previous page*

Heart Size *see* Esophagram *on page 296*

Hysterosalpingogram

CPT 74741

Synonyms Uterogram

Abstract **PROCEDURE COMMONLY INCLUDES:** Injection of a contrast agent into the uterus and fallopian tubes **INDICATIONS:** Examination allows demonstration and radiographic documentation of the outline of the uterine cavity. It also facilitates opacification of the fallopian tubes. Because of this, it is commonly part of the work-up in cases of infertility. Also used to evaluate the tubes subsequent to tubal ligation and to evaluate the results of reconstructive surgery. **CONTRAINDICATIONS:** Pregnancy, active pelvic inflammatory disease (PID).

Patient Care/Scheduling **COMPLICATIONS:** While some procedural discomfort pain is frequently encountered, it is usually transient. Tubule granulomas are occasionally encountered and are thought to be more commonly related to the use of oil based contrast material.

Specimen **CAUSES FOR REJECTION:** Incorrect time in menstrual cycle. The exam is best performed following menstruation but before ovulation. This is usually between the 7th and 14th day of the menstrual cycle.

References

Wolf DM and Spataro RF, "The Current State of Hysterosalpingography," *Radiographics*, 1988, 8:1041.

Infusion Pyelogram *see* Urography *on page 305*

Intraoperative Cholangiogram *see* Cholangiogram, Operative *on page 293*

Intravenous Pyelogram *see* Urography *on page 305*

IVP *see* Urography *on page 305*

KUB *see* Abdomen X-ray *on page 289*

Laryngogram

CPT 70373 (laryngography, contrast: supervision and interpretation only); 70374 (complete procedure)

Abstract **PROCEDURE COMMONLY INCLUDES:** Fluoroscopic and radiographic evaluation of the larynx utilizing positive contrast material. CT scanning has replaced the use of tomography, xeroradiography, and laryngography for the radiologic evaluation of laryngeal tumors. This modality compliments direct laryngoscopy. Computed tomography demonstrates the status of the cartilage, tumor extension into the extralaryngeal and paralaryngeal spaces, and subglottic extensions.

(Continued)

Laryngogram *(Continued)*

References

Mancuso AA and Hanafee WN, "A Comparative Evaluation of Computed Tomography and Laryngography," *Radiology*, 1979, 133:131-8.

Loop-O-Gram, X-ray

CPT 74420 (urogram retrograde with/without KUB)

Abstract PROCEDURE COMMONLY INCLUDES: Introduction of a catheter into the ileal conduit, injection of contrast material to reflux up the ureters and into the renal collecting systems. INDICATIONS: Evaluation of the collecting systems and ureters in patients who have previously undergone a urinary diversion.

Patient Care/Scheduling PATIENT PREPARATION: Views on the necessity and the usefulness of cathartics in the preparation of patients for loop-o-grams vary. Some patients advocate the routine use of 10 oz of magnesium citrate the evening before the examination. Alternatives would include a mild laxative such as 1 1/4 oz of a standard extract of senna fruit the evening before the examination. Others feel cathartics are not indicated. SPECIAL INSTRUCTIONS: Schedule this test before barium studies of the GI tract.

Specimen CAUSES FOR REJECTION: Residual barium TURNAROUND TIME: Reports are mailed out within 24 hours after the examination is performed. If a preliminary reading is desired, please specify on the completed and signed requisition.

Lumbar Venogram *see* Epidural Venogram *on page 296*

Lumbosacral Spine

CPT 72100 (AP/lateral); 72110 (complete with obliques)

Abstract PROCEDURE COMMONLY INCLUDES: AP view of the lumbosacral spine obtained with the patient in the supine position and the knee flexed. Lateral view of the lumbosacral spine obtained with the patient recumbent. Oblique views of the lumbosacral spine are obtained, when requested, for demonstration of the pars interarticulares and the apophyseal joints to best advantage. INDICATIONS: Evaluate the bones for the presence of metastatic and primary neoplasms, trauma, infectious disease, degenerative, reactive, and postsurgical changes. Intervertebral disc spaces are also well evaluated by this method.

Mammogram

CPT 76090 (unilateral); 76091 (bilateral)

Synonyms Breast, X-ray

Abstract PROCEDURE COMMONLY INCLUDES: A minimum of two views of the breast INDICATIONS: A mammogram is indicated in the evaluation of any newly appearing breast lump considered suspicious for tumor. Because of the high incidence of breast cancer among the female population, the American Cancer Society recommends screening mammography for detection of cancer in the asymptomatic patient. The American Cancer Society sets down the following guidelines for screening. The society recommends a baseline mammogram be obtained in all females between the ages of 35 and 39. Between the ages of 40 and 49 they recommend a mammogram every 1-2 years. Patients 50 years of age or older are recommended to have a mammogram on an annual basis.

Patient Care/Scheduling PATIENT PREPARATION: Cleansing of the skin surface over both breasts and in the axilla is recommended prior to the examination. It should be noted that talcum powder and some deodorants may produce significant artifact on the film. Cleansing is therefore of the utmost importance to ensure no unnecessary repeat examinations.

Method EQUIPMENT: While the examination may be performed utilizing either xeromammographic equipment or film screen mammography, there is a growing body of opinion that the film screen mammogram is the best available method for radiographic examination of the breast.

Interpretation ADDITIONAL INFORMATION: Nonpalpable breast lesions considered suspicious for malignancy should be excised. These abnormalities may be localized for the surgeon prior to surgery by the radiologist utilizing a localization needle. There are various localization markers commercially available. Subsequent to placement of the localization needle, its position within the abnormality is confirmed mammographically. The patient is then transported to the operating room. Once resected, the specimen is returned to Radiology where a further film is obtained to ensure that all the tissue believed to be suspicious in nature has been removed from the patient's breast.

References

"1989 Survey of Physicians Attitudes and Practices in Early Cancer Detection," *CA – A Cancer Journal for Clinicians*, 1990, 40:77.

Mandible, Complete or Partial *see* Skull, X-ray *on page 305*

Mastoids Complete *see* Skull, X-ray *on page 305*

Maxilla *see* Skull, X-ray *on page 305*

Metastatic Series Plus Long Bones *see* Skeletal Survey *on page 304*

Nasal Bones *see* Skull, X-ray *on page 305*

Oral Cholecystogram, Gallbladder Series

CPT 74290; 74291 (additional or repeat examination or multiple day examination)

Synonyms Cholecystography; Gallbladder Series; Gallbladder X-ray

Abstract PROCEDURE COMMONLY INCLUDES: Radiographic examination of the gallbladder is performed subsequent to opacification of this organ by orally ingested contrast material. Patient ingests oral contrast material the evening prior to the radiographic examination. Radiographs of the right upper quadrant are obtained for evaluation of the opacified gallbladder. INDICATIONS: Cholelithiasis, cholecystitis, right upper quadrant pain CONTRAINDICATIONS: Prior cholecystectomy, iodine allergy, severe diarrhea.

Patient Care/Scheduling PATIENT PREPARATION: Various oral contrast preparations are available. These are ingested the evening before the study and the dosage and timing of ingestion will be provided with the tablets. Some physicians advocate ingestion of a high fat lunch the day before the study. This stimulates evacuation of the gallbladder and refilling with opacified bile. The patient is to ingest nothing by mouth after midnight. SPECIAL INSTRUCTIONS: By appointment only COMPLICATIONS: The gallbladder may not be visualized for a number of reasons. These include a lack of absorption of the contrast material from the patient's bowel. This may require an additional, repeat, or multiple day examination.

Method EQUIPMENT: Standard radiography equipment.

Interpretation ADDITIONAL INFORMATION: This radiographic examination is rarely requested, having been almost totally supplanted by ultrasonography of the gallbladder. It is generally maintained among the radiology community that sonography warrants the pre-eminent position in the diagnosis of gallbladder disease.

References

Amberg JR and Leopold GR, "Is Oral Cholecystography Still Useful?" *AJR*, 1988, 151:73-4.

Gelfand DW, Wolfman NT, Ott DJ, et al, "Oral Cholecystography vs Gallbladder Sonography: A Prospective, Blinded Reappraisal," *AJR*, 1988, 151(1):69-72.

PA *see* Chest Films *on page 292*

PA and Lateral CXR *see* Chest Films *on page 292*

Paranasal Sinuses

CPT 70210 (paranasal sinuses less than 3 views); 70220 (paranasal sinuses minimum of 3 views)

Related Information

Computed Transaxial Tomography, Paranasal Sinuses *on page 280*

Synonyms Sinuses

Abstract PROCEDURE COMMONLY INCLUDES: In the adult, the paranasal sinus radiographic evaluation usually includes four films. The first of these is obtained with the nose and forehead against the cassette and the x-ray beam passing in a posterior to anterior projection. The x-ray tube is tilted 15° caudally (Caldwell's projection). This projection demonstrates

(Continued)

Paranasal Sinuses *(Continued)*

the frontal and ethmoid sinuses to best advantage. The maxillary sinuses are obscured by the petrous ridges in this projection. The maxillary antra are shown to best advantage with the Waters' projection. Here the beam again passes from a posterior to anterior direction and the patient's chin rests on the cassette. The nose is positioned 2-3 cm from the cassette. This view is generally obtained in both the recumbent and upright positions. The upright position allows demonstration of air fluid levels within the maxillary antra. The series is completed with a lateral projection of the paranasal sinuses. The sphenoid sinuses are seen to best advantage in this projection. The lateral projection also affords a good demonstration of the frontal sinuses. **INDICATIONS:** The examination is most commonly employed for the diagnosis of sinusitis. Films may demonstrate complete opacification of the sinuses, thickening of the mucoperiosteal lining of the sinuses, or air fluid levels. In addition to inflammatory conditions, this series of films may reveal congenital abnormalities, traumatic and neoplastic diseases. See also Computed Transaxial Tomography, Paranasal Sinuses.

Patient Care/Scheduling **PATIENT PREPARATION:** No special preparation is required for this examination. **SPECIAL INSTRUCTIONS:** Relevant information pertinent to the examination should be indicated on the requisition which should accompany the patient to the Radiology Department.

Interpretation **ADDITIONAL INFORMATION:** In the pediatric age group, the paranasal sinuses are difficult to evaluate due to variability in patterns of development. The maxillary and ethmoid sinuses are present and aerated at birth. The frontal sinuses usually do not develop until 7-10 years of age. The sphenoid sinuses develop shortly after the maxillary and ethmoid sinus cavities. The modified Waters' view and the lateral view suffice for evaluation of the paranasal sinuses in the pediatric population. In the pediatric population, the nose should be placed closer to the cassette for the Waters' projection. If the angulation is too steep, the sinuses may not be visualized or may appear falsely obliterated.

References

Lloyd GA, "Diagnostic Imaging of the Nose and Paranasal Sinuses," *J Laryngol Otol*, 1989, 103(5):453-60.

Swischuk LE, Hayden CK, and Dillard RA, "Sinusitis in Children," *Radiographics*, 1982, 2:241-52.

Pelvimetry

CPT 74710

Abstract **PROCEDURE COMMONLY INCLUDES:** Traditionally, pelvimetry has been performed utilizing the Colcher-Sussman pelvimeter with AP and lateral views of the pelvis. More recently, digital radiography has been effectively utilized in the performance of pelvimetry with a reduction in the radiation dose. **INDICATIONS:** Pelvimetry may be of value in breech presentation since it may demonstrate hyperextension of the fetal head. The main indication is in the diagnosis of cephalopelvic disproportion. Used to evaluate the maternal pelvis for size in relation to the fetal presenting part.

Patient Care/Scheduling **PATIENT PREPARATION:** Send patient with requisition to Radiology. Patient must wear x-ray gown to department.

References

Federle MP, Cohen HA, Rosenwein MF, et al, "Pelvimetry by Digital Radiography: A Low Dose Examination," *Radiology*, 1982, 143:733-5.

Philpott RH, "The Recognition of Cephalopelvic Disproportion," *Clin Obstet Gynecol*, 1982, 9:3.

Percutaneous Biopsy of Musculoskeletal Lesions and Synovial Membranes *see* Bone Biopsy *on page 290*

Positive Contrast Examinations of the Pharynx and Esophagus *see* Esophagram *on page 296*

Postoperative Cholangiography *see* Cholangiography, Postoperative, T-Tube *on page 293*

Pyelogram, Retrograde

CPT 74420 (urography retrograde with/without KUB)

Related Information

Urography *on page 305*

Applies to Retrograde Pyelogram Generally Performed in the Operating Room

Abstract PROCEDURE COMMONLY INCLUDES: AP view of the abdomen obtained prior to the introduction of any contrast material. Further films of the abdomen exposed subsequent to opacification of the ureters and renal collecting systems. INDICATIONS: Evaluation of renal collecting systems and ureters in cases where urography is unsatisfactory.

Patient Care/Scheduling PATIENT PREPARATION: Obtain signed procedure permit for retrograde pyelogram. If the examination is to be done under general anesthesia, patient should have nothing by mouth after midnight. Bowel preparation recommendations are the same as those for urography. SPECIAL INSTRUCTIONS: Schedule this test before barium studies of the gastrointestinal tract.

Method EQUIPMENT: When performed in the operating room, the room should be equipped with a standard overhead x-ray tube. If this is unavailable, portable radiographs may be obtained.

Retrograde Pyelogram Generally Performed in the Operating Room *see* Pyelogram, Retrograde *on this page*

Scoliosis *see* Scoliosis Series, X-ray *on this page*

Scoliosis, Multiple Films *see* Scoliosis Series, X-ray *on this page*

Scoliosis Series, X-ray

CPT 72010 (radiologic examination of spine, entire, survey study, AP and lateral); 72020 (radiologic examination of spine, single view, specify level)

Synonyms Scoliosis; Scoliosis, Multiple Films

Abstract PROCEDURE COMMONLY INCLUDES: AP and lateral views of the spine are obtained at a standard 6 ft distance. INDICATIONS: Documentation of the type of curvature deformity and evaluation of the site and magnitude of deformity, assessment of the patient's skeletal maturity. Films of the spine are obtained for documentation of type and etiology of curvature deformity.

Method TECHNIQUE: Films are generally taken in the AP and lateral projections with the patient upright. Ideally, a 14" x 36" cassette is utilized so that the whole spine may be included. Film is exposed at standard 6 ft focal spot film distance to allow accurate measurement of growth. Ideally, an aluminum filter may be employed to achieve uniform radiographic density over the exposure. DATA ACQUIRED: The angular deformity may be measured by the Cobb-Lippman technique of measurement. These measurements are made by the orthopedist or orthopedic radiologist.

Specimen TURNAROUND TIME: Reports are mailed out within 24 hours after the examination is performed. If a preliminary reading is desired, please specify on the completed and signed requisition.

References

Bradford DS, Lonstein JE, Moe JH, et al, *Textbook of Scoliosis and Other Spinal Deformities*, Philadelphia, PA: WB Saunders Co, 1987.

Sella Turcica *see* Skull, X-ray *on page 305*

Sialogram

CPT 70391 (complete procedure)

Abstract PROCEDURE COMMONLY INCLUDES: Placement of small catheter in the salivary duct and injection of contrast material with films is obtained both preinjection and postinjection. While conventional radiography and sialography have proved very useful in the diagnosis of inflammatory salivary gland disease and were once the method of choice in the evaluation of salivary gland tumors, the last decade has seen computed tomography emerge as the method of choice for evaluation of salivary gland neoplasms. INDICATIONS: These in-

(Continued)

Sialogram *(Continued)*

clude recurrent sialoadenitis, pain, dryness of the mouth, postoperative or post-traumatic salivary fistula or soft fluctuant swelling suggesting a sialocele. Sudden acute swelling of the gland especially during eating. **CONTRAINDICATIONS:** Acute infection, known sensitivity to iodine compounds.

Patient Care/Scheduling **PATIENT PREPARATION:** The patient should be informed of the purpose of the study and its impact in determination of therapy. The patient should also be warned that the gland may enlarge as a result of this study but should return to normal size in the subsequent 24-48 hours. **AFTERCARE:** Evacuation of contrast material from the salivary glands may be facilitated by having the patient suck on a lemon or suck some citrate tablets. This will stimulate the flow of saliva and thus aid in the clearance of contrast material from the gland.

Interpretation **LIMITATIONS:** Cannot do bilateral sialogram; one side per day.

References

Casselman JW and Mancuso AA, "Major Salivary Gland Masses: Comparison of MR Imaging and CT," *Radiology*, 1987, 165:183-9.

Rabinov K and Weber AL, *Radiology of the Salivary Glands*, Boston, MA: GK Hall Medical Publishers, 1985.

Sinuses *see* Paranasal Sinuses *on page 301*

Skeletal Survey

CPT 76061 (limited); 76062 (complete [axial and appendicular])

Synonyms Metastatic Series Plus Long Bones

Abstract **PROCEDURE COMMONLY INCLUDES:** Lateral skull, AP long bones, AP thorax with rib detail, AP lumbar with pelvis to include femoral heads, lateral cervical, dorsal, and lumbar spines **INDICATIONS:** Survey for metastatic disease, survey for battered child.

Patient Care/Scheduling **PATIENT PREPARATION:** Any area to be radiographically examined should bare the lightest possible dressing and only if absolutely necessary.

Method **EQUIPMENT:** Examination may be performed on commercially available radiography equipment.

Specimen **TURNAROUND TIME:** Report will be mailed out within 24 hours after the examination has been performed. If a preliminary reading is desired, please specify on the completed and signed requisition.

Interpretation **LIMITATIONS:** These examinations should be performed prior to barium studies of the gastrointestinal tract. Barium may obscure portions of the axial skeleton. **ADDITIONAL INFORMATION:** A nuclear medicine bone scan is usually a more sensitive method of determining the presence of metastatic disease involving the skeleton. Whereas plain films of the bone may show no abnormality in the presence of considerable destruction. The bone scan reflects metabolic activity within the bone itself and is thus more sensitive in the detection of bone destruction. Rarely a tumor such as myeloma may be so aggressive as to produce a "cold spot" on the bone scan. In these cases a skeletal survey may be more effective in demonstrating the disseminated disease.

Skull AP and Lateral *see* Skull, X-ray *on next page*

Skull Basilar View Only *see* Skull, X-ray *on next page*

Skull Series Complete *see* Skull, X-ray *on next page*

Skull, X-ray

CPT 70100 (mandible, partial); 70110 (complete mandible, minimum 4 views); 70120 (mastoids, less than 3 views per side); 70130 (minimum 3 views per side); 70134 (internal auditory meatus complete); 70140 (radiologic examination, facial bones); 70150 (complete facial bones, minimum 3 views); 70190 (optic foramina); 70200 (orbits complete, minimum 4 views); 70250 (radiologic exam skull, partial, with or without stereo); 70260 (complete examination, minimum 4 views with or without stereo)

Related Information

Facial Bones *on page 297*

Applies to Mandible, Complete or Partial; Mastoids Complete; Maxilla; Nasal Bones; Sella Turcica; Skull AP and Lateral; Skull Basilar View Only; Skull Series Complete; Temporomandibular Joints

Abstract PROCEDURE COMMONLY INCLUDES: A series of radiographs, variable in number, obtained in projections designed to demonstrate the area of interest to maximum advantage. INDICATIONS: Establish the presence of fractures, infection, neoplastic destruction, degenerative and reactive processes of the skull, congenital anomalies.

Patient Care/Scheduling PATIENT PREPARATION: Remove all jewelry, hairpins, glass eyes, braids, contact lenses, glasses, dentures, and dressings where possible. SPECIAL INSTRUCTIONS: Indicate if there is suspicion of neck injury since positioning requires considerable flexion and extension of neck.

Method EQUIPMENT: Dedicated skull radiography unit desirable.

References

Masters SJ, "Evaluation of Head Trauma: Efficacy of Skull Films," *AJR*, 1980, 135:539-47.

Small Bowel Enema *see* Enteroclysis *on page 295*

Surgical Cholangiogram *see* Cholangiogram, Operative *on page 293*

Temporomandibular Joints *see* Skull, X-ray *on this page*

Thoracic Spine *see* Dorsal Spine *on page 295*

T-Tube *see* Cholangiography, Postoperative, T-Tube *on page 293*

Upper GI Examination *see* Gastrointestinal Series *on page 298*

Urography

CPT 74400 (with or without KUB)

Related Information

Pyelogram, Retrograde *on page 303*

Synonyms Infusion Pyelogram; Intravenous Pyelogram; IVP

Abstract PROCEDURE COMMONLY INCLUDES: Intravenous administration of a contrast material. The contrast material is concentrated and excreted by the kidneys. Appropriate radiographs are exposed during the concentration and excretion of the contrast material for evaluation of the morphology and function of the urinary tract. INDICATIONS: This examination accurately demonstrates normal anatomy and a wide range of abnormalities involving the urinary tract. CONTRAINDICATIONS: Allergy to iodine or a previous serious adverse reaction, advanced renal failure. A known diagnosis of multiple myeloma constitutes a relative contraindication. Every attempt should be made to hydrate patients with this diagnosis or with the diagnosis of diabetes mellitus prior to performance of a urogram as these patients run an increased risk of acute renal failure.

Patient Care/Scheduling PATIENT PREPARATION: Patients are encouraged to take nothing by mouth after midnight the night before the examination. This degree of fluid restriction will not produce significant dehydration but will improve the overall quality of the examination. If the urography examination is to be performed in the afternoon, a light liquid breakfast may be consumed. Views on the necessity and the usefulness of cathartics in the preparation of patients for urography vary. Some physicians advocate the routine use of 10 oz of magnesium citrate the evening before the examination. Alternatives would include a mild laxative such as 1 1/4 oz of a standard extract of senna fruit the evening before the examination. AFTERCARE: Encourage hydration by fluid ingestion. SPECIAL INSTRUCTIONS: All patients undergoing this examination should be questioned specifically with regard to

(Continued)

Urography *(Continued)*

drug allergies, particularly iodine. A recent serum creatinine is requested on patients 60 years of age or older, those with significant atherosclerotic disease, those with a known diagnosis of diabetes mellitus or with known pre-existing renal disease. **COMPLICATIONS:** Reactions to contrast material and specific treatment for such reactions are beyond the scope of this handbook. An appropriately equipped emergency cart should be immediately available should resuscitation be necessary.

Method **EQUIPMENT:** Overhead radiography tube with float top table. Tomographic capabilities are desirable.

Interpretation **LIMITATIONS:** Urography should be performed prior to barium studies of the gastrointestinal tract. The presence of barium within the abdomen will compromise the urographic examination.

References

Hattery RR, Williamson B, Hartman GW, et al, "Intravenous Urographic Technique," *Radiology*, 1988, 167(3):593-9.

Miller DL, Chang R, Wells WT, et al, "Intravascular Contrast Media: Effect of Dose on Renal Function," *Radiology*, 1988, 167(3):607-11.

Uterogram *see* Hysterosalpingogram *on page 299*

Voiding Cystourethrogram *see* Cystourethrogram *on page 294*

Zygomatic Arch, Left and Right *see* Facial Bones *on page 297*

INVASIVE RADIOLOGY

Michael A. Geisinger, MD

While it is usually difficult to date the beginning of any subspecialty, the field of Invasive Radiology probably began in 1952 when Sven-Ivar Seldinger presented his revolutionary technique of percutaneously placing a catheter within the vascular system for the injection of contrast material. Catheter angiography quickly became commonplace and has come to represent the "gold standard" for the depiction of the vascular system. The past two decades have seen the further evolution of the Seldinger technique resulting in the development of catheters for balloon angioplasty of stenotic arteries and for therapeutic embolization of tumors, arteriovenous malformations, and bleeding sites.

Over the years these catheter techniques have also been modified for use in the biliary and urinary tracts. Under fluoroscopy or one of the other imaging modalities, percutaneous access to the bile ducts or renal collecting system can be obtained, permitting placement of drainage catheters, removal of stones, and balloon dilation of strictures. Other procedures in the field of invasive radiology include needle biopsies, arthrograms, myelograms, and basically any procedure where an imaging modality is used to guide a needle accurately.

Since these procedures are by nature invasive, the risk of complication is higher than for a noninvasive radiologic examinations. Communication between the clinician and the invasive radiologist is important in order to minimize the risk of complication and to maximize the amount of information obtained from the procedure. All of these procedures require careful informed patient consent.

Abdominal Aortogram *see* Arteriogram, Transaxillary or Transbrachial Approach *on page 312*

Abdominal Aortogram *see* Arteriogram, Transfemoral Approach *on page 313*

Abscess Drainage Under Fluoroscopic, Ultrasonic, or CT Guidance

CPT 75990

Synonyms Catheter Drainage; External Decompression; Percutaneous Drainage

Applies to Drainage of Fluid Collection

Abstract **PROCEDURE COMMONLY INCLUDES:** Placement of a catheter to drain or decompress an abscess or fluid collection. These examinations are typically performed under fluoroscopic, ultrasonic, or computed tomographic guidance. Aspirated material is usually sent for Gram stain and culture. **INDICATIONS:** Presence of an intra-abdominal, intrathoracic, or pelvic abscess or presence of a symptomatic fluid collection such as a hematoma, hygroma, lymphocele, urinoma, biloma, or pseudocyst. **CONTRAINDICATIONS:** A fluid or abscess collection which is inaccessible to percutaneous needle puncture, bleeding abnormalities, elevated prothrombin or partial thromboplastin times.

Patient Care/Scheduling **PATIENT PREPARATION:** Informed consent is obtained from the patient. The patient is placed on a clear liquid diet starting 4 hours before the procedure. Recent coagulation parameters (PT, PTT, and platelet count) are recorded on the chart. In cases of abscesses and infected fluid collections, broad spectrum antibiotics are administered. **AFTERCARE:** Patient is placed on bedrest for approximately 4 hours after the procedure. Vital signs should be obtained every 30 minutes for 2 hours, then every hour for 4 hours. During this time, the patient should be closely observed for any evidence of internal or external bleeding. The drainage catheters should be connected to a collection bag. Appropriate precautions should be made that the catheter is not inadvertently pulled out. **SPECIAL INSTRUCTIONS:** These examinations are usually arranged by the requesting physician in consultation with the interventional radiologist. Any previous imaging studies of the area to be drained should be made available to the interventional radiologist. Any bleeding abnormalities should be corrected beforehand. **COMPLICATIONS:** Most complications are related to either bleeding or sepsis. Delayed complications include fistula formation, plugging, or dislodgment of the drainage catheter.

Method **EQUIPMENT:** Fluoroscopy, computed tomography, or ultrasonography; appropriate interventional needles, wires, and catheters **TECHNIQUE:** The abscess or fluid collection is localized with ultrasound, CT, or occasionally fluoroscopy and the appropriate entry path is determined. Local anesthesia is instilled at the appropriate site and a needle with or without a sheath is guided into the collection. Fluid is aspirated and sent to the laboratory for appropriate bacteriological, cytological, and/or chemical analysis. If a sheathed needle system has been used, the sheath is advanced over the needle into the fluid collection. Otherwise, a wire is passed through the needle, the needle is removed, and a catheter is then inserted over the wire into the fluid collection. The catheter is then secured in place and connected to an external drainage bag.

Interpretation **LIMITATIONS:** Some fluid collections do not lend themselves to percutaneous drainage due to the presence of multiple septations within the collection. Some collections are inaccessible to percutaneous drainage secondary to overlying bony structures or close approximation to a vascular structure. If the material to be drained is very viscous, it may be necessary to place progressively larger drainage catheters.

References

Mueller PR, van Sonnenberg E, and Ferrucci JT Jr, "Percutaneous Drainage of 250 Abdominal Abscesses and Fluid Collections. Part II: Current Procedural Concepts," *Radiology*, 1984, 151:343-7.

Sones PJ, "Percutaneous Drainage of Abdominal Abscesses," *AJR*, 1984, 142:35-9.

van Sonnenberg E, Mueller PR, and Ferrucci JT Jr, "Percutaneous Drainage of 250 Abdominal Abscesses and Fluid Collections. Part I: Results, Failures, and Complications," *Radiology*, 1984, 151:337-41.

Adrenal Arteriogram *see* Arteriogram, Transfemoral Approach *on page 313*

Adrenal Venogram *see* Venogram, Transfemoral or Transjugular Approach *on page 331*

Angiogram *see* Arteriogram, Transfemoral Approach *on page 313*

Angioinfarction *see* Embolization, Percutaneous Transcatheter *on page 321*

Angioplasty, Percutaneous Transluminal (PTA)

CPT 75963

Synonyms Balloon Dilatation; Dotter Procedure; Transluminal Angioplasty (TLA)

Applies to Atherectomy, Percutaneous; Laser Angioplasty

Abstract PROCEDURE COMMONLY INCLUDES: Dilatation of a narrowed segment of an artery usually by means of a balloon catheter which has been inserted through the femoral artery or, less commonly, the axillary artery. INDICATIONS: Treatment of symptomatic arterial stenoses (such as angina in the case of coronary artery stenosis; hypertension or renal failure in the case of renal artery stenosis; and claudication, ischemic rest pain, or ulceration in the case of lower extremity stenosis) CONTRAINDICATIONS: Acute renal failure, bleeding abnormalities, elevated prothrombin or partial thromboplastin times, extremely high blood pressure, or inability to cross the stenosis with an angiographic wire.

Patient Care/Scheduling PATIENT PREPARATION: Informed consent is obtained from the patient. The patient is placed on a clear liquid diet on the morning of the procedure. All medications are continued. Some physicians will begin the patient on antiplatelet agents, such as aspirin, before the procedure. An intravenous line is begun before the procedure in order to ensure that the patient is well hydrated (thus decreasing the risk of acute renal failure) and to facilitate the administration of any medications required during the procedure. Recent laboratory results (BUN, creatinine, platelet count, PT, and PTT) should be recorded on the chart. Some physicians will request blood typing beforehand. AFTERCARE: The patient is placed on bedrest for the remainder of the day. During this time, the patient should be flat in bed with the legs straight. Vital signs should be obtained at every 30 minutes for 2 hours, then every hour for 4 hours. At these times, the femoral puncture site should be examined for any evidence of bleeding or swelling and the legs should be evaluated for any change in pulses, color, or warmth. SPECIAL INSTRUCTIONS: These examinations are often arranged by the requesting physician in consultation with the physician performing the procedure. The physician should be alerted to any potential problem areas in the patient's condition, such as a significant elevation in blood pressure, renal insufficiency, bleeding abnormalities or a history of severe contrast reaction. Since larger catheters tend to be used in angioplasty compared to routine arteriography, particular attention should be given to the possibility of hematoma formation or bleeding at the puncture site. COMPLICATIONS: Immediate complications include contrast reaction, acute renal failure, bleeding or hematoma formation at the puncture site, vessel dissection or occlusion, and distal embolization of any clots which may have formed on the catheter. Delayed complications consist of formation of either a false aneurysm or arteriovenous fistula at the puncture site.

Method EQUIPMENT: Fluoroscopy, balloon catheters, and angiographic catheters and wires. Some laboratories now have a variety of atherectomy catheters as well as laser potential. TECHNIQUE: Local anesthetic agent is instilled over the common femoral artery. The artery is percutaneously punctured and a catheter is inserted and fluoroscopically guided to the area of arterial stenosis. The stenosis is carefully crossed with an angiographic wire. A balloon catheter is placed over the wire and the balloon is inflated to dilate the lesion. Alternate methods now include use of a laser to cross the stenosis or occlusion. Also, atherectomy catheters are now being used in some instances to extract the atheroma causing the stenosis rather than dilating it with a balloon. After the angioplasty procedure, an arteriogram is performed to visualize the results. DATA ACQUIRED: Angiograms of the stenosis and systolic pressure gradients across the stenosis are obtained both before and after the dilatation procedure in order to help assess the degree of improvement.

Interpretation NORMAL FINDINGS: After the angioplasty procedure, there should be significant improvement in the caliber of the artery. There is often a small dissection at the angioplasty site which will usually heal in the ensuing weeks. There should be no evidence of extravasation of contrast outside the arterial wall and no evidence of distal embolization.

(Continued)

Angioplasty, Percutaneous Transluminal (PTA) *(Continued)*

LIMITATIONS: The primary limitation is an inability to cross a very tight stenosis or an occlusion. In general, success rates are lower for lesions that are long or calcified as opposed to ones that are short or noncalcified.

References

Athanasoulis CA, "Percutaneous Transluminal Angioplasty: General Principles," *AJR*, 1980, 135:893-900.

Becker GJ, Katzen BT, and Dake MD, "Noncoronary Angioplasty," *Radiology*, 1989, 170(3 Pt 2):921-40.

Ankle Arthrogram *see* Arthrogram *on page 314*

Antegrade Nephrostogram, Percutaneous

CPT 74476

Synonyms Antegrade Pyelogram, Percutaneous

Abstract **PROCEDURE COMMONLY INCLUDES:** Visualization of the upper urinary tract by the injection of contrast medium through a needle which has been percutaneously placed into a calix or the pelvis of the kidney. **INDICATIONS:** Determination of the cause and location of an obstruction of the upper urinary tract when an intravenous pyelogram or a retrograde pyelogram has not been helpful. Possible causes of obstruction include stone, neoplasm, compression from an extrinsic mass, retroperitoneal fibrosis, or an inflammatory, posttraumatic, or postsurgical stricture.

Patient Care/Scheduling **PATIENT PREPARATION:** Informed consent is obtained from the patient. The patient is placed on a clear diet or NPO 4 hours before the procedure. Medications can be continued. An intravenous line is begun before the procedure to facilitate the administration of any medications or antibiotics required during the procedure. Most physicians will prescribe coverage with a broad spectrum antibiotic. Recent laboratory results (BUN, creatinine, platelet count, PT, and PTT) should be recorded on the chart. **AFTERCARE:** The patient is placed on bedrest for approximately 4 hours. Vital signs should be obtained every 30 minutes for 2 hours, then every hour for 4 hours. The patient should be observed closely for any signs of sepsis or internal bleeding. **SPECIAL INSTRUCTIONS:** Any previous imaging study of the urinary tract should be made available to the interventional radiologist. Any bleeding abnormality should be corrected beforehand. **COMPLICATIONS:** Sepsis, shock, urinoma formation, hemorrhage.

Method **EQUIPMENT:** Fluoroscopy, ultrasound, needle, contrast medium, and method of x-ray film recording **TECHNIQUE:** The patient is placed prone and a percutaneous entry site is chosen, usually with the assistance of ultrasound and/or fluoroscopy. If the kidney to be studied still functions adequately, contrast material can be injected intravenously to help localize the collecting system. Local anesthetic agent is instilled at the entry site which is usually located along the posterolateral aspect of the patient at approximately the level of the second lumbar vertebrae. A 21-gauge needle is then inserted into a calix or the pelvis of the kidney under fluoroscopic or ultrasonic guidance. Urine is aspirated and can be sent for Gram stain, culture, or cytology if desired. Contrast medium is then injected and x-ray films are obtained. **DATA ACQUIRED:** Opacification of an upper urinary tract.

Interpretation **NORMAL FINDINGS:** The pelvocalyceal system of the kidney and the ureter should be of normal caliber and configuration. There should be no evidence for any dilatation, filling defect, extrinsic compression, stricture formation, or extravasation. Contrast should flow freely down the ureter into the urinary bladder. **LIMITATIONS:** It can be difficult to successfully cannulate a urinary collection system which is both nondilated and not visualized from an intravenous injection of contrast medium.

References

Newhouse JH and Pfister RC, "Antegrade Pyelography," *Interventional Radiology*, Athanasoulis CA, Pfister RC, Green RE, et al, eds, Philadelphia, PA: WB Saunders Co, 1982, 437-54.

Antegrade Pyelogram, Percutaneous *see* Antegrade Nephrostogram, Percutaneous *on this page*

Aortogram, Translumbar Approach

CPT 75626

Synonyms Translumbar Abdominal Aortogram; Translumbar Aortogram

Abstract **PROCEDURE COMMONLY INCLUDES:** Visualization of the infrarenal abdominal aorta and iliac arteries by the injection of contrast medium through a needle which has been percutaneously placed through the lumbar region. **INDICATIONS:** Evaluation of the abdominal aorta and iliac vessels for aneurysmal dilatation, atherosclerotic irregularity, stenosis, or occlusion **CONTRAINDICATIONS:** Acute renal failure, known aneurysm at the projected site of puncture, bleeding abnormalities, elevated prothrombin or partial thromboplastin times, extremely high blood pressure, shock.

Patient Care/Scheduling **PATIENT PREPARATION:** Informed consent is obtained from the patient. If the procedure is to be performed under general anesthesia, the patient should be NPO; otherwise, the patient is placed on a clear liquid diet on the morning of the procedure. An intravenous line is begun before the procedure in order to ensure that the patient is well hydrated and to facilitate the administration of any medications required during the procedure. Recent laboratory results should be recorded on the chart. **AFTERCARE:** Continued hydration is recommended. The patient is placed on bedrest for at least 6 hours after the procedure and often for the remainder of the day. Vital signs should be obtained every 30 minutes for 2 hours then every hour for 4 hours. The patient should be observed for any signs of retroperitoneal hemorrhage, such as an unexplained decrease in blood pressure with an increase in pulse rate. Many physicians will obtain a follow-up hematocrit 12-24 hours after the procedure. **SPECIAL INSTRUCTIONS:** These examinations are often arranged by the requesting physician in consultation with the physician performing the procedure. Depending on the institution, the procedure may be performed in the operating room or in the angiography suite. Any previous imaging studies of the abdominal aorta or iliac arteries should be made available to the physician performing the procedure. Any patient problems such as renal insufficiency, bleeding abnormalities, diabetes, or history of severe contrast reaction should be noted. **COMPLICATIONS:** Retroperitoneal or para-aortic hemorrhage, dissection of the abdominal aorta or one of its branches, hemothorax or pneumothorax, pseudoaneurysm, paraplegia, or osteomyelitis of the adjacent vertebral body or disc.

Method **EQUIPMENT:** 18-gauge needle with or without a sheath, fluoroscopy, x-ray machine **TECHNIQUE:** With the patient lying prone, local anesthesia is instilled in the lumbar region beneath the 12th rib and to the left of the mid line. Under fluoroscopic guidance, the needle is inserted into the abdominal aorta at the level of the L2-3 lumbar vertebral bodies. Contrast is injected and films are obtained. **DATA ACQUIRED:** Visualization of the infrarenal abdominal aorta and of the iliac arteries.

Interpretation **NORMAL FINDINGS:** The abdominal aorta should be smooth and normal in caliber without evidence for irregularity, aneurysm, stenosis, or occlusion. **LIMITATIONS:** Anything which would obscure the blood vessels, such as overlying barium or patient motion.

References

Johnsrude IS, "Catheterization Techniques," *A Practical Approach to Angiography*, 2nd ed, Johnsrude IS, Jackson DC, and Dunnick NR, eds, Boston, MA: Little, Brown and Co, 1987, 44-70.

Arm Arteriogram *see* Arteriogram, Transaxillary or Transbrachial Approach *on next page*

Arm Arteriogram *see* Arteriogram, Transfemoral Approach *on page 313*

Arm Venogram *see* Venogram, Extremity *on page 330*

Arterial Study *see* Arteriogram, Transfemoral Approach *on page 313*

Arterial Study via Upper Extremity Approach *see* Arteriogram, Transaxillary or Transbrachial Approach *on next page*

Arteriogram, Transaxillary or Transbrachial Approach

CPT 75606 (thoracic aorta); 75627 (abdominal aorta); 75673 (cerebral); 75682 (carotid); 75697 (vertebral); 75718 (extremities); 75725 (renal); 75727 (mesenteric); 75728 (hepatic/splenic); 75737 (pelvic); 75755 (coronary)

Synonyms Arterial Study via Upper Extremity Approach; Brachial Cut-Down; Transaxillary Angiogram; Transbrachial Angiogram

Applies to Abdominal Aortogram; Arm Arteriogram; Carotid Arteriogram; Cerebral Arteriogram; Coronary Arteriogram; Hepatic Arteriogram; Leg Arteriogram; Mesenteric Arteriogram; Pelvic Arteriogram; Renal Arteriogram; Splenic Arteriogram; Thoracic Aortogram; Vertebral Arteriogram

Abstract **PROCEDURE COMMONLY INCLUDES:** Visualization of the arteries in the area of clinical concern by injection of contrast medium through a catheter which has been placed through the brachial or axillary artery. This upper extremity approach is an alternative to the femoral artery approach, especially when the femoral artery approach is not feasible secondary to femoral artery occlusion, aneurysm, or infection. **INDICATIONS:** Evaluation of the arteries in the area of clinical interest for abnormalities such as arterial aneurysm, atherosclerosis, embolism, fistula, hemorrhage, neoplasm, occlusion, arteriovenous shunting, stenosis, thrombosis, trauma, vasculitis. **CONTRAINDICATIONS:** Absence of axillary pulses, acute renal failure, bleeding abnormalities, elevated prothrombin or partial thromboplastin times, extremely high blood pressure, shock.

Patient Care/Scheduling **PATIENT PREPARATION:** Informed consent is obtained from the patient. The patient is placed on a clear liquid diet (not NPO) on the morning of the procedure. All medications are continued. If the axillary approach is to be used, the appropriate axilla should be shaved. Similarly, if a brachial approach is anticipated, the antecubital fossa should be shaved if necessary. An intravenous line is begun in the opposite arm before the procedure in order to ensure that the patient is well hydrated (thus decreasing the risk of acute renal failure) and to facilitate the administration of any medications required during the procedure. Recent laboratory results (BUN, creatinine, platelet count, PT, and PTT) should be appropriately recorded on the chart. The patient with chart is sent on a stretcher to the angiography suite when notified. **AFTERCARE:** The patient need be on bedrest for only 3-4 hours after the procedure. The patient should keep the upper extremity used for the procedure at rest at his side for the remainder of the day. Eating and other activity should be performed with the opposite arm. Vital signs should be obtained every 30 minutes for the first 2 hours, then every hour for the next 4 hours. At these times, the axilla or brachial entry site should be examined for any evidence of bleeding or swelling and the arm should be evaluated for any change in pulses, color, or warmth. Also, the hand grasp should be evaluated at these times to evaluate for any potential nerve damage. No blood pressure should be obtained using that arm for the following 48 hours. If the procedure has been performed via a cut-down, skin sutures must be removed in 5-6 days. **SPECIAL INSTRUCTIONS:** These examinations are often arranged by the requesting physician in consultation with the cardiovascular radiologist. The requisition should state clearly the reason for the study as well as the specific vessels to be examined. Any previous imaging studies of the area to be examined should be made available to the cardiovascular radiologist. The cardiovascular radiologist should be alerted to any potential problem areas in the patient's condition, such as renal insufficiency, bleeding abnormalities, or history of severe contrast reaction. **COMPLICATIONS:** Immediate complications include contrast reaction, acute renal failure, bleeding or hematoma formation at the puncture site or the site of cut-down, vessel dissection or occlusion, and distal embolization of any clots which may have formed on the catheter. A complication unique to the axillary approach is the potential for brachial plexus neuropathy secondary to hematoma formation within the brachial plexus sheath.

Method **EQUIPMENT:** Fluoroscopy, angiographic catheters and wires, a cut-down tray if a brachial artery cut-down approach is anticipated, and a method of film recording (either conventional cut-film or digital subtraction films). **TECHNIQUE:** A local anesthetic agent is instilled over either the axillary artery or the brachial artery. For the axillary approach, the artery is percutaneously punctured. For the brachial approach, the artery can be either percutaneously punctured or a cut-down can be performed. After the catheter is inserted, it is fluoroscopically guided into the artery of interest. Contrast medium is injected and the films are obtained. **DATA ACQUIRED:** Visualization of the arteries in the area of clinical concern on either conventional x-ray film or on digitally subtracted images, sometimes referred to as intra-arterial DSA.

Interpretation NORMAL FINDINGS: The opacified arteries should be smooth and gradually taper as they continue to branch. There should be no evidence of vessel wall irregularity, aneurysm, narrowing, occlusion, extravasation, or arteriovenous shunting. LIMITATIONS: Anything which would obscure the blood vessels, such as overlying barium or patient motion.

References

Johnsrude IS, "Catheterization Techniques," *A Practical Approach to Angiography*, 2nd ed, Johnsrude IS, Jackson DC, and Dunnick NR, eds, Boston, MA: Little, Brown and Co, 1987, 47-70.

Arteriogram, Transfemoral Approach

CPT 75606 (thoracic aorta); 75627 (abdominal aorta); 75673 (cerebral); 75682 (carotid); 75697 (vertebral); 75718 (extremities); 75725 (renal); 75727 (mesenteric); 75728 (hepatic/splenic); 75734 (adrenal); 75737 (pelvic); 75755 (coronary)

Synonyms Angiogram; Arterial Study; Percutaneous Transfemoral Angiogram

Applies to Abdominal Aortogram; Adrenal Arteriogram; Arm Arteriogram; Bronchial Arteriogram; Carotid Arteriogram; Cerebral Arteriogram; Coronary Arteriogram; Hepatic Arteriogram; Leg Arteriogram; Mesenteric Arteriogram; Pelvic Arteriogram; Renal Arteriogram; Splenic Arteriogram; Thoracic Aortogram; Vertebral Arteriogram

Abstract PROCEDURE COMMONLY INCLUDES: Visualization of the arteries in the area of clinical concern by injection of contrast medium through a catheter which has been percutaneously placed through the femoral artery. INDICATIONS: Evaluation of the arteries in the area of clinical interest for abnormalities such as arterial aneurysm, atherosclerosis, embolism, fistula, hemorrhage, neoplasm, occlusion, arteriovenous shunting, stenosis, thrombosis, trauma, vasculitis. CONTRAINDICATIONS: Inability of the patient to lie supine, absence of femoral pulses, acute renal failure, bleeding abnormalities, elevated prothrombin or partial thromboplastin times, extremely high blood pressure, shock.

Patient Care/Scheduling PATIENT PREPARATION: Informed consent is obtained from the patient. The patient is placed on a clear liquid diet (not NPO) on the morning of the procedure. All medications are continued. An intravenous line is begun before the procedure in order to ensure that the patient is well hydrated (thus decreasing the risk of acute renal failure) and to facilitate the administration of any medications required during the procedure. Recent laboratory results (BUN, creatinine, platelets, PT, and PTT) should be appropriately recorded on the chart. The patient with chart is sent on a stretcher to the angiography suite when notified. AFTERCARE: The patient is placed on bedrest for at least 6 hours after the procedure and often for the remainder of the day. During this time, the patient should be flat in bed with the legs straight. Vital signs should be obtained every 30 minutes for the first 2 hours, then every hour for the next 4 hours. At these times, the femoral puncture site should be examined for any evidence of bleeding or swelling and the leg should be examined for any change in pulses, color, or warmth. SPECIAL INSTRUCTIONS: These examinations are often arranged by the requesting physician in consultation with the cardiovascular radiologist. The requisition should state clearly the reason for the study as well as the specific vessels to be examined. Any previous imaging studies of the area to be examined should be made available to the cardiovascular radiologist. The cardiovascular radiologist should be alerted to any potential problem areas in the patient's condition, such as renal insufficiency, bleeding abnormalities, or history of severe contrast reaction. COMPLICATIONS: Immediate complications include contrast reaction, acute renal failure, bleeding or hematoma formation at the puncture site, vessel dissection or occlusion, and distal embolization of any clots which may have formed on the catheter. Delayed complications consist of formation of either a false aneurysm or arteriovenous fistula at the puncture site.

Method EQUIPMENT: Fluoroscopy, angiographic catheter and wires, and a method of film recording (either conventional cut-film or digital subtraction films). TECHNIQUE: Local anesthetic agent is instilled over the common femoral artery. The artery is percutaneously punctured and a catheter is inserted and fluoroscopically guided into the artery of interest. Contrast medium is injected and the films are obtained. DATA ACQUIRED: Visualization of the arteries in the area of clinical concern on either conventional x-ray film or on digitally subtracted images, sometimes referred to as intra-arterial DSA.

(Continued)

Arteriogram, Transfemoral Approach *(Continued)*

Interpretation NORMAL FINDINGS: The opacified arteries should be smooth and gradually taper as they continue to branch. There should be no evidence of vessel wall irregularity, aneurysm, narrowing, occlusion, extravasation, or arteriovenous shunting. LIMITATIONS: Anything which would obscure the blood vessels, such as overlying barium or patient motion.

References

Johnsrude IS, "Catheterization Techniques," *A Practical Approach to Angiography*, 2nd ed, Johnsrude IS, Jackson DC, and Dunnick NR, eds, Boston, MA: Little, Brown and Co, 1987, 33-44, 58-70.

Arteriovenous Fistulogram *see* Dialysis Fistulogram *on page 319*

Arteriovenous Malformation Embolization *see* Embolization, Percutaneous Transcatheter *on page 321*

Arthrogram

CPT 70333 (TMJ); 73041 (shoulder); 73086 (elbow); 73116 (wrist); 73526 (hip); 73581 (knee); 73616 (ankle)

Synonyms Joint Study

Applies to Ankle Arthrogram; Elbow Arthrogram; Hip Arthrogram; Knee Arthrogram; Shoulder Arthrogram; Temporomandibular Joint Arthrogram; Wrist Arthrogram

Abstract INDICATIONS: Evaluation of any damage to the cartilage, ligaments, and bony structures composing the joint CONTRAINDICATIONS: Bleeding abnormalities.

Patient Care/Scheduling PATIENT PREPARATION: Informed consent is obtained AFTERCARE: No strenuous activity involving the joint of interest for 24 hours.

Method EQUIPMENT: 22-gauge needle, contrast medium, and fluoroscopic and x-ray equipment TECHNIQUE: Local anesthesia is instilled at the appropriate site. A small gauge needle is inserted into the joint space. Any fluid within the joint space is aspirated and sent for appropriate chemical or bacteriologic analysis. Contrast medium and air are then inserted into the joint space under fluoroscopic guidance. Radiographs and occasionally tomograms are then obtained in multiple projections. DATA ACQUIRED: Visualization of the components of the joint space including the cartilage, ligaments, menisci, and connecting bursa.

Interpretation NORMAL FINDINGS: The joint space should not contain fluid. The cartilaginous surfaces and menisci should be smooth without evidence for erosions, tears, or disintegration. LIMITATIONS: Large joint effusions can be difficult to aspirate completely, thus resulting in dilution of the contrast material and poor visualization of the joint space structures.

References

Resnick D, "Arthrography, Tenography and Bursography," *Diagnosis of Bone and Joint Disorders*, 2nd ed, Resnick D and Niwayama G, eds, Philadelphia, PA: WB Saunders Co, 1988, 302-444.

Atherectomy, Percutaneous *see* Angioplasty, Percutaneous Transluminal (PTA) *on page 309*

Balloon Dilatation *see* Angioplasty, Percutaneous Transluminal (PTA) *on page 309*

Basket Extraction of Biliary Stones *see* Biliary Stone Extraction, Percutaneous *on next page*

Biliary Decompression *see* Biliary Drainage, Percutaneous Transhepatic *on this page*

Biliary Drainage, Percutaneous Transhepatic

CPT 75981

Synonyms Biliary Decompression; External Biliary Drainage

Applies to Biliary Stent Placement, Percutaneous; Biliary Stricture Dilatation, Percutaneous; Cholecystotomy, Percutaneous; Gallbladder Drainage, Percutaneous

Abstract PROCEDURE COMMONLY INCLUDES: Percutaneous placement of a drainage catheter in an obstructed biliary system INDICATIONS: Biliary obstruction resulting in jaundice, cholangitis, sepsis, or pain. The site of the obstruction should be in one of the larger ducts (such as the right hepatic, left hepatic, common hepatic or common bile duct). The cause of obstruction can be secondary to malignancy, stone, pancreatitis, or stricture related to surgery, trauma, or infection. Drainage of the gallbladder can be performed in cases of cholecystitis and/or calculi when patients are at too high a risk for surgery. CONTRAINDICATIONS: Tense ascites, bleeding abnormalities, elevated prothrombin and partial thromboplastin times, low platelet count.

Patient Care/Scheduling PATIENT PREPARATION: Informed consent is obtained from the patient. The patient is placed on a clear liquid diet or NPO 4 hours before the procedure. All medications are continued. An intravenous line is begun before the procedure in order to ensure that the patient is well hydrated (thus decreasing the risk of acute renal failure) and to facilitate the administration of any medications required during the procedure. If the patient is not already on antibiotics, a broad spectrum antibiotic should be administered intravenously 30 minutes before the procedure. AFTERCARE: The patient is placed on bedrest for approximately 4 hours. Vital signs should be obtained every 30 minutes for 2 hours, then every hour for 4 hours. The patient should be observed closely for any signs of internal bleeding or sepsis. SPECIAL INSTRUCTIONS: The volume of output from the biliary drain should be recorded. While the drainage may be blood tinged, any profuse bleeding from the catheter should be attended to promptly. If the drainage ceases completely, the catheter may be irrigated to remove blood clot or debris. Drainage of bile around the catheter at the skin site is usually a sign that the catheter is at least partially obstructed. COMPLICATIONS: Bleeding and sepsis are the most common complications, occurring in as many as 5% to 10% of cases. Delayed complications include dislodgment or plugging of the drainage catheter, infection at the skin entry site, development of a biloma, or erosion of a hepatic blood vessel by the catheter resulting in hemobilia or pseudoaneurysm formation.

Method EQUIPMENT: Fluoroscopy, steerable wires, and catheters TECHNIQUE: The site of entry is determined using fluoroscopy and/or ultrasound. Local anesthetic agent is instilled at the entry site and a needle is inserted into the biliary system. After the ducts have been opacified with contrast, a steerable wire is maneuvered to the point of obstruction. A drainage catheter is then passed over this wire. The catheter is affixed to the skin to prevent dislodgment. This percutaneous access route can later be used for placement of a stent across the obstruction or for balloon dilatation of an obstructing stricture. Essentially the same technique is used for drainage of the gallbladder. DATA ACQUIRED: A bile specimen can be sent for Gram stain and culture.

Interpretation LIMITATIONS: Obstructions cephalad to the level of the porta hepatis are usually not amenable to drainage.

References

Ferrucci JT Jr, Mueller PR, and Harbin WP, "Percutaneous Transhepatic Biliary Drainage," *Radiology*, 1980, 135:1-13.

McLean GK, Ring EJ, and Freiman DB, "Therapeutic Alternatives in the Treatment of Intrahepatic Biliary Obstruction," *Radiology*, 1982, 145:289-95.

Biliary Stent Placement, Percutaneous *see* Biliary Drainage, Percutaneous Transhepatic *on previous page*

Biliary Stone Extraction, Percutaneous

CPT 47630

Synonyms Basket Extraction of Biliary Stones; Biliary Stone Extraction Via T-Tube Track

Applies to Percutaneous Extraction of Gallbladder Calculi

Abstract PROCEDURE COMMONLY INCLUDES: Removal of a retained calculi within the biliary system after surgery through the T-tube track. The procedure can also be performed through a percutaneous biliary drainage track. INDICATIONS: Removal of retained calculi within the biliary system, typically after a cholecystectomy CONTRAINDICATIONS: An immature track (T-tube in place less than 6 weeks).

Patient Care/Scheduling PATIENT PREPARATION: The procedure can be performed on an outpatient basis. Informed consent is obtained from the patient. The patient is placed on

(Continued)

Biliary Stone Extraction, Percutaneous *(Continued)*

a clear liquid diet or NPO 4 hours before the procedure. An intravenous line is begun to ensure adequate hydration and to facilitate the administration of any sedatives during the procedure. Most physicians will administer a broad spectrum antibiotic intravenously before the procedure. **AFTERCARE:** The patient is observed for 30-60 minutes. After that time, the patient can be discharged if no untoward symptoms are reported. **SPECIAL INSTRUCTIONS:** Any prior cholangiograms which demonstrate the calculi which are to be removed should be made available to the interventional radiologist beforehand. **COMPLICATIONS:** Complications are very infrequent and are usually secondary to subsequent cholangitis or pancreatitis.

Method **EQUIPMENT:** Fluoroscopy, steerable catheters, basket retrieval catheters, flexible forceps **TECHNIQUE:** When the procedure is to be performed via a T-tube track, the T-tube must have been in place for 6 weeks. By this time, a mature track has been established and the T-tube can be removed. A steerable catheter is advanced through the mature T-tube track into the biliary system and up to the retained calculus. A collapsible wire basket is advanced through the steerable catheter and the stone is engaged in the basket. The steerable catheter and the basket with the stone are removed as a unit through the T-tube track. If the stone is larger than the track, it is fragmented first and then the pieces are removed percutaneously. Alternatively, the stones can be pushed down the common bile duct and into the duodenum and allowed to pass through the GI tract. When many stones or fragments are present, several extraction sessions may be necessary to remove all the particles. When no T-tube track is available, it is also possible to remove stones via a percutaneous drainage catheter or percutaneous cholecystostomy.

Interpretation **NORMAL FINDINGS:** After stone extraction, a repeat cholangiogram should show no evidence of any retained particles. Contrast should flow freely through the biliary system into the duodenum. **LIMITATIONS:** The T-tube track must be in place for at least 6 weeks beforehand. It is possible to lose access to the biliary system when attempts are made to remove calculi through an immature track.

References

Burhenne HJ, "Percutaneous Extraction of Retained Biliary Tract Stones: 661 Patients," *AJR*, 1980, 134:888-98.

Biliary Stone Extraction Via T-Tube Track *see* Biliary Stone Extraction, Percutaneous *on previous page*

Biliary Stricture Dilatation, Percutaneous *see* Biliary Drainage, Percutaneous Transhepatic *on page 314*

Biopsy, Percutaneous Needle, Under Fluoroscopic, CT or Ultrasound Guidance

CPT 76003 (fluoroscopy); 76361 (CT); 76943 (ultrasound)

Synonyms Needle Aspiration Biopsy

Applies to Needle Biopsy Under CT Guidance; Needle Biopsy Under Ultrasound Guidance; Needle Localization; Transthoracic Needle Aspiration Biopsy

Abstract **PROCEDURE COMMONLY INCLUDES:** Obtaining a sample of cells from a mass via a percutaneously placed needle. The needle placement can be performed using fluoroscopic, ultrasonic, or computed tomographic guidance. The specimen is then sent for cytologic, pathologic, or bacteriologic analysis. **INDICATIONS:** Presence of a mass of unknown origin **CONTRAINDICATIONS:** Masses of vascular origin (aneurysm, pseudoaneurysm, arteriovenous malformation, etc) are absolute contraindications for biopsy. Neoplasms that are highly vascular (hemangioma, meningioma, hypervascular malignant neoplasms, etc) are relative contraindications. Other contraindications are bleeding abnormalities, elevated prothrombin or partial thromboplastin times, low platelet count.

Patient Care/Scheduling **PATIENT PREPARATION:** Informed consent is obtained from the patient. The patient is placed on a clear liquid diet or NPO 4 hours before the procedure. Recent coagulation parameters (PT, PTT, and platelet count) are recorded on the chart. An intravenous line is begun before the procedure to facilitate the administration of any medications or sedation required during the procedure. **AFTERCARE:** The patient is placed on bedrest for approximately 4 hours after the procedure. Vital signs should be obtained every 30 minutes for 2 hours, then every hour for 4 hours. During this time, the patient should be closely observed for any evidence of internal or external bleeding. If biopsy has involved the thoracic region, the patient should be observed for any signs of a pneumothorax or hemothorax. **SPECIAL INSTRUCTIONS:** These examinations are usually arranged by the requesting physician in consultation with the interventional radiologist. Any previous imaging studies of the mass to be biopsied should be made available to the interventional radiologist. Any bleeding abnormalities should be corrected beforehand. **COMPLICATIONS:** Most complications are related to either bleeding, pneumothorax, or sepsis.

Method **EQUIPMENT:** Fluoroscopy, computed tomography, or ultrasonography; aspiration or cutting biopsy needles; appropriate fixatives or culture media **TECHNIQUE:** The mass or region to be biopsied is localized with ultrasound, CT, or fluoroscopy and the appropriate entry path is determined. Local anesthesia is instilled at the appropriate site and the aspiration or cutting biopsy needle is guided into the mass. The specimen is then sent to the laboratory for appropriate cytological, pathological, or bacteriological analysis. If a sufficient amount of cellular material is not obtained and the patient remains stable, the procedure can be repeated. **DATA ACQUIRED:** Cytologic, pathologic, or bacteriologic analysis of the cells within a mass.

Interpretation **LIMITATIONS:** Some masses are inaccessible to percutaneous biopsy secondary to overlying bony structures or close approximation to vascular structures.

References

Bernardino ME, "Percutaneous Biopsy," *AJR*, 1984, 142:41-5.

Bipedal Lymphangiography *see* Lymphangiogram *on page 322*

Brachial Cut-Down *see* Arteriogram, Transaxillary or Transbrachial Approach *on page 312*

Bronchial Arteriogram *see* Arteriogram, Transfemoral Approach *on page 313*

Bronchial Artery Embolization *see* Embolization, Percutaneous Transcatheter *on page 321*

Carotid Arteriogram *see* Arteriogram, Transaxillary or Transbrachial Approach *on page 312*

Carotid Arteriogram *see* Arteriogram, Transfemoral Approach *on page 313*

Catheter Drainage *see* Abscess Drainage Under Fluoroscopic, Ultrasonic, or CT Guidance *on page 308*

Catheter Placement for Infusion of Drugs or Chemotherapy

CPT 75897

Synonyms Intra-arterial Catheter Placement; Intra-arterial Infusion Therapy

Applies to Chemotherapy Infusion by Catheter; Papaverine Infusion by Catheter; Pitressin® Infusion by Catheter; Streptokinase Infusion by Catheter; Thrombolytic Therapy Infusion by Catheter; Tissue Plasminogen Activator Infusion by Catheter; Urokinase Infusion by Catheter; Vasopressin Infusion by Catheter

Abstract **PROCEDURE COMMONLY INCLUDES:** Placement of a catheter into a specific artery for the purposes of infusing a therapeutic drug **INDICATIONS:** Treatment of localized tumor by infusion of chemotherapy, control of gastrointestinal bleeding with vasopressin (Pitressin®), alleviation of ischemia with papaverine, or dissolution of thromboembolism with thrombolytic therapy (urokinase, streptokinase, or tissue plasminogen activator) **CONTRAINDICATIONS:** Inability of the patient to lie supine, acute renal failure, bleeding abnormalities, extremely high blood pressure.

Patient Care/Scheduling **PATIENT PREPARATION:** Informed consent is obtained from the patient. The patient is placed on a clear liquid diet before the procedure. An intravenous line is begun to ensure that the patient is well hydrated and to facilitate the administration of any medications during the procedure. Recent laboratory results (BUN, creatinine, platelet count, PT, and PTT) should be recorded on the chart. The patient with chart is sent on a stretcher to the angiography suite when notified. **AFTERCARE:** While the catheter is in place and the drug or chemotherapy is being infused, the patient must remain in a su-

(Continued)

Catheter Placement for Infusion of Drugs or Chemotherapy *(Continued)*

pine position and the leg in which the catheter has been inserted must remain straight. This leg should be observed regularly for any evidence of ischemia (decreased pulses, pallor, or coolness) or for any evidence of bleeding at the catheter entry site. At times when no drug or chemotherapy is being infused through the catheter, the catheter should be infused with normal saline or heparinized saline to prevent the catheter from becoming clotted. **SPECIAL INSTRUCTIONS:** The reason for the catheter placement and drug infusion should be discussed beforehand in consultation with the cardiovascular radiologist. The requisition should state clearly the drug to be infused and the specific vessel to be catheterized. **COMPLICATIONS:** Complications which occur at the catheter entry site include bleeding, hematoma formation, thrombosis, false aneurysm, or arteriovenous fistula. Complications which can occur at the specific vessel that is catheterized include vessel dissection, occlusion, or distal embolization of any clots which may have formed on the catheter. The contrast material which is used during the procedure may result in a contrast reaction or acute renal failure. Complications can also occur from the specific drug which is infused.

Method **EQUIPMENT:** Fluoroscopy and angiographic catheters and wires **TECHNIQUE:** Local anesthetic agent is instilled over the common femoral artery. The artery is percutaneously punctured and a catheter is inserted and fluoroscopically guided into the artery of interest. Contrast medium is injected and films are obtained to document the abnormality and the catheter position. The catheter is left in place while the appropriate drug is infused.

Interpretation **NORMAL FINDINGS:** The preliminary angiogram should document the abnormality to be treated, such as the neoplasm for chemotherapy, the gastrointestinal bleed for Pitressin® infusion, the thromboembolism for thrombolytic therapy, etc. **LIMITATIONS:** It may not be appropriate to infuse the drug if the underlying abnormality cannot be demonstrated angiographically. Occasionally, the appropriate vessel cannot be catheterized because of anatomical considerations, atherosclerotic disease, or vessel occlusion.

Catheter Portography *see* Portal Venogram, Percutaneous Transhepatic *on page 326*

Cerebral Arteriogram *see* Arteriogram, Transaxillary or Transbrachial Approach *on page 312*

Cerebral Arteriogram *see* Arteriogram, Transfemoral Approach *on page 313*

Cervical Myelogram *see* Myelogram *on page 323*

Chemotherapy Infusion by Catheter *see* Catheter Placement for Infusion of Drugs or Chemotherapy *on previous page*

Cholangiogram, Percutaneous Transhepatic (PTC)

CPT 74321

Applies to Cholecystogram, Percutaneous

Abstract **PROCEDURE COMMONLY INCLUDES:** Visualization of the biliary system by the injection of contrast medium through a needle which has been percutaneously placed into the intrahepatic biliary system or, occasionally, the gallbladder **INDICATIONS:** Determination of the cause and location of an obstruction of the biliary system. Possible causes include stones, pancreatitis, sclerosing cholangitis, inflammatory or traumatic stricture, pancreatic carcinoma, cholangiocarcinoma, gallbladder carcinoma, and metastases. **CONTRAINDICATIONS:** Inability of the patient to lie supine, bleeding abnormalities, elevated prothrombin or partial thromboplastin times, acute renal failure.

Patient Care/Scheduling **PATIENT PREPARATION:** Informed consent is obtained from the patient. The patient is placed on a clear liquid diet or NPO 4 hours before the procedure. All medications are continued. An intravenous line is begun before the procedure in order to ensure that the patient is well hydrated (thus decreasing the risk of acute renal failure) and to facilitate the administration of any medications required during the procedure. Most physicians will prescribe coverage with broad spectrum antibiotics. Blood typing is often requested beforehand. Recent laboratory results (BUN, creatinine, platelet count, PT, and

PTT) are recorded on the chart. **AFTERCARE:** The patient is placed on bedrest for approximately 4 hours. Vital signs should be obtained every 30 minutes for 2 hours, then every hour for 4 hours. The patient should be observed closely for any signs of internal bleeding or sepsis. **SPECIAL INSTRUCTIONS:** Any previous imaging study of the hepatobiliary system should be made available to the interventional radiologist. Any potential problem areas should be noted, such as renal insufficiency, bleeding abnormalities, or a history of severe contrast reaction. **COMPLICATIONS:** Most complications are secondary to either sepsis or hemorrhage.

Method **EQUIPMENT:** Fluoroscopy, ultrasound, needle, contrast medium, and a method of x-ray film recording **TECHNIQUE:** A percutaneous entry site is chosen, usually with the assistance of ultrasound and/or fluoroscopy. Local anesthetic agent is instilled at the entry site. A 20-gauge needle is inserted into the liver until a bile duct is encountered. This may require several passages with the needle until a duct is successfully cannulated. Contrast medium is then injected and x-ray films are obtained. A sample of bile is often sent for Gram stain and culture. **DATA ACQUIRED:** Opacification of the biliary system.

Interpretation **NORMAL FINDINGS:** The bile duct should be smooth and of normal caliber. There should be no evidence of any dilatation, filling defects, bile duct narrowing, or extravasation. Contrast should flow freely into the duodenum. **LIMITATIONS:** It can be difficult to successfully cannulate intrahepatic bile ducts which are not dilated, especially in cases of sclerosing cholangitis where the ducts are narrower than normal.

References

Mueller PR, Harbin WP, Ferrucci JT, et al, "Fine Needle Transhepatic Cholangiography: Reflections After 450 Cases," *AJR*, 1981, 136:85-90.

Turner MA, Cho SR, and Messmer JM, "Pitfalls in Cholangiographic Interpretation," *Radiographics*, 1987, 7:1067-105.

Cholecystogram, Percutaneous *see* Cholangiogram, Percutaneous Transhepatic (PTC) *on previous page*

Cholecystotomy, Percutaneous *see* Biliary Drainage, Percutaneous Transhepatic *on page 314*

Coronary Arteriogram *see* Arteriogram, Transaxillary or Transbrachial Approach *on page 312*

Coronary Arteriogram *see* Arteriogram, Transfemoral Approach *on page 313*

Dialysis Fistulogram

CPT 75790

Synonyms Arteriovenous Fistulogram; Dialysis Shuntogram

Abstract **PROCEDURE COMMONLY INCLUDES:** Visualization of an arteriovenous fistula or graft which has been constructed as a vascular access for dialysis **INDICATIONS:** Evaluation of the cause for poor flow through or loss of pulse in a dialysis fistula or graft **CONTRAINDICATIONS:** Bleeding abnormalities, elevated prothrombin or partial thromboplastin times, low platelet count.

Patient Care/Scheduling **PATIENT PREPARATION:** Informed consent is obtained from the patient. The patient is placed on a clear liquid diet 2-4 hours before the procedure. Recent laboratory studies (platelet count, PT, and PTT) should be appropriately recorded on the chart. **AFTERCARE:** The needle entry site should be observed for bleeding or hematoma formation. **COMPLICATIONS:** Bleeding or hematoma formation at the needle entry site, thrombosis of the graft or fistula, extravasation of contrast material into the surrounding soft tissues.

Method **EQUIPMENT:** Fluoroscopy, angiographic catheter or needle, and a method of film recording **TECHNIQUE:** Local anesthetic agent is instilled over the fistula or graft. The fistula is palpated and punctured with a needle. Blood return will confirm that the needle tip is intraluminal. If desired, the needle can be exchanged for an angiographic catheter. Contrast material is injected and the films are obtained. **DATA ACQUIRED:** Visualization of the arteriovenous fistula, the surgical anastomoses, the artery supplying the fistula or graft and the veins draining it.

(Continued)

Dialysis Fistulogram *(Continued)*

Interpretation **NORMAL FINDINGS:** The surgical anastomoses should be patent without evidence for stenosis. The artery supplying the fistula as well as the veins draining it should be normal in caliber without evidence of stricture or occlusion. **LIMITATIONS:** Inability to adequately and securely cannulate the fistula will preclude contrast injection.

References

Gilula L, Staple TW, Anderson CB, et al, "Venous Angiography of Hemodialysis Fistulas, Experience With 52 Cases," *Radiology*, 1975, 115:555-62.

Dialysis Shuntogram *see* Dialysis Fistulogram *on previous page*

Digital Subtraction Angiogram, Intravenous

Synonyms DSA; IV-DSA

Abstract **PROCEDURE COMMONLY INCLUDES:** Visualization of the arteries in the area of clinical concern by injection of contrast medium into a catheter placed in an arm vein and recording the subsequent x-ray images using digital computer technology **INDICATIONS:** Screening evaluation of arteries for stenoses or occlusions, typically renal arteries for hypertension and carotid arteries for transient ischemic attacks (TIA). Also useful for follow-up evaluation of angioplasty sites and surgical grafts. **CONTRAINDICATIONS:** Inability of the patient to lie flat and motionless, acute renal failure.

Patient Care/Scheduling **PATIENT PREPARATION:** Informed consent is obtained from the patient. The patient is placed on a clear liquid diet 2-4 hours before the procedure. Recent laboratory studies (BUN, creatinine) should be appropriately recorded on the chart. **AFTERCARE:** A small compression dressing is applied to the venous catheter entry site for the remainder of the day. **COMPLICATIONS:** Contrast reaction, acute renal failure, upper extremity vein thrombosis.

Method **EQUIPMENT:** An intracath or angiographic catheter, fluoroscopy, and a digital subtraction angiographic unit **TECHNIQUE:** An intracath or an angiographic catheter is placed into a vein of the upper extremity, typically in the antecubital fossa. Most angiographers will advance the catheter under fluoroscopy into the superior vena cava or right atrium; others will merely place an angiocath through the vein up to the upper arm. Approximately 40-50 mL contrast material is then injected into the vein or right atrium and a series of x-rays are obtained over the area of clinical interest. The computer will then "subtract" an image of the area obtained after the arrival of contrast material from an image obtained before the arrival of contrast material, leaving only an image of the contrast material in the blood vessels. **DATA ACQUIRED:** Visualization of the arteries in the area of clinical concern in the form of digitally subtracted images.

Interpretation **NORMAL FINDINGS:** The opacified arteries should be smooth and gradually taper as they continue to branch. There should be no evidence of vessel wall irregularity, aneurysm, narrowing, occlusion, extravasation, neovascularity, or arteriovenous shunting. **LIMITATIONS:** Because the computer subtracts x-ray images after the arrival of contrast material from an image obtained before the arrival of contrast material, any patient motion which has occurred in the interval will create an artifact. This includes respiratory motion, bowel motion, or patient motion. These artifacts can considerably obscure the image. Also, there is global opacification of all arteries in the area, often resulting in overlapping of multiple arterial structures which can obscure an area of interest. Finally, image quality is considerably degraded in patients who have poor cardiac output.

References

Meaney TF, Weinstein MA, Buonocore E, et al, "Digital Subtraction Angiography of the Human Cardiovascular System," *AJR*, 1980, 135:1153-60.

Direct Portography *see* Portal Venogram, Percutaneous Transhepatic *on page 326*

Direct Splenoportography *see* Splenoportogram, Percutaneous *on page 328*

Dotter Procedure *see* Angioplasty, Percutaneous Transluminal (PTA) *on page 309*

Drainage of Fluid Collection *see* Abscess Drainage Under Fluoroscopic, Ultrasonic, or CT Guidance *on page 308*

DSA *see* Digital Subtraction Angiogram, Intravenous *on previous page*

Elbow Arthrogram *see* Arthrogram *on page 314*

Embolization of Gastroesophageal Varices *see* Portal Venogram, Percutaneous Transhepatic *on page 326*

Embolization, Percutaneous Transcatheter

CPT 75895 (embolization using particulate or liquid); 75956 (embolization using balloon, coil, or methacrylate, permanent)

Synonyms Angioinfarction; Vessel Occlusion, Transcatheter

Applies to Arteriovenous Malformation Embolization; Bronchial Artery Embolization; Gastrointestinal (GI Bleed) Embolization; Tumor Embolization; Varicocele Embolization

Abstract **PROCEDURE COMMONLY INCLUDES:** Occlusion of an artery or branch which is bleeding or which supplies a tumor, arteriovenous malformation, or other vascular abnormality by expelling embolic material or a sclerosing agent through a catheter **INDICATIONS:** Possible indications for transcatheter embolization include nonresectable tumors, upper gastrointestinal bleeding, genitourinary bleeding, bronchial artery bleeding, traumatic bleeds, intractable nasal bleeds, certain intracranial aneurysms and fistulas, arteriovenous malformations, varicoceles **CONTRAINDICATIONS:** Bacteremia, sepsis.

Patient Care/Scheduling **PATIENT PREPARATION:** Informed consent is obtained from the patient. The patient is placed on a clear liquid diet on the morning of the procedure when possible, although many of these procedures are done on an emergent basis. Any coagulation abnormalities are corrected to the extent possible. An intravenous line is begun before the procedure in order to optimize hydration and to facilitate the administration of any medications required during the procedure. Recent laboratory results (BUN, creatinine, platelet count, PT, and PTT) should be recorded on the chart. Some physicians will administer a broad spectrum antibiotic intravenously before the procedure. **AFTERCARE:** The patient is placed on bedrest for at least 8 hours after the procedure and often for the remainder of the day. During this time, the patient should be flat in bed with the legs straight. Vital signs should be obtained every 30 minutes for the first 2 hours, then every hour for the next 6 hours. At these times, the femoral puncture site should be examined for any evidence of bleeding or swelling and the legs should be examined for any change in pulses, color, or warmth. The patient may require parental pain medication and/or antinauseants for the pain and nausea related to the postinfarction syndrome. **SPECIAL INSTRUCTIONS:** These examinations are usually arranged by the requesting physician in consultation with the cardiovascular radiologist. The requisition should state clearly the reason for the procedure as well as the specific vessels to be embolized. Any previous imaging study of the area should be made available to the physician performing the procedure. Notation should be made of any conditions which may increase the risk of the procedure, such as renal insufficiency, bleeding abnormalities, or a history of severe contrast reaction. **COMPLICATIONS:** Inadvertent embolization of a nontarget artery, contrast reaction, acute renal failure, bleeding or hematoma formation at the puncture site, abscess formation at the target site. A postinfarction syndrome is not uncommon and consists of pain, fever, nausea, and vomiting.

Method **EQUIPMENT:** Fluoroscopy, angiographic catheter and wires, a method of film recording (either conventional cut films or digital subtraction films) and embolic or sclerosing agents such as Gelfoam® particles, Ivalon® particles, coils, detachable balloons, absolute alcohol, and cyanobucrylate **TECHNIQUE:** Local anesthetic agent is instilled over the common femoral artery. The artery is percutaneously punctured and a catheter is inserted and fluoroscopically guided into the artery of interest. An angiogram is then performed by injecting contrast through the catheter in order to demonstrate the abnormality. An embolic or sclerosing agent is chosen on the basis of the size of the vessel to be occluded, the desired duration of occlusion, and the type of abnormality to be treated. The embolic or sclerosing agent is deposited through the catheter. A follow-up angiogram is performed to determine the effectiveness of the embolization procedure.

(Continued)

Embolization, Percutaneous Transcatheter *(Continued)*

Interpretation NORMAL FINDINGS: After the embolization procedure, the appropriate vessels should be occluded. There should be no occlusion of any nontarget artery. LIMITATIONS: The primary limitation is an inability to maneuver the catheter into the appropriate artery or branch when the vessels are tortuous, stenotic, or occluded.

References

Feldman L, Greenfield AJ, Waltman AC, et al, "Transcatheter Vessel Occlusion: Angiographic Results Versus Clinical Success," *Radiology*, 1983, 147:1-5.

White RI, "Embolotherapy in Vascular Disease," *AJR*, 1984, 142:27-30.

External Biliary Drainage *see* Biliary Drainage, Percutaneous Transhepatic *on page 314*

External Decompression *see* Abscess Drainage Under Fluoroscopic, Ultrasonic, or CT Guidance *on page 308*

Filter Insertion *see* Vena Caval Filter Placement *on page 329*

Gallbladder Drainage, Percutaneous *see* Biliary Drainage, Percutaneous Transhepatic *on page 314*

Gastrointestinal (GI Bleed) Embolization *see* Embolization, Percutaneous Transcatheter *on previous page*

Greenfield Filter Placement *see* Vena Caval Filter Placement *on page 329*

Hepatic Arteriogram *see* Arteriogram, Transaxillary or Transbrachial Approach *on page 312*

Hepatic Arteriogram *see* Arteriogram, Transfemoral Approach *on page 313*

Hepatic Venogram *see* Venogram, Transfemoral or Transjugular Approach *on page 331*

Hip Arthrogram *see* Arthrogram *on page 314*

Iliofemoral Venogram *see* Venogram, Transfemoral or Transjugular Approach *on page 331*

Inferior Vena Cava Filter Placement *see* Vena Caval Filter Placement *on page 329*

Inferior Vena Cavogram *see* Venogram, Transfemoral or Transjugular Approach *on page 331*

Intra-arterial Catheter Placement *see* Catheter Placement for Infusion of Drugs or Chemotherapy *on page 317*

Intra-arterial Infusion Therapy *see* Catheter Placement for Infusion of Drugs or Chemotherapy *on page 317*

IV-DSA *see* Digital Subtraction Angiogram, Intravenous *on page 320*

Joint Study *see* Arthrogram *on page 314*

Knee Arthrogram *see* Arthrogram *on page 314*

Laser Angioplasty *see* Angioplasty, Percutaneous Transluminal (PTA) *on page 309*

Leg Arteriogram *see* Arteriogram, Transaxillary or Transbrachial Approach *on page 312*

Leg Arteriogram *see* Arteriogram, Transfemoral Approach *on page 313*

Leg Venogram *see* Venogram, Extremity *on page 330*

Lower Extremity Venogram *see* Venogram, Extremity *on page 330*

Lumbar Myelogram *see* Myelogram *on next page*

Lymphangiogram

CPT 75808

Synonyms Bipedal Lymphangiography

Abstract PROCEDURE COMMONLY INCLUDES: Visualization of the lymphatic vessels and associated lymph nodes in the extremities, the pelvis, and the retroperitoneum, as well as the thoracic duct in the thorax **INDICATIONS:** Evaluation of the lymph nodes for possible involvement with primary or metastatic cancer or for occlusion or interruption of the lymphatic vessels secondary to a traumatic, surgical, or congenital cause.

Patient Care/Scheduling **PATIENT PREPARATION:** Informed consent is obtained from the patient. There are no dietary restrictions. **AFTERCARE:** Dressings are placed on the incision sites on the dorsum of the feet. The feet should not be emersed in water until the stitches are removed approximately 7 days after the procedure. The patient should be informed that his urine will have a blue-green color for several days. **SPECIAL INSTRUCTIONS:** The patient should be informed that the procedure will require a second set of x-rays the day following the actual injection of contrast material. **COMPLICATIONS:** Infection at the incision site, contrast reaction.

Method **EQUIPMENT:** A surgical cut down tray, small gauge needles (27- to 30-gauge), fluoroscopy and an x-ray unit **TECHNIQUE:** The dorsa of both feet are sterilely prepared and draped. A blue dye (Lymphazurin®) is injected intradermally into the webs between the toes. Within 30 minutes, this dye is picked up by the lymphatic system and the lymphatic channels on the dorsum of the foot become evident. Local anesthetic is then instilled over one of these lymphatic channels and a small surgical cut-down is performed. The lymphatic channel is isolated and a small gauge needle is inserted into it under direct vision. Approximately 7-10 mL oil based contrast material (eg, Ethiodol®) is then injected over a 30- to 60-minute period using an automated pump device. The needles are then removed and the incision sites are sutured. Radiographs are then obtained of the pelvis and abdomen to display the major lymphatic channels. Repeat films are then performed 24 hours later after the contrast material has been picked up by the lymph nodes themselves. **DATA ACQUIRED:** The first day films demonstrate the lymphatic channels within the extremity, pelvis, and retroperitoneum as well as the thoracic duct. The second day films demonstrate the lymph nodes in these regions.

Interpretation **NORMAL FINDINGS:** The appropriate lymphatic channels should be visualized without evidence for occlusion, displacement, or leakage. The lymph nodes themselves should be of normal size and architecture without evidence for enlargement or partial or complete replacement by neoplasm. **LIMITATIONS:** Inability to isolate and cannulate a lymph vessel (a process which is more difficult in children and patients with swollen feet, lymphangiectasia or small, frail lymphatic vessels).

References

Fuchs WA, "Technique and Complications of Lymphography," *Abrams Angiography, Vascular and Interventional Radiology*, 3rd ed, Abrams HL, ed, Boston, MA: Little, Brown and Co, 1983, 1979-86.

Jing B, Wallace S, and Zornoza J, "Metastases to Retroperitoneal and Pelvic Lymph Nodes, Computed Tomography and Lymphangiography," *Radiol Clin North Am*, 1982, 20:511-30.

Mesenteric Arteriogram *see* Arteriogram, Transaxillary or Transbrachial Approach *on page 312*

Mesenteric Arteriogram *see* Arteriogram, Transfemoral Approach *on page 313*

Myelogram

CPT 72241 (cervical); 72256 (thoracic); 72266 (lumbar); 72271 (entire spinal canal)

Related Information

Lumbar Puncture *on page 165*

Synonyms Cervical Myelogram; Lumbar Myelogram; Thoracic Myelogram

Applies to Spinal Tap Under Fluoroscopy

Abstract **PROCEDURE COMMONLY INCLUDES:** Visualization of the cervical, thoracic, and/or lumbar spinal cord by the injection of contrast material into the subarachnoid space through a percutaneously placed spinal needle. Spinal fluid is usually aspirated before the contrast is instilled and sent for appropriate laboratory analysis. **INDICATIONS:** Visualization of spinal cord abnormalities; evaluation of signs and/or symptoms of compression of the spinal nerve roots or spinal cord by a herniated disc, degenerative spur, traumatic injury, neoplasm, or other mass **CONTRAINDICATIONS:** Evidence of raised intracranial pressure, such as papilledema; bleeding abnormalities, such as elevated prothrombin or partial thromboplastin times, decreased platelet count, or patients on anticoagulation.

(Continued)

Myelogram *(Continued)*

Patient Care/Scheduling PATIENT PREPARATION: Informed consent is obtained from the patient. Patient is made NPO 2-4 hours before the procedure. Any bleeding abnormality is corrected beforehand. The patient with chart is sent on a stretcher to the myelography suite. AFTERCARE: The patient is placed on bedrest with the head of the bed elevated at least 30° to 45° for 12 hours. Oral fluids are encouraged and the diet is as tolerated. Any nausea or vomiting which occurs should not be treated with phenothiazine antinauseants. The patient is advised to remain still in bed in a head up position for the remainder of the day. SPECIAL INSTRUCTIONS: Any previous spine x-rays or any prior CT or MR studies of the spine should be made available to the radiologist. The patient should not be on phenothiazines at the time of the procedure. COMPLICATIONS: Seizure, arachnoiditis, subarachnoid bleeding, spinal infection; nausea and vomiting are not infrequent side effects.

Method EQUIPMENT: Spinal needle, nonionic contrast material, fluoroscopy, and x-ray equipment with a tilting table TECHNIQUE: Under fluoroscopy, an appropriate entry site is selected over the lumbar spine or, occasionally, over the upper cervical spine. Local anesthetic is instilled and a 21-gauge spinal needle is fluoroscopically guided into the subarachnoid space. If desired, spinal fluid can be obtained and sent for appropriate laboratory analysis (eg, cell count, cytology, Gram stain, culture, protein, immunoglobulins). Approximately 10 mL nonionic contrast material is injected into the subarachnoid space of the spinal canal with the patient in a reverse Trendelenburg position and films of the lumbar area are obtained. Since the contrast material is heavier than spinal fluid, the patient is slowly tilted downward to obtain films of the thoracic and spinal regions. Care is made not to allow the contrast material to enter the intracranial region. DATA ACQUIRED: Visualization of the subarachnoid space of the lumbar, thoracic, and/or cervical spine.

Interpretation NORMAL FINDINGS: There should be no evidence for any filling defect within or extrinsic compression on the subarachnoid space. There should be no impingement upon or displacement of the nerve roots or the spinal cord. LIMITATIONS: Adhesions from arachnoiditis or areas of marked compression may impede the flow of contrast material. Severe kyphosis, scoliosis, or ankylosing spondylitis can make the examination technically difficult.

References

Benson JE and Han JS, "Examination of the Spine," *Radiology: Diagnosis – Imaging – Intervention*, Vol 3, Chapter 102, Taveras JM and Ferrucci JT, eds, Philadelphia, PA: JB Lippincott Co, 1986, 7-12.

Needle Aspiration Biopsy *see* Biopsy, Percutaneous Needle, Under Fluoroscopic, CT or Ultrasound Guidance *on page 316*

Needle Biopsy Under CT Guidance *see* Biopsy, Percutaneous Needle, Under Fluoroscopic, CT or Ultrasound Guidance *on page 316*

Needle Biopsy Under Ultrasound Guidance *see* Biopsy, Percutaneous Needle, Under Fluoroscopic, CT or Ultrasound Guidance *on page 316*

Needle Localization *see* Biopsy, Percutaneous Needle, Under Fluoroscopic, CT or Ultrasound Guidance *on page 316*

Nephrostomy, Percutaneous

CPT 74476

Synonyms Percutaneous Renal Drainage

Applies to Ureteral Stent Placement, Percutaneous; Ureteral Stricture Dilatation, Percutaneous; Whittaker Test

Abstract PROCEDURE COMMONLY INCLUDES: Percutaneous placement of a drainage catheter in an obstructed kidney INDICATIONS: Partial or complete ureteral obstruction resulting in pain, infection, hydronephrosis, pyohydronephrosis, sepsis, or decreased renal function. The cause of obstruction may be secondary to stone, neoplasm, fibrosis, extrinsic compression, or a stricture related to surgery, trauma, infection, or radiation. CONTRAINDICATIONS: Bleeding abnormalities, elevated prothrombin or partial thromboplastin times, low platelet count.

Patient Care/Scheduling PATIENT PREPARATION: Informed consent is obtained from the patient. The patient is placed on a clear liquid diet or NPO 4 hours before the procedure.

Medications may be continued. An intravenous line is begun before the procedure to facilitate the administration of any antibiotics or medications during the procedure. If the patient is not already on antibiotics and the kidney is obstructed, most physicians will prescribe a broad spectrum antibiotic to be administered intravenously 30 minutes before the procedure. **AFTERCARE:** The patient is placed on bedrest for approximately 4 hours. Vital signs should be obtained every 30 minutes for 2 hours, then every hour for the 4 hours. The patient should be observed closely for any signs of internal bleeding or sepsis. **SPECIAL INSTRUCTIONS:** The volume of output from the nephrostomy tube should be recorded. While the urine from the drainage tube may be blood tinged, any profuse bleeding from the catheter should be attended to promptly. If the drainage ceases completely, the catheter may be irrigated to remove blood clot or debris. Drainage of urine around the catheter at the skin site is usually a sign that the catheter is at least partially obstructed. **COMPLICATIONS:** Bleeding and sepsis are the most common complications occurring in the first several hours after the procedure. Delayed complications include infection at the skin entry site and dislodgment or plugging of the drainage catheter.

Method **EQUIPMENT:** Ultrasound, fluoroscopy, steerable wires, and catheters **TECHNIQUE:** The patient is placed prone and a percutaneous entry site is chosen with the assistance of ultrasound or fluoroscopy. If the kidney to be drained still functions adequately, contrast material can be injected intravenously to help localize the collecting system. Local anesthetic is instilled at the entry site which is usually located along the posterolateral aspect of the patient at approximately the level of the second lumbar vertebrae. A needle is then percutaneously inserted into a posterolateral calix or infundibulum of the renal collecting system. A guidewire is placed through the needle and advanced into the renal pelvis. The needle is then removed and a drainage catheter is passed over the guidewire. The drainage catheter is fixed to the skin to prevent dislodgment. This percutaneous access route can later be used for placement of a ureteral stent across the point of obstruction or for balloon dilatation of an obstructing stricture. Also, a Whittaker test can be performed to determine if a narrowing is urodynamically significant by measuring pressures in the renal pelvis and the urinary bladder simultaneously as saline is instilled through the nephrostomy catheter. **DATA ACQUIRED:** A urine specimen from the obstructed urinary tract can be sent for culture, Gram stain, and cytology.

Interpretation **LIMITATIONS:** It can be technically difficult to place a drainage catheter into a renal collecting system which is completely occupied by a staghorn calculus.

References

Lang EK and Price ET, "Redefinitions of Indications for Percutaneous Nephrostomy," *Radiology*, 1983, 147:419-26.

Pfister RC and Newhouse JH, "Interventional Percutaneous Pyeloureteral Techniques. II. Percutaneous Nephrostomy and Other Procedures," *Radiol Clin North Am*, 1979, 17:351-63.

Papaverine Infusion by Catheter *see* Catheter Placement for Infusion of Drugs or Chemotherapy *on page 317*

Pelvic Arteriogram *see* Arteriogram, Transaxillary or Transbrachial Approach *on page 312*

Pelvic Arteriogram *see* Arteriogram, Transfemoral Approach *on page 313*

Percutaneous Drainage *see* Abscess Drainage Under Fluoroscopic, Ultrasonic, or CT Guidance *on page 308*

Percutaneous Extraction of Gallbladder Calculi *see* Biliary Stone Extraction, Percutaneous *on page 315*

Percutaneous Renal Drainage *see* Nephrostomy, Percutaneous *on previous page*

Percutaneous Transfemoral Angiogram *see* Arteriogram, Transfemoral Approach *on page 313*

Percutaneous Transfemoral Venogram *see* Venogram, Transfemoral or Transjugular Approach *on page 331*

Percutaneous Transjugular Venogram *see* Venogram, Transfemoral or Transjugular Approach *on page 331*

Pitressin® Infusion by Catheter *see* Catheter Placement for Infusion of Drugs or Chemotherapy *on page 317*

Portal or Mesenteric Venous Sampling *see* Portal Venogram, Percutaneous Transhepatic *on this page*

Portal Venogram, Percutaneous Transhepatic

CPT 75888

Synonyms Catheter Portography; Direct Portography

Applies to Embolization of Gastroesophageal Varices; Portal or Mesenteric Venous Sampling

Abstract PROCEDURE COMMONLY INCLUDES: Visualization of the portal vein and its connecting veins (eg, splenic, superior mesenteric, inferior mesenteric, gastroduodenal, or coronary veins) by the injection of contrast material through a catheter which has been placed through a percutaneous puncture of the liver. This catheter technique can also be used for obtaining venous samples from various regions to help localize an endocrine-secreting pancreatic tumor or for embolizing gastroesophageal varices in an attempt to control variceal bleeding. INDICATIONS: Elevation of the portal venous system, localization of endocrine pancreatic tumor, embolization of bleeding varices CONTRAINDICATIONS: Tense ascites, bleeding abnormalities, elevated prothrombin or partial thromboplastin times, low platelet count, acute renal failure.

Patient Care/Scheduling PATIENT PREPARATION: Informed consent is obtained from the patient. The patient is placed on a clear liquid diet or NPO 4 hours before the procedure. All medications are continued. An intravenous line is begun before the procedure in order to ensure adequate hydration and to facilitate the administration of any medications required during the procedure. Blood typing is often requested beforehand. Recent laboratory results (BUN, creatinine, platelet count, PT, and PTT) are recorded on the chart. AFTERCARE: The patient is placed on bedrest for approximately 4 hours. Vital signs should be obtained every 30 minutes for 2 hours, then every hour for 4 hours. The patient should be observed closely for any signs of internal bleeding or sepsis. Many physicians will routinely check a hematocrit 6-8 hours after the procedure. SPECIAL INSTRUCTIONS: Any previous imaging study of the upper abdomen should be made available to the interventional radiologist. Any bleeding abnormalities should be corrected beforehand. Any problem areas should be called attention to, such as renal insufficiency or a history of severe contrast reaction. COMPLICATIONS: Most complications are secondary to internal hemorrhage or sepsis.

Method EQUIPMENT: Fluoroscopy, x-ray equipment, and angiographic needles, wires, and catheters TECHNIQUE: An appropriate entry site is determined with fluoroscopy or ultrasound. Typically, this is in a low intercostal space along the right midaxillary line. Local anesthesia is instilled and a 10-15 cm 21-gauge needle or sheathed needle is advanced through the liver into a intrahepatic portal vein. A guide wire is then placed through the needle or sheath, the needle or sheath is removed leaving the wire in place and then an angiographic catheter is advanced over the wire into the portal vein. The angiographic catheter is then guided under fluoroscopy into the vein of interest. Contrast material is injected and x-rays are obtained to demonstrate the portal venous system. When searching for an endocrine-secreting tumor (eg, insulinoma, gastrinoma, glucagonoma, APUDoma) venous samples are obtained at various sites. For embolization of bleeding varices, the catheter is advanced into the varices and embolic material is discharged through the catheter. DATA ACQUIRED: Visualization of the portal venous system.

Interpretation NORMAL FINDINGS: The portal veins and the veins draining into it should be of normal caliber without evidence for occlusion, filling defect, compression, displacement or variceal formation. LIMITATIONS: Anything which would obscure the portal veins, such as overlying barium or patient motion. Also, a small, very firm, or cirrhotic liver can make the procedure technically difficult and increase the risk for complication.

References

L'Hermine CL, Chastanet P, Delemazure O, et al, "Percutaneous Transhepatic Embolization of Gastroesophageal Varices: Results in 400 Patients," *AJR*, 1989, 152(4):755-60.

Lunderquist A, Hoevels J, and Owman T, "Transhepatic Portal Venography," *Abrams Angiography, Vascular and Interventional Radiology*, 3rd ed, Abrams HL, ed, Boston, MA: Little, Brown and Co, 1983, 1505-29.

Pulmonary Angiogram *see* Pulmonary Arteriogram, Transfemoral or Transjugular Approach *on this page*

Pulmonary Arteriogram, Transfemoral or Transjugular Approach

CPT 75742 (unilateral); 75744 (bilateral)

Synonyms Pulmonary Angiogram

Abstract **PROCEDURE COMMONLY INCLUDES:** Visualization of the pulmonary arteries and their branches by the injection of contrast material through a catheter which has been percutaneously placed through a common femoral or internal jugular vein **INDICATIONS:** Evaluation of the pulmonary arteries for the presence of pulmonary embolism, stenosis, arteriovenous malformation, or aneurysm **CONTRAINDICATIONS:** Inability of the patient to lie supine, acute renal failure.

Patient Care/Scheduling **PATIENT PREPARATION:** Informed consent is obtained from the patient. The patient is placed on a clear liquid diet (not NPO) on the morning of the procedure if possible, although this procedure is often done on an emergency basis. All medications are continued. An intravenous line is begun before the procedure in order to ensure that the patient is well hydrated and to facilitate the administration of any medications required during the procedure. Recent laboratory results (BUN, creatinine, platelet count, PT, and PTT) should be appropriately recorded on the chart. The patient with chart is sent on a stretcher to the angiography suite when notified. **AFTERCARE:** If a femoral approach was used, the patient is placed on bedrest for 4 hours after the procedure. During this time, the patient should remain flat in bed with the legs straight. Vital signs should be observed every 30 minutes for the first 2 hours, then every hour for the next 2 hours. At these times, the femoral puncture site should be examined for any evidence of bleeding or swelling and legs should be examined for any changes in color or warmth. If the jugular approach was used, the head of the bed should be elevated and the site should be observed for any signs of bleeding. **SPECIAL INSTRUCTIONS:** These examinations are often arranged by the requesting physician in consultation with the cardiovascular radiologist. Any prior chest x-rays or lung scans should be made available. Any potential problem areas such as renal insufficiency or a history of severe contrast reaction should be noted. **COMPLICATIONS:** Contrast reaction; acute renal failure; cardiopulmonary arrest; or venous thrombosis, bleeding, or hematoma formation at the puncture site.

Method **EQUIPMENT:** Fluoroscopy, angiographic catheters and wires, and a method of film recording (either conventional cut films or digital subtraction films) **TECHNIQUE:** Local anesthetic agent is instilled over the entry site, either the common femoral vein or the internal jugular vein. The vein is percutaneously punctured and a catheter is inserted and fluoroscopically maneuvered through the vena cava, right atrium, and right ventricle and then into the pulmonary arteries. Contrast medium is injected and the films are obtained. **DATA ACQUIRED:** Visualization of the pulmonary arterial tree. Also, pulmonary arterial pressures and pressures in the right atrium and ventricle can be obtained at this time.

Interpretation **NORMAL FINDINGS:** The pulmonary arteries should taper gradually as they continue to branch. There should be no radiolucent filling defects (representing pulmonary emboli) and no evidence for vessel stenosis, aneurysm, arteriovenous malformation, or fistula. **LIMITATIONS:** Since these patients are often short of breath, breathing artifact may be present on the films and this can result in a considerable degradation of the image quality.

References

Alderson PO and Martin EC, "Pulmonary Embolism: Diagnosis With Multiple Imaging Modalities," *Radiology*, 1987, 164:297-312.

Renal Arteriogram *see* Arteriogram, Transaxillary or Transbrachial Approach *on page 312*

Renal Arteriogram *see* Arteriogram, Transfemoral Approach *on page 313*

Renal Vein Renin Sampling *see* Venogram, Transfemoral or Transjugular Approach *on page 331*

Renal Venogram *see* Venogram, Transfemoral or Transjugular Approach *on page 331*

Shoulder Arthrogram *see* Arthrogram *on page 314*

Spinal Tap Under Fluoroscopy *see* Myelogram *on page 323*

Splenic Arteriogram *see* Arteriogram, Transaxillary or Transbrachial Approach *on page 312*

Splenic Arteriogram *see* Arteriogram, Transfemoral Approach *on page 313*

Splenoportogram, Percutaneous

CPT 75811

Synonyms Direct Splenoportography

Abstract **PROCEDURE COMMONLY INCLUDES:** Visualization of the splenic veins and portal venous system by the injection of contrast material through a needle which has been percutaneously placed into the pulp of the spleen **INDICATIONS:** Evaluation of the status of the splenic or portal veins when they are not adequately visualized on the venous phase of a celiac or splenic arteriogram. Most commonly used for cases of suspected splenic vein or portal vein thrombosis **CONTRAINDICATIONS:** Bleeding abnormalities, elevated prothrombin or partial thromboplastin times, low platelet count, ascites, acute renal failure.

Patient Care/Scheduling **PATIENT PREPARATION:** Informed consent is obtained from the patient. The patient is placed on a clear liquid diet or NPO 4 hours before the procedure. All medications can be continued. An intravenous line is begun before the procedure in order to ensure adequate hydration and to facilitate the administration of any medications or blood products required during the procedure. Blood typing should be performed beforehand. Recent laboratory results (BUN, creatinine, platelet count, PT, and PTT) are recorded on the chart. **AFTERCARE:** The patient is placed on bedrest for approximately 6 hours. Vital signs should be obtained every 30 minutes for 2 hours, then every hour for 4 hours. The patient should be observed closely for any signs of internal bleeding or sepsis. Many physicians will routinely check a hematocrit 6-8 hours after the procedure. **SPECIAL INSTRUCTIONS:** Any previous imaging study of the upper abdomen should be made available to the interventional radiologist. Any bleeding abnormality should be corrected. Potential problem areas should be noted, such as renal insufficiency or a history of severe contrast reaction. **COMPLICATIONS:** Internal hemorrhage, shock, splenic rupture.

Method **EQUIPMENT:** Fluoroscopy, x-ray equipment, and a sheathed needle **TECHNIQUE:** The appropriate entry site is localized with fluoroscopy and/or ultrasound. Typically, this is in a low intercostal space along the left midaxillary line. A sheathed needle is inserted into the splenic pulp and the needle is removed leaving only the sheath in place. Contrast material is injected at a rate of approximately 5-6 mL/second for 5-7 seconds and x-rays are obtained. **DATA ACQUIRED:** Opacification of the splenic and portal veins as well as any collaterals or varices.

Interpretation **NORMAL FINDINGS:** The splenic and portal veins should be smooth and of normal caliber without evidence of occlusion, thrombosis, compression, filling defect, displacement, portosystemic shunting, or variceal formation. **LIMITATIONS:** Anything which would obscure the splenic or portal veins, such as overlying barium or patient motion.

References

Bergstrand I, "Splenoportography," *Abrams Angiography, Vascular and Interventional Radiology*, 3rd ed, Abrams HL, ed, Boston, MA: Little, Brown and Co, 1983, 1573-1604.

Brazzini A, Hunter DW, Darcy MD, et al, "Safe Splenoportography," *Radiology*, 1987, 162:607-9.

Streptokinase Infusion by Catheter *see* Catheter Placement for Infusion of Drugs or Chemotherapy *on page 317*

Superior Vena Cavogram *see* Venogram, Transfemoral or Transjugular Approach *on page 331*

Temporomandibular Joint Arthrogram *see* Arthrogram *on page 314*

Thoracic Aortogram *see* Arteriogram, Transaxillary or Transbrachial Approach *on page 312*

Thoracic Aortogram *see* Arteriogram, Transfemoral Approach *on page 313*

Vena Caval Filter Placement

CPT 75941

Synonyms Filter Insertion; Greenfield Filter Placement; Inferior Vena Cava Filter Placement; Umbrella Insertion

Abstract PROCEDURE COMMONLY INCLUDES: Placement of a filtering device (sometimes referred to as an umbrella filter) into the inferior vena cava through a common femoral vein or internal jugular vein approach either percutaneously or via a surgical cut-down INDICATIONS: Prevention of pulmonary emboli in patients with lower extremity deep venous thrombosis (DVT) or pelvic thrombosis and for whom anticoagulation is contraindicated or ineffective CONTRAINDICATIONS: Complete thrombosis of the inferior vena cava.

Patient Care/Scheduling PATIENT PREPARATION: Informed consent is obtained from the patient. The patient is placed on a clear liquid diet on the morning of the procedure if possible, although the procedure is often performed on an emergent basis. An intravenous line is begun before the procedure in order to ensure that the patient is well hydrated and to facilitate the administration of any medications required during the procedure. Recent laboratory results (BUN, creatinine, platelet count, PT, and PTT) should be recorded on the chart. AFTERCARE: If the procedure was performed via a common femoral vein approach, the patient is placed on bedrest for approximately 4 hours. During this time, the patient should be flat in bed with the legs straight. Vital signs should be obtained every 30 minutes for 2 hours and then every hour for the next 2 hours. At these times, the femoral puncture site should be examined for any evidence of bleeding or swelling. If an internal jugular vein approach was utilized, bedrest is not mandatory. If a surgical cut-down was per-

(Continued)

Vena Caval Filter Placement *(Continued)*

formed, sutures need to be removed in approximately 7 days. **SPECIAL INSTRUCTIONS:** These examinations are usually arranged by the requesting physician in consultation with the physician performing the procedure. There should be a clear reason why the patient cannot be treated with anticoagulation rather than placement of a caval filter. The physician performing the procedure should be alerted to any potential problem areas such as a history of severe contrast reaction, renal insufficiency, or bleeding abnormalities. **COMPLICATIONS:** Vein thrombosis at the insertion site, caval thrombosis at the filter site, filter migration or inadvertent placement of the filter in an inappropriate location, hematoma formation at the entry site, contrast reaction.

Method **EQUIPMENT:** Caval filter (several varieties are now available) and its delivery system, angiographic catheters and wires, fluoroscopy and x-ray equipment **TECHNIQUE:** Local anesthetic agent is instilled over either the common femoral vein or the internal jugular vein. The vein is percutaneously punctured or, alternatively, a surgical cut-down can be performed. A catheter is inserted and carefully advanced into the inferior vena cava. An inferior vena cavogram is performed in order to depict the anatomy and to assess for any thrombus within the cava. The catheter is then removed and the filter delivery system is advanced into the cava. The filter is then extruded into the inferior vena cava, usually below the level of the renal veins and above the level of the confluence of the common iliac veins.

Interpretation **NORMAL FINDINGS:** The caval filter should be expanded appropriately at the expected location without excessive tilting. **LIMITATIONS:** When thrombus is present within the inferior vena cava itself, there may not be sufficient room to place a filter if the thrombus extends into the intrahepatic segment of the inferior vena cava.

References

Greenfield LJ and Michna BA, "Twelve-Year Clinical Experience With the Greenfield Vena Caval Filter," *Surgery*, 1988, 104(4):706-12.

Pais SO and Tobin KD, "Percutaneous Insertion of the Greenfield Filter," *AJR*, 1989, 152(5):933-8.

Venogram, Extremity

CPT 75821

Synonyms Arm Venogram; Leg Venogram; Lower Extremity Venogram; Upper Extremity Venogram

Abstract **PROCEDURE COMMONLY INCLUDES:** Visualization of the veins of an extremity by injection of contrast material through a needle which has been inserted into a vein on the dorsum of the foot or hand **INDICATIONS:** Suspicion of deep vein thrombosis, occlusion or compression, usually manifested by extremity swelling and/or pain; search for a source of pulmonary emboli **CONTRAINDICATIONS:** Acute renal failure.

Patient Care/Scheduling **PATIENT PREPARATION:** Patient is placed on a clear liquid diet for 4 hours prior to the procedure if possible, although the procedure is often performed on an emergent basis. Recent renal functions (BUN, creatinine) should be available. **COMPLICATIONS:** Contrast reaction, contrast-induced acute renal failure, contrast-induced venous thrombosis, extravasation of contrast at the needle puncture site.

Method **EQUIPMENT:** 19-gauge butterfly needle, contrast material, fluoroscopy, and x-ray equipment **TECHNIQUE:** A butterfly needle is inserted into a vein on the dorsum of the foot or distal calf for a lower extremity venogram, or on the dorsum of the hand or in the forearm for an upper extremity venogram. Approximately 50-75 mL contrast is injected and films of the extremity are obtained. If necessary, the procedure is repeated in multiple projections. Tourniquets may be used to help better visualize the deep veins. **DATA ACQUIRED:** Depiction of venous anatomy.

Interpretation **NORMAL FINDINGS:** There should be good opacification of the deep venous system. There should be no evidence of any radiolucent filling defects (representing clots) or venous occlusion or compression. **LIMITATIONS:** Inability to adequately cannulate a vein of the affected extremity. Also, prior venous thromboses may have resulted in chronic occlusions which can make visualization of any superimposed acute thrombi difficult.

References

Naidich JB, Feinberg AW, Karp-Harman H, et al, "Contrast Venography: Reassessment of Its Role," *Radiology*, 1988, 168(1):97-100.

Rabinov K and Paulin S, "Roentgen Diagnosis of Venous Thrombosis in the Leg," *Arch Surg*, 1972, 104:134-44.

Venogram, Transfemoral or Transjugular Approach

CPT 75826 (inferior vena cava); 75828 (superior vena cava); 75834 (renal); 75843 (adrenal); 75892 (hepatic); 75893 (venous sampling)

Synonyms Percutaneous Transfemoral Venogram; Percutaneous Transjugular Venogram

Applies to Adrenal Venogram; Hepatic Venogram; Iliofemoral Venogram; Inferior Vena Cavogram; Renal Vein Renin Sampling; Renal Venogram; Superior Vena Cavogram; Venous Sampling

Abstract PROCEDURE COMMONLY INCLUDES: Visualization of the veins of the pelvis, abdomen (excluding the portal venous system), thorax, or cervical region by the injection of contrast material through a catheter which has been percutaneously placed through the common femoral vein or, less frequently, the internal jugular vein. This catheter can also be used to obtain venous samples for endocrine assay (eg, renin levels from the renal veins, parathormone levels from the cervical veins or aldosterone, catechol, and cortisol levels from the adrenal veins.) INDICATIONS: Evaluation of the pelvic, abdominal, or thoracic venous systems for thrombus formation, occlusion, compression, stenosis, trauma, or aneurysm CONTRAINDICATIONS: Inability to lie supine, acute renal failure, bleeding abnormalities or abnormal coagulation parameters.

Patient Care/Scheduling PATIENT PREPARATION: Informed consent is obtained from the patient. The patient is placed on a clear liquid diet (not NPO) on the morning of the procedure. All medications are continued. An intravenous line is begun before the procedure in order to ensure that the patient is well hydrated (thus decreasing the risk of acute renal failure) and to facilitate the administration of any medications required during the procedure. Recent laboratory results (BUN, creatinine, platelet count, PT, and PTT) should be appropriately recorded on the chart. The patient with chart is sent on a stretcher to the angiography suite when notified. AFTERCARE: If a femoral approach was used, the patient is placed on bedrest for 4 hours after the procedure. During this time, the patient should remain flat in bed with the legs straight. Vital signs should be observed every 30 minutes for the first 2 hours, then every hour for the next 2 hours. At these times, the femoral puncture site should be examined for any evidence of bleeding or swelling and the leg should be examined for any changes in color or warmth. If the jugular approach was used, the head of the bed should be elevated and the site should be observed for bleeding. SPECIAL INSTRUCTIONS: These examinations are often arranged by the requesting physician in consultation with the cardiovascular radiologist. The requisition should state clearly the reason for the study as well as the specific vessels to be examined or the specific veins which should be sampled for endocrine assays. The cardiovascular radiologist should be alerted to any potential problem areas such as renal insufficiency or a history of severe contrast reaction. COMPLICATIONS: Contrast reaction; acute renal failure; venous thrombosis, bleeding, or hematoma formation at the puncture site.

Method EQUIPMENT: Fluoroscopy, angiographic catheters and wires, and a method of film recording (either conventional cut films or digital subtraction films) TECHNIQUE: Local anesthetic agent is instilled over the common femoral vein or, less frequently, the internal jugular vein. The vein is percutaneously punctured and a catheter is inserted and fluoroscopically guided into the vein of interest. Contrast medium is injected and the films are obtained. DATA ACQUIRED: Visualization of the venous systems in the areas of clinical concern on either conventional x-ray film or on digitally subtracted images. If desired, venous samples can be assayed for the appropriate endocrine levels.

Interpretation NORMAL FINDINGS: The veins should be smooth and of normal caliber. There should be no radiolucent filling defects (representing thrombi) and no evidence for vessel stenosis, occlusion, compression, extravasation, or aneurysm. LIMITATIONS: Anything which would obscure the blood vessels, such as overlying barium or patient motion.

References

Johnsrude IS, "Catheterization Techniques," *A Practical Approach to Angiography*, 2nd ed, Johnsrude IS, Jackson DC, and Dunnick NR, eds, Boston, MA: Little, Brown and Co, 1987, 55-7.

MAGNETIC RESONANCE IMAGING

Jeffrey S. Ross, MD

Magnetic resonance was first described in the 1940's, but it was not until the early 1970's that the first MR image was produced. There was subsequently rapid development and integration of MR into the radiologic diagnostic armamentarium, particularly in the case of brain, spine, and musculoskeletal imaging. The advantages of MR over other imaging modalities include high contrast ionizing radiation. The process employs the magnetic properties of the hydrogen nucleus (proton) and its interaction with strong external magnetic fields and radiofrequency pulses. The patient is placed in a strong magnetic field and radiofrequency pulses are transmitted into the patient in an extremely controlled and defined manner. The protons within the patient will subsequently emit a radiofrequency signal which is processed by computer to produce the image. The images are placed onto film as in other conventional imaging techniques or onto videotape in the case of cine motion studies.

Discogram *replaced by* Magnetic Resonance Scan, Cervical Spinal Canal and Contents *on page 342*

Magnetic Resonance Angiography *see* Magnetic Resonance Scan, Vascular *on page 355*

Magnetic Resonance Scan, Abdomen

CPT 74181

Abstract INDICATIONS: Evaluation of the liver, spleen, pancreas, kidneys, adrenal glands, and the remainder of the upper abdomen. In addition to similar information gained from computed tomography (CT) of the upper abdomen, MRI has been found to be useful in certain instances in differentiating benign from malignant pathology. CONTRAINDICATIONS: Patients weighing more than 300 lb and patients unable to squeeze into the magnet cannot undergo MRI. An absolute contraindication for MRI is a cardiac pacemaker. Relative contraindications to magnetic resonance imaging include intracranial aneurysm clips, cochlear implants, insulin infusion and chemotherapy pumps, neurocutaneous stimulators and prosthetic heart valves, depending on date of manufacture and metallurgical composition. Please consult MRI physician if questions arise. Patients who have metallic foreign bodies within the eye or who have undergone recent surgery within the last 6 weeks requiring placement of a vascular surgical clip, should also not undergo MRI. The safety of MRI in pregnant patients has not been determined. In such cases, prior consultation with the MRI physician is required. Generally, patients who have undergone recent surgery not requiring vascular clips or who have had coronary artery bypass surgery in the past may undergo MRI. Patients who have shrapnel wounds or orthopedic prostheses can generally safely undergo MRI unless the metallic device is in the anatomic region to be scanned which results in degradation of the images. Patients with surgically implanted intravascular vena cava filters to prevent pulmonary embolism can usually be scanned if the device has been in place for at least 6 weeks. Patients requiring life support equipment including ventilators require special preparation. Please contact MRI physician ahead of time. Central venous lines, Swan-Ganz catheters, and nasogastric (NG) tubes usually present no problems. If the patient is positive when screened for metallic devices and you are uncertain of their significance, the MRI radiologist will provide additional information to assist you.

Patient Care/Scheduling PATIENT PREPARATION: Patients should remain NPO at least 4 hours prior to the exam. Inpatient: Patient must be able to lie quietly while the scan is performed. The patient should be screened for metallic devices by nursing personnel. (See Contraindications.) This includes metal introduced into the patient either surgically or by trauma. All metallic objects must be removed from the patient including jewelry or any other metal objects which may be in the patient's bedding. Please remove dentures or other dental appliances. I.V.s which contain no metal are fine, but infusion pumps must be removed. Oxygen tanks and metallic backboards may come with the patient but will be removed prior to the patient entering the magnet room. Oxygen may be provided in the magnet room. Trauma, ICU, or CCU patients should be accompanied by a nurse. The patient needs to be NPO for abdominal MRI exams. If the patient is restless, combative, or claustrophobic, proper sedation may be administered on the floor prior to the MRI, or at the MRI Center. Consult the MRI radiologists with questions on proper sedation. Outpatient: The patient should be screened for metallic devices. (See Contraindications.) If a question exists as to the patient's suitability for MRI, the MRI radiologist will assist you with your questions. If the patient is claustrophobic, oral or parenteral sedation may be necessary. If so, the patient should be accompanied by another adult to provide transportation home after the examination. AFTERCARE: If the patient received an MRI contrast agent (Magnevist®) and develops a delayed hypersensitivity reaction (ie, hives or shortness of breath), the referring physician or MRI radiologist should be contacted immediately.

Method DATA ACQUIRED: Digital information with film reproduction.

Interpretation LIMITATIONS: Generally, the greatest limitation of magnetic resonance imaging results from the patient's fear of the procedure. The patient must remain quiet and still for several scans, each lasting from several minutes to 10 minutes in length. Total examination time is usually 30-45 minutes and occasionally up to 1 hour. If the patient is restless during the examination, motion artifacts will be present on the images limiting their diagnostic value. If the patient is claustrophobic, mild oral sedation or occasionally parenteral sedation may be needed. Also the patient can be accompanied by a family member or friend during the examination which helps calm the patient's anxiety in many cases. Patients requiring life support equipment such as ventilators require special preparation. Please refer to Contraindications for further causes for rejection. **ADDITIONAL INFORMATION:** In some cases, an MRI contrast agent (Magnevist®) may be needed to increase the diagnostic accuracy of the MRI. This contrast agent can be administered to patients with a previous history of allergies to conventional iodinated x-ray agents as it contains no iodine. Contraindications to its use include previous allergy to the contrast agent itself, renal failure, certain types of anemia, and Wilson's disease. The contrast agent is generally very safe and increases the diagnostic efficacy of the MRI. Intramuscular or subcutaneous injection of glucagon may be given to decrease motion artifacts from peristalsis.

References

Glazer GM, "MR Imaging of the Liver, Kidneys, and Adrenal Glands," *Radiology*, 1988, 166(2):303-12.

Mattrey R, Trambert M, and Edelman RR, "MR Imaging of the Upper Abdomen and Adrenal Glands," *Clinical Magnetic Resonance Imaging*, Philadelphia, PA: WB Saunders Co, 1990, 845-98.

Magnetic Resonance Scan, Aorta

CPT 71550

Abstract **INDICATIONS:** Evaluation of the aorta for aneurysm, dissection, tumor **CONTRAINDICATIONS:** Patients weighing more than 300 lb and patients unable to squeeze into the magnet cannot undergo MRI. An absolute contraindication for MRI is a cardiac pacemaker. Relative contraindications to magnetic resonance imaging include intracranial aneurysm clips, cochlear implants, insulin infusion and chemotherapy pumps, neurocutaneous stimulators and prosthetic heart valves, depending on date of manufacture and metallurgical composition. Please consult MRI physician if questions arise. Patients who have metallic foreign bodies within the eye or who have undergone recent surgery within the last 6 weeks requiring placement of a vascular surgical clip, should also not undergo MRI. The safety of MRI in pregnant patients has not been determined. In such cases, prior consultation with the MRI physician is required. Generally, patients who have undergone recent surgery not requiring vascular clips or who have had coronary artery bypass surgery in the past may undergo MRI. Patients who have shrapnel wounds or orthopedic prostheses can generally safely undergo MRI unless the metallic device is in the anatomic region to be scanned which results in degradation of the images. Patients with surgically implanted intravascular vena cava filters to prevent pulmonary embolism can usually be scanned if the device has been in place for at least 6 weeks. Patients requiring life support equipment including ventilators require special preparation. Please contact MRI physician ahead of time. Central venous lines, Swan-Ganz catheters, and nasogastric (NG) tubes usually present no problems. If the patient is positive when screened for metallic devices and you are uncertain of their significance, the MRI radiologist will provide additional information to assist you.

Patient Care/Scheduling **PATIENT PREPARATION:** Inpatient: Patient must be able to lie quietly while the scan is performed. The patient should be screened for metallic devices by nursing personnel. (See Contraindications.) This includes metal introduced into the patient either surgically or by trauma. All metallic objects must be removed from the patient including jewelry or any other metal objects which may be in the patient's bedding. Please remove dentures or other dental appliances. I.V.s which contain no metal are fine, but infusion pumps must be removed. Oxygen tanks and metallic backboards may come with the patient but will be removed prior to the patient entering the magnet room. Oxygen may be provided in the magnet room. Trauma, ICU, or CCU patients should be accompanied by a nurse. If the patient is restless, combative, or claustrophobic, proper sedation may be administered on the floor prior to the MRI, or at the MRI Center. Consult the MRI radiologists with questions on proper sedation. Outpatient: The patient should be screened for metallic devices. (See Contraindications.) If a question exists as to the patient's suitability for MRI, the MRI radiologist will assist you with your questions. If the patient is claustrophobic, oral or parenteral sedation may be necessary. If so, the patient should be accompa-

(Continued)

Magnetic Resonance Scan, Aorta *(Continued)*

nied by another adult to provide transportation home after the examination. **AFTERCARE:** If the patient received an MRI contrast agent (Magnevist®) and develops a delayed hypersensitivity reaction (ie, hives or shortness of breath), the referring physician or MRI radiologist should be contacted immediately.

Method **DATA ACQUIRED:** Digital information with film reproduction.

Interpretation **LIMITATIONS:** Patient motion and cardiac rhythm abnormalities will degrade the study, limiting interpretation. Generally, the greatest limitation of magnetic resonance imaging results from the patient's fear of the procedure. The patient must remain quiet and still for several scans, each lasting from several minutes to 10 minutes in length. Total examination time is usually up to 1 hour. If the patient is restless during the examination, motion artifacts will be present on the images limiting their diagnostic value. If the patient is claustrophobic, oral or parenteral sedation may be needed. Patients requiring life support equipment such as ventilators require special preparation. Please refer to Contraindications for further causes for rejection. **ADDITIONAL INFORMATION:** In some cases, an MRI contrast agent (Magnevist®) may be needed to increase the diagnostic accuracy of the MRI. This contrast agent can be administered to patients with a previous history of allergies to conventional iodinated x-ray agents as it contains no iodine. Contraindications to its use include previous allergy to the contrast agent itself, renal failure, certain types of anemia, and Wilson's disease. The contrast agent is generally very safe and increases the diagnostic efficacy of the MRI.

References

Dinsmore R, "Examination of the Adult Heart and Great Vessels," *Clinical Magnetic Resonance Imaging*, Philadelphia, PA: WB Saunders Co, 1990, 773-829.

Magnetic Resonance Scan, Bone

CPT 76400

Abstract **INDICATIONS:** Evaluation of bone anatomy and pathology including marrow throughout the body including the wrists and hips **CONTRAINDICATIONS:** Patients weighing more than 300 lb and patients unable to squeeze into the magnet cannot undergo MRI. An absolute contraindication for MRI is a cardiac pacemaker. Relative contraindications to magnetic resonance imaging include intracranial aneurysm clips, cochlear implants, insulin infusion and chemotherapy pumps, neurocutaneous stimulators and prosthetic heart valves, depending on date of manufacture and metallurgical composition. Please consult MRI physician if questions arise. Patients who have metallic foreign bodies within the eye or who have undergone recent surgery within the last 6 weeks requiring placement of a vascular surgical clip, should also not undergo MRI. The safety of MRI in pregnant patients has not been determined. In such cases, prior consultation with the MRI physician is required. Generally, patients who have undergone recent surgery not requiring vascular clips or who have had coronary artery bypass surgery in the past may undergo MRI. Patients who have shrapnel wounds or orthopedic prostheses can generally safely undergo MRI unless the metallic device is in the anatomic region to be scanned which results in degradation of the images. Patients with surgically implanted intravascular vena cava filters to prevent pulmonary embolism can usually be scanned if the device has been in place for at least 6 weeks. Patients requiring life support equipment including ventilators require special preparation. Please contact MRI physician ahead of time. Central venous lines, Swan-Ganz catheters, and nasogastric (NG) tubes usually present no problems. If the patient is positive when screened for metallic devices and you are uncertain of their significance, the MRI radiologist will provide additional information to assist you.

Patient Care/Scheduling **PATIENT PREPARATION:** Inpatient: Patient must be able to lie quietly while the scan is performed. The patient should be screened for metallic devices by nursing personnel. (See Contraindications.) This includes metal introduced into the patient either surgically or by trauma. All metallic objects must be removed from the patient including jewelry or any other metal objects which may be in the patient's bedding. Please remove dentures or other dental appliances. I.V.s which contain no metal are fine, but infusion pumps must be removed. Oxygen tanks and metallic backboards may come with the patient but will be removed prior to the patient entering the magnet room. Oxygen may be provided in the magnet room. Trauma, ICU, or CCU patients should be accompanied by a nurse. If the patient is restless, combative, or claustrophobic, proper sedation may be administered on the floor prior to the MRI, or at the MRI Center. Consult the MRI radiologists with questions on proper sedation. Outpatient: The patient should be screened for metallic devices. (See Contraindications.) If a question exists as to the patient's suitability for MRI, the MRI radiologist will assist you with your questions. If the patient is claustrophobic, oral or parenteral sedation may be necessary. If so, the patient should be accompanied by another adult to provide transportation home after the examination. **AFTERCARE:** If the patient received an MRI contrast agent (Magnevist®) and develops a delayed hypersensitivity reaction (ie, hives or shortness of breath), the referring physician or MRI radiologist should be contacted immediately.

Method **DATA ACQUIRED:** Digital information with film reproduction.

Specimen **CAUSES FOR REJECTION:** See Contraindications.

Interpretation **LIMITATIONS:** Implanted orthopedic devices in the anatomical area being imaged may limit the usefulness of the test. Generally, the greatest limitation of magnetic resonance imaging results from the patient's fear of the procedure. The patient must remain quiet and still for several scans, each lasting from several minutes to 10 minutes in length. Total examination time is usually 30-45 minutes and occasionally up to 1 hour. If the patient is restless during the examination, motion artifacts will be present on the images limiting their diagnostic value. If the patient is claustrophobic, mild oral sedation or occasionally parenteral sedation may be needed. Also the patient can be accompanied by a family member or friend during the examination which helps calm the patient's anxiety in many cases. Patients requiring life support equipment such as ventilators require special preparation. Please refer to Contraindications for further causes for rejection. **ADDITIONAL INFORMATION:** In some cases, an MRI contrast agent (Magnevist®) may be needed to increase the diagnostic accuracy of the MRI. This contrast agent can be administered to patients with a previous history of allergies to conventional iodinated x-ray agents as it contains no iodine. Contraindications to its use include previous allergy to the contrast agent itself, renal failure, certain types of anemia, and Wilson's disease. The contrast agent is generally very safe and increases the diagnostic efficacy of the MRI.

References

Deutsch AL and Mink JH, "Magnetic Resonance Imaging of Musculoskeletal Injuries," *Radiol Clin North Am*, 1989, 27(5):983.

Kursunoglu-Brahme S, Gundry CR, and Resnick D, "Advanced Imaging of the Wrist," *Radiol Clin North Am*, 1990, 28(2):307-20.

Magnetic Resonance Scan, Bone Marrow

CPT 76400

Abstract **INDICATIONS:** To define marrow anatomy and assess its morphologic appearance. Primary/metastatic tumor involvement can be evaluated as well as inflammatory processes (vertebral osteomyelitis). **CONTRAINDICATIONS:** Patients weighing more than 300 lb and patients unable to squeeze into the magnet cannot undergo MRI. An absolute contraindication for MRI is a cardiac pacemaker. Relative contraindications to magnetic resonance imaging include intracranial aneurysm clips, cochlear implants, insulin infusion and chemotherapy pumps, neurocutaneous stimulators and prosthetic heart valves, depending on date of manufacture and metallurgical composition. Please consult MRI physician if questions arise. Patients who have metallic foreign bodies within the eye or who have undergone recent surgery within the last 6 weeks requiring placement of a vascular surgical clip, should also not undergo MRI. The safety of MRI in pregnant patients has not been determined. In such cases, prior consultation with the MRI physician is required. Generally, patients who have undergone recent surgery not requiring vascular clips or who have had coronary artery bypass surgery in the past may undergo MRI. Patients who have shrapnel wounds or orthopedic prostheses can generally safely undergo MRI unless the metallic device is in the anatomic region to be scanned which results in degradation of the images. Patients with surgically implanted intravascular vena cava filters to prevent pulmonary embolism can usually be scanned if the device has been in place for at least 6 weeks. Patients requiring life support equipment including ventilators require special preparation. Please contact MRI physician ahead of time. Central venous lines, Swan-Ganz catheters, and nasogastric (NG) tubes usually present no problems. If the patient is positive when screened for metallic devices and you are uncertain of their significance, the MRI radiologist will provide additional information to assist you.

(Continued)

Magnetic Resonance Scan, Bone Marrow *(Continued)*

Patient Care/Scheduling PATIENT PREPARATION: Inpatient: Patient must be able to lie quietly while the scan is performed. The patient should be screened for metallic devices by nursing personnel. (See Contraindications.) This includes metal introduced into the patient either surgically or by trauma. All metallic objects must be removed from the patient including jewelry or any other metal objects which may be in the patient's bedding. Please remove dentures or other dental appliances. I.V.s which contain no metal are fine, but infusion pumps must be removed. Oxygen tanks and metallic backboards may come with the patient but will be removed prior to the patient entering the magnet room. Oxygen may be provided in the magnet room. Trauma, ICU, or CCU patients should be accompanied by a nurse. If the patient is restless, combative, or claustrophobic, proper sedation may be administered on the floor prior to the MRI, or at the MRI Center. Consult the MRI radiologists with questions on proper sedation. Outpatient: The patient should be screened for metallic devices. (See Contraindications.) If a question exists as to the patient's suitability for MRI, the MRI radiologist will assist you with your questions. If the patient is claustrophobic, oral or parenteral sedation may be necessary. If so, the patient should be accompanied by another adult to provide transportation home after the examination. AFTERCARE: If the patient received an MRI contrast agent (Magnevist®) and develops a delayed hypersensitivity reaction (ie, hives or shortness of breath), the referring physician or MRI radiologist should be contacted immediately.

Method DATA ACQUIRED: Digital information with film reproduction.

Interpretation LIMITATIONS: Generally, the greatest limitation of magnetic resonance imaging results from the patient's fear of the procedure. The patient must remain quiet and still for several scans, each lasting from several minutes to 10 minutes in length. Total examination time is usually 30-45 minutes and occasionally up to 1 hour. If the patient is restless during the examination, motion artifacts will be present on the images limiting their diagnostic value. If the patient is claustrophobic, mild oral sedation or occasionally parenteral sedation may be needed. Also the patient can be accompanied by a family member or friend during the examination which helps calm the patient's anxiety in many cases. Patients requiring life support equipment such as ventilators require special preparation. Please refer to Contraindications for further causes for rejection. Implanted orthopedic appliances may limit the usefulness of the scan in the area being imaged. ADDITIONAL INFORMATION: In some cases, an MRI contrast agent (Magnevist®) may be needed to increase the diagnostic accuracy of the MRI. This contrast agent can be administered to patients with a previous history of allergies to conventional iodinated x-ray agents as it contains no iodine. Contraindications to its use include previous allergy to the contrast agent itself, renal failure, certain types of anemia, and Wilson's disease. The contrast agent is generally very safe and increases the diagnostic efficacy of the MRI.

References

Carmody RF, Yang PJ, Seeley GW, et al, "Spinal Cord Compression Due to Metastatic Disease: Diagnosis With MR Imaging Versus Myelography," *Radiology*, 1989, 173(1):225-9.

Genez BM, Wilson MR, Houk RW, et al, "Early Osteonecrosis of the Femoral Head: Detection in High Risk Patients With MR Imaging," *Radiology*, 1988, 168(2):521-4.

Magnetic Resonance Scan, Brachial Plexus

Abstract INDICATIONS: Clinical concern of brachial plexus lesion including primary or secondary neoplasms, especially superior sulcus tumors CONTRAINDICATIONS: Patients weighing more than 300 lb and patients unable to squeeze into the magnet cannot undergo MRI. An absolute contraindication for MRI is a cardiac pacemaker. Relative contraindications to magnetic resonance imaging include intracranial aneurysm clips, cochlear implants, insulin infusion and chemotherapy pumps, neurocutaneous stimulators and prosthetic heart valves, depending on date of manufacture and metallurgical composition. Please consult MRI physician if questions arise. Patients who have metallic foreign bodies within the eye or who have undergone recent surgery within the last 6 weeks requiring placement of a vascular surgical clip, should also not undergo MRI. The safety of MRI in pregnant patients has not been determined. In such cases, prior consultation with the MRI physician is required. Generally, patients who have undergone recent surgery not requiring vascular clips or who have had coronary artery bypass surgery in the past may undergo MRI. Patients who have shrapnel wounds or orthopedic prostheses can generally safely undergo MRI unless the metallic device is in the anatomic region to be scanned which results in degradation of the images. Patients with surgically implanted intravascular vena cava filters to prevent pulmonary embolism can usually be scanned if the device has been in place for at least 6 weeks. Patients requiring life support equipment including ventilators require special preparation. Please contact MRI physician ahead of time. Central venous lines, Swan-Ganz catheters, and nasogastric (NG) tubes usually present no problems. If the patient is positive when screened for metallic devices and you are uncertain of their significance, the MRI radiologist will provide additional information to assist you.

Patient Care/Scheduling PATIENT PREPARATION: Inpatient: Patient must be able to lie quietly while the scan is performed. The patient should be screened for metallic devices by nursing personnel. (See Contraindications.) This includes metal introduced into the patient either surgically or by trauma. All metallic objects must be removed from the patient including jewelry or any other metal objects which may be in the patient's bedding. Please remove dentures or other dental appliances. I.V.s which contain no metal are fine, but infusion pumps must be removed. Oxygen tanks and metallic backboards may come with the patient but will be removed prior to the patient entering the magnet room. Oxygen may be provided in the magnet room. Trauma, ICU, or CCU patients should be accompanied by a nurse. If the patient is restless, combative, or claustrophobic, proper sedation may be administered on the floor prior to the MRI, or at the MRI Center. Consult the MRI radiologists with questions on proper sedation. Outpatient: The patient should be screened for metallic devices. (See Contraindications.) If a question exists as to the patient's suitability for MRI, the MRI radiologist will assist you with your questions. If the patient is claustrophobic, oral or parenteral sedation may be necessary. If so, the patient should be accompanied by another adult to provide transportation home after the examination. AFTERCARE: If the patient received an MRI contrast agent (Magnevist®) and develops a delayed hypersensitivity reaction (ie, hives or shortness of breath), the referring physician or MRI radiologist should be contacted immediately.

Method DATA ACQUIRED: Digital information with film reproduction.

Interpretation LIMITATIONS: Generally, the greatest limitation of magnetic resonance imaging results from the patient's fear of the procedure. The patient must remain quiet and still for several scans, each lasting from several minutes to 10 minutes in length. Total examination time is usually up to 1 hour. If the patient is restless during the examination, motion artifacts will be present on the images limiting their diagnostic value. If the patient is claustrophobic, oral or parenteral sedation may be needed. Patients requiring life support equipment such as ventilators require special preparation. Please refer to Contraindications for further causes for rejection. ADDITIONAL INFORMATION: In some cases, an MRI contrast agent (Magnevist®) may be needed to increase the diagnostic accuracy of the MRI. This contrast agent can be administered to patients with a previous history of allergies to conventional iodinated x-ray agents as it contains no iodine. Contraindications to its use include previous allergy to the contrast agent itself, renal failure, certain types of anemia, and Wilson's disease. The contrast agent is generally very safe and increases the diagnostic efficacy of the MRI.

References

Rapoport S, Blair DN, McCarthy SM, et al, "Brachial Plexus: Correlation of MR Imaging With CT and Pathologic Findings," *Radiology*, 1988, 167(1):161-5.

Magnetic Resonance Scan, Brain

CPT 70551

Applies to Magnetic Resonance Scan, Head

Abstract INDICATIONS: To diagnose intracranial abnormalities including tumors, ischemia, infection, multiple sclerosis or any abnormalities relating to the brain or calvarium. MRI is an excellent modality for assessment of congenital brain abnormalities or relating to the status of brain maturation in the pediatric population. CONTRAINDICATIONS: Patients weighing more than 300 lb and patients unable to squeeze into the magnet cannot undergo MRI. An absolute contraindication for MRI is a cardiac pacemaker. Relative contraindications to magnetic resonance imaging include intracranial aneurysm clips, cochlear implants, insulin infusion and chemotherapy pumps, neurocutaneous stimulators and prosthetic heart

(Continued)

Magnetic Resonance Scan, Brain *(Continued)*

valves, depending on date of manufacture and metallurgical composition. Please consult MRI physician if questions arise. Patients who have metallic foreign bodies within the eye or who have undergone recent surgery within the last 6 weeks requiring placement of a vascular surgical clip, should also not undergo MRI. The safety of MRI in pregnant patients has not been determined. In such cases, prior consultation with the MRI physician is required. Generally, patients who have undergone recent surgery not requiring vascular clips or who have had coronary artery bypass surgery in the past may undergo MRI. Patients who have shrapnel wounds or orthopedic prostheses can generally safely undergo MRI unless the metallic device is in the anatomic region to be scanned which results in degradation of the images. Patients with surgically implanted intravascular vena cava filters to prevent pulmonary embolism can usually be scanned if the device has been in place for at least 6 weeks. Patients requiring life support equipment including ventilators require special preparation. Please contact MRI physician ahead of time. Central venous lines, Swan-Ganz catheters, and nasogastric (NG) tubes usually present no problems. If the patient is positive when screened for metallic devices and you are uncertain of their significance, the MRI radiologist will provide additional information to assist you.

Patient Care/Scheduling **PATIENT PREPARATION:** Inpatient: Patient must be able to lie quietly while the scan is performed. The patient should be screened for metallic devices by nursing personnel. (See Contraindications.) This includes metal introduced into the patient either surgically or by trauma. All metallic objects must be removed from the patient including jewelry or any other metal objects which may be in the patient's bedding. Please remove dentures or other dental appliances. I.V.s which contain no metal are fine, but infusion pumps must be removed. Oxygen tanks and metallic backboards may come with the patient but will be removed prior to the patient entering the magnet room. Oxygen may be provided in the magnet room. Trauma, ICU, or CCU patients should be accompanied by a nurse. If the patient is restless, combative, or claustrophobic, proper sedation may be administered on the floor prior to the MRI, or at the MRI Center. Consult the MRI radiologists with questions on proper sedation. Outpatient: The patient should be screened for metallic devices. (See Contraindications.) If a question exists as to the patient's suitability for MRI, the MRI radiologist will assist you with your questions. If the patient is claustrophobic, oral or parenteral sedation may be necessary. If so, the patient should be accompanied by another adult to provide transportation home after the examination. **AFTERCARE:** If the patient received an MRI contrast agent (Magnevist®) and develops a delayed hypersensitivity reaction (ie, hives or shortness of breath), the referring physician or MRI radiologist should be contacted immediately.

Method **DATA ACQUIRED:** Digital information with film reproduction.

Interpretation **LIMITATIONS:** Generally, the greatest limitation of magnetic resonance imaging results from the patient's fear of the procedure. The patient must remain quiet and still for several scans, each lasting from several minutes to 10 minutes in length. Total examination time is usually 30-45 minutes and occasionally up to 1 hour. If the patient is restless during the examination, motion artifacts will be present on the images limiting their diagnostic value. If the patient is claustrophobic, mild oral sedation or occasionally parenteral sedation may be needed. Also the patient can be accompanied by a family member or friend during the examination which helps calm the patient's anxiety in many cases. Patients requiring life support equipment such as ventilators require special preparation. Please refer to Contraindications for further causes for rejection. **ADDITIONAL INFORMATION:** In some cases, an MRI contrast agent (Magnevist®) may be needed to increase the diagnostic accuracy of the MRI. This contrast agent can be administered to patients with a previous history of allergies to conventional iodinated x-ray agents as it contains no iodine. Contraindications to its use include previous allergy to the contrast agent itself, renal failure, certain types of anemia, and Wilson's disease. The contrast agent is generally very safe and increases the diagnostic efficacy of the MRI.

References

Topics in Magnetic Resonance Imaging, Rockville, MD: Aspen Publishers, Inc, 1989.

Magnetic Resonance Scan, Cardiac

CPT 75552

Abstract **INDICATIONS:** To assess congenital malformations (right ventricular outflow obstruction, septal defects, transposition); aortic valve evaluation (AS or AI); constrictive pericarditis; restrictive cardiomyopathy; cardiac tumors **CONTRAINDICATIONS:** Patients weighing more than 300 lb and patients unable to squeeze into the magnet cannot undergo MRI. An absolute contraindication for MRI is a cardiac pacemaker. Relative contraindications to magnetic resonance imaging include intracranial aneurysm clips, cochlear implants, insulin infusion and chemotherapy pumps, neurocutaneous stimulators and prosthetic heart valves, depending on date of manufacture and metallurgical composition. Please consult MRI physician if questions arise. Patients who have metallic foreign bodies within the eye or who have undergone recent surgery within the last 6 weeks requiring placement of a vascular surgical clip, should also not undergo MRI. The safety of MRI in pregnant patients has not been determined. In such cases, prior consultation with the MRI physician is required. Generally, patients who have undergone recent surgery not requiring vascular clips or who have had coronary artery bypass surgery in the past may undergo MRI. Patients who have shrapnel wounds or orthopedic prostheses can generally safely undergo MRI unless the metallic device is in the anatomic region to be scanned which results in degradation of the images. Patients with surgically implanted intravascular vena cava filters to prevent pulmonary embolism can usually be scanned if the device has been in place for at least 6 weeks. Patients requiring life support equipment including ventilators require special preparation. Please contact MRI physician ahead of time. Central venous lines, Swan-Ganz catheters, and nasogastric (NG) tubes usually present no problems. If the patient is positive when screened for metallic devices and you are uncertain of their significance, the MRI radiologist will provide additional information to assist you.

Patient Care/Scheduling PATIENT PREPARATION: Inpatient: Patient must be able to lie quietly while the scan is performed. The patient should be screened for metallic devices by nursing personnel. (See Contraindications.) This includes metal introduced into the patient either surgically or by trauma. All metallic objects must be removed from the patient including jewelry or any other metal objects which may be in the patient's bedding. Please remove dentures or other dental appliances. I.V.s which contain no metal are fine, but infusion pumps must be removed. Oxygen tanks and metallic backboards may come with the patient but will be removed prior to the patient entering the magnet room. Oxygen may be provided in the magnet room. Trauma, ICU, or CCU patients should be accompanied by a nurse. If the patient is restless, combative, or claustrophobic, proper sedation may be administered on the floor prior to the MRI, or at the MRI Center. Consult the MRI radiologists with questions on proper sedation. Outpatient: The patient should be screened for metallic devices. (See Contraindications.) If a question exists as to the patient's suitability for MRI, the MRI radiologist will assist you with your questions. If the patient is claustrophobic, oral or parenteral sedation may be necessary. If so, the patient should be accompanied by another adult to provide transportation home after the examination. AFTERCARE: If the patient received an MRI contrast agent (Magnevist®) and develops a delayed hypersensitivity reaction (ie, hives or shortness of breath), the referring physician or MRI radiologist should be contacted immediately.

Method DATA ACQUIRED: Digital information displayed as static film based images and cine loop. Data is EKG gated.

Interpretation LIMITATIONS: Patient motion and cardiac rhythm abnormalities will degrade the study, limiting interpretation. Generally, the greatest limitation of magnetic resonance imaging results from the patient's fear of the procedure. The patient must remain quiet and still for several scans, each lasting from several minutes to 10 minutes in length. Total examination time is usually up to 1 hour. If the patient is restless during the examination, motion artifacts will be present on the images limiting their diagnostic value. If the patient is claustrophobic, oral or parenteral sedation may be needed. Patients requiring life support equipment such as ventilators require special preparation. Please refer to Contraindications for further causes for rejection. ADDITIONAL INFORMATION: In some cases, an MRI contrast agent (Magnevist®) may be needed to increase the diagnostic accuracy of the MRI. This contrast agent can be administered to patients with a previous history of allergies to conventional iodinated x-ray agents as it contains no iodine. Contraindications to its use include previous allergy to the contrast agent itself, renal failure, certain types of anemia, and Wilson's disease. The contrast agent is generally very safe and increases the diagnostic efficacy of the MRI.

References

Bouchard A, Woods G, Cranney G, et al, "Uses of Magnetic Resonance Imaging in Cardiovascular Disease," *Am J Cardiac Imaging*, 1989, 3:75-87.

Magnetic Resonance Scan, Cervical Spinal Canal and Contents

CPT 72141

Replaces Discogram

Abstract INDICATIONS: For assessment of intramedullary spinal cord disease including tumors, infection, ischemia, and demyelination. Extramedullary-intradural disease including tumors, infection, disc degeneration, and herniation. The skull base including the cervicomedullary junction can be evaluated. Congenital abnormalities are also well evaluated. CONTRAINDICATIONS: Patients weighing more than 300 lb and patients unable to squeeze into the magnet cannot undergo MRI. An absolute contraindication for MRI is a cardiac pacemaker. Relative contraindications to magnetic resonance imaging include intracranial aneurysm clips, cochlear implants, insulin infusion and chemotherapy pumps, neurocutaneous stimulators and prosthetic heart valves, depending on date of manufacture and metallurgical composition. Please consult MRI physician if questions arise. Patients who have metallic foreign bodies within the eye or who have undergone recent surgery within the last 6 weeks requiring placement of a vascular surgical clip, should also not undergo MRI. The safety of MRI in pregnant patients has not been determined. In such cases, prior consultation with the MRI physician is required. Generally, patients who have undergone recent surgery not requiring vascular clips or who have had coronary artery bypass surgery in the past may undergo MRI. Patients who have shrapnel wounds or orthopedic prostheses can generally safely undergo MRI unless the metallic device is in the anatomic region to be scanned which results in degradation of the images. Patients with surgically implanted intravascular vena cava filters to prevent pulmonary embolism can usually be scanned if the device has been in place for at least 6 weeks. Patients requiring life support equipment including ventilators require special preparation. Please contact MRI physician ahead of time. Central venous lines, Swan-Ganz catheters, and nasogastric (NG) tubes usually present no problems. If the patient is positive when screened for metallic devices and you are uncertain of their significance, the MRI radiologist will provide additional information to assist you.

Patient Care/Scheduling PATIENT PREPARATION: Inpatient: Patient must be able to lie quietly while the scan is performed. The patient should be screened for metallic devices by nursing personnel. (See Contraindications.) This includes metal introduced into the patient either surgically or by trauma. All metallic objects must be removed from the patient including jewelry or any other metal objects which may be in the patient's bedding. Please remove dentures or other dental appliances. I.V.s which contain no metal are fine, but infusion pumps must be removed. Oxygen tanks and metallic backboards may come with the patient but will be removed prior to the patient entering the magnet room. Oxygen may be provided in the magnet room. Trauma, ICU, or CCU patients should be accompanied by a nurse. If the patient is restless, combative, or claustrophobic, proper sedation may be administered on the floor prior to the MRI, or at the MRI Center. Consult the MRI radiologists with questions on proper sedation. Outpatient: The patient should be screened for metallic devices. (See Contraindications.) If a question exists as to the patient's suitability for MRI, the MRI radiologist will assist you with your questions. If the patient is claustrophobic, oral or parenteral sedation may be necessary. If so, the patient should be accompanied by another adult to provide transportation home after the examination. AFTERCARE: If the patient received an MRI contrast agent (Magnevist®) and develops a delayed hypersensitivity reaction (ie, hives or shortness of breath), the referring physician or MRI radiologist should be contacted immediately.

Interpretation LIMITATIONS: Generally, the greatest limitation of magnetic resonance imaging results from the patient's fear of the procedure. The patient must remain quiet and still for several scans, each lasting from several minutes to 10 minutes in length. Total examination time is usually 30-45 minutes and occasionally up to 1 hour. If the patient is restless during the examination, motion artifacts will be present on the images limiting their diagnostic value. If the patient is claustrophobic, mild oral sedation or occasionally parenteral sedation may be needed. Also the patient can be accompanied by a family member or friend during the examination which helps calm the patient's anxiety in many cases. Patients requiring life support equipment such as ventilators require special preparation. Please refer to Contraindications for further causes for rejection. ADDITIONAL INFORMATION: In some cases, an MRI contrast agent (Magnevist®) may be needed to increase the diagnostic accuracy of the MRI. This contrast agent can be administered to patients with a previous history of allergies to conventional iodinated x-ray agents as it contains no iodine. Contraindications to its use include previous allergy to the contrast agent itself, renal failure, certain types of anemia, and Wilson's disease. The contrast agent is generally very safe and increases the diagnostic efficacy of the MRI.

References

Simon JE and Lukin RR, "Discogenic Disease of the Cervical Spine," *Semin Roentgenol*, 1988, 23:118-24.

Magnetic Resonance Scan, Chest

CPT 71550

Applies to Magnetic Resonance Scan, Thorax

Abstract INDICATIONS: Evaluation of the chest for pathology including the heart, major vessels, mediastinum, lungs, and chest wall CONTRAINDICATIONS: Patients weighing more than 300 lb and patients unable to squeeze into the magnet cannot undergo MRI. An absolute contraindication for MRI is a cardiac pacemaker. Relative contraindications to magnetic resonance imaging include intracranial aneurysm clips, cochlear implants, insulin infusion and chemotherapy pumps, neurocutaneous stimulators and prosthetic heart valves, depending on date of manufacture and metallurgical composition. Please consult MRI physician if questions arise. Patients who have metallic foreign bodies within the eye or who have undergone recent surgery within the last 6 weeks requiring placement of a vascular surgical clip, should also not undergo MRI. The safety of MRI in pregnant patients has not been determined. In such cases, prior consultation with the MRI physician is required. Generally, patients who have undergone recent surgery not requiring vascular clips or who have had coronary artery bypass surgery in the past may undergo MRI. Patients who have shrapnel wounds or orthopedic prostheses can generally safely undergo MRI unless the metallic device is in the anatomic region to be scanned which results in degradation of the images. Patients with surgically implanted intravascular vena cava filters to prevent pulmonary embolism can usually be scanned if the device has been in place for at least 6 weeks. Patients requiring life support equipment including ventilators require special preparation. Please contact MRI physician ahead of time. Central venous lines, Swan-Ganz catheters, and nasogastric (NG) tubes usually present no problems. If the patient is positive when screened for metallic devices and you are uncertain of their significance, the MRI radiologist will provide additional information to assist you.

Patient Care/Scheduling PATIENT PREPARATION: Inpatient: Patient must be able to lie quietly while the scan is performed. The patient should be screened for metallic devices by nursing personnel. (See Contraindications.) This includes metal introduced into the patient either surgically or by trauma. All metallic objects must be removed from the patient including jewelry or any other metal objects which may be in the patient's bedding. Please remove dentures or other dental appliances. I.V.s which contain no metal are fine, but infusion pumps must be removed. Oxygen tanks and metallic backboards may come with the patient but will be removed prior to the patient entering the magnet room. Oxygen may be provided in the magnet room. Trauma, ICU, or CCU patients should be accompanied by a nurse. If the patient is restless, combative, or claustrophobic, proper sedation may be administered on the floor prior to the MRI, or at the MRI Center. Consult the MRI radiologists with questions on proper sedation. Outpatient: The patient should be screened for metallic devices. (See Contraindications.) If a question exists as to the patient's suitability for MRI, the MRI radiologist will assist you with your questions. If the patient is claustrophobic, oral or parenteral sedation may be necessary. If so, the patient should be accompanied by another adult to provide transportation home after the examination. AFTERCARE: If the patient received an MRI contrast agent (Magnevist®) and develops a delayed hypersensitivity reaction (ie, hives or shortness of breath), the referring physician or MRI radiologist should be contacted immediately.

Method DATA ACQUIRED: Digital information with film reproduction.

Interpretation LIMITATIONS: Generally, the greatest limitation of magnetic resonance imaging results from the patient's fear of the procedure. The patient must remain quiet and still for several scans, each lasting from several minutes to 10 minutes in length. Total examination time is usually 30-45 minutes and occasionally up to 1 hour. If the patient is restless during the examination, motion artifacts will be present on the images limiting their diag-

(Continued)

Magnetic Resonance Scan, Chest *(Continued)*

nostic value. If the patient is claustrophobic, mild oral sedation or occasionally parenteral sedation may be needed. Also the patient can be accompanied by a family member or friend during the examination which helps calm the patient's anxiety in many cases. Patients requiring life support equipment such as ventilators require special preparation. Please refer to Contraindications for further causes for rejection. **ADDITIONAL INFORMATION:** In some cases, an MRI contrast agent (Magnevist®) may be needed to increase the diagnostic accuracy of the MRI. This contrast agent can be administered to patients with a previous history of allergies to conventional iodinated x-ray agents as it contains no iodine. Contraindications to its use include previous allergy to the contrast agent itself, renal failure, certain types of anemia, and Wilson's disease. The contrast agent is generally very safe and increases the diagnostic efficacy of the MRI.

References

Gefter WB, "Chest Applications of Magnetic Resonance Imaging: An Update," *Radiol Clin North Am*, 1988, 26(3):573-88

Swensen SJ, Ehman RL, Brown LR, et al, "Magnetic Resonance Imaging of the Thorax," *J Thorac Imaging*, 1989, 4(2):19-33.

Magnetic Resonance Scan, Dorsal Spine *see* Magnetic Resonance Scan, Thoracic Spinal Canal and Contents *on page 354*

Magnetic Resonance Scan, Extremities (Lower)

CPT 73720

Abstract **INDICATIONS:** Evaluation and characterization of the anatomy and pathology of the lower extremities **CONTRAINDICATIONS:** Patients weighing more than 300 lb and patients unable to squeeze into the magnet cannot undergo MRI. An absolute contraindication for MRI is a cardiac pacemaker. Relative contraindications to magnetic resonance imaging include intracranial aneurysm clips, cochlear implants, insulin infusion and chemotherapy pumps, neurocutaneous stimulators and prosthetic heart valves, depending on date of manufacture and metallurgical composition. Please consult MRI physician if questions arise. Patients who have metallic foreign bodies within the eye or who have undergone recent surgery within the last 6 weeks requiring placement of a vascular surgical clip, should also not undergo MRI. The safety of MRI in pregnant patients has not been determined. In such cases, prior consultation with the MRI physician is required. Generally, patients who have undergone recent surgery not requiring vascular clips or who have had coronary artery bypass surgery in the past may undergo MRI. Patients who have shrapnel wounds or orthopedic prostheses can generally safely undergo MRI unless the metallic device is in the anatomic region to be scanned which results in degradation of the images. Patients with surgically implanted intravascular vena cava filters to prevent pulmonary embolism can usually be scanned if the device has been in place for at least 6 weeks. Patients requiring life support equipment including ventilators require special preparation. Please contact MRI physician ahead of time. Central venous lines, Swan-Ganz catheters, and nasogastric (NG) tubes usually present no problems. If the patient is positive when screened for metallic devices and you are uncertain of their significance, the MRI radiologist will provide additional information to assist you.

Patient Care/Scheduling **PATIENT PREPARATION:** Inpatient: Patient must be able to lie quietly while the scan is performed. The patient should be screened for metallic devices by nursing personnel. (See Contraindications.) This includes metal introduced into the patient either surgically or by trauma. All metallic objects must be removed from the patient including jewelry or any other metal objects which may be in the patient's bedding. Please remove dentures or other dental appliances. I.V.s which contain no metal are fine, but infusion pumps must be removed. Oxygen tanks and metallic backboards may come with the patient but will be removed prior to the patient entering the magnet room. Oxygen may be provided in the magnet room. Trauma, ICU, or CCU patients should be accompanied by a nurse. If the patient is restless, combative, or claustrophobic, proper sedation may be administered on the floor prior to the MRI, or at the MRI Center. Consult the MRI radiologists with questions on proper sedation. Outpatient: The patient should be screened for metallic devices. (See Contraindications.) If a question exists as to the patient's suitability for MRI, the MRI radiologist will assist you with your questions. If the patient is claustrophobic, oral or parenteral sedation may be necessary. If so, the patient should be accompanied by another adult to provide transportation home after the examination. **AFTERCARE:** If the patient received an MRI contrast agent (Magnevist®) and develops a delayed hypersensitivity reaction (ie, hives or shortness of breath), the referring physician or MRI radiologist should be contacted immediately.

Method **DATA ACQUIRED:** Digital information with film reproduction.

Interpretation **LIMITATIONS:** Generally, the greatest limitation of magnetic resonance imaging results from the patient's fear of the procedure. The patient must remain quiet and still for several scans, each lasting from several minutes to 10 minutes in length. Total examination time is usually 30-45 minutes and occasionally up to 1 hour. If the patient is restless during the examination, motion artifacts will be present on the images limiting their diagnostic value. If the patient is claustrophobic, mild oral sedation or occasionally parenteral sedation may be needed. Also the patient can be accompanied by a family member or friend during the examination which helps calm the patient's anxiety in many cases. Patients requiring life support equipment such as ventilators require special preparation. Please refer to Contraindications for further causes for rejection. **ADDITIONAL INFORMATION:** In some cases, an MRI contrast agent (Magnevist®) may be needed to increase the diagnostic accuracy of the MRI. This contrast agent can be administered to patients with a previous history of allergies to conventional iodinated x-ray agents as it contains no iodine. Contraindications to its use include previous allergy to the contrast agent itself, renal failure, certain types of anemia, and Wilson's disease. The contrast agent is generally very safe and increases the diagnostic efficacy of the MRI.

References

Dalinka MK, Zlatkin MB, Chao P, et al, "Use of Magnetic Resonance Imaging in the Evaluation of Bone and Soft-Tissue Tumors," *Radiol Clin North Am*, 1990, 28(2):461-70.

Magnetic Resonance Scan, Extremities (Upper)

CPT 73220

Abstract **INDICATIONS:** Evaluation and characterization of the anatomy and pathology of the upper extremities **CONTRAINDICATIONS:** Patients weighing more than 300 lb and patients unable to squeeze into the magnet cannot undergo MRI. An absolute contraindication for MRI is a cardiac pacemaker. Relative contraindications to magnetic resonance imaging include intracranial aneurysm clips, cochlear implants, insulin infusion and chemotherapy pumps, neurocutaneous stimulators and prosthetic heart valves, depending on date of manufacture and metallurgical composition. Please consult MRI physician if questions arise. Patients who have metallic foreign bodies within the eye or who have undergone recent surgery within the last 6 weeks requiring placement of a vascular surgical clip, should also not undergo MRI. The safety of MRI in pregnant patients has not been determined. In such cases, prior consultation with the MRI physician is required. Generally, patients who have undergone recent surgery not requiring vascular clips or who have had coronary artery bypass surgery in the past may undergo MRI. Patients who have shrapnel wounds or orthopedic prostheses can generally safely undergo MRI unless the metallic device is in the anatomic region to be scanned which results in degradation of the images. Patients with surgically implanted intravascular vena cava filters to prevent pulmonary embolism can usually be scanned if the device has been in place for at least 6 weeks. Patients requiring life support equipment including ventilators require special preparation. Please contact MRI physician ahead of time. Central venous lines, Swan-Ganz catheters, and nasogastric (NG) tubes usually present no problems. If the patient is positive when screened for metallic devices and you are uncertain of their significance, the MRI radiologist will provide additional information to assist you.

Patient Care/Scheduling **PATIENT PREPARATION:** Inpatient: Patient must be able to lie quietly while the scan is performed. The patient should be screened for metallic devices by nursing personnel. (See Contraindications.) This includes metal introduced into the patient either surgically or by trauma. All metallic objects must be removed from the patient including jewelry or any other metal objects which may be in the patient's bedding. Please remove dentures or other dental appliances. I.V.s which contain no metal are fine, but infusion pumps must be removed. Oxygen tanks and metallic backboards may come with the

(Continued)

Magnetic Resonance Scan, Extremities (Upper) *(Continued)*

patient but will be removed prior to the patient entering the magnet room. Oxygen may be provided in the magnet room. Trauma, ICU, or CCU patients should be accompanied by a nurse. If the patient is restless, combative, or claustrophobic, proper sedation may be administered on the floor prior to the MRI, or at the MRI Center. Consult the MRI radiologists with questions on proper sedation. Outpatient: The patient should be screened for metallic devices. (See Contraindications.) If a question exists as to the patient's suitability for MRI, the MRI radiologist will assist you with your questions. If the patient is claustrophobic, oral or parenteral sedation may be necessary. If so, the patient should be accompanied by another adult to provide transportation home after the examination. **AFTERCARE:** If the patient received an MRI contrast agent (Magnevist®) and develops a delayed hypersensitivity reaction (ie, hives or shortness of breath), the referring physician or MRI radiologist should be contacted immediately.

Method **DATA ACQUIRED:** Digital information with film reproduction.

Interpretation **LIMITATIONS:** Generally, the greatest limitation of magnetic resonance imaging results from the patient's fear of the procedure. The patient must remain quiet and still for several scans, each lasting from several minutes to 10 minutes in length. Total examination time is usually 30-45 minutes and occasionally up to 1 hour. If the patient is restless during the examination, motion artifacts will be present on the images limiting their diagnostic value. If the patient is claustrophobic, mild oral sedation or occasionally parenteral sedation may be needed. Also the patient can be accompanied by a family member or friend during the examination which helps calm the patient's anxiety in many cases. Patients requiring life support equipment such as ventilators require special preparation. Please refer to Contraindications for further causes for rejection. Implanted orthopedic appliances may limit the usefulness of the scan in the area being imaged. **ADDITIONAL INFORMATION:** In some cases, an MRI contrast agent (Magnevist®) may be needed to increase the diagnostic accuracy of the MRI. This contrast agent can be administered to patients with a previous history of allergies to conventional iodinated x-ray agents as it contains no iodine. Contraindications to its use include previous allergy to the contrast agent itself, renal failure, certain types of anemia, and Wilson's disease. The contrast agent is generally very safe and increases the diagnostic efficacy of the MRI.

References

Dalinka MK, Zlatkin MB, Chao P, et al, "Use of Magnetic Resonance Imaging in the Evaluation of Bone and Soft-Tissue Tumors," *Radiol Clin North Am*, 1990, 28(2):461-70.

Magnetic Resonance Scan, Head *see* Magnetic Resonance Scan, Brain *on page 339*

Magnetic Resonance Scan, Knee

CPT 73721

Abstract **INDICATIONS:** Diagnose internal derangements of the knee including meniscal tears and degeneration, assess ligament morphology, articular cartilage, bones and bone marrow of the knee joint as well as surrounding tissue **CONTRAINDICATIONS:** Patients weighing more than 300 lb and patients unable to squeeze into the magnet cannot undergo MRI. An absolute contraindication for MRI is a cardiac pacemaker. Relative contraindications to magnetic resonance imaging include intracranial aneurysm clips, cochlear implants, insulin infusion and chemotherapy pumps, neurocutaneous stimulators and prosthetic heart valves, depending on date of manufacture and metallurgical composition. Please consult MRI physician if questions arise. Patients who have metallic foreign bodies within the eye or who have undergone recent surgery within the last 6 weeks requiring placement of a vascular surgical clip, should also not undergo MRI. The safety of MRI in pregnant patients has not been determined. In such cases, prior consultation with the MRI physician is required. Generally, patients who have undergone recent surgery not requiring vascular clips or who have had coronary artery bypass surgery in the past may undergo MRI. Patients who have shrapnel wounds or orthopedic prostheses can generally safely undergo MRI unless the metallic device is in the anatomic region to be scanned which results in degradation of the images. Patients with surgically implanted intravascular vena cava filters to prevent pulmonary embolism can usually be scanned if the device has been in place for at least 6 weeks. Patients requiring life support equipment including ventilators require special preparation. Please contact MRI physician ahead of time. Central venous lines, Swan-Ganz catheters, and nasogastric (NG) tubes usually present no problems. If the patient is positive when screened for metallic devices and you are uncertain of their significance, the MRI radiologist will provide additional information to assist you.

Patient Care/Scheduling PATIENT PREPARATION: Inpatient: Patient must be able to lie quietly while the scan is performed. The patient should be screened for metallic devices by nursing personnel. (See Contraindications.) This includes metal introduced into the patient either surgically or by trauma. All metallic objects must be removed from the patient including jewelry or any other metal objects which may be in the patient's bedding. Please remove dentures or other dental appliances. I.V.s which contain no metal are fine, but infusion pumps must be removed. Oxygen tanks and metallic backboards may come with the patient but will be removed prior to the patient entering the magnet room. Oxygen may be provided in the magnet room. Trauma, ICU, or CCU patients should be accompanied by a nurse. If the patient is restless, combative, or claustrophobic, proper sedation may be administered on the floor prior to the MRI, or at the MRI Center. Consult the MRI radiologists with questions on proper sedation. Outpatient: The patient should be screened for metallic devices. (See Contraindications.) If a question exists as to the patient's suitability for MRI, the MRI radiologist will assist you with your questions. If the patient is claustrophobic, oral or parenteral sedation may be necessary. If so, the patient should be accompanied by another adult to provide transportation home after the examination. AFTERCARE: If the patient received an MRI contrast agent (Magnevist®) and develops a delayed hypersensitivity reaction (ie, hives or shortness of breath), the referring physician or MRI radiologist should be contacted immediately.

Method DATA ACQUIRED: Digital information with film reproduction.

Interpretation LIMITATIONS: Generally, the greatest limitation of magnetic resonance imaging results from the patient's fear of the procedure. The patient must remain quiet and still for several scans, each lasting from several minutes to 10 minutes in length. Total examination time is usually 30-45 minutes and occasionally up to 1 hour. If the patient is restless during the examination, motion artifacts will be present on the images limiting their diagnostic value. If the patient is claustrophobic, mild oral sedation or occasionally parenteral sedation may be needed. Also the patient can be accompanied by a family member or friend during the examination which helps calm the patient's anxiety in many cases. ADDITIONAL INFORMATION: In some cases, an MRI contrast agent (Magnevist®) may be needed to increase the diagnostic accuracy of the MRI. This contrast agent can be administered to patients with a previous history of allergies to conventional iodinated x-ray agents as it contains no iodine. Contraindications to its use include previous allergy to the contrast agent itself, renal failure, certain types of anemia, and Wilson's disease. The contrast agent is generally very safe and increases the diagnostic efficacy of the MRI.

References

Burk Jr DL, Mitchell DG, Rifkin MD, "Recent Advances in Magnetic Resonance Imaging of the Knee," *Radiol Clin North Am*, 1990, 28(2):379-93.

Mink JH, Reicher MA, Crues JV III, *Magnetic Resonance Imaging of the Knee*, New York, NY: Raven Press, 1987.

Magnetic Resonance Scan, Lumbar Spinal Canal and Contents

CPT 72148 (without contrast); 72149 (with contrast)

Abstract INDICATIONS: Diagnose degenerative disk disease (herniation, canal stenosis), tumor, infection, and other processes affecting the lumbar spine CONTRAINDICATIONS: Patients weighing more than 300 lb and patients unable to squeeze into the magnet cannot undergo MRI. An absolute contraindication for MRI is a cardiac pacemaker. Relative contraindications to magnetic resonance imaging include intracranial aneurysm clips, cochlear implants, insulin infusion and chemotherapy pumps, neurocutaneous stimulators and prosthetic heart valves, depending on date of manufacture and metallurgical composition. Please consult MRI physician if questions arise. Patients who have metallic foreign bodies within the eye or who have undergone recent surgery within the last 6 weeks requiring placement of a vascular surgical clip, should also not undergo MRI. The safety of MRI in pregnant patients has not been determined. In such cases, prior consultation with the MRI

(Continued)

Magnetic Resonance Scan, Lumbar Spinal Canal and Contents *(Continued)*

physician is required. Generally, patients who have undergone recent surgery not requiring vascular clips or who have had coronary artery bypass surgery in the past may undergo MRI. Patients who have shrapnel wounds or orthopedic prostheses can generally safely undergo MRI unless the metallic device is in the anatomic region to be scanned which results in degradation of the images. Patients with surgically implanted intravascular vena cava filters to prevent pulmonary embolism can usually be scanned if the device has been in place for at least 6 weeks. Patients requiring life support equipment including ventilators require special preparation. Please contact MRI physician ahead of time. Central venous lines, Swan-Ganz catheters, and nasogastric (NG) tubes usually present no problems. If the patient is positive when screened for metallic devices and you are uncertain of their significance, the MRI radiologist will provide additional information to assist you.

Patient Care/Scheduling PATIENT PREPARATION: Inpatient: Patient must be able to lie quietly while the scan is performed. The patient should be screened for metallic devices by nursing personnel. (See Contraindications.) This includes metal introduced into the patient either surgically or by trauma. All metallic objects must be removed from the patient including jewelry or any other metal objects which may be in the patient's bedding. Please remove dentures or other dental appliances. I.V.s which contain no metal are fine, but infusion pumps must be removed. Oxygen tanks and metallic backboards may come with the patient but will be removed prior to the patient entering the magnet room. Oxygen may be provided in the magnet room. Trauma, ICU, or CCU patients should be accompanied by a nurse. If the patient is restless, combative, or claustrophobic, proper sedation may be administered on the floor prior to the MRI, or at the MRI Center. Consult the MRI radiologists with questions on proper sedation. Outpatient: The patient should be screened for metallic devices. (See Contraindications.) If a question exists as to the patient's suitability for MRI, the MRI radiologist will assist you with your questions. If the patient is claustrophobic, oral or parenteral sedation may be necessary. If so, the patient should be accompanied by another adult to provide transportation home after the examination. AFTERCARE: If the patient received an MRI contrast agent (Magnevist®) and develops a delayed hypersensitivity reaction (ie, hives or shortness of breath), the referring physician or MRI radiologist should be contacted immediately.

Method DATA ACQUIRED: Digital information with film reproduction.

Interpretation LIMITATIONS: Generally, the greatest limitation of magnetic resonance imaging results from the patient's fear of the procedure. The patient must remain quiet and still for several scans, each lasting from several minutes to 10 minutes in length. Total examination time is usually 30-45 minutes and occasionally up to 1 hour. If the patient is restless during the examination, motion artifacts will be present on the images limiting their diagnostic value. If the patient is claustrophobic, mild oral sedation or occasionally parenteral sedation may be needed. Also the patient can be accompanied by a family member or friend during the examination which helps calm the patient's anxiety in many cases. Patients requiring life support equipment such as ventilators require special preparation. Please refer to Contraindications for further causes for rejection. Patients with intraspinal metallic rods may be scanned; however, images may not be optimal due to metallic distortion artifacts. ADDITIONAL INFORMATION: In some cases, an MRI contrast agent (Magnevist®) may be needed to increase the diagnostic accuracy of the MRI. This contrast agent can be administered to patients with a previous history of allergies to conventional iodinated x-ray agents as it contains no iodine. Contraindications to its use include previous allergy to the contrast agent itself, renal failure, certain types of anemia, and Wilson's disease. The contrast agent is generally very safe and increases the diagnostic efficacy of the MRI.

References

Enzman DR, DeLaPaz RL, and Rubin JB, *Magnetic Resonance of the Spine*, St Louis, MO: CV Mosby Co, 1990.

Magnetic Resonance Scan, Orbit/Face

CPT 70540

Abstract INDICATIONS: Diagnose pathology of the orbit and of the face CONTRAINDICATIONS: Patients weighing more than 300 lb and patients unable to squeeze into the magnet cannot undergo MRI. An absolute contraindication for MRI is a cardiac pacemaker. Relative contraindications to magnetic resonance imaging include intracranial aneurysm clips, cochlear implants, insulin infusion and chemotherapy pumps, neurocutaneous stimulators and prosthetic heart valves, depending on date of manufacture and metallurgical composition. Please consult MRI physician if questions arise. Patients who have metallic foreign bodies within the eye or who have undergone recent surgery within the last 6 weeks requiring placement of a vascular surgical clip, should also not undergo MRI. The safety of MRI in pregnant patients has not been determined. In such cases, prior consultation with the MRI physician is required. Generally, patients who have undergone recent surgery not requiring vascular clips or who have had coronary artery bypass surgery in the past may undergo MRI. Patients who have shrapnel wounds or orthopedic prostheses can generally safely undergo MRI unless the metallic device is in the anatomic region to be scanned which results in degradation of the images. Patients with surgically implanted intravascular vena cava filters to prevent pulmonary embolism can usually be scanned if the device has been in place for at least 6 weeks. Patients requiring life support equipment including ventilators require special preparation. Please contact MRI physician ahead of time. Central venous lines, Swan-Ganz catheters, and nasogastric (NG) tubes usually present no problems. If the patient is positive when screened for metallic devices and you are uncertain of their significance, the MRI radiologist will provide additional information to assist you.

Patient Care/Scheduling **PATIENT PREPARATION:** All cosmetic make-up must be removed prior to the scan in addition to contact lenses. Inpatient: Patient must be able to lie quietly while the scan is performed. The patient should be screened for metallic devices by nursing personnel. (See Contraindications.) This includes metal introduced into the patient either surgically or by trauma. All metallic objects must be removed from the patient including jewelry or any other metal objects which may be in the patient's bedding. Please remove dentures or other dental appliances. I.V.s which contain no metal are fine, but infusion pumps must be removed. Oxygen tanks and metallic backboards may come with the patient but will be removed prior to the patient entering the magnet room. Oxygen may be provided in the magnet room. Trauma, ICU, or CCU patients should be accompanied by a nurse. If the patient is restless, combative, or claustrophobic, proper sedation may be administered on the floor prior to the MRI, or at the MRI Center. Consult the MRI radiologists with questions on proper sedation. Outpatient: The patient should be screened for metallic devices. (See Contraindications.) If a question exists as to the patient's suitability for MRI, the MRI radiologist will assist you with your questions. If the patient is claustrophobic, oral or parenteral sedation may be necessary. If so, the patient should be accompanied by another adult to provide transportation home after the examination. **AFTERCARE:** If the patient received an MRI contrast agent (Magnevist®) and develops a delayed hypersensitivity reaction (ie, hives or shortness of breath), the referring physician or MRI radiologist should be contacted immediately.

Method **DATA ACQUIRED:** Digital information with film reproduction.

Interpretation **LIMITATIONS:** Generally, the greatest limitation of magnetic resonance imaging results from the patient's fear of the procedure. The patient must remain quiet and still for several scans, each lasting from several minutes to 10 minutes in length. Total examination time is usually 30-45 minutes and occasionally up to 1 hour. If the patient is restless during the examination, motion artifacts will be present on the images limiting their diagnostic value. If the patient is claustrophobic, mild oral sedation or occasionally parenteral sedation may be needed. Also the patient can be accompanied by a family member or friend during the examination which helps calm the patient's anxiety in many cases. Patients requiring life support equipment such as ventilators require special preparation. Please refer to Contraindications for further causes for rejection. **ADDITIONAL INFORMATION:** In some cases, an MRI contrast agent (Magnevist®) may be needed to increase the diagnostic accuracy of the MRI. This contrast agent can be administered to patients with a previous history of allergies to conventional iodinated x-ray agents as it contains no iodine. Contraindications to its use include previous allergy to the contrast agent itself, renal failure, certain types of anemia, and Wilson's disease. The contrast agent is generally very safe and increases the diagnostic efficacy of the MRI.

References

Atlas SW, "MR Imaging of the Orbit: Current Status," *Magnetic Resonance Q*, 1989, 5:39-96.

Magnetic Resonance Scan, Oropharynx/Nasopharynx/Neck

CPT 70540

Abstract **INDICATIONS:** Diagnose and characterize pathology of the nasopharynx, oropharynx and neck including tumors, infection, and congenital abnormalities **CONTRAINDICATIONS:** Patients weighing more than 300 lb and patients unable to squeeze into the magnet cannot undergo MRI. An absolute contraindication for MRI is a cardiac pacemaker. Relative contraindications to magnetic resonance imaging include intracranial aneurysm clips, cochlear implants, insulin infusion and chemotherapy pumps, neurocutaneous stimulators and prosthetic heart valves, depending on date of manufacture and metallurgical composition. Please consult MRI physician if questions arise. Patients who have metallic foreign bodies within the eye or who have undergone recent surgery within the last 6 weeks requiring placement of a vascular surgical clip, should also not undergo MRI. The safety of MRI in pregnant patients has not been determined. In such cases, prior consultation with the MRI physician is required. Generally, patients who have undergone recent surgery not requiring vascular clips or who have had coronary artery bypass surgery in the past may undergo MRI. Patients who have shrapnel wounds or orthopedic prostheses can generally safely undergo MRI unless the metallic device is in the anatomic region to be scanned which results in degradation of the images. Patients with surgically implanted intravascular vena cava filters to prevent pulmonary embolism can usually be scanned if the device has been in place for at least 6 weeks. Patients requiring life support equipment including ventilators require special preparation. Please contact MRI physician ahead of time. Central venous lines, Swan-Ganz catheters, and nasogastric (NG) tubes usually present no problems. If the patient is positive when screened for metallic devices and you are uncertain of their significance, the MRI radiologist will provide additional information to assist you.

Patient Care/Scheduling **PATIENT PREPARATION:** Inpatient: Patient must be able to lie quietly while the scan is performed. The patient should be screened for metallic devices by nursing personnel. (See Contraindications.) This includes metal introduced into the patient either surgically or by trauma. All metallic objects must be removed from the patient including jewelry or any other metal objects which may be in the patient's bedding. Please remove dentures or other dental appliances. I.V.s which contain no metal are fine, but infusion pumps must be removed. Oxygen tanks and metallic backboards may come with the patient but will be removed prior to the patient entering the magnet room. Oxygen may be provided in the magnet room. Trauma, ICU, or CCU patients should be accompanied by a nurse. If the patient is restless, combative, or claustrophobic, proper sedation may be administered on the floor prior to the MRI, or at the MRI Center. Consult the MRI radiologists with questions on proper sedation. Outpatient: The patient should be screened for metallic devices. (See Contraindications.) If a question exists as to the patient's suitability for MRI, the MRI radiologist will assist you with your questions. If the patient is claustrophobic, oral or parenteral sedation may be necessary. If so, the patient should be accompanied by another adult to provide transportation home after the examination. **AFTERCARE:** If the patient received an MRI contrast agent (Magnevist®) and develops a delayed hypersensitivity reaction (ie, hives or shortness of breath), the referring physician or MRI radiologist should be contacted immediately.

Method **DATA ACQUIRED:** Digital information with film reproduction.

Interpretation **LIMITATIONS:** Generally, the greatest limitation of magnetic resonance imaging results from the patient's fear of the procedure. The patient must remain quiet and still for several scans, each lasting from several minutes to 10 minutes in length. Total examination time is usually 30-45 minutes and occasionally up to 1 hour. If the patient is restless during the examination, motion artifacts will be present on the images limiting their diagnostic value. If the patient is claustrophobic, mild oral sedation or occasionally parenteral sedation may be needed. Also the patient can be accompanied by a family member or friend during the examination which helps calm the patient's anxiety in many cases. Patients requiring life support equipment such as ventilators require special preparation. Please refer to Contraindications for further causes for rejection. **ADDITIONAL INFORMATION:** In some cases, an MRI contrast agent (Magnevist®) may be needed to increase the diagnostic accuracy of the MRI. This contrast agent can be administered to patients with a previous history of allergies to conventional iodinated x-ray agents as it contains no iodine. Contraindications to its use include previous allergy to the contrast agent itself, renal failure, certain types of anemia, and Wilson's disease. The contrast agent is generally very safe and increases the diagnostic efficacy of the MRI.

Magnetic Resonance Scan, Pelvis

CPT 74181

Abstract **INDICATIONS:** Define and characterize pathology of the pelvis including lymphadenopathy, bladder, prostate, uterus, and adnexa **CONTRAINDICATIONS:** Patients weighing more than 300 lb and patients unable to squeeze into the magnet cannot undergo MRI. An absolute contraindication for MRI is a cardiac pacemaker. Relative contraindications to magnetic resonance imaging include intracranial aneurysm clips, cochlear implants, insulin infusion and chemotherapy pumps, neurocutaneous stimulators and prosthetic heart valves, depending on date of manufacture and metallurgical composition. Please consult MRI physician if questions arise. Patients who have metallic foreign bodies within the eye or who have undergone recent surgery within the last 6 weeks requiring placement of a vascular surgical clip, should also not undergo MRI. The safety of MRI in pregnant patients has not been determined. In such cases, prior consultation with the MRI physician is required. Generally, patients who have undergone recent surgery not requiring vascular clips or who have had coronary artery bypass surgery in the past may undergo MRI. Patients who have shrapnel wounds or orthopedic prostheses can generally safely undergo MRI unless the metallic device is in the anatomic region to be scanned which results in degradation of the images. Patients with surgically implanted intravascular vena cava filters to prevent pulmonary embolism can usually be scanned if the device has been in place for at least 6 weeks. Patients requiring life support equipment including ventilators require special preparation. Please contact MRI physician ahead of time. Central venous lines, Swan-Ganz catheters, and nasogastric (NG) tubes usually present no problems. If the patient is positive when screened for metallic devices and you are uncertain of their significance, the MRI radiologist will provide additional information to assist you.

Patient Care/Scheduling **PATIENT PREPARATION:** Inpatient: Patient must be able to lie quietly while the scan is performed. The patient should be screened for metallic devices by nursing personnel. (See Contraindications.) This includes metal introduced into the patient either surgically or by trauma. All metallic objects must be removed from the patient including jewelry or any other metal objects which may be in the patient's bedding. Please remove dentures or other dental appliances. I.V.s which contain no metal are fine, but infusion pumps must be removed. Oxygen tanks and metallic backboards may come with the patient but will be removed prior to the patient entering the magnet room. Oxygen may be provided in the magnet room. Trauma, ICU, or CCU patients should be accompanied by a nurse. If the patient is restless, combative, or claustrophobic, proper sedation may be administered on the floor prior to the MRI, or at the MRI Center. Consult the MRI radiologists with questions on proper sedation. Outpatient: The patient should be screened for metallic devices. (See Contraindications.) If a question exists as to the patient's suitability for MRI, the MRI radiologist will assist you with your questions. If the patient is claustrophobic, oral or parenteral sedation may be necessary. If so, the patient should be accompanied by another adult to provide transportation home after the examination. **AFTERCARE:** If the patient received an MRI contrast agent (Magnevist®) and develops a delayed hypersensitivity reaction (ie, hives or shortness of breath), the referring physician or MRI radiologist should be contacted immediately.

Method **DATA ACQUIRED:** Digital information with film reproduction.

Interpretation **LIMITATIONS:** Generally, the greatest limitation of magnetic resonance imaging results from the patient's fear of the procedure. The patient must remain quiet and still for several scans, each lasting from several minutes to 10 minutes in length. Total examination time is usually 30-45 minutes and occasionally up to 1 hour. If the patient is restless during the examination, motion artifacts will be present on the images limiting their diagnostic value. If the patient is claustrophobic, mild oral sedation or occasionally parenteral sedation may be needed. Also the patient can be accompanied by a family member or friend during the examination which helps calm the patient's anxiety in many cases. Patients requiring life support equipment such as ventilators require special preparation. Please refer to Contraindications for further causes for rejection. **ADDITIONAL INFORMATION:** In some cases, an MRI contrast agent (Magnevist®) may be needed to increase the diagnostic accuracy of the MRI. This contrast agent can be administered to patients with a previous history of allergies to conventional iodinated x-ray agents as it contains no iodine. Contraindications to its use include previous allergy to the contrast agent itself, renal failure, certain types of anemia, and Wilson's disease. The contrast agent is generally very

(Continued)

Magnetic Resonance Scan, Pelvis *(Continued)*

safe and increases the diagnostic efficacy of the MRI. Air insufflation in the rectum may be used to improve image contrast. Intramuscular or subcutaneous glucagon injection may be used to decrease motion artifacts from peristalsis. Use of a vaginal tampon in female patients may be required.

References

Cohen EK and Kressel HY, "MR Imaging of the Pelvis," *Clinical Magnetic Resonance Imaging*, Edelman R and Hesselink J, eds, Philadelphia, PA: WB Saunders Co, 1990, 915-37.

Magnetic Resonance Scan, Shoulder

CPT 73221

Abstract INDICATIONS: Diagnose internal derangements of the shoulder joint including tears of the rotator cuff tendons, musculoskeletal injury, and/or involvement by tumor or infection CONTRAINDICATIONS: Patients weighing more than 300 lb and patients unable to squeeze into the magnet cannot undergo MRI. An absolute contraindication for MRI is a cardiac pacemaker. Relative contraindications to magnetic resonance imaging include intracranial aneurysm clips, cochlear implants, insulin infusion and chemotherapy pumps, neurocutaneous stimulators and prosthetic heart valves, depending on date of manufacture and metallurgical composition. Please consult MRI physician if questions arise. Patients who have metallic foreign bodies within the eye or who have undergone recent surgery within the last 6 weeks requiring placement of a vascular surgical clip, should also not undergo MRI. The safety of MRI in pregnant patients has not been determined. In such cases, prior consultation with the MRI physician is required. Generally, patients who have undergone recent surgery not requiring vascular clips or who have had coronary artery bypass surgery in the past may undergo MRI. Patients who have shrapnel wounds or orthopedic prostheses can generally safely undergo MRI unless the metallic device is in the anatomic region to be scanned which results in degradation of the images. Patients with surgically implanted intravascular vena cava filters to prevent pulmonary embolism can usually be scanned if the device has been in place for at least 6 weeks. Patients requiring life support equipment including ventilators require special preparation. Please contact MRI physician ahead of time. Central venous lines, Swan-Ganz catheters, and nasogastric (NG) tubes usually present no problems. If the patient is positive when screened for metallic devices and you are uncertain of their significance, the MRI radiologist will provide additional information to assist you.

Patient Care/Scheduling PATIENT PREPARATION: Inpatient: Patient must be able to lie quietly while the scan is performed. The patient should be screened for metallic devices by nursing personnel. (See Contraindications.) This includes metal introduced into the patient either surgically or by trauma. All metallic objects must be removed from the patient including jewelry or any other metal objects which may be in the patient's bedding. Please remove dentures or other dental appliances. I.V.s which contain no metal are fine, but infusion pumps must be removed. Oxygen tanks and metallic backboards may come with the patient but will be removed prior to the patient entering the magnet room. Oxygen may be provided in the magnet room. Trauma, ICU, or CCU patients should be accompanied by a nurse. If the patient is restless, combative, or claustrophobic, proper sedation may be administered on the floor prior to the MRI, or at the MRI Center. Consult the MRI radiologists with questions on proper sedation. Outpatient: The patient should be screened for metallic devices. (See Contraindications.) If a question exists as to the patient's suitability for MRI, the MRI radiologist will assist you with your questions. If the patient is claustrophobic, oral or parenteral sedation may be necessary. If so, the patient should be accompanied by another adult to provide transportation home after the examination. AFTERCARE: If the patient received an MRI contrast agent (Magnevist®) and develops a delayed hypersensitivity reaction (ie, hives or shortness of breath), the referring physician or MRI radiologist should be contacted immediately.

Method DATA ACQUIRED: Digital information with film reproduction.

Interpretation LIMITATIONS: Generally, the greatest limitation of magnetic resonance imaging results from the patient's fear of the procedure. The patient must remain quiet and still for several scans, each lasting from several minutes to 10 minutes in length. Total examination time is usually 30-45 minutes and occasionally up to 1 hour. If the patient is restless during the examination, motion artifacts will be present on the images limiting their diagnostic value. If the patient is claustrophobic, mild oral sedation or occasionally parenteral sedation may be needed. Also the patient can be accompanied by a family member or friend during the examination which helps calm the patient's anxiety in many cases. Patients requiring life support equipment such as ventilators cannot undergo MRI. Please refer to Contraindications for further causes for rejection. The exam may be somewhat limited if orthopedic appliances have been placed previously on the affected shoulder. **ADDITIONAL INFORMATION:** In some cases, an MRI contrast agent (Magnevist®) may be needed to increase the diagnostic accuracy of the MRI. This contrast agent can be administered to patients with a previous history of allergies to conventional iodinated x-ray agents as it contains no iodine. Contraindications to its use include previous allergy to the contrast agent itself, renal failure, certain types of anemia, and Wilson's disease. The contrast agent is generally very safe and increases the diagnostic efficacy of the MRI.

References

Tsai JC and Zlatkin MB, "Magnetic Resonance Imaging of the Shoulder," *Radiol Clin North Am*, 1990, 28(2):279-91.

Magnetic Resonance Scan, Temporomandibular Joint

CPT 70540

Abstract **INDICATIONS:** Diagnose pathology and function of the temporomandibular joint including surgically implanted prosthesis **CONTRAINDICATIONS:** Patients weighing more than 300 lb and patients unable to squeeze into the magnet cannot undergo MRI. An absolute contraindication for MRI is a cardiac pacemaker. Relative contraindications to magnetic resonance imaging include intracranial aneurysm clips, cochlear implants, insulin infusion and chemotherapy pumps, neurocutaneous stimulators and prosthetic heart valves, depending on date of manufacture and metallurgical composition. Please consult MRI physician if questions arise. Patients who have metallic foreign bodies within the eye or who have undergone recent surgery within the last 6 weeks requiring placement of a vascular surgical clip, should also not undergo MRI. The safety of MRI in pregnant patients has not been determined. In such cases, prior consultation with the MRI physician is required. Generally, patients who have undergone recent surgery not requiring vascular clips or who have had coronary artery bypass surgery in the past may undergo MRI. Patients who have shrapnel wounds or orthopedic prostheses can generally safely undergo MRI unless the metallic device is in the anatomic region to be scanned which results in degradation of the images. Patients with surgically implanted intravascular vena cava filters to prevent pulmonary embolism can usually be scanned if the device has been in place for at least 6 weeks. Patients requiring life support equipment including ventilators require special preparation. Please contact MRI physician ahead of time. Central venous lines, Swan-Ganz catheters, and nasogastric (NG) tubes usually present no problems. If the patient is positive when screened for metallic devices and you are uncertain of their significance, the MRI radiologist will provide additional information to assist you.

Patient Care/Scheduling **PATIENT PREPARATION:** Inpatient: Patient must be able to lie quietly while the scan is performed. The patient should be screened for metallic devices by nursing personnel. (See Contraindications.) This includes metal introduced into the patient either surgically or by trauma. All metallic objects must be removed from the patient including jewelry or any other metal objects which may be in the patient's bedding. Please remove dentures or other dental appliances. I.V.s which contain no metal are fine, but infusion pumps must be removed. If the patient is restless, combative, or claustrophobic, proper sedation may be administered on the floor prior to the MRI, or at the MRI Center. Consult the MRI radiologists with questions on proper sedation. Outpatient: The patient should be screened for metallic devices. (See Contraindications.) If a question exists as to the patient's suitability for MRI, the MRI radiologist will assist you with your questions. If the patient is claustrophobic, oral or parenteral sedation may be necessary. If so, the patient should be accompanied by another adult to provide transportation home after the examination.

Method **DATA ACQUIRED:** Digital information with film reproduction.

Interpretation **LIMITATIONS:** Generally, the greatest limitation of magnetic resonance imaging results from the patient's fear of the procedure. The patient must remain quiet and still

(Continued)

Magnetic Resonance Scan, Temporomandibular Joint *(Continued)*

for several scans, each lasting from several minutes to 10 minutes in length. Total examination time is usually 30-45 minutes and occasionally up to 1 hour. If the patient is restless during the examination, motion artifacts will be present on the images limiting their diagnostic value. If the patient is claustrophobic, mild oral sedation or occasionally parenteral sedation may be needed. Also the patient can be accompanied by a family member or friend during the examination which helps calm the patient's anxiety in many cases.

References

Harms SE and Wilk RM, "Magnetic Resonance of the Temporomandibular Joint," *Radiographics*, 1987, 7:521-42.

Rao VM, Farole A, and Karasick D, "Temporomandibular Joint Dysfunction: Correlation of MR Imaging, Arthrography, and Arthroscopy," *Radiology*, 1990, 174(3 Pt 1):663-7.

Magnetic Resonance Scan, Thoracic Spinal Canal and Contents

CPT 72146 (without contrast material); 72147 (with contrast material)

Applies to Magnetic Resonance Scan, Dorsal Spine

Abstract **INDICATIONS:** Diagnose intramedullary, extramedullary-intradural, extradural disease of the thoracic spine. This includes degenerative disk disease (herniation), tumor, infection, ischemia, and demyelination processes. **CONTRAINDICATIONS:** Patients weighing more than 300 lb and patients unable to squeeze into the magnet cannot undergo MRI. An absolute contraindication for MRI is a cardiac pacemaker. Relative contraindications to magnetic resonance imaging include intracranial aneurysm clips, cochlear implants, insulin infusion and chemotherapy pumps, neurocutaneous stimulators and prosthetic heart valves, depending on date of manufacture and metallurgical composition. Please consult MRI physician if questions arise. Patients who have metallic foreign bodies within the eye or who have undergone recent surgery within the last 6 weeks requiring placement of a vascular surgical clip, should also not undergo MRI. The safety of MRI in pregnant patients has not been determined. In such cases, prior consultation with the MRI physician is required. Generally, patients who have undergone recent surgery not requiring vascular clips or who have had coronary artery bypass surgery in the past may undergo MRI. Patients who have shrapnel wounds or orthopedic prostheses can generally safely undergo MRI unless the metallic device is in the anatomic region to be scanned which results in degradation of the images. Patients with surgically implanted intravascular vena cava filters to prevent pulmonary embolism can usually be scanned if the device has been in place for at least 6 weeks. Patients requiring life support equipment including ventilators require special preparation. Please contact MRI physician ahead of time. Central venous lines, Swan-Ganz catheters, and nasogastric (NG) tubes usually present no problems. If the patient is positive when screened for metallic devices and you are uncertain of their significance, the MRI radiologist will provide additional information to assist you.

Patient Care/Scheduling **PATIENT PREPARATION:** Inpatient: Patient must be able to lie quietly while the scan is performed. The patient should be screened for metallic devices by nursing personnel. (See Contraindications.) This includes metal introduced into the patient either surgically or by trauma. All metallic objects must be removed from the patient including jewelry or any other metal objects which may be in the patient's bedding. Please remove dentures or other dental appliances. I.V.s which contain no metal are fine, but infusion pumps must be removed. Oxygen tanks and metallic backboards may come with the patient but will be removed prior to the patient entering the magnet room. Oxygen may be provided in the magnet room. Trauma, ICU, or CCU patients should be accompanied by a nurse. If the patient is restless, combative, or claustrophobic, proper sedation may be administered on the floor prior to the MRI, or at the MRI Center. Consult the MRI radiologists with questions on proper sedation. Outpatient: The patient should be screened for metallic devices. (See Contraindications.) If a question exists as to the patient's suitability for MRI, the MRI radiologist will assist you with your questions. If the patient is claustrophobic, oral or parenteral sedation may be necessary. If so, the patient should be accompanied by another adult to provide transportation home after the examination. **AFTERCARE:** If the patient received an MRI contrast agent (Magnevist®) and develops a delayed hypersensitivity reaction (ie, hives or shortness of breath), the referring physician or MRI radiologist should be contacted immediately.

Method DATA ACQUIRED: Digital information with film reproduction.

Interpretation LIMITATIONS: Generally, the greatest limitation of magnetic resonance imaging results from the patient's fear of the procedure. The patient must remain quiet and still for several scans, each lasting from several minutes to 10 minutes in length. Total examination time is usually 30-45 minutes and occasionally up to 1 hour. If the patient is restless during the examination, motion artifacts will be present on the images limiting their diagnostic value. If the patient is claustrophobic, mild oral sedation or occasionally parenteral sedation may be needed. Also the patient can be accompanied by a family member or friend during the examination which helps calm the patient's anxiety in many cases. Patients requiring life support equipment such as ventilators cannot undergo MRI. Please refer to Contraindications for further causes for rejection. Patients with intraspinal metallic rods may be scanned, however, images may not be optimal due to metallic distortion artifacts. ADDITIONAL INFORMATION: In some cases, an MRI contrast agent (Magnevist®) may be needed to increase the diagnostic accuracy of the MRI. This contrast agent can be administered to patients with a previous history of allergies to conventional iodinated x-ray agents as it contains no iodine. Contraindications to its use include previous allergy to the contrast agent itself, renal failure, certain types of anemia, and Wilson's disease. The contrast agent is generally very safe and increases the diagnostic efficacy of the MRI.

References

New PFJ and Shoukimas GM, "Thoracic Spine and Spinal Cord," *Magnetic Resonance Imaging*, Stark D and Bradley W, eds, St Louis, MO: CV Mosby Co, 1988, 632-65.

Magnetic Resonance Scan, Thorax *see* Magnetic Resonance Scan, Chest *on page 343*

Magnetic Resonance Scan, Vascular

CPT 76400

Synonyms Magnetic Resonance Angiography; Magnetic Resonance Venography

Abstract INDICATIONS: Diagnose and characterize vascular abnormalities throughout the body but particularly intracranial abnormalities and cervical carotid lesions. These include vascular malformations, aneurysms, vertebrovascular and carotid atherosclerosis and thrombosis, dissection. CONTRAINDICATIONS: Patients weighing more than 300 lb and patients unable to squeeze into the magnet cannot undergo MRI. An absolute contraindication for MRI is a cardiac pacemaker. Relative contraindications to magnetic resonance imaging include intracranial aneurysm clips, cochlear implants, insulin infusion and chemotherapy pumps, neurocutaneous stimulators and prosthetic heart valves, depending on date of manufacture and metallurgical composition. Please consult MRI physician if questions arise. Patients who have metallic foreign bodies within the eye or who have undergone recent surgery within the last 6 weeks requiring placement of a vascular surgical clip, should also not undergo MRI. The safety of MRI in pregnant patients has not been determined. In such cases, prior consultation with the MRI physician is required. Generally, patients who have undergone recent surgery not requiring vascular clips or who have had coronary artery bypass surgery in the past may undergo MRI. Patients who have shrapnel wounds or orthopedic prostheses can generally safely undergo MRI unless the metallic device is in the anatomic region to be scanned which results in degradation of the images. Patients with surgically implanted intravascular vena cava filters to prevent pulmonary embolism can usually be scanned if the device has been in place for at least 6 weeks. Patients requiring life support equipment including ventilators require special preparation. Please contact MRI physician ahead of time. Central venous lines, Swan-Ganz catheters, and nasogastric (NG) tubes usually present no problems. If the patient is positive when screened for metallic devices and you are uncertain of their significance, the MRI radiologist will provide additional information to assist you.

Patient Care/Scheduling PATIENT PREPARATION: Inpatient: Patient must be able to lie quietly while the scan is performed. The patient should be screened for metallic devices by nursing personnel. (See Contraindications.) This includes metal introduced into the patient either surgically or by trauma. All metallic objects must be removed from the patient including jewelry or any other metal objects which may be in the patient's bedding. Please remove dentures or other dental appliances. I.V.s which contain no metal are fine, but infu-

(Continued)

Magnetic Resonance Scan, Vascular *(Continued)*

sion pumps must be removed. Oxygen tanks and metallic backboards may come with the patient but will be removed prior to the patient entering the magnet room. Oxygen may be provided in the magnet room. Trauma, ICU, or CCU patients should be accompanied by a nurse. If the patient is restless, combative, or claustrophobic, proper sedation may be administered on the floor prior to the MRI, or at the MRI Center. Consult the MRI radiologists with questions on proper sedation. Outpatient: The patient should be screened for metallic devices. (See Contraindications.) If a question exists as to the patient's suitability for MRI, the MRI radiologist will assist you with your questions. If the patient is claustrophobic, oral or parenteral sedation may be necessary. If so, the patient should be accompanied by another adult to provide transportation home after the examination. **AFTERCARE:** If the patient received an MRI contrast agent (Magnevist®) and develops a delayed hypersensitivity reaction (ie, hives or shortness of breath), the referring physician or MRI radiologist should be contacted immediately.

Method **DATA ACQUIRED:** Digital information with film reproduction.

Interpretation **LIMITATIONS:** Generally, the greatest limitation of magnetic resonance imaging results from the patient's fear of the procedure. The patient must remain quiet and still for several scans, each lasting from several minutes to 10 minutes in length. Total examination time is usually 30-45 minutes and occasionally up to 1 hour. If the patient is restless during the examination, motion artifacts will be present on the images limiting their diagnostic value. If the patient is claustrophobic, mild oral sedation or occasionally parenteral sedation may be needed. Also the patient can be accompanied by a family member or friend during the examination which helps calm the patient's anxiety in many cases. Patients requiring life support equipment such as ventilators require special preparation. Please refer to Contraindications for further causes for rejection. **ADDITIONAL INFORMATION:** In some cases, an MRI contrast agent (Magnevist®) may be needed to increase the diagnostic accuracy of the MRI. This contrast agent can be administered to patients with a previous history of allergies to conventional iodinated x-ray agents as it contains no iodine. Contraindications to its use include previous allergy to the contrast agent itself, renal failure, certain types of anemia, and Wilson's disease. The contrast agent is generally very safe and increases the diagnostic efficacy of the MRI.

References

Masaryk TJ and Ross JS, "MR Angiography: Clinical Applications," *Magnetic Resonance Imaging of the Brain and Spine*, Atlas SW, ed, New York, NY: Raven Press, 1991, 1079-97.

Magnetic Resonance Venography *see* Magnetic Resonance Scan, Vascular *on previous page*

NUCLEAR MEDICINE

James K. O'Donnell, MD

Nuclear medicine procedures routinely involve the generation of images that depict the functional status of various body organs. Similar to conventional radiographic images (x-rays), but also distinctly different from them, scintigrams or scans in nuclear medicine result from the detection of gamma rays in an organ after the noninvasive administration of a mildly radioactive pharmaceutical, usually intravenously. The radiation dose to the patient is usually less than that from a corresponding radiographic procedure.

Nuclear medicine images differ from conventional radiographs in that they depict organ physiology or function rather than just anatomy. Especially when interfaced to current state-of-the-art computer systems, information regarding dynamic physiologic parameters such as organ perfusion, metabolism, excretion, and the presence or absence of obstruction can be obtained.

Additional nonimaging nuclear medicine procedures such as thyroid uptakes, Schilling test for vitamin B_{12} absorption, and measurements of blood volume components can also provide important physiologic information for clinical decision making.

Rapid and ongoing developments in both new technology and new radiopharmaceuticals promise to further refine the ability of nuclear medicine to provide increasingly accurate and sophisticated physiologic information to correlate with other diagnostic tests in the clinical management of our patients.

Nuclear Medicine Physiologic Imaging Applications

Procedure	Agent	Physiologic Action	Clinical Application
Biliary	^{99m}Tc IDA	Liver excretion into bile	Obstruction, cholecystitis
Bone	^{99m}Tc MDP	Uptake in bone	Metastases, infection, trauma
Brain	^{99m}Tc HMPAO ^{123}I IMP	Cerebral perfusion	Stroke, TIA, seizures, psychiatry
Heart	^{201}Tl	Myocardial perfusion	Myocardial ischemia or scarring
	^{99m}Tc RBC	Blood pool label	Ventricular function
	^{99m}Tc PYP	Uptake in recent necrosis	Recent myocardial infarct
Liver/spleen	^{99m}Tc SC	Uptake in RE cells	Hepatocellular dysfunction, focal liver disease
Lung	^{99m}Tc MAA	Particles trapped in small arterioles	Pulmonary perfusion, emboli
	^{99m}Tc DTPA	Aerosol	Pulmonary ventilation, emboli
Thyroid	^{99m}Tc TcO_4^-	Thyroid trapping	Thyroid function, masses
	^{123}I NaI	Thyroid trapping/organification	Thyroid function, masses
Renal	^{99m}Tc DTPA	Glomerular filtration analogue	Renal differential function, obstruction, quantitative GFR
	^{99m}Tc GHA	Bound in renal cortex	Renal cortical anatomy, scarring
	^{123}I OIH	Renal plasma flow analogue	Renal differential function, obstruction, quantitative ERPF

Acute Myocardial Infarction Scan *see* Myocardial Infarction Scan *on page 374*
Aerosol Lung Scan *see* Lung Scan, Ventilation *on page 373*

Angiogram, Radionuclide

CPT 78445

Related Information

Cardiac Blood Pool Scan, First Pass *on page 364*
Renal Scan *on page 381*

Synonyms Arterial Flow Study; Vascular Dynamic Study; Vascular Flow Study

Applies to Brain Flow Only; Superior Venacavagram

Abstract **PROCEDURE COMMONLY INCLUDES:** The patient receives an intravenous injection of a technetium-99m (^{99m}Tc) compound. During and immediately following injection, rapid sequence images of the vascular structures and/or organs of interest are acquired. With computer assistance, a cine display of initial perfusion through major vascular structures can be made. Additional computer analysis can generate flow/perfusion curves and other quantitative information. **INDICATIONS:** Radionuclide angiograms are helpful in noninvasively evaluating perfusion to many organ systems. They are often used to assess the functional significance of known or suspected anatomic abnormalities such as vascular stenoses or obstructions. They are a routine part of many dynamic organ imaging procedures (see Cardiac Blood Pool Scan, First Pass and Renal Scan). Additional applications include the detection of superior vena cava obstruction or documentation of absent cerebral perfusion (brain death).

Patient Care/Scheduling **PATIENT PREPARATION:** The patient does not need to be fasting or NPO for this procedure. Patient should have all RIA blood work performed, or at least drawn, prior to the injection of any radioactive material. **SPECIAL INSTRUCTIONS:** Requisition must state the current patient diagnosis in order to select the most appropriate radiopharmaceutical and/or imaging technique. **DURATION OF PROCEDURE**: 30 minutes **RADIOPHARMACEUTICAL** ^{99m}Tc DTPA or other ^{99m}Tc compound.

Specimen **CAUSES FOR REJECTION:** Other recent Nuclear Medicine procedure may interfere. **TURNAROUND TIME:** A written report will be sent to the patient's chart and/or to the referring physician.

Interpretation **NORMAL FINDINGS:** Prompt transit of the radionuclide bolus through arterial vascular structures and homogeneous perfusion of the organs supplied by these vessels **LIMITATIONS:** Radionuclide angiograms provide accurate screening for functional aspects of vascular flow and organ perfusion. However, image resolution is not good enough to accurately assess the exact anatomy, eg, the precise location and the extent of an obstruction. Radionuclide angiography is best used as a screening test to better select patients who may need a more invasive contrast angiographic procedure.

References

Coltart RS and Wraight EP, "The Value of Radionuclide Venography in Superior Vena Caval Obstruction," *Clin Radiol*, 1985, 36:415-8.

Rudavsky AZ, "Radionuclide Angiography in the Evaluation of Arterial and Venous Grafts," *Semin Nucl Med*, 1988, 18(3):261-8.

Taki J, Bunko H, Tonami, N, et al, "Shunt Between Right Subclavian Vein and the Left Heart in Superior Vena Cava Obstruction Due to Lung Cancer," *Clin Nucl Med*, 1990, 15:251-3.

Arterial Flow Study *see* Angiogram, Radionuclide *on this page*
Biliary Patency Scan *see* Biliary Scan *on this page*
Biliary Reflux Scan *see* Biliary Scan *on this page*

Biliary Scan

CPT 78220 (liver function study); 78223 (hepatobiliary imaging)

Synonyms Biliary Patency Scan; Choletec® Scan; DISIDA® Scan; Disofenin Scan; Gallbladder Ejection Fraction Scan; Gallbladder Scan; Hepatobiliary Scan; Hepatobiliary Scintigraphy; HIDA® Liver Scan; Mebrofenin® Scan

Applies to Biliary Reflux Scan
Replaces Rose Bengal Liver Scan
Abstract PROCEDURE COMMONLY INCLUDES: The patient receives an intravenous injection of a technetium-99m (^{99m}Tc) IDA radiopharmaceutical which is excreted through the biliary system. Multiple images are acquired serially until appearance of the radiopharmaceutical in the gallbladder and small bowel or a sufficient period of time has passed. INDICATIONS: Biliary imaging has become the procedure of choice in evaluating patients with suspected acute cholecystitis because in virtually all cases of acute cholecystitis there is obstruction of the cystic duct with no passage of radionuclide into the gallbladder. The test can also be used to detect enterogastric reflux of bile and neonatal biliary atresia as well as to assess biliary kinetics (gallbladder ejection fraction) in suspected chronic cholecystitis.
Patient Care/Scheduling PATIENT PREPARATION: Patient should have all RIA blood work performed, or at least drawn, prior to injection of any radioactive material. Patient must be fasting (NPO) 2-3 hours before scan. SPECIAL INSTRUCTIONS: Requisition must state the current patient diagnosis in order to select the most appropriate radiopharmaceutical and/or imaging technique. A serum bilirubin level is needed and should be noted on request form in order to administer the proper dose of radiopharmaceutical. DURATION OF PROCEDURE: 1-4 hours although additional delayed images for up to 24 hours may be required. RADIOPHARMACEUTICAL: ^{99m}Tc IDA or related compound.
Method TECHNIQUE: The application of single-photon emission tomography (SPECT) techniques may contribute significantly to the diagnostic accuracy of this imaging study.
Specimen CAUSES FOR REJECTION: Nonfasting patient, other recent Nuclear Medicine procedure may interfere. If uncertain, call the Nuclear Medicine Department. TURNAROUND TIME: A written report will be sent to the patient's chart and/or to the referring physician.
Interpretation NORMAL FINDINGS: Early tracer accumulation within the liver and subsequent visualization of the gallbladder and small bowel within 1 hour after injection LIMITATIONS: Sensitivity/specificity for acute cholecystitis decrease as bilirubin levels rise $>$5 mg/dL. ADDITIONAL INFORMATION: Intravenous injection of cholecystokinin (CCK), or its synthetic form sincalide, may improve diagnostic accuracy in patients fasted for prolonged periods who can demonstrate a false-positive study. This intervention is also employed in selected patients to assess biliary kinetics quantitatively (gallbladder ejection fraction).
References

Cooperberg PL and Gibney RG, "Imaging of the Gallbladder," *Radiology*, 1987, 163:605-13.
Freitas JE, Coleman RE, Nagle CE, et al, "Influence of Scan and Pathologic Criteria on the Specificity of Cholescintigraphy," *J Nucl Med*, 1983, 24:876-9.
Kloiber R, AuCoin R, Hershfield NB, et al, "Biliary Obstruction After Cholecystectomy: Diagnosis With Quantitative Cholescintigraphy," *Radiology*, 1988, 169(3):643-7.
Krishnamurthy GT and Turner FE, "Pharmacokinetics and Clinical Applications of Technetium-99m Labeled Hepatobiliary Agents," *Semin Nucl Med*, 1990, 20(2):130-49.
Meekin GK, Ziessman HA, and Klappenbach RS, "Prognostic Value and Pathophysiologic Significance of the Rim Sign in Cholescintigraphy," *J Nucl Med*, 1987, 28:1679-82.
Shih WJ, Coupal JJ, Domstad PA, et al, "Disorders of Gallbladder Function Related to Duodenogastric Reflux in Technetium-99m DISIDA Hepatobiliary Scintigraphy," *Clin Nucl Med*, 1987, 12:857-60.

Bladder Reflux Study *see* Voiding Cystourethrogram, Radionuclide *on page 389*

Blood Loss Localization Study *see* Gastrointestinal Bleed Localization Study *on page 368*

Blood Volume

CPT 78110 (plasma volume); 78120 (red cell volume)
Related Information
Red Cell Volume *on page 380*
Synonyms Plasma/Blood Volume; Total Blood Volume
Applies to Plasma Volume Measurement; Red Cell Mass; Red Cell Mass Measurement
Abstract PROCEDURE COMMONLY INCLUDES: Determinations of red blood cell and plasma volumes are nonimaging procedures in which the patient receives intravenous injections of radiolabeled autologous red cells followed later by radiolabeled albumin (RISA). The re-
(Continued)

Blood Volume *(Continued)*

spective volumes in the circulation are measured in subsequent timed blood samples. **INDICATIONS:** Red cell volume measurement is helpful in the differential diagnosis of polycythemia. Plasma volumes assist in therapeutic management of patients with fluid losses such as from burns, severe diarrhea, or surgery. **CONTRAINDICATIONS:** Active bleeding, edema.

Patient Care/Scheduling **PATIENT PREPARATION:** Patient should have all RIA blood work performed, or at least drawn, prior to injection of any radioactive material. The patient does not need to be fasting or NPO for this procedure. Other blood samples should not be taken during this procedure nor should transfusions of blood products be given. **SPECIAL INSTRUCTIONS:** Requisition must state the current patient diagnosis in order to select the most appropriate radiopharmaceutical and/or imaging technique. Before the test is ordered it should be verified that the patient has **not** recently received an isotope *in vivo* (eg, bone scans, liver scans, brain scans). Include patient's height and weight on requisition because it is needed for calculations. **DURATION OF PROCEDURE:** 2-4 hours. **RADIOPHARMACEUTICAL:** Chromium-51 chromate for RBC label and iodine-131 or iodine-125 human serum albumin.

Specimen **CAUSES FOR REJECTION:** Active bleeding or recent blood transfusions, other recent Nuclear Medicine procedure may interfere. If uncertain, call the Nuclear Medicine Department. **TURNAROUND TIME:** A written report will be sent to the patient's chart and/or to the referring physician.

Interpretation **NORMAL FINDINGS:** Normal blood volumes are a function of the size and sex of the patient. Expected blood volumes are estimated based on body surface area. Measured volumes are compared to the expected results and normally can vary ±20%. Obese patients may have volumes somewhat less than expected. **LIMITATIONS:** Any *in vivo* isotope test will affect blood volume (eg, bone scans, liver scans, brain scans). The procedure is technically difficult with multiple laboratory steps which tend to introduce errors.

References

Benedetto AR and Nusynowitz ML, "Correlation of Right and Left Ventricular Ejection Fraction and Volume Measurements," *J Nucl Med*, 1988, 29(6):1114-7.

Pollycove M and Tono M, "Blood Volume," *Diagnostic Nuclear Medicine*, Gottschalk A, Hoffer PB, and Potchen EJ, eds, Baltimore, MD: Williams & Wilkins, 1988, 690-8.

Srivastava SC and Chervu LR, "Radionuclide-Labeled Red Blood Cells: Current Status and Future Prospects," *Semin Nucl Med*, 1984, 14:68-82.

Bone Marrow Function Scan *see* Bone Marrow Scan *on this page*

Bone Marrow Scan

CPT 78102 (limited area); 78103 (multiple areas); 78104 (whole body)

Synonyms Bone Marrow Function Scan; Marrow Scan

Abstract **PROCEDURE COMMONLY INCLUDES:** The patient receives an intravenous injection of a technetium-99m (^{99m}Tc) colloid compound which localizes in the reticuloendothelial cells of the bone marrow. Whole body or appropriate regional images of active marrow sites in the skeleton are acquired. **INDICATIONS:** Bone marrow imaging is helpful in detecting the presence and distribution of active functioning marrow versus alterations due to a variety of hematologic disorders such as myelofibrosis, leukemia, lymphoma, and anemia including sickle cell anemia with marrow infarction. Additional applications include estimation of bone marrow function in oncology before or after radiation or chemotherapy, determining the best site for bone marrow biopsy, and assessment of blood supply to the femoral head in possible avascular necrosis.

Patient Care/Scheduling **PATIENT PREPARATION:** Patient should have all RIA blood work performed, or at least drawn, prior to injection of any radioactive material. The patient does not need to be fasting or NPO for this procedure. **SPECIAL INSTRUCTIONS:** Requisition must state the current patient diagnosis in order to select the most appropriate radiopharmaceutical and/or imaging technique. **DURATION OF PROCEDURE:** 1-2 hours. **RADIOPHARMACEUTICAL:** ^{99m}Tc sulfur colloid.

Specimen **CAUSES FOR REJECTION:** Other recent Nuclear Medicine procedure may interfere. If uncertain, call the Nuclear Medicine Department. **TURNAROUND TIME:** A written report will be sent to the patient's chart and/or to the referring physician.

Interpretation NORMAL FINDINGS: Homogenous and symmetric distribution of activity in sites of functioning marrow reticuloendothelial cells. In adults this includes the skull, axial skeleton, and proximal third of the humeral and femoral shafts. Active marrow extends more distally in children. LIMITATIONS: Reticuloendothelial cell distribution varies somewhat from that of functioning hematopoietic cells. Asymmetric activity patterns are nonspecific and should be correlated with other radiographic and clinical findings.

References

Alavi A and Heyman S, "Bone Marrow Imaging," *Diagnostic Nuclear Medicine*, Gottschalk A, Hoffer PB, and Potchen EJ, eds, Baltimore, MD: Williams & Wilkins, 1988, 707-24.

Linden A, Zankovich R, Theissen P, et al, "Malignant Lymphoma: Bone Marrow Imaging Versus Biopsy," *Radiology*, 1989, 173(2):335-9.

Vogler JB and Murphy WA, "Bone Marrow Imaging," *Radiology*, 1988, 168(3):679-93.

Bone Scan

CPT 78300 (limited area); 78305 (multiple areas); 78306 (whole body)

Synonyms Bone Scintigraphy; Radionuclide Bone Scan; Whole Body Bone Scan

Applies to Bone Scan With Flow; Three-Phase Bone Scan

Abstract PROCEDURE COMMONLY INCLUDES: The patient receives an intravenous injection of a technetium-99m (^{99m}Tc) phosphonate radiopharmaceutical which localizes in bone with intensity proportional to the degree of metabolic activity present. Three hours after the injection, whole body and appropriate regional skeletal images are acquired. An initial dynamic flow study and/or early images may also be acquired if osteomyelitis, osteonecrosis, Legg-Calvé-Perthes disease, septic arthritis, or other inflammatory disease is suspected (three-phase technique). INDICATIONS: Bone imaging is extremely sensitive for the detection of infection or malignancy involving any part of the skeleton. It is the most appropriate screening test for these conditions, since scan abnormalities are present long before structural defects develop radiographically. Bone scans are also accurate for localizing lesions for biopsy, excision, or debridement. Stress fractures can be diagnosed by bone scan when radiographs are completely normal.

Patient Care/Scheduling PATIENT PREPARATION: Patient should have all RIA blood work performed, or at least drawn, prior to injection of any radioactive material. The patient does not need to be fasting or NPO for this procedure. Patient should be encouraged to drink fluids during the waiting period before scanning and will be asked to void just before scanning begins. SPECIAL INSTRUCTIONS: Requisition must state the current patient diagnosis in order to select the most appropriate radiopharmaceutical and/or imaging technique. When ordering liver and bone scans for the same patient, schedule liver scan at least 1 day before the bone scan. DURATION OF PROCEDURE: 3-4.5 hours. This includes a 2-3 hour delay after tracer injection to allow adequate localization in bone. RADIOPHARMACEUTICAL: ^{99m}Tc phosphonate compound.

Method TECHNIQUE: The application of single-photon emission tomography (SPECT) techniques may contribute significantly to the diagnostic accuracy of this imaging study.

Specimen CAUSES FOR REJECTION: Other recent Nuclear Medicine procedure may interfere. If uncertain, call the Nuclear Medicine Department. TURNAROUND TIME: A written report will be sent to the patient's chart and/or to the referring physician.

Interpretation NORMAL FINDINGS: Homogeneous and symmetric distribution of activity throughout all skeletal structures LIMITATIONS: In postoperative orthopedic patients and diabetics, additional imaging with gallium or indium-labeled white blood cells may help to confirm the presence of active infection and serve as a baseline for later comparison.

References

Datz FL, "Radionuclide Imaging of Joint Inflammation in the 90s," *J Nucl Med*, 1990, 31(5):684-7.

Gupta NC and Prezio JA, "Radionuclide Imaging in Osteomyelitis," *Semin Nucl Med*, 1988, 18(4):287-99.

Jacobson AF, Cronin EB, Stomper PC, et al, "Bone Scans With One or Two Abnormalities in Cancer Patients With No Known Metastases: Frequency and Serial Scintigraphic Behavior of Benign and Malignant Lesions," *Radiology*, 1990, 175(1):229-32.

Lusins JO, Danielski EF, and Goldsmith SJ, "Bone SPECT in Patients With Persistent Back Pain After Lumbar Spine Surgery," *J Nucl Med*, 1989, 30(4):490-6.

(Continued)

Bone Scan *(Continued)*

Matin P, "Basic Principles of Nuclear Medicine Techniques for Detection and Evaluation of Trauma and Sports Medicine Injuries," *Semin Nucl Med*, 1988, 18(2):90-112.

McDougall IR and Keeling CA, "Complications of Fractures and Their Healing," *Semin Nucl Med*, 1988, 18(2):113-25.

McNeil BJ, "Value of Bone Scanning in Neoplastic Disease," *Semin Nucl Med*, 1985, 14:277-86.

Palmer E, Henrikson B, McKusick K, et al, "Pain as an Indicator of Bone Metastasis," *Acta Radiol*, 1988, 29:445-9.

Bone Scan With Flow *see* Bone Scan *on previous page*

Bone Scintigraphy *see* Bone Scan *on previous page*

Brain Flow Only *see* Angiogram, Radionuclide *on page 358*

Brain Perfusion Scan *see* Brain Scan *on this page*

Brain Scan

CPT 78600 (limited procedure); 78601 (limited with vascular flow); 78605 (complete study); 78606 (complete with vascular flow); 78607 (tomography - SPECT)

Synonyms Brain Scintigraphy; Ceretec® Brain Scan; Spectamine® Brain Scan

Applies to Brain Perfusion Scan; Brain Scan With Flow

Abstract **PROCEDURE COMMONLY INCLUDES:** Use of radiopharmaceuticals that do not cross the blood-brain barrier. The patient receives an intravenous injection of a radiopharmaceutical which crosses the blood-brain barrier and localizes in the brain proportionate to regional brain perfusion. Images are then obtained which demonstrate the presence and symmetry of perfusion and metabolism within the brain. **INDICATIONS:** Brain imaging is useful for the early diagnosis of cerebrovascular disease. Stroke and/or transient ischemic episodes can be detected before anatomic abnormalities develop on CT or MR scans. Other indications include localization of seizure foci, detection of tumors, and the assessment of neuropsychiatric disorders such as schizophrenia, depression, organic brain syndromes, and dementias including Alzheimer's.

Patient Care/Scheduling **PATIENT PREPARATION:** Patient should have all RIA blood work performed, or at least drawn, prior to injection of any radioactive material. The patient will lie in a quiet area with low lighting for several minutes before tracer injection. Motion during image acquisition will degrade the quality and accuracy of the procedure. If sedation is necessary, it is preferable to administer it after tracer injection. **SPECIAL INSTRUCTIONS:** Requisition must state the current patient diagnosis in order to select the most appropriate radiopharmaceutical and/or imaging technique. **DURATION OF PROCEDURE:** 1 hour. Additional delayed images may be required. **RADIOPHARMACEUTICAL:** Technetium-99m (^{99m}Tc) HMPAO (Ceretec®) or iodine-123 iodoamphetamine (Spectamine®).

Method **TECHNIQUE:** The application of single-photon emission tomography (SPECT) techniques may contribute significantly to the diagnostic accuracy of this imaging study.

Specimen **CAUSES FOR REJECTION:** Other recent Nuclear Medicine procedure may interfere. If uncertain, call the Nuclear Medicine Department. **TURNAROUND TIME:** A written report will be sent to the patient's chart and/or to the referring physician.

Interpretation **NORMAL FINDINGS:** Homogeneous and symmetric distribution of activity throughout the brain. Cerebellar activity is usually somewhat greater than in other structures.

References

Biersack NJ, Grünwald F, Reichmann K, et al, "Functional Brain Imaging With Single-Photon Emission Computed Tomography Using ^{99m}Tc-Labeled HM-PAO," *Nucl Med Ann*, 1990, 59-94.

Mountz JM, Modell JG, Foster NL, et al, "Prognostication of Recovery Following Stroke Using the Comparison of CT and Technetium-99m HM-PAO SPECT," *J Nucl Med*, 1990, 31(1):61-6.

O'Connell RA, VanHeertum RL, Billick SB, et al, "Single Photon Emission Computed Tomography (SPECT) With (^{123}I) IMP in the Differential Diagnosis of Psychiatric Disorders," *J Neuropsych*, 1989, 1:145-53.

Reid RH, Gulenchyn KY, Ballinger JR, et al, "Cerebral Perfusion Imaging With Technetium-99m HMPAO Following Cerebral Trauma - Initial Experience," *Clin Nucl Med*, 1990, 15:383-8.

Brain Scan With Flow *see* Brain Scan *on previous page*

Brain Scintigraphy *see* Brain Scan *on previous page*

Cardiac Blood Pool Scan, ECG-Gated

CPT 78471 (with gated equilibrium, at rest, wall motion study plus ejection fraction); 78472 (with regional ejection fraction)

Related Information

Cardiac Blood Pool Scan, First Pass *on next page*

Venogram, Radionuclide *on page 389*

Synonyms Ejection Fraction Study; Gated Cardiac Scan, Rest and/or Exercise; Gated Study; MUGA; Radionuclide Angiography; Radionuclide Ventriculogram; Wall Motion Study

Applies to Exercise Radionuclide Angiography; Radionuclide Angiography, Stress; Stress Gated Study

Abstract PROCEDURE COMMONLY INCLUDES: The patient receives an intravenous injection of either technetium-99m (^{99m}Tc) pertechnetate in a technique to radiolabel circulating erythrocytes (^{99m}Tc RBC) or ^{99m}Tc albumin (HSA). Multiple images of the heart synchronized to the electrocardiographic RR interval (ECG-gated) are then acquired several minutes later at equilibrium. These images are acquired into a Nuclear Medicine computer to achieve a cine display of cardiac chamber wall motion, calculation of ventricular ejection fractions (global and regional), and functional images based on mathematical manipulation of the initially acquired data. Repetitive data acquisition is possible during graded levels of exercise, usually either bicycle ergometer or handgrip, to assess ventricular functional response to exercise. INDICATIONS: Cardiac blood pool imaging is used to assess the functional status of the heart at rest and/or in response to physiologic stress. Quantification of ventricular ejection fractions calculated by this technique are quite accurate and are independent of chamber geometry, relying on the proportionality of blood volume with the amount of radioactivity in the cardiac chambers. Routine uses include evaluation of effects of coronary artery disease, heart failure, cardiomyopathies, and cardiotoxic drugs. Repetitive studies to assess response to therapeutic interventions can give accurate follow-up information. CONTRAINDICATIONS: Cardiac arrhythmia, especially atrial fibrillation, will degrade image resolution.

Patient Care/Scheduling PATIENT PREPARATION: The patient does not need to be fasting or NPO for this procedure. Patient should have all RIA blood work performed, or at least drawn, prior to the injection of any radioactive material. SPECIAL INSTRUCTIONS: Requisition must state the current patient diagnosis in order to select the most appropriate radiopharmaceutical and/or imaging technique. DURATION OF PROCEDURE: 1 hour. RADIOPHARMACEUTICAL: ^{99m}Tc labeled RBC or ^{99m}Tc HSA (albumin).

Method TECHNIQUE: The application of single-photon emission tomography (SPECT) techniques may contribute significantly to the diagnostic accuracy of this imaging study.

Specimen CAUSES FOR REJECTION: Other recent Nuclear Medicine procedure may interfere. If uncertain, call the Nuclear Medicine Department. TURNAROUND TIME: A written report will be sent to the patient's chart and/or to the referring physician.

Interpretation NORMAL FINDINGS: Normal biventricular size and regional wall motion with ejection fractions >50% (left) and/or >45% (right). LIMITATIONS: The technique of gating involves synchronization of image acquisition with the patient's electrocardiographic rhythm. Patients who have arrhythmias will have degraded image resolution and calculations of ejection fraction and other parameters will only be approximate. Rapid atrial fibrillation will give particularly poor results. When arrhythmias are severe, a first-pass technique may provide more accurate information. Right ventricular ejection fractions by a gated technique are limited by underlying right atrial isotope activity and sometimes by poor separation from left ventricular activity. A more accurate right ventricular ejection fraction may be gained from a first pass study. This can often be performed dynamically during isotope injection for the equilibrium ECG-gated study.

(Continued)

Cardiac Blood Pool Scan, ECG-Gated *(Continued)*

References

Dilsizian V, Rocco TP, Bonow RO, et al, "Cardiac Blood-Pool Imaging II: Applications in Noncoronary Heart Disease," *J Nucl Med*, 1990, 31(1):10-22.

Fischman AJ, Moore RH, Gill JB, et al, "Gated Blood Pool Tomography: A Technology Whose Time Has Come," *Semin Nucl Med*, 1989, 19(1):13-21.

Lazor L, Russell JC, DaSilva J, et al, "Use of the Multiple Gated Acquisition Scan for the Preoperative Assessment of Cardiac Risk," *Surg Gynecol Obstet*, 1988, 167(3):234-8.

Rocco TP, Dilsizian V, Fischman AJ, et al, "Evaluation of Ventricular Function in Patients With Coronary Artery Disease," *J Nucl Med*, 1989, 30(7):1149-65.

Cardiac Blood Pool Scan, First Pass

CPT 78481 (at rest, wall motion study with ejection fraction); 78484 (wall motion study plus ejection fraction plus ventricular volume determination)

Related Information

Angiogram, Radionuclide *on page 358*

Cardiac Blood Pool Scan, ECG-Gated *on previous page*

Synonyms Cardiac Scan, First Pass; First Pass Ejection Fraction; Radionuclide Cineangiography; Radionuclide Ventriculogram, First Pass

Applies to Exercise Radionuclide Angiography, First Pass

Abstract **PROCEDURE COMMONLY INCLUDES:** The patient receives an intravenous injection of a technetium-99m (^{99m}Tc) radiopharmaceutical with acquisition of image data on computer in a rapid sequence as the isotope first passes through the cardiac chambers. Similar information to ECG-gated procedures (see Cardiac Blood Pool Scan, ECG-Gated) can be obtained without the need for synchronization with the patient's ECG. **INDICATIONS:** First pass cardiac blood pool imaging can provide information about the functional status of the heart at rest and/or in response to physiologic stress. Quantification of both right and left ventricular ejection fractions is possible. A first pass right ventricular ejection fraction is usually more accurate than by ECG-gated technique (see Cardiac Blood Pool Scan, ECG-Gated).

Patient Care/Scheduling **PATIENT PREPARATION:** Patient should have all RIA blood work performed, or at least drawn, prior to injection of any radioactive material. The patient does not need to be fasting or NPO for this procedure. **SPECIAL INSTRUCTIONS:** Requisition must state the current patient diagnosis in order to select the most appropriate radiopharmaceutical and/or imaging technique. **DURATION OF PROCEDURE:** 30 minutes **RADIOPHARMACEUTICAL:** ^{99m}Tc DTPA, pertechnetate, or other compound.

Specimen **CAUSES FOR REJECTION:** Other recent Nuclear Medicine procedure may interfere. If uncertain, call the Nuclear Medicine Department. **TURNAROUND TIME:** A written report will be sent to the patient's chart and/or to the referring physician at the completion of the procedure.

Interpretation **NORMAL FINDINGS:** Normal biventricular size and regional wall motion with ejection fractions >50% (left) and/or >45% (right).

References

Benedetto AR and Nusynowitz ML, "Correlation of Right and Left Ventricular Ejection Fraction and Volume Measurements," *J Nucl Med*, 1988, 29(6):1114-7.

Brill DM and Konstam MA, "RV Function in Ischemic and Nonischemic Heart Disease," *Cardiology*, 1988, 6:57-66.

DePuey EG, "Evaluation of Cardiac Function With Radionuclides," *Diagnostic Nuclear Medicine*, Gottschalk A, Hoffer PB, and Potchen EJ, eds, Baltimore, MD: Williams & Wilkins, 1988, 383-7.

Cardiac Scan, First Pass *see* Cardiac Blood Pool Scan, First Pass *on this page*

Cerebrospinal Fluid Scan *see* Cisternogram *on next page*

Ceretec® Brain Scan *see* Brain Scan *on page 362*

Choletec® Scan *see* Biliary Scan *on page 358*

Chromium-51 Red Cell Survival

CPT 78130 (red cell survival study); 78135 (with splenic and/or hepatic sequestration)

Synonyms Erythrocyte Survival; RBC Survival Test; Red Blood Cell Sequestration; Red Cell Survival; Survival of Red Blood Cells

Applies to Splenic Sequestration Study

Abstract PROCEDURE COMMONLY INCLUDES: Determinations of red blood cell survival and splenic sequestration are nonimaging procedures in which the patient receives an intravenous injection of radiolabeled autologous red cells. Blood samples are then drawn after 24 hours and periodically for approximately 3 weeks. The half-life of the circulating radiolabeled red cells is then calculated. Additionally, periodic external measurements of radioactivity from the heart (blood pool), liver, and spleen help to assess the role of the spleen in a possible hemolytic condition. INDICATIONS: This procedure is helpful in the differential diagnosis and management of hemolytic anemia including conditions such as spherocytosis, red cell enzyme deficiency, and various hemoglobinopathies. Occult blood loss can also be evaluated. Evaluation of red cell sequestration within the spleen demonstrates the possible role of the spleen in the hemolytic process and may predict the therapeutic value of splenectomy.

Patient Care/Scheduling PATIENT PREPARATION: Patient should have all RIA blood work performed, or at least drawn, prior to injection of any radioactive material. The patient does not need to be fasting or NPO for this procedure. Transfusions of blood products should be avoided during this procedure. The Nuclear Medicine Department will provide a schedule for drawing of serial blood samples. SPECIAL INSTRUCTIONS: Requisition must state the current patient diagnosis in order to select the most appropriate radiopharmaceutical technique. At least 21 days should be allowed for this study. When selective splenic sequestration as cause of hemolysis is suspected, liver and spleen readings are performed in conjunction with chromium-51 RBC survival test. Please notify the Nuclear Medicine Department if the patient is to be discharged. DURATION OF PROCEDURE: 3-4 weeks. RADIOPHARMACEUTICAL: Chromium-51 chromate for RBC label.

Specimen CAUSES FOR REJECTION: Active or known intermittent bleeding, recent blood transfusions, other recent Nuclear Medicine procedure may interfere. TURNAROUND TIME: A written report will be sent to the patient's chart and/or to the referring physician.

Interpretation NORMAL FINDINGS: The normal red cell survival half-time (50% survival) range is 25-30 days. Shorter half-times indicate excessive red cell destruction and/or blood loss. The normal spleen to liver (or spleen to precordium) ratio is 1:1. Splenomegaly alone may show a ratio of 1 to 2:1. Ratios >2.5:1 indicate significant splenic sequestration of red cells. LIMITATIONS: This procedure cannot discriminate between red cell loss due to intravascular hemolysis and red cell loss due to bleeding. The procedure is also technically difficult and requires a prolonged period of time to obtain results.

References

Baker WJ and Datz FL, "Preparation and Clinical Utility of Labeled Blood Products," *Essentials of Nuclear Medicine Science*, Hladik WB, Saha GB, and Study KT, eds, Baltimore, MD: Williams & Wilkins, 1987, 91-2.

Price DC and McIntyre PA, "The Hematopoietic System," *Textbook of Nuclear Medicine*, Vol II, Harbert J and DaRocha AFG, eds, Philadelphia, PA: Lea & Febiger, 1984, 536-50.

Srivastava SC and Chervu LR, "Radionuclide-Labeled Red Blood Cells: Current Status and Future Prospects," *Semin Nucl Med*, 1984, 14:68-82.

Chromium-Labeled Red Cell Volume *see* Red Cell Volume *on page 380*

Cisternogram

CPT 78630; 78635 (ventriculography); 78645 (shunt evaluation); 78650 (CSF leakage detection and localization); 78652 (tomographic – ECT)

Synonyms Cerebrospinal Fluid Scan; CSF Scan; CSF Scintigraphy; Radionuclide Cisternography

Abstract PROCEDURE COMMONLY INCLUDES: The patient undergoes a lumbar puncture under sterile conditions with subarachnoid injection of a water-soluble radiopharmaceutical which distributes into the cerebrospinal fluid (CSF). For patients with ventricular shunts or implanted CSF reservoirs, the radiopharmaceutical may be injected into these directly by

(Continued)

Cisternogram *(Continued)*

appropriate personnel. Images of the spinal canal and CSF spaces of the brain are acquired intermittently for up to 72 hours to assess CSF pathways and/or shunt patency. **INDICATIONS:** Cisternography is helpful in the differential diagnosis of hydrocephalus. In normal pressure hydrocephalus (NPH) there is a typical pattern of abnormal CSF movement. Additional indications are the detection of traumatic or postoperative CSF leaks as well as determination of CSF shunt patency.

Patient Care/Scheduling **PATIENT PREPARATION:** Patient should have all RIA blood work performed, at least drawn, prior to injection of any radioactive material. The patient does not need to be fasting or NPO for this procedure. **SPECIAL INSTRUCTIONS:** Requisition must state the current patient diagnosis in order to select the most appropriate radiopharmaceutical and/or imaging technique. **DURATION OF PROCEDURE:** 4-72 hours. **RADIOPHARMACEUTICAL:** Pyrogen-free indium-111 DTPA or ^{169}Y6 DTPA.

Method **TECHNIQUE:** CSF samples should not be taken during the lumbar puncture for this procedure. This would lower CSF volume and alter the physiologic flow pattern.

Specimen **CAUSES FOR REJECTION:** Other recent Nuclear Medicine procedure may interfere. If uncertain, call the Nuclear Medicine Department. **TURNAROUND TIME:** A written report will be sent to the patient's chart and/or to the referring physician.

Interpretation **NORMAL FINDINGS:** The normal CSF pattern of flow is from the lumbar region to the basal cisterns within 2-4 hours. There is progressive passage symmetrically over the cerebral convexities during the first 24 hours with no reflux into the lateral ventricles. From 24-72 hours there should be gradual clearance from the CSF via the choroid plexus. **LIMITATIONS:** Inadequate images may result from other than a true subarachnoid injection of tracer. Early images of the injection site confirm the technique success or failure. **ADDITIONAL INFORMATION:** For detection of CSF rhinorrhea or otorrhea, cotton pledgets may be placed in the nasal turbinates or external ear canals. These are removed within 4-6 hours for weighing and counting the radioactivity present. Notify the Nuclear Medicine Department when scheduling the procedure if a CSF leak is suspected.

References

Krasnow AZ, Collier BD, Isitman AT, et al, "The Use of Radionuclide Cisternography in the Diagnosis of Pleural Cerebrospinal Fluid Fistulae," *J Nucl Med*, 1989, 30(1):120-3.

Lyons MK and Meyer FB, "Cerebrospinal Fluid Physiology and the Management of Increased Intracranial Pressure," *Mayo Clin Proc*, 1990, 65(5):684-707.

Sandler MP, Price AC, Runge VM, et al, "Cerebrospinal Fluid Cisternography," *Diagnostic Nuclear Medicine*, Gottschalk A, Hoffer PB, and Potchen EJ, eds, Baltimore, MD: Williams & Wilkins, 1988, 888-98.

CSF Scan *see* Cisternogram *on previous page*

CSF Scintigraphy *see* Cisternogram *on previous page*

DISIDA® Scan *see* Biliary Scan *on page 358*

Disofenin Scan *see* Biliary Scan *on page 358*

Diuretic Renal Scan *see* Renal Scan *on page 381*

Ectopic Gastric Mucosa Scan *see* Meckel's Diverticulum Scan *on page 374*

Ejection Fraction Study *see* Cardiac Blood Pool Scan, ECG-Gated *on page 363*

Erythrocyte Survival *see* Chromium-51 Red Cell Survival *on previous page*

Exercise Radionuclide Angiography *see* Cardiac Blood Pool Scan, ECG-Gated *on page 363*

Exercise Radionuclide Angiography, First Pass *see* Cardiac Blood Pool Scan, First Pass *on page 364*

First Pass Ejection Fraction *see* Cardiac Blood Pool Scan, First Pass *on page 364*

Gallbladder Ejection Fraction Scan *see* Biliary Scan *on page 358*

Gallbladder Scan *see* Biliary Scan *on page 358*

Gallium Abscess Scan *see* Gallium Scan, Abscess and/or Tumor *on next page*

Gallium Scan, Abscess and/or Tumor

CPT 78800 (tumor); 78801 (tumor, multiple areas); 78802 (whole body); 78803 (tumor localization - SPECT); 78805 (abscess, limited areas); 78806 (abscess, multiple areas)

Applies to Gallium Abscess Scan; Gallium Tumor Scan; Soft Tissue Scan

Abstract PROCEDURE COMMONLY INCLUDES: The patient receives an intravenous injection of gallium-67 citrate. Images are then acquired for some combination of 24, 48, and 72 hours after injection. INDICATIONS: Gallium localizes at sites of active inflammation or infection as well as in some neoplasms. Gallium imaging is very sensitive in detection of abscesses, pneumonia, pyelonephritis, active sarcoidosis, and active tuberculosis. Even in immunocompromised patients, eg, those with AIDS, gallium imaging can detect early complications such as *Pneumocystis carinii* pneumonitis. The nonspecificity of gallium activity, however, requires that correlation with other radiographic studies and clinical findings be given close attention. Gallium imaging is very useful in the differential diagnosis and staging of some neoplasms, notably Hodgkin's disease, lymphoma, hepatocellular carcinoma, bronchogenic carcinoma, melanoma, and leukemia. Recent evidence has shown a correlation of gallium localization in the lungs with the activity of disease in pulmonary fibrosis and asbestosis. Gallium is also used in addition to bone scintigraphy for detecting osteomyelitis, especially in its chronic stages. A common indication for gallium imaging is as a screening procedure for infection in fever of unknown origin (FUO).

Patient Care/Scheduling PATIENT PREPARATION: Patient should have all RIA blood work performed, or at least drawn, prior to injection of any radioactive material. The patient does not need to be fasting or NPO for this procedure. SPECIAL INSTRUCTIONS: Requisition must state the current patient diagnosis in order to select the most appropriate radiopharmaceutical and/or imaging technique. Other Nuclear Medicine procedures (bone, liver, lung) should be completed prior to gallium injection. If abdominal abscess/infection is suspected, laxatives, and/or enemas may be ordered for the patient prior to delayed imaging at 48 or 72 hours. This will help clear normal intestinal gallium activity from the colon. DURATION OF PROCEDURE: 24-72 hours RADIOPHARMACEUTICAL: Gallium-67 citrate.

Method TECHNIQUE: The application of single-photon emission tomography (SPECT) techniques may contribute significantly to the diagnostic accuracy of this imaging study.

Specimen TURNAROUND TIME: A written report will be sent to the patient's chart and/or to the referring physician.

Interpretation NORMAL FINDINGS: Gallium will localize to some degree in liver and spleen, bone, nasopharynx, lacrimal glands, and breast tissue. There is normally some secretion of gallium into the bowel. This may require laxatives and/or enemas for the patient to evacuate this normal activity before additional imaging of possible abdominal infection or abscess. Abnormal accumulation of gallium will usually be asymmetric, increase in later images, and remain in the same location (normal bowel luminal gallium activity will transit). LIMITATIONS: There is variable normal excretion of gallium via the intestinal tract. This contributes to the nonspecificity of gallium imaging in suspected abdominal or pelvic infections. Previous treatment with antibiotics or high doses of steroids may decrease the inflammatory response and result in false-negative gallium imaging. ADDITIONAL INFORMATION: Other isotope studies may need to be postponed up to 7 days after a gallium scan has been done due to its slow elimination from soft tissue.

References

Bisson G, Lamoureux G, and Bégin R, "Quantitative Gallium-67 Lung Scan to Assess the Inflammatory Activity in the Pneumoconioses," *Semin Nucl Med*, 1987, 17:72-80.

Israel O, Front D, Epelbaum R, et al, "Residual Mass and Negative Gallium Scintigraphy in Treated Lymphoma," *J Nucl Med*, 1990, 31(3):365-8.

Maderazo EG, Hickingbotham NB, Woronick CL, et al, "The Influence of Various Factors on the Accuracy of Gallium-67 Imaging for Occult Infection," *J Nucl Med*, 1988, 29(5):608-15.

Rossleigh MA, Murray IP, Mackey DW, et al, "Pediatric Solid Tumors: Evaluation by Gallium-67 SPECT Studies," *J Nucl Med*, 1990, 31(2):168-72.

Gallium Tumor Scan *see* Gallium Scan, Abscess and/or Tumor *on this page*

Gastric Emptying Quantitation *see* Gastric Emptying Scan *on next page*

Gastric Emptying Scan

CPT 78264

Synonyms Gastric Emptying Quantitation; Gastric Emptying Scintigraphy

Abstract **PROCEDURE COMMONLY INCLUDES:** The patient receives an oral radiolabeled solid-phase meal. Sequential computer assisted images of the gastric region are acquired over the next 2 hours. Gastric emptying lines are calculated based on the decrease in radioactivity with time after ingestion of the meal. If emptying of solids is abnormally prolonged, a repeat procedure assessing the emptying of a liquid radiolabeled bolus can be performed 1-2 days later. Some departments employ a dual isotope technique (eg, technetium-99m (^{99m}Tc) solid and indium-111 liquid) to quantify solid and liquid emptying simultaneously. **INDICATIONS:** Quantification of gastric emptying physiology is helpful in evaluating patients with suspected gastric motility disorders. These include diagnoses of diabetic gastroparesis, anorexia nervosa, gastric outlet obstruction syndromes, postvagotomy, and postgastrectomy syndromes, and other systemic diseases known to affect motility. Treatment responses can also be assessed.

Patient Care/Scheduling **PATIENT PREPARATION:** The patient should be NPO from midnight the night before this procedure. The procedure itself should be scheduled for the early AM time period. The patient should also abstain from alcohol and smoking for the previous 24 hours. Other medications should be noted. The patient should have all RIA blood work performed, or at least drawn, prior to administration of any radioactive material. **SPECIAL INSTRUCTIONS:** Requisition must state the current patient diagnosis in order to select the most appropriate radiopharmaceutical and/or imaging technique. **DURATION OF PROCEDURE:** 2 hours **RADIOPHARMACEUTICAL:** ^{99m}Tc sulfur colloid (solid), ^{99m}Tc DTPA (liquid), indium-111 DTPA (liquid if simultaneous with solid).

Method **TECHNIQUE:** Routinely, ^{99m}Tc sulfur colloid is mixed with two eggs and then cooked as scrambled eggs in a microwave oven. This is then served as a sandwich. Multiple alternative "recipes" exist but many do not sufficiently bind the isotope to a true solid phase to assess emptying accurately. If a simultaneous dual isotope technique is utilized, the usual liquid phase is indium-111 DTPA mixed in 6 oz orange juice.

Specimen **CAUSES FOR REJECTION:** Other recent Nuclear Medicine procedure may interfere. If uncertain, call the Nuclear Medicine Department. **TURNAROUND TIME:** A written report will be sent to the patient's chart and/or to the referring physician.

Interpretation **NORMAL FINDINGS:** Normal half-emptying (T 1/2) times for gastric contents are 45-90 minutes for solids and 5-30 minutes for a liquid phase. **LIMITATIONS:** These are approximations for the meals described above in a sitting patient. Results will vary markedly as a function of alternative meals, patient positioning, and the medication status of the patient.

References

Datz FL, Christian PE, and Moore J, "Gender-Related Differences in Gastric Emptying," *J Nucl Med*, 1987, 28:1204-7.

Urbain JL, Vantrappen G, Janssens J, et al, "Intravenous Erythromycin Dramatically Accelerates Gastric Emptying in Gastroparesis Diabeticorum and Normals and Abolishes the Emptying Discrimination Between Solids and Liquids," *J Nucl Med*, 1990, 31(9):1490-3.

Velchik MG, Reynolds JC, and Alavi A, "The Effect of Meal Energy Content on Gastric Emptying," *J Nucl Med*, 1989, 30(6):1106-10.

Gastric Emptying Scintigraphy *see* Gastric Emptying Scan *on this page*

Gastrointestinal Bleed Localization Study

CPT 78278

Synonyms Blood Loss Localization Study; Gastrointestinal Blood Loss Scan; GI Bleed Scintigraphy; Lower GI Blood Loss Scan

Abstract **PROCEDURE COMMONLY INCLUDES:** The patient receives an intravenous injection of a technetium-99m (^{99m}Tc) radiopharmaceutical which remains in the circulation for sufficient time to extravasate and accumulate within the bowel lumen at the site of active bleeding. Depending on the radiopharmaceutical used, delayed images or repetitive injections may demonstrate intermittent bleeding. **INDICATIONS:** Gastrointestinal bleeding, even severe hemorrhage, is intermittent. Scintigraphy is a noninvasive method of detecting and localizing active lower (and sometimes upper) GI tract bleeding in order to better direct endoscopic or angiographic studies. Two scan techniques are available. ^{99m}Tc labeled red blood cells are accurate in detecting intermittent bleeding if serial images are acquired for up to 24 hours. ^{99m}Tc sulfur colloid, which rapidly localizes in the liver and spleen, is very sensitive for detecting active bleeding at the time of injection. Very small amounts of extravasated activity in the bowel lumen can be detected. Repetitive injections can detect intermittent bleeding.

Patient Care/Scheduling **PATIENT PREPARATION:** Patient should have all RIA blood work performed, or at least drawn, prior to the injection of any radioactive material. The patient does not need to be fasting or NPO for this procedure. **SPECIAL INSTRUCTIONS:** Requisition must state the current patient diagnosis in order to select the most appropriate radiopharmaceutical and/or imaging technique. **DURATION OF PROCEDURE:** 1-2 hours. Additional delayed images may be required. **RADIOPHARMACEUTICAL:** ^{99m}Tc sulfur colloid or ^{99m}Tc labeled RBC.

Specimen **CAUSES FOR REJECTION:** Recent radiographic barium studies within 24-48 hours, other recent Nuclear Medicine procedure may interfere. If uncertain, call the Nuclear Medicine Department. **TURNAROUND TIME:** A written report will be sent to the patient's chart and/or to the referring physician.

Interpretation **NORMAL FINDINGS:** Uptake by the liver and spleen (^{99m}Tc colloid) or circulating activity in the large vessels (^{99m}Tc RBC) with no ectopic extravascular activity **LIMITATIONS:** The scan only detects intermittent active bleeding. It is of little use in the patient with chronic anemia or slowly decreasing hematocrit. The scan is less accurate for bleeding in the upper gastrointestinal tract, ie, stomach or small bowel.

References

Avali A, "Detection of Gastrointestinal Bleeding With ^{99m}Tc Sulfur Colloid," *Semin Nucl Med*, 1982, 12:126-38.

Alavi A, "Scintigraphic Detection and Localization of Gastrointestinal Bleeding Sites," *Diagnostic Nuclear Medicine*, Gottschalk A, Hoffer PB, and Potchen EJ, eds, Baltimore, MD: Williams & Wilkins, 1988, 631-62.

Dorfman GS, Cronan JJ, and Staudinger KM, "Scintigraphic Signs and Pitfalls in Lower Gastrointestinal Hemorrhage: The Continued Necessity of Angiography," *Radiographics*, 1987, 7:543-62.

Smith R, Copely DJ, and Bolen FH, "^{99m}Tc RBC Scintigraphy: Correlation of Gastrointestinal Bleeding Rates With Scintigraphic Findings," *Am J Roentgenol*, 1987, 148:869-74.

Winzelberg GG, McKusick KA, Froelich JW, et al, "Detection of Gastrointestinal Bleeding With ^{99m}Tc Labeled Red Blood Cells," *Semin Nucl Med*, 1982, 12:139-46.

Gastrointestinal Blood Loss Scan *see* Gastrointestinal Bleed Localization Study *on previous page*

Gated Cardiac Scan, Rest and/or Exercise *see* Cardiac Blood Pool Scan, ECG-Gated *on page 363*

Gated Study *see* Cardiac Blood Pool Scan, ECG-Gated *on page 363*

GI Bleed Scintigraphy *see* Gastrointestinal Bleed Localization Study *on previous page*

Hepatobiliary Scan *see* Biliary Scan *on page 358*

Hepatobiliary Scintigraphy *see* Biliary Scan *on page 358*

HIDA® Liver Scan *see* Biliary Scan *on page 358*

Hippuran Scan *see* Renal Scan *on page 381*

^{131}I Body Scan *see* Thyroid Metastatic Survey, Iodine-131 *on page 385*

^{131}I Metastatic Survey *see* Thyroid Metastatic Survey, Iodine-131 *on page 385*

Indium-111 Labeled Leukocyte Scan *see* Indium Leukocyte Scan *on next page*

Indium Leukocyte Scan

CPT 78192 (white blood cell localization; limited area scanning) 78193 (whole body)

Synonyms Indium-111 Labeled Leukocyte Scan; Infection Scan; Infection Scintigraphy; Leukocyte Scintigraphy; WBC Scan; White Blood Cell Scan

Abstract **PROCEDURE COMMONLY INCLUDES:** The patient receives an intravenous reinjection of radiolabeled leukocytes. The patient initially has a 60-80 mL sample of blood drawn for an *in vitro* process of labeling and separating the leukocyte component. Images are acquired at intervals between 2-24 hours after subsequent reinjection of radiolabeled cells. **INDICATIONS:** Radiolabeled leukocyte imaging is useful either in determining the site of an occult infection or in confirming the presence or absence of infection at a suspected site. This technique has largely replaced gallium-67 imaging for acute infections because of the better image resolution and greater specificity. Some chronic infections, eg, chronic osteomyelitis, may be better imaged with gallium-67. Radiolabeled leukocyte imaging is especially helpful in detecting postoperative infection sites and in documenting lack of residual infection after a course of therapy.

Patient Care/Scheduling **PATIENT PREPARATION:** The patient does not need to be fasting or NPO for this procedure. Patient should have all RIA blood work performed, or at least drawn, prior to injection of any radioactive material. **SPECIAL INSTRUCTIONS:** Requisition must state the current patient diagnosis in order to select the most appropriate radiopharmaceutical and/or imaging technique. **DURATION OF PROCEDURE:** Two hours from blood draw to reinjection of labeled cells. 2-24 hours for imaging at intervals. **RADIOPHARMACEUTICAL:** Indium-111 labeled leukocytes.

Specimen **CAUSES FOR REJECTION:** Other recent Nuclear Medicine procedure may interfere. If uncertain, call the Nuclear Medicine Department. **TURNAROUND TIME:** A written report will be sent to the patient's chart and/or to the referring physician.

Interpretation **NORMAL FINDINGS:** Radiolabeled leukocytes will localize to some degree in the liver, spleen, and bone marrow. Focal accumulations in soft tissue or asymmetric uptake in bone will be seen in infected or inflamed sites. For osteomyelitis, a bone scan is usually performed first for comparison with the radiolabeled leukocyte scan findings. **LIMITATIONS:** Leukocyte radiolabeling is a complex process and is usually performed on-site only where there are dedicated radiopharmacy laboratories. Most commercial radiopharmacies will also provide this service locally. **ADDITIONAL INFORMATION:** An alternative method of leukocyte radiolabeling with technetium-99m (^{99m}Tc) HMPAO is now available. Early reports show possible advantages with earlier imaging times and better sensitivity for infections in extremities with utilization of higher doses of ^{99m}Tc versus indium-111.

References

Abreu SH, "Skeletal Uptake of Indium-111 Labeled White Blood Cells," *Semin Nucl Med*, 1989, 19:152-5.

Datz FL and Thorne DA, "Effect of Antibiotic Therapy on the Sensitivity of Indium-111 Labeled Leukocyte Scans," *J Nucl Med*, 1986, 27:1849-53.

Froelich JW and Field SA, "The Role of Indium-111 White Blood Cells in Inflammatory Bowel Disease," *Semin Nucl Med*, 1988, 18(4):300-7.

Laitinen R, Tähtinen J, Lantto T, et al, "^{99m}Tc Labeled Leukocytes in Imaging of Patients With Suspected Acute Abdominal Inflammation," *Clin Nucl Med*, 1990, 15:597-602.

Roddie ME, Peters AM, Danpure HJ, et al, "Inflammation: Imaging With ^{99m}Tc HMPAO-Labeled Leukocytes," *Radiology*, 1988, 166(3):767-72.

Infarct-Avid Scan *see* Myocardial Infarction Scan *on page 374*

Infection Scan *see* Indium Leukocyte Scan *on this page*

Infection Scintigraphy *see* Indium Leukocyte Scan *on this page*

Iodine Therapy *see* Radioactive Iodine Therapy *on page 377*

Iodine Thyroid Scan *see* Thyroid Scan *on page 386*

Isotope Venogram *see* Venogram, Radionuclide *on page 389*

^{131}I Therapy *see* Radioactive Iodine Therapy *on page 377*

^{131}I Whole Body Survey *see* Thyroid Metastatic Survey, Iodine-131 *on page 385*

Kidney Scan *see* Renal Scan *on page 381*

Leukocyte Scintigraphy *see* Indium Leukocyte Scan *on previous page*

Liver and Spleen Scan

CPT 78215 (liver and spleen, static); 78216 (liver and spleen, with vascular flow)

Synonyms Liver Scintigraphy; Liver-Spleen Scan; Radioisotope Hepatic Scan; Radionuclide Liver Scan; Spleen Scan

Abstract **PROCEDURE COMMONLY INCLUDES:** The patient receives an intravenous injection of a technetium-99m (^{99m}Tc) colloidal radiopharmaceutical which is rapidly accumulated in reticuloendothelial cells of the liver and spleen. Shortly after the injection, multiple images of the liver and spleen are acquired. An initial dynamic flow study may also be acquired to assess hepatic and/or splenic perfusion, especially in cases of trauma. **INDICATIONS:** Liver and spleen imaging is an accurate noninvasive method to delineate overall organ size, the presence of focal lesions, and/or the degree of hepatocellular dysfunction in diffuse liver disease. It has been used to detect and document later resolution of traumatic splenic hematomas or infarcts.

Patient Care/Scheduling **PATIENT PREPARATION:** Patient should have all RIA blood work performed, or at least drawn, prior to injection of any radioactive material. The patient does not need to be fasting or NPO for this procedure. **SPECIAL INSTRUCTIONS:** Requisition must state the current patient diagnosis in order to select the most appropriate radiopharmaceutical and/or imaging technique. Schedule a liver scan at least 1 day before a bone scan if both are ordered for the same patient. **DURATION OF PROCEDURE:** 30 minutes to 1 hour **RADIOPHARMACEUTICAL:** ^{99m}Tc sulfur colloid or other microcolloid compound.

Method **TECHNIQUE:** The application of single-photon emission tomography (SPECT) techniques may contribute significantly to the diagnostic accuracy of this imaging study.

Specimen **CAUSES FOR REJECTION:** Residual barium in GI tract from recent x-rays, other recent Nuclear Medicine procedure may interfere. If uncertain, call the Nuclear Medicine Department. **TURNAROUND TIME:** A written report will be sent to the patient's chart and/or to the referring physician.

Interpretation **NORMAL FINDINGS:** Homogeneous distribution of activity throughout both liver and spleen with no organomegaly or focal defects. The ratio of spleen:liver activity should be about equal. Increased relative splenic uptake, especially if accompanied by visualization of bone marrow reticuloendothelial uptake, indicates at least some degree of hepatocellular dysfunction.

References

Krishnamurthy S and Krishnamurthy GT, "Nuclear Hepatology: Where Is it Heading Now?" *J Nucl Med*, 1988, 29(6):1144-9.

Oppenheim BE, Wellman HN, and Hoffer PB, "Liver Imaging," *Diagnostic Nuclear Medicine*, Gottschalk A, Hoffer PB, and Potchen EJ, eds, Baltimore, MD: Williams & Wilkins, 1988, 538-65.

Van Heertum RL, Brunetti JC, and Yudd AP, "Abdominal SPECT Imaging," *Semin Nucl Med*, 1987, 17:230-46.

Liver Scintigraphy *see* Liver and Spleen Scan *on this page*

Liver-Spleen Scan *see* Liver and Spleen Scan *on this page*

Lower Extremity Venogram, Radionuclide *see* Venogram, Radionuclide *on page 389*

Lower GI Blood Loss Scan *see* Gastrointestinal Bleed Localization Study *on page 368*

Lung-Liver Scan for Subdiaphragmatic Abscesses *see* Radioisotope Liver-Lung Scan for Subdiaphragmatic Abscesses *on page 379*

Lung Perfusion Scintigraphy *see* Lung Scan, Perfusion *on next page*

Lung Scan, Perfusion

CPT 78580 (particulate); 78581 (gaseous)

Related Information

Lung Scan, Ventilation *on next page*

Synonyms Lung Perfusion Scintigraphy; Perfusion Lung Scan; Perfusion-Ventilation Scan; Pulmonary Scan; Radionuclide Perfusion Lung Scan; V/2 Scan

Applies to Quantitative Perfusion Lung Scan; Ventilation-Perfusion Lung Scan

Abstract PROCEDURE COMMONLY INCLUDES: The patient receives an intravenous injection of a technetium-99m (^{99m}Tc) macroaggregated albumin radiopharmaceutical which is trapped by the small arterioles of the pulmonary circulation. Multiple images of the lungs are then acquired to assess lung perfusion. **Special note:** This procedure is almost always combined with a lung ventilation scan to detect a characteristic pattern of segmental perfusion deficits with normal corresponding regional ventilation that is the hallmark of pulmonary emboli. (See Lung Scan, Ventilation.) A perfusion scan performed alone or in conjunction with a ventilation scan, but with computer image acquisition and quantification of regional perfusion and ventilation, is sometimes used to predict the prognosis in patients under consideration for pneumonectomy or lobectomy surgery. INDICATIONS: The primary indication for lung perfusion and ventilation imaging is the detection of acute pulmonary emboli. These procedures together provide an accurate noninvasive screening test both for the detection of emboli and for documentation of resolution during and after therapy. Perfusion lung scans are also used to assess regional pulmonary perfusion preoperatively in patients undergoing lung resection surgery. CONTRAINDICATIONS: Caution should be exercised in performing this procedure for patients with known primary or secondary pulmonary hypertension. The microembolization with the ^{99m}Tc macroaggregated albumin may worsen the underlying condition temporarily. The procedure can usually still be performed with a lower dose.

Patient Care/Scheduling PATIENT PREPARATION: Patient should have all RIA blood work performed, or at least drawn, prior to injection of any radioactive material. The patient does not need to be fasting or NPO for this procedure. The patient should have a routine chest radiograph performed within 12 hours prior to imaging or receive one immediately after. SPECIAL INSTRUCTIONS: Requisition must state the current patient diagnosis in order to select the most appropriate radiopharmaceutical and/or imaging technique. DURATION OF PROCEDURE: 30 minutes to 1 hour RADIOPHARMACEUTICAL: ^{99m}Tc macroaggregated albumin (MAA) or albumin microspheres (HAM).

Method TECHNIQUE: The application of single-photon emission tomography (SPECT) techniques may contribute significantly to the diagnostic accuracy of this imaging study.

Specimen CAUSES FOR REJECTION: Other recent Nuclear Medicine procedure may interfere. If uncertain, call the Nuclear Medicine Department. TURNAROUND TIME: A written report will be sent to the patient's chart and/or to the referring physician.

Interpretation NORMAL FINDINGS: Homogeneous distribution of activity throughout the lungs LIMITATIONS: The procedure is somewhat nonspecific in the presence of underlying lung conditions such as pneumonia or chronic obstructive disease. A same day chest radiograph is necessary for review and comparison with scan findings.

References

Kahn D, Bushnell DL, Dean R, et al, "Clinical Outcome of Patients With a "Low Probability" of Pulmonary Embolism on Ventilation-Perfusion Lung Scan," *Arch Intern Med*, 1989, 149(2):377-9.

PIOPED Investigators, "Value of the Ventilation/Perfusion Scan in Acute Pulmonary Embolism, Results of the Prospective Investigation of Pulmonary Embolism Diagnosis (PIOPED)," *JAMA*, 1990, 263(20):2753-9.

Touya JJ, Corbus HF, Savala KM, et al, "Single-Photon Emission Computed Tomography in the Diagnosis of Pulmonary Thromboembolism," *Semin Nucl Med*, 1986, 16:306-36.

Wellman HN, "Pulmonary Thromboembolism: Current Status Report on the Role of Nuclear Medicine," *Semin Nucl Med*, 1986, 16:236-74.

Lung Scan, Ventilation

CPT 78587 (aerosol, multiple projections); 78594 (gaseous, multiple projections)

Related Information

Lung Scan, Perfusion *on previous page*

Synonyms Aerosol Lung Scan; Radionuclide Ventilation Lung Scan; Ventilation Lung Scan; Xenon Lung Scan

Applies to Quantitative Ventilation Lung Scan; Ventilation-Perfusion Lung Scan

Abstract **PROCEDURE COMMONLY INCLUDES:** The patient inhales a radioactive gas or nebulized aerosol and multiple images of the lungs are then acquired to assess lung ventilation. **Special note:** This procedure is almost always combined with a lung perfusion scan to detect a characteristic pattern of segmental perfusion deficits with normal corresponding regional ventilation that is the hallmark of pulmonary emboli. (See Lung Scan, Perfusion.) **INDICATIONS:** The primary indication for lung ventilation and perfusion imaging is the detection of acute pulmonary emboli. These procedures together provide an accurate noninvasive screening test both for the detection of emboli and for documentation of resolution during and after therapy. Lung ventilation imaging is also helpful in quantifying regional pulmonary ventilation in patients with severe obstructive lung disease or who are being considered for lung resection surgery.

Patient Care/Scheduling **PATIENT PREPARATION:** Patient should have all RIA blood work performed, or at least drawn, prior to injection of any radioactive material. The patient does not need to be fasting or NPO for this procedure. The patient should have a routine chest radiograph performed within 12 hours prior to imaging or receive one immediately after. Notify the Nuclear Medicine Department if patients require high flow oxygen or respirator assistance. **SPECIAL INSTRUCTIONS:** Requisition must state the current patient diagnosis in order to select the most appropriate radiopharmaceutical and/or imaging technique. **DURATION OF PROCEDURE:** 30 minutes to 1 hour **RADIOPHARMACEUTICAL:** See table.

Radiopharmaceuticals for Lung Ventilation Imaging

Agent	Isotope Half-Life	Timing vs Perfusion Scan	Advantages	Disadvantages
^{99m}Tc DTPA aerosol	6 hours	Before	Multiple views of ventilation	Turbulent air flow can cause patchy distribution; no washout phase
^{133}Xe gas	5 days	Before	Single view with equilibrium and washout phases	Requires good single-breath effort; single view (usually posterior)
^{127}Xe gas	36 days	After	Single view with equilibrium and washout phases; may be performed after perfusion scan	
^{81m}Kr gas	13 seconds	During	Multiple views of ventilation; no gas trap required	Nonavailability on 24-hour basis; expense

Specimen **CAUSES FOR REJECTION:** Other recent Nuclear Medicine procedure may interfere. If uncertain, call the Nuclear Medicine Department. **TURNAROUND TIME:** A written report will be sent to the patient's chart and/or to the referring physician.

Interpretation **NORMAL FINDINGS:** Homogeneous distribution of activity throughout the lungs **LIMITATIONS:** Patients must be able to cooperate in performing this test. They will be required to breathe through a mouthpiece, remain still for approximately 15 minutes, (usually in the supine position) and if xenon gas is used, hold their breath for 10 seconds or longer. The procedure is somewhat nonspecific in the presence of underlying lung conditions such as pneumonia or chronic obstructive disease. A same day chest radiograph is necessary for review and comparison with scan findings. **ADDITIONAL INFORMATION:** Patients on high flow oxygen or respirator assistance can undergo ventilation scans with radioactive aerosols using special nebulizer adaptors.

References

Butler SP, Alderson PO, Greenspan RL, et al, "The Utility of Technetium-99m DTPA Inhalational Scans in Artificially Ventilated Patients," *J Nucl Med*, 1990, 31(1):46-51.

Kahn D, Bushnell DL, Dean R, et al, "Clinical Outcome of Patients With a "Low Probability" of Pulmonary Embolism on Ventilation-Perfusion Lung Scan," *Arch Intern Med*, 1989, 149(2):377-9.

(Continued)

Lung Scan, Ventilation *(Continued)*

PIOPED Investigators, "Value of the Ventilation/Perfusion Scan in Acute Pulmonary Embolism, Results of the Prospective Investigation of Pulmonary Embolism Diagnosis (PIOPED)," *JAMA*, 1990, 263(20):2753-9.

Marrow Scan *see* Bone Marrow Scan *on page 360*

Mebrofenin® Scan *see* Biliary Scan *on page 358*

Meckel's Diverticulum Scan

CPT 78290

Synonyms Ectopic Gastric Mucosa Scan; Meckel's Scan; Meckel's Scintigraphy

Abstract **PROCEDURE COMMONLY INCLUDES:** The patient receives an intravenous injection of technetium-99m (^{99m}Tc) pertechnetate which is quickly secreted by gastric mucosa cells including sites of ectopic tissue, the Meckel's diverticulum. Sequential images of the abdomen are then acquired. The abnormality usually visualizes early, but delayed images are sometimes necessary. **INDICATIONS:** The procedure is useful in detecting the presence and location of a Meckel's diverticulum, a collection of functioning ectopic gastric mucosa usually located in the ileum and in the right lower quadrant of the abdomen. The abnormality usually occurs in young children and 50% of cases that bleed symptomatically will present before the age of 2 years.

Patient Care/Scheduling **PATIENT PREPARATION:** Patient should have all RIA blood work performed, or at least drawn, prior to injection of any radioactive material. Patient must be fasting at least 4 hours before scan. **SPECIAL INSTRUCTIONS:** Requisition must state the current patient diagnosis in order to select the most appropriate radiopharmaceutical and/or imaging technique. **DURATION OF PROCEDURE:** 30 minutes to 1 hour although additional delayed images may be required. **RADIOPHARMACEUTICAL:** ^{99m}Tc pertechnetate.

Specimen **CAUSES FOR REJECTION:** Residual barium in GI tract from recent x-rays, other recent Nuclear Medicine procedure may interfere. If uncertain, call the Nuclear Medicine Department. **TURNAROUND TIME:** A written report will be sent to the patient's chart and/or to the referring physician.

Interpretation **NORMAL FINDINGS:** Lack of any focal secreted activity in the abdomen. Patients are often placed in a left lateral decubitus position to slow transit of normal secreted activity from the stomach into the small bowel. **LIMITATIONS:** A Meckel's diverticulum without functioning gastric mucosa will not visualize. However, those lacking mucosa are also unlikely to bleed. Some false-positives may result from nondiverticular bleeding, intussusception, duplication cysts, or inflammatory bowel disease.

References

Cooney DR, Duszynski DO, Camboa E, et al, "The Abdominal Technetium Scan (A Decade of Experience)," *J Pediatr Surg*, 1982, 17:611-9.

Dutro JA, Santanello SA, Unger F, et al, "Rectal Bleeding in a 4-Month Old Boy," *JAMA*, 1986, 255:2239-40.

Gilday DL, Eng B, and Pui M, "Specific Problems in Children," *Diagnostic Nuclear Medicine*, Gottschalk A, Hoffer PB, and Potchen EJ, eds, Baltimore, MD: Williams & Wilkins, 1988, 997-8.

Sfakianakis GN and Conway JJ, "Detection of Ectopic Gastric Mucosa in Meckel's Diverticulum and in Other Aberrations by Scintigraphy: II. Indications and Methods – A 10-Year Experience," *J Nucl Med*, 1981, 22:732-8.

Meckel's Scan *see* Meckel's Diverticulum Scan *on this page*

Meckel's Scintigraphy *see* Meckel's Diverticulum Scan *on this page*

MUGA *see* Cardiac Blood Pool Scan, ECG-Gated *on page 363*

Myocardial Infarction Scan

CPT 78466 (qualitative); 78467 (quantitative)

Synonyms Acute Myocardial Infarction Scan; Infarct-Avid Scan; PYP Cardiac Scan; Pyrophosphate Cardiac Scan

Abstract **PROCEDURE COMMONLY INCLUDES:** The patient receives an intravenous injection of a ^{99m}Tc pyrophosphate radiopharmaceutical which localizes in recently infarcted myocardial tissue. Multiple images of the heart are acquired at 1-3 hours after isotope injection. **INDICATIONS:** The primary indication for pyrophosphate cardiac imaging is the detection of recent myocardial infarction. Pyrophosphate will localize in damaged myocardium as a result of necrosis and disruption of myocardial cell membranes. This procedure is not useful in the first 24 hours after acute infarction. Maximum localization will occur from 24-72 hours after an acute event and then gradually diminish over the next 10-14 days. Vary rarely, especially in elderly patients, pyrophosphate will continue to localize indefinitely. Positive scans in patients with unstable angina indicate a higher risk of subsequent infarction. Pyrophosphate imaging has also been used to detect non-necrotic damage in cardiac contusions as well as some cardiomyopathies, amyloidosis, and sarcoidosis.

Patient Care/Scheduling **PATIENT PREPARATION:** The patient does not need to be fasting or NPO for this procedure. Patient should have all RIA blood work performed, or at least drawn, prior to injection of any radioactive material. If not contraindicated by the cardiac status, patients should be encouraged to ingest fluids and to void frequently in order to enhance renal excretion of isotope and decrease background activity. **SPECIAL INSTRUCTIONS:** Requisition must state the current patient diagnosis in order to select the most appropriate radiopharmaceutical and/or imaging technique. **DURATION OF PROCEDURE:** 2-4 hours **RADIOPHARMACEUTICAL:** ^{99m}Tc pyrophosphate.

Method **TECHNIQUE:** The application of single-photon emission tomography (SPECT) techniques may contribute significantly to the diagnostic accuracy of this imaging study.

Specimen **CAUSES FOR REJECTION:** Other recent Nuclear Medicine procedure may interfere. If uncertain, call the Nuclear Medicine Department. **TURNAROUND TIME:** A written report will be sent to the patient's chart and/or to the referring physician.

Interpretation **NORMAL FINDINGS:** The radiopharmaceutical normally localizes in bone. There should be no uptake above background activity in the myocardium. When there is localization in the myocardium it is usually graded (1+ to 4+) relative to rib uptake. **LIMITATIONS:** The timing of this procedure is important and should be from 1-3 days after an acute onset of symptoms. Earlier or later timing may give false-negative results. Cardioversion causing localized chest wall burns or cracked ribs may complicate interpretation. Use in other conditions such as cardiomyopathy or amyloidosis is less specific. False-positive scans may result from pericarditis or myocarditis, cardiac neoplasms, aneurysms, or calcifications in valves and coronary arteries.

References

Antunes ML, Seldin DW, Wall RM, et al, "Measurement of Acute Q-Wave Myocardial Infarct Size With Single Photon Emission Computed Tomography Imaging of Indium-111 Antimyosin," *Am J Cardiol*, 1989, 63(12):777-83.

Botvinick EH, "Hot Spot Imaging Agents for Acute Myocardial Infarction," *J Nucl Med*, 1990, 31(2):143-6.

Lewis SE, Parkey RW, Bonte FJ, et al, "Infarct-Avid Imaging in Acute Myocardial Infarction," *Diagnostic Nuclear Medicine*, Gottschalk A, Hoffer PB, and Potchen EJ, eds, Baltimore, MD: Williams & Wilkins, 1988, 399-413.

Myocardial Perfusion Scan

CPT 78460 (resting, quantitative or qualitative); 78461 (exercise and redistribution)

Synonyms Stress Thallium Scan; Thallium-201 Scan, Thallium Stress Test

Applies to Rest Thallium Scan; Thallium Scan, Rest Only

Abstract **PROCEDURE COMMONLY INCLUDES:** The patient undergoes either physiologic stress with routine treadmill exercise or pharmacologic "stress" with an infusion of a vasodilator such as dipyridamole or adenosine. At maximum stress, the patient receives an intravenous injection of thallium-201 chloride, a potassium analog which localizes in muscle tissue, including the myocardium, in proportion to regional blood flow and cell viability. Images of the heart are acquired immediately after stress and again in the thallium redistribution (resting) phase 2-4 hours later. An early defect which normalizes in the redistribution phase implies ischemia. A persistent defect indicates scarring. **INDICATIONS:** Myocardial perfusion imaging is employed to evaluate patients with known or suspected coronary artery stenoses. Regional areas of stress-induced myocardial ischemia or residual scarring (infarction) can be identified. Routine applications are in the differential diagnosis of chest pain and in the follow-up of patients who have had myocardial infarctions and/or who have undergone interventions such as coronary bypass surgery or balloon angioplasty.

(Continued)

Myocardial Perfusion Scan *(Continued)*

Patient Care/Scheduling **PATIENT PREPARATION:** Must be fasting from midnight the night before the test. The patient should have all RIA blood work performed, or at least drawn, prior to the injection of any radioactive material. **SPECIAL INSTRUCTIONS:** Requisition must state the current patient diagnosis in order to select the most appropriate radiopharmaceutical and/or imaging technique. **DURATION OF PROCEDURE:** 4 hours **RADIOPHARMACEUTICAL:** Thallium-201 thallous chloride.

Method **TECHNIQUE:** The application of single-photon emission tomography (SPECT) techniques may contribute significantly to the diagnostic accuracy of this imaging study.

Specimen **CAUSES FOR REJECTION:** Other recent Nuclear Medicine procedure may interfere. If uncertain, call the Nuclear Medicine Department. **TURNAROUND TIME:** A written report will be sent to the patient's chart and/or to the referring physician.

Interpretation **NORMAL FINDINGS:** Homogeneous distribution of isotope throughout all segments of the left ventricle with no transient or fixed thallium defects **LIMITATIONS:** Some false-positive results occur in females, patients with valvular disease, and patients with hypertrophic cardiomyopathies. Inadequate submaximal treadmill stress may result in false-negative results. Many quantitative computer processing techniques have been developed to improve the diagnostic accuracy of thallium imaging. These techniques need to be validated and compared with a normal population at each clinical site for optimum application. Recent studies have shown that severe ischemia may cause a persistent defect at 2-4 hours of redistribution. Additional delayed images at 6-24 hours may demonstrate the reversible pattern of ischemia. Thallium imaging is unable to distinguish the age of a persistent defect (scarring or infarction), ie, between old or new infarction. **ADDITIONAL INFORMATION:** This procedure is normally performed in conjunction with a standard stress electrocardiogram test.

References

Fintel DJ, Links JM, Brinker JA, et al, "Improved Diagnostic Performance of Exercise Thallium-201 Single Photon Emission Computed Tomography Over Planar Imaging in the Diagnosis of Coronary Artery Disease: A Receiver Operating Characteristic Analysis," *J Am Coll Cardiol*, 1989, 13(3):600-12.

Freeman MR, Chisholm RJ, and Armstrong PW, "Usefulness of Exercise Electrocardiography and Thallium Scintigraphy in Unstable Angina Pectoris in Predicting the Extent and Severity of Coronary Artery Disease," *Am J Cardiol*, 1988, 62(17):1164-70.

Hör G, Kober G, Maul F-D, et al, "Assessing Coronary Angioplasty With Myocardial Perfusion Imaging," *Nucl Med Ann*, 1990, 95-112.

Nunn AD, "Radiopharmaceuticals for Imaging Myocardial Perfusion," *Semin Nucl Med*, 1990, 20(2):111-8.

Ranhosky A and Kempthorne-Rawson J, "The Safety of Intravenous Dipyridamole Thallium Myocardial Perfusion Imaging," *Circulation*, 1990, 81(4):1205-9.

Parathyroid Localization Scan *see* Parathyroid Scan *on this page*

Parathyroid Scan

CPT 78070

Synonyms Parathyroid Localization Scan; Parathyroid Scintigraphy

Replaces Selenium-75 Parathyroid Scan

Abstract **PROCEDURE COMMONLY INCLUDES:** The patient receives intravenous injections of thallium-201 chloride and technetium-99m (^{99m}Tc) pertechnetate in a sequence with computer acquisition of images to enable an appropriate image subtraction technique. This allows for identification of a hyperemic (thallium-201) parathyroid adenoma after separation of normal thyroid (^{99m}Tc) activity. **INDICATIONS:** Parathyroid imaging with a dual-isotope subtraction technique is useful in the preoperative localization of overactive parathyroid glands, especially in differentiating a solitary adenoma from a generalized parathyroid hyperplasia. The sensitivity of the technique is approximately 85%.

Patient Care/Scheduling **PATIENT PREPARATION:** Patient should have all RIA blood work performed, or at least drawn, prior to injection of any radioactive material. The patient does not need to be fasting or NPO for this procedure. **SPECIAL INSTRUCTIONS:** Requisition must state the current patient diagnosis in order to select the most appropriate radiopharmaceutical and/or imaging technique. **DURATION OF PROCEDURE:** 30 minutes to 1 hour **RADIOPHARMACEUTICAL:** Thallium-201 thallous chloride and ^{99m}Tc pertechnetate.

Specimen **CAUSES FOR REJECTION:** Other recent Nuclear Medicine procedure may interfere. Recent radiographic procedure involving iodinated contrast administration may preclude thyroid localization of ^{99m}Tc pertechnetate. If uncertain, call the Nuclear Medicine Department. **TURNAROUND TIME:** A written report will be sent to the patient's chart and/or to the referring physician.

Interpretation **NORMAL FINDINGS:** No thallium-201 activity above background in the computer-subtracted images of the thyroid/parathyroid region of the neck. **LIMITATIONS:** Poor localization of ^{99m}Tc pertechnetate in the thyroid gland due to exogenous iodine or hypothyroidism may give erroneous results. Nodular disease, eg, multinodular goiter, neoplasm, and cysts will also frequently give false-positive results.

References

Krubsack AJ, Wilson SD, Lawson TL, et al, "Prospective Comparison of Radionuclide, Computed Tomographic, and Sonographic Localization of Parathyroid Tumors," *World J Surg*, 1986, 10:579-85.

Miller DL, Doppman JL, Shawker TH, et al, "Localization of Parathyroid Adenomas in Patients Who Have Undergone Surgery. Part I. Noninvasive Imaging Methods," *Radiology*, 1987, 162:133-7.

Okerlund M, "Scintigraphy Finds Tumors in Parathyroid Glands," *Diagnostic Imaging*, 1988, 6:130-4.

Statz E and Oates E, "Scintigraphic Demonstration of an Ectopic Parathyroid Adenoma," *Clin Nucl Med*, 1988, 13:130-1.

Parathyroid Scintigraphy *see* Parathyroid Scan *on previous page*

Parotid Scan *see* Salivary Gland Scan *on page 383*

^{32}P Chromate Therapy *see* Radioactive Phosphorus Treatment of Metastatic Cavitary Effusions *on page 379*

Perchlorate Discharge Test *see* Thyroid Uptake *on page 387*

Perfusion Lung Scan *see* Lung Scan, Perfusion *on page 372*

Perfusion-Ventilation Scan *see* Lung Scan, Perfusion *on page 372*

Phlebothrombogram, Radionuclide *see* Venogram, Radionuclide *on page 389*

Phosphorus Treatment for Polycythemia Vera *see* Radioactive Phosphorus Treatment for Polycythemia Vera *on next page*

Plasma/Blood Volume *see* Blood Volume *on page 359*

Plasma Volume Measurement *see* Blood Volume *on page 359*

Polycythemia Vera, Radioactive Phosphorus Therapy *see* Radioactive Phosphorus Treatment for Polycythemia Vera *on next page*

^{32}P Phosphate Treatment for Thrombocytosis *see* Radioactive Phosphorus Treatment for Polycythemia Vera *on next page*

Pulmonary Scan *see* Lung Scan, Perfusion *on page 372*

PYP Cardiac Scan *see* Myocardial Infarction Scan *on page 374*

Pyrophosphate Cardiac Scan *see* Myocardial Infarction Scan *on page 374*

Quantitative Perfusion Lung Scan *see* Lung Scan, Perfusion *on page 372*

Quantitative Ventilation Lung Scan *see* Lung Scan, Ventilation *on page 373*

Radioactive Iodine Therapy

CPT 79000 (initial); 79001 (subsequent)

Synonyms Iodine Therapy; ^{131}I Therapy; Radioiodine Therapy

Abstract **PROCEDURE COMMONLY INCLUDES:** The patient receives an oral dose of iodine-131 sodium iodide which localizes in thyroid tissue and/or iodine-avid sites of metastases from

(Continued)

Radioactive Iodine Therapy *(Continued)*

thyroid carcinoma. The radioiodine partially or fully ablates these tissues. **INDICATIONS:** Radioiodine therapy is used in the treatment of hyperthyroidism, Graves' disease, toxic multinodular goiters, and some thyroid carcinoma.

Patient Care/Scheduling **PATIENT PREPARATION:** Patient should have all RIA blood work performed, or at least drawn, prior to ingestion of radioiodine. Patients should be fasting for at least 2 hours before receiving the oral radioiodine dose. They may resume their normal diet 1 hour after the dose is given. Any recently ingested iodine or radiographic procedures using iodinated contrast may suppress proper localization of radioiodine. Refer to Limitations. **Note**: Any patient receiving 30 mCi or more of iodine-131 sodium iodide must be admitted to the hospital until the calculated residual body burden is <30 mCi. Other radiation safety regulations also govern high doses of radioiodine. Call Nuclear Medicine for current requirements. **SPECIAL INSTRUCTIONS:** Requisition must state the current patient diagnosis in order to select the most appropriate radiopharmaceutical and/or imaging technique. Special instructions governing radioiodine therapy will be discussed with the patient by Nuclear Medicine personnel.

Specimen **CAUSES FOR REJECTION:** Other recent Nuclear Medicine procedure may interfere. If uncertain, call the Nuclear Medicine Department. **TURNAROUND TIME:** A written report will be sent to the patient's chart and/or to the referring physician at the completion of the procedure.

Interpretation **LIMITATIONS:** Iodine-containing compounds and foods interfere with any tests using radioactive iodine. The following exogenous iodine sources may suppress uptake measurements or scans for the time indicated:

- iodine compounds (Lugol's, tincture, potassium iodide, kelp): 1-2 weeks
- seafood, Ovaltine®, vitamin pills, Ornade®, Combid® cough syrups: 3-5 days
- Diodrast, Hypaque®, Renografin®, (ie, intravenous pyelograms, CT with contrast and arteriograms): 4-6 weeks
- lipiodol (ie, bronchograms), Oragrafin® (ie, gallbladder exams), Pantopaque® (ie, myelograms): at least 6 months
- antithyroid drugs (ie, propylthiouracil, Tapazole®): 7 days
- thyroid hormone (ie, desiccated thyroid, thyroxine): 4 weeks
- tri-iodothyronine (Cytomel®): 10-12 day

Call the Nuclear Medicine Department for further information.

References

Becker DV and Hurley JR, "Radioiodine Treatment of Hyperthyroidism," *Diagnostic Nuclear Medicine*, Gottschalk A, Hoffer PB, and Potchen EJ, eds, Baltimore, MD: Williams & Wilkins, 1988, 778-91.

Simpson WJ, Panzarella T, Carruthers JS, et al, "Papillary and Follicular Thyroid Cancer: Impact of Treatment in 1578 Patients," *Int J Radiat Oncol Biol Phys*, 1988, 14:1063.

Velkeniers B, Cytryn R, Vanhaelst L, et al, "Treatment of Hyperthyroidism With Radioiodine: Adjunctive Therapy With Antithyroid Drugs Reconsidered," *Lancet*, 1988, 1(8595):1127-9.

Radioactive Iodine Uptake *see* Thyroid Uptake *on page 387*

Radioactive Phosphorus Treatment for Polycythemia Vera

CPT 79100

Synonyms Polycythemia Vera, Radioactive Phosphorus Therapy; Phosphorus Treatment for Polycythemia Vera

Applies to ^{32}P Phosphate Treatment for Thrombocytosis

Abstract **PROCEDURE COMMONLY INCLUDES:** The patient receives an intravenous injection of soluble phosphorus-32 (^{32}P) phosphate as a therapeutic intervention for polycythemia vera. **INDICATIONS:** Intravenous ^{32}P phosphate is useful in controlling the thrombocytosis of polycythemia vera.

Patient Care/Scheduling **PATIENT PREPARATION:** Patient should have all RIA blood work performed, or at least drawn, prior to injection of any radioactive material. The patient does not need to be fasting or NPO for this procedure. **SPECIAL INSTRUCTIONS:** Requisition must state the current patient diagnosis in order to select the most appropriate radiopharmaceutical and/or imaging technique. **RADIOPHARMACEUTICAL:** ^{32}P sodium phosphate (soluble).

References

Price DC and McIntyre PA, "The Hematopoietic System," *Textbook of Nuclear Medicine*, Vol II, Harbert J and DaRocha AFG, eds, Philadelphia, PA: Lea & Febiger, 1984, 588-96.

Wagner S, Waxman J, and Sikora K, "Treatment of Essential Thrombocythemia With Radioactive Phosphorus," *Clin Radiol*, 1989, 40(2):190-2.

Radioactive Phosphorus Treatment of Metastatic Cavitary Effusions

CPT 79200

Synonyms ^{32}P Chromate Therapy

Abstract PROCEDURE COMMONLY INCLUDES: A colloidal suspension of phosphorus-32 (^{32}P) chromate is injected into the peritoneal or pleural cavity. INDICATIONS: Intracavitary ^{32}P chromate is useful in treating peritoneal or pleural cavity metastatic implants and/or effusions.

Patient Care/Scheduling PATIENT PREPARATION: Patient should have all RIA blood work performed, or at least drawn, prior to injection of any radioactive material. The patient does not need to be fasting or NPO for this procedure. SPECIAL INSTRUCTIONS: Requisition must state the current patient diagnosis in order to select the most appropriate radiopharmaceutical and/or imaging technique. Paracentesis or thoracocentesis usually precedes the administration procedure. Sufficient fluid should be left in the cavity so that the space can be located RADIOPHARMACEUTICAL: ^{32}P chromic phosphate (colloidal). **Note:** Not for intravascular use.

References

Reddy S, Sutton GP, Stehman FB, et al, "Ovarian Cancer: Adjuvant Treatment With Phosphorus-32," *Radiology*, 1987, 165:275-8.

Taasan V, Shapiro B, Taren JA, et al, "Phosphorus-32 Therapy of Cystic Grade IV Astrocytomas: Technique and Preliminary Application," *J Nucl Med*, 1985, 26:1335-8.

Radioactive Renogram *see* Renal Scan *on page 381*

Radioactive Venogram *see* Venogram, Radionuclide *on page 389*

Radioactive Vitamin B_{12} Absorption Test, With or Without Intrinsic Factor *see* Schilling Test *on page 383*

Radioiodine Therapy *see* Radioactive Iodine Therapy *on page 377*

Radioiodine Thyroid Uptake and/or Scan *see* Thyroid Uptake *on page 387*

Radioisotope Hepatic Scan *see* Liver and Spleen Scan *on page 371*

Radioisotope Liver-Lung Scan *see* Radioisotope Liver-Lung Scan for Subdiaphragmatic Abscesses *on this page*

Radioisotope Liver-Lung Scan for Subdiaphragmatic Abscesses

CPT 78225

Synonyms Lung-Liver Scan for Subdiaphragmatic Abscesses; Radioisotope Liver-Lung Scan

Abstract PROCEDURE COMMONLY INCLUDES: The patient receives intravenous injections of technetium-99m (^{99m}Tc) macroaggregated albumin (MAA) and ^{99m}Tc sulfur colloid to localize the lungs and liver. Multiple images are acquired centered over the right hemidiaphragm to detect any abnormal spaces or loculations between the right lung and liver. INDICATIONS: Liver-lung imaging may be helpful in the detection of subdiaphragmatic abscesses and in differentiating between lung and liver lesions adjacent to the diaphragm.

Patient Care/Scheduling PATIENT PREPARATION: Patient should have all RIA blood work performed, or at least drawn, prior to injection of any radioactive material. The patient does not need to be fasting or NPO for this procedure. SPECIAL INSTRUCTIONS: Requisition must state the current patient diagnosis in order to select the most appropriate radiopharmaceutical and/or imaging technique. DURATION OF PROCEDURE: 1 hour RADIOPHARMACEUTICALS: ^{99m}Tc MAA and ^{99m}Tc sulfur colloid.

(Continued)

Radioisotope Liver-Lung Scan for Subdiaphragmatic Abscesses *(Continued)*

Method TECHNIQUE: The application of single-photon emission tomography (SPECT) techniques may contribute significantly to the diagnostic accuracy of this imaging study.

Specimen CAUSES FOR REJECTION: Barium radiographic procedures within 24 hours prior to isotope. Other recent Nuclear Medicine procedure may interfere. If uncertain, call the Nuclear Medicine Department. TURNAROUND TIME: A written report will be sent to the patient's chart and/or to the referring physician.

Interpretation LIMITATIONS: This study may also be able to delineate a left sided subdiaphragmatic abscess. It is most useful in detecting space occupying lesions between the top of the liver and the right hemidiaphragm. ADDITIONAL INFORMATION: Abdominal CT scanning and radionuclide procedures using gallium-67 or indium-111 leukocytes have largely replaced this procedure.

References

Halvorsen RA Jr, Foster WL Jr, Wilkinson RH Jr, et al, "Hepatic Abscess: Sensitivity of Imaging Tests and Clinical Findings," *Gastrointest Radiol*, 1988, 13(2):135-41.

Oppenheim BE, Wellman HN, and Hoffer PB, "Liver Imaging," *Diagnostic Nuclear Medicine*, Gottschalk A, Hoffer PB, and Potchen EJ, eds, Baltimore, MD: Williams & Wilkins, 1988, 549-50.

Sangar VK, Gini A, Fuentes RT, et al, "Diagnosis of a Liver Abscess With Gallium-67 and Radiocolloid Tomography," *Clin Nucl Med*, 1989, 14:443-5.

Radionuclide Angiography *see* Cardiac Blood Pool Scan, ECG-Gated *on page 363*

Radionuclide Angiography, Stress *see* Cardiac Blood Pool Scan, ECG-Gated *on page 363*

Radionuclide Bone Scan *see* Bone Scan *on page 361*

Radionuclide Cineangiography *see* Cardiac Blood Pool Scan, First Pass *on page 364*

Radionuclide Cisternography *see* Cisternogram *on page 365*

Radionuclide Liver Scan *see* Liver and Spleen Scan *on page 371*

Radionuclide Perfusion Lung Scan *see* Lung Scan, Perfusion *on page 372*

Radionuclide Ventilation Lung Scan *see* Lung Scan, Ventilation *on page 373*

Radionuclide Ventriculogram *see* Cardiac Blood Pool Scan, ECG-Gated *on page 363*

Radionuclide Ventriculogram, First Pass *see* Cardiac Blood Pool Scan, First Pass *on page 364*

RAI Uptake and/or Scan *see* Thyroid Uptake *on page 387*

RBC Survival Test *see* Chromium-51 Red Cell Survival *on page 365*

Red Blood Cell Sequestration *see* Chromium-51 Red Cell Survival *on page 365*

Red Cell Mass *see* Blood Volume *on page 359*

Red Cell Mass *see* Red Cell Volume *on this page*

Red Cell Mass Measurement *see* Blood Volume *on page 359*

Red Cell Survival *see* Chromium-51 Red Cell Survival *on page 365*

Red Cell Volume

CPT 78120

Related Information

Blood Volume *on page 359*

Synonyms Chromium-Labeled Red Cell Volume; Red Cell Mass

Abstract PROCEDURE COMMONLY INCLUDES: Determination of red cell volume is a nonimaging procedure in which the patient receives an intravenous injection of a known volume of his red cells which are labeled with a known amount of chromium (^{51}Cr). A sample of the patient's blood is drawn after equilibration of the radiolabeled cells and the circulating red cell volume can then be calculated. **INDICATIONS:** Red cell volume measurement is helpful in the differential diagnosis of polycythemia. The procedure is also helpful in monitoring the effects of some antineoplastic drugs. Red cell volume measurement is routinely combined with plasma volume measurements to determine total blood volume (see Blood Volume). **CONTRAINDICATIONS:** Patient actively bleeding, edema.

Patient Care/Scheduling **PATIENT PREPARATION:** Patient should have all RIA blood work performed, or at least drawn, prior to injection of any radioactive material. The patient does not need to be fasting or NPO for this procedure. Other blood samples should not be taken during this procedure. Nor should transfusions of blood products be given. **SPECIAL INSTRUCTIONS:** Requisition must state the current patient diagnosis in order to select the most appropriate radiopharmaceutical and/or imaging technique. Also include the patient's accurate height and weight. **DURATION OF PROCEDURE:** 2-3 hours **RADIOPHARMACEUTICAL:** Chromium-51 chromate for RBC label.

Specimen **CAUSES FOR REJECTION:** Other recent Nuclear Medicine procedure may interfere. If uncertain, call the Nuclear Medicine Department. **TURNAROUND TIME:** A written report will be sent to the patient's chart and/or to the referring physician.

Interpretation **NORMAL FINDINGS:** Normal RBC and blood volumes are a function of the size and sex of the patient. Expected volumes are estimated based on body surface area. Measured volumes are compared to the expected results and normally can vary ±20%. Obese patients may have volumes somewhat less than expected. **LIMITATIONS:** The procedure is technically difficult with multiple laboratory steps which tend to introduce errors. **ADDITIONAL INFORMATION:** The assessment of anemia and polycythemia (assessment of whether or not one of these conditions truly exists) depends foremost upon a reliable and direct determination of red cell volume. RBC count, Hgb level, and Hct provide only concentration parameters, the measured number or amount relative to the solution in which it exists. In a number of clinical situations (eg, acute blood loss) the RBC count, Hgb, and Hct will not indicate the actual decrease or increase in circulating red cell mass. In the majority of clinical situations CBC components (RBC count, etc) do correlate with RBC volume. Due to technical complexity (resulting in high cost and prolonged turnaround time), CBC is usually used, especially for follow-up or monitoring situations, even though RBC mass study would provide a more meaningful result. Nevertheless, some clinical situations (eg, polycythemia, complicated fluid, and electrolyte management problems) will benefit from at least initial red cell volume determination.

References

Dawry FP, "Splenic Sequestration of Red Blood Cells: A Computerized Approach Using Two Radionuclides," *J Nucl Med Tech*, 1988, 16:185-6.

Pollycove M and Tono M, "Blood Volume," *Diagnostic Nuclear Medicine*, Gottschalk A, Hoffer PB, and Potchen EJ, eds, Baltimore, MD: Williams & Wilkins, 1988, 690-8.

Srivastava SC and Chervu LR, "Radionuclide-Labeled Red Blood Cells: Current Status and Future Prospects," *Semin Nucl Med*, 1984, 14:68-82.

Renal Scan

CPT 78700 (static only); 78701 (with vascular flow)

Related Information

Angiogram, Radionuclide *on page 358*

Synonyms Kidney Scan; Radioactive Renogram; Renal Scintigraphy; Renogram

Applies to Diuretic Renal Scan; Hippuran Scan; Triple Phase Renal Scan (Renogram, Renal Flow and Scan)

Abstract **PROCEDURE COMMONLY INCLUDES:** The patient receives an intravenous injection of the appropriate renal radiopharmaceutical (see following table). Initial rapid sequence images are acquired to assess renal perfusion if a technetium-99m (^{99m}Tc) compound is used. Sequential static images are then acquired for the next 30-45 minutes to evaluate renal cortical uptake, excretion, and parenchymal clearance. Delayed images may be required to evaluate patients with obstruction or renal insufficiency. **INDICATIONS:** Renal imaging is an accurate technique for evaluating multiple parameters of renal function to compare and correlate with the anatomic information gained by ultrasound or other radio-

(Continued)

Renal Scan *(Continued)*

Radiopharmaceuticals for Renal Imaging

Isotope	Compound	Physiology	Measurement
^{99m}Tc	DMSA	Cortical binding	Renal function; cortical imaging
	DTPA	Glomerular filtration	Renal perfusion and function; quantitative GFR
	Glucoheptonate	Cortical binding	Renal perfusion and function; cortical imaging
	Mertiatide (MAG_3)	Effective renal plasma flow	Renal function; quantitative ERPF
^{123}I ^{131}I	Hippuran	Effective renal plasma flow	Renal function; quantitative ERPF

^{99m}Tc DTPA or glucoheptonate can be given in sufficient dose (10–15 mCi) to accurately assess renal arterial perfusion.
^{123}I hippuran provides better image resolution and technical statistical information than the higher energy ^{131}I form.

graphic procedures. With computer acquisition of images, differential estimates of left and right kidney contributions to glomerular filtration rate and effective renal plasma flow can be calculated. With the use of diuretic stimulation during the functional phase, it is possible to differentiate between anatomic obstruction and nonobstructive residual dilatation from previous hydronephrosis. By using one of the cortical imaging agents (^{99m}Tc GHA or DMSA) high resolution delayed images of isotope activity in the renal cortex can be obtained. These help in evaluating suspected renal masses, scarring, cysts, infarcts, or cortical irregularities such as a column of Bertin. Renal perfusion imaging with ^{99m}Tc DTPA or iodine-131/iodine-123 hippuran after an oral dose of captopril has recently been demonstrated to be a useful screening test for renovascular hypertension.

Patient Care/Scheduling **PATIENT PREPARATION:** Patient should have all RIA blood work performed, or at least drawn, prior to the injection of any radioactive material. The patient does not need to be fasting or NPO for this procedure. In fact, fluid intake should be encouraged during the 2 hours prior to renal imaging unless the patient has a restricted fluid intake for other reasons. **SPECIAL INSTRUCTIONS:** Requisition must state the current patient diagnosis in order to select the most appropriate radiopharmaceutical and/or imaging technique. **DURATION OF PROCEDURE:** 1 to 1 1/2 hour **RADIOPHARMACEUTICAL:** See table.

Specimen **CAUSES FOR REJECTION:** Other recent Nuclear Medicine procedure may interfere. If uncertain, call the Nuclear Medicine Department. **TURNAROUND TIME:** A written report will be sent to the patient's chart and/or to the referring physician.

Interpretation **NORMAL FINDINGS:** Prompt symmetric bilateral perfusion; good early cortical accumulation bilaterally with visualization of the collecting systems by 3-5 minutes postinjection; rapid excretion into the bladder with no delay to indicate a partial or complete obstruction **LIMITATIONS:** At serum creatinine levels >3 mg/dL, renal insufficiency will produce apparent decreases in renal perfusion and function. Hippuran may be the better radiopharmaceutical for imaging in these cases.

References

Conway JJ, "The Role of Scintigraphy in Urinary Tract Infection," *Semin Nucl Med*, 1988, 18(4):308-19.

Eshima D, Fritzberg AR, and Taylor A Jr, "^{99m}Tc Renal Tubular Function Agents: Current Status," *Semin Nucl Med*, 1990, 20(1):28-40.

Fine EJ and Sarkar S, "Differential Diagnosis and Management of Renovascular Hypertension Through Nuclear Medicine Techniques," *Semin Nucl Med*, 1989, 19(2):101-15.

Russell CD and Dubovsky EV, "Measurement of Renal Function With Radionuclides," *J Nucl Med*, 1989, 30(12):2053-7.

Summerville DA, Potter CS, and Treves ST, "The Use of Radiopharmaceuticals in the Measurement of Glomerular Filtration Rate: A Review," *Nucl Med Ann*, 1990, 191-221.

Renal Scintigraphy *see* Renal Scan *on previous page*

Renogram *see* Renal Scan *on previous page*

Rest Thallium Scan *see* Myocardial Perfusion Scan *on page 375*

Rose Bengal Liver Scan *replaced by* Biliary Scan *on page 358*

Salivary Gland Scan

CPT 78230 (salivary gland imaging); 78231 (with serial images); 78232 (function study)

Synonyms Parotid Scan

Abstract PROCEDURE COMMONLY INCLUDES: The patient receives an intravenous injection of technetium-99m (^{99m}Tc) pertechnetate which is taken up and secreted by the salivary glands. Immediate magnified images of the glands are acquired. Repeat images are acquired after the patient ingests lemon juice to stimulate salivary secretion. INDICATIONS: This procedure is helpful in the differential diagnosis of dry mouth conditions, eg, Sjögren's syndrome, salivary duct obstructions, and other parotid conditions such as asymmetric hypertrophy and mass lesions, especially Warthin's tumors.

Patient Care/Scheduling PATIENT PREPARATION: The patient does not need to be fasting or NPO for this procedure. Patient should have all RIA blood work performed, or at least drawn, prior to the injection of any radioactive material. SPECIAL INSTRUCTIONS: Requisition must state the current patient diagnosis in order to select the most appropriate radiopharmaceutical and/or imaging technique. DURATION OF PROCEDURE: 1 hour RADIOPHARMACEUTICAL: ^{99m}Tc pertechnetate.

Specimen CAUSES FOR REJECTION: Other recent Nuclear Medicine procedure may interfere. If uncertain, call the Nuclear Medicine Department. TURNAROUND TIME: A written report will be sent to the patient's chart and/or to the referring physician.

Interpretation LIMITATIONS: The procedure will not definitely differentiate benign lesions from malignant ones. ADDITIONAL INFORMATION: Computer acquisition of scintigraphic data is acquired over time and analysis is performed which is useful for determining salivary flow kinetics. Conditions in which this would be useful are in the diagnosis of Sjögren's syndrome, obstruction with calculi, and sialadenitis.

References

Copely DJ and Smith R, "Salivary Scintigraphy: Unilateral Increased Activity," *Semin Nucl Med*, 1986, 16:222-3.

Dosoretz C and Lieberman LM, "Increased Uptake of Technetium-99M Pertechnetate in a Salivary Gland Cancer," *Clin Nucl Med*, 1987, 12:944-6.

Higashi T, Shinds J, Everhart FR, et al, "Technetium-99M Pertechnetate and Gallium-67 Imaging in Salivary Gland Disease," *Clin Nucl Med*, 1989, 14:504.

Schilling Test

CPT 78270 (without intrinsic factor); 78271 (with intrinsic factor)

Synonyms Radioactive Vitamin B_{12} Absorption Test, With or Without Intrinsic Factor; Schilling Test, Stages 1 and 2; Vitamin B_{12} Absorption Test

Abstract PROCEDURE COMMONLY INCLUDES: The patient ingests an oral dose of radiolabeled vitamin B_{12}. An intramuscular injection of nonradioactive vitamin B_{12} is then given which is rapidly absorbed and saturates any available hepatic binding sites. The radiolabeled vitamin B_{12}, once absorbed in the terminal ileum, is then promptly excreted in the urine. The patient's urine is collected for a 24-hour period and the percent of the original dose present in the urine is calculated. INDICATIONS: The Schilling test measures the patient's ability to absorb vitamin B_{12} from the intestinal tract and to excrete absorbed vitamin into the urine. The stage 1 test employs radiolabeled vitamin B_{12} alone (see table). If abnormal, stage 2, radiolabeled vitamin B_{12} with intrinsic factor is performed. These tests are useful for evaluating any macrocytic anemia to detect pernicious anemia. It helps in the differentiation of intrinsic factor deficiency from other causes of vitamin B_{12} malabsorption. In inflammatory bowel disease the Schilling test helps to determine the presence and severity of involvement in the distal small bowel. On rare occasions, a stage 3 test may be useful. This employs vitamin B_{12} alone but after a 7-10 day course of oral tetracycline. This serves to distinguish bacterial overgrowth in the small bowel from other causes of vitamin B_{12} malabsorption.

Patient Care/Scheduling PATIENT PREPARATION: Patient should have all RIA blood work performed, or at least drawn, prior to injection of any radioactive material. Also, any mea-

(Continued)

Schilling Test *(Continued)*

Schilling Test

Stage	Content	Application
I	Vitamin B_{12}	Screening test for normal absorption vs malabsorption of vitamin
II	Vitamin B_{12} + intrinsic factor	Differentiates conditions of intrinsic factor deficiency (eg, congenital or postgastrectomy) from other causes of malabsorption
III	Vitamin B_{12} after P.O. tetracycline course	Differentiates syndrome of bacterial overgrowth from other causes of malabsorption

surement of serum vitamin B_{12} and folate should be drawn before beginning this test. The patient must be fasting overnight and should remain fasting for an hour after receiving the oral dose of radiolabeled vitamin B_{12}. The patient will be instructed to collect all urine for 24 hours. In some departments, a 48-hour collection is routine, ie, two sequential 24-hour collections. An incomplete urine collection will invalidate the test results. **SPECIAL INSTRUCTIONS:** Requisition must state the current patient diagnosis in order to select the most appropriate radiopharmaceutical and/or imaging technique. **DURATION OF PROCEDURE:** 24-48 hours. **RADIOPHARMACEUTICAL:** Cobalt-57 labeled vitamin B_{12}.

Specimen 24-hour urine collection **CAUSES FOR REJECTION:** Other recent Nuclear Medicine procedure may interfere. If uncertain, call the Nuclear Medicine Department. **TURNAROUND TIME:** A written report will be sent to the patient's chart and/or to the referring physician following submission of urine specimen.

Interpretation **NORMAL FINDINGS:** The normal stage 1 result is an excretion >10% of the originally administered oral dose into the urine within 24 hours. A result <10% excretion should be followed by a stage 2 test. Normalization of excretion in stage 2 confirms a lack of intrinsic factor as the cause of malabsorption. An incomplete urine collection, even the loss of a single specimen in the 24-hour collection, may give an artifactually low result. **LIMITATIONS:** The test without intrinsic factor must be completed before testing with intrinsic factor. If other isotope tests are to be performed, schedule the Schilling tests first. The presence of renal dysfunction, pancreatic insufficiency, myxedema, liver disease, or any other condition resulting in the decreased absorption of B_{12} from the GI tract, its concentration in the liver, or its excretion in the urine may result in abnormal values. This procedure presumes normal renal function. In renal insufficiency or in elderly males with possible prostatic hypertrophy and high bladder residual volumes, urine collections are sometimes continued for 48-72 hours.

References

Cohen MB, "Gamut: Vitamin B_{12} Deficiency," *Semin Nucl Med*, 1981, 11:226.

Fish MB, "Measurement of Gastrointestinal Absorption of Vitamin B_{12}," *Diagnostic Nuclear Medicine*, Gottschalk A, Hoffer PB, and Potchen EJ, eds, Baltimore, MD: Williams & Wilkins, 1988, 699-706.

Schilling Test, Stages 1 and 2 *see* Schilling Test *on previous page*

Scrotal Scan *see* Testicular Scan *on next page*

Selenium-75 Parathyroid Scan *replaced by* Parathyroid Scan *on page 376*

Soft Tissue Scan *see* Gallium Scan, Abscess and/or Tumor *on page 367*

Spectamine® Brain Scan *see* Brain Scan *on page 362*

Spleen Scan *see* Liver and Spleen Scan *on page 371*

Splenic Sequestration Study *see* Chromium-51 Red Cell Survival *on page 365*

Stress Gated Study *see* Cardiac Blood Pool Scan, ECG-Gated *on page 363*

Stress Thallium Scan *see* Myocardial Perfusion Scan *on page 375*

Superior Venacavagram *see* Angiogram, Radionuclide *on page 358*

Survival of Red Blood Cells *see* Chromium-51 Red Cell Survival *on page 365*

Technetium Thyroid Scan *see* Thyroid Scan *on next page*

Testicular Scan

CPT 78760 (testicular imaging); 78761 (with vascular flow)

Synonyms Scrotal Scan; Testicular Torsion Scan

Abstract PROCEDURE COMMONLY INCLUDES: The patient receives an intravenous injection of technetium-99m (^{99m}Tc) pertechnetate. Dynamic serial perfusion images of the scrotal and perineal area are acquired to assess testicular blood flow. Additional static images are also acquired. INDICATIONS: The primary use of testicular imaging is the differentiation between testicular torsion and epididymitis in cases of acute scrotal pain. Other conditions such as hematoma, abscess, tumor, hydrocele, and spermatocele may be detected but the procedure is less accurate for these conditions.

Patient Care/Scheduling PATIENT PREPARATION: Patient should have all RIA blood work performed, or at least drawn, prior to the injection of any radioactive material. The patient does not need to be fasting or NPO for this procedure. SPECIAL INSTRUCTIONS: Requisition must state the current patient diagnosis in order to select the most appropriate radiopharmaceutical and/or imaging technique. DURATION OF PROCEDURE: 30 minutes RADIOPHARMACEUTICAL: ^{99m}Tc pertechnetate.

Specimen TURNAROUND TIME: A written report will be sent to the patient's chart and/or to the referring physician.

Interpretation NORMAL FINDINGS: Homogenous and symmetric distribution of activity in the testes with no focal decreases or increases.

References

Lowry PA, Pjura GA, Kim EE, et al, "Radionuclide Imaging of the Lower Genitourinary Tract," *Diagnostic Nuclear Medicine*, Gottschalk A, Hoffer PB, and Potchen EJ, eds, Baltimore, MD: Williams & Wilkins, 1988, 973-84.

Lutzker LG and Zuckier LS, "Testicular Scanning and Other Applications of Radionuclide Imaging of the Genital Tract," *Semin Nucl Med*, 1990, 20(2):159-88.

Testicular Torsion Scan *see* Testicular Scan *on this page*

Thallium-201 Scan, Thallium Stress Test *see* Myocardial Perfusion Scan *on page 375*

Thallium Scan, Rest Only *see* Myocardial Perfusion Scan *on page 375*

Three-Phase Bone Scan *see* Bone Scan *on page 361*

Thrombophlebogram, Radionuclide *see* Venogram, Radionuclide *on page 389*

Thyroid Metastatic Survey, Iodine-131

CPT 78015 (limited areas); 78017 (multiple areas); 78018 (whole body)

Related Information

Thyroid Scan *on next page*

Synonyms ^{131}I Body Scan; ^{131}I Metastatic Survey; ^{131}I Whole Body Survey

Abstract PROCEDURE COMMONLY INCLUDES: The patient receives an oral dose of iodine-131 sodium iodide which localizes in residual thyroid tissue or in iodine-avid metastatic sites from thyroid carcinoma. Images of the neck, thorax, and other body areas are acquired between 24-72 hours later. INDICATIONS: Radioiodine surveys are used to delineate residual thyroid tissue after surgical procedures for thyroid carcinoma and to detect regional or distant metastases.

Patient Care/Scheduling PATIENT PREPARATION: Patient should have all RIA blood work performed, or at least drawn, prior to injection of any radioactive material. The patient should be fasting (NPO) for 4 hours prior to receiving the oral dose. The patient should avoid ingesting iodine-containing foods or medications for at least 2 weeks prior to the procedure. Any thyroid hormone medications should also be discontinued for at least 2 weeks (T_3) or 4 weeks (T_4). SPECIAL INSTRUCTIONS: Requisition must state the current patient diagnosis in order to select the most appropriate radiopharmaceutical and/or imaging technique. DURATION OF PROCEDURE: 30 minutes RADIOPHARMACEUTICAL: technetium-99m (^{99m}Tc) pertechnetate.

(Continued)

Thyroid Metastatic Survey, Iodine-131 *(Continued)*

Specimen TURNAROUND TIME: A written report will be sent to the patient's chart and/or to the referring physician.

Interpretation NORMAL FINDINGS: There may be normal uptake of radioiodine in residual remnants of tissue after thyroidectomy. There is also excretion of iodine by the salivary glands, stomach, and kidneys/bladder. LIMITATIONS: Administration of iodine-containing foods and medications as well as radiographic contrast media will suppress radioiodine uptake in tissue. Residual functioning thyroid tissue will usually prevent sufficient uptake in metastatic sites to allow visualization. Thus, residual tissue must be ablated with high-dose radioiodine before adequate later investigation for metastases can be undertaken.

References

Hurley JR and Becker DV, "Treatment of Thyroid Carcinoma With Radioiodine," *Diagnostic Nuclear Medicine*, Gottschalk A, Hoffer PB, and Potchen EJ, eds, Baltimore, MD: Williams & Wilkins, 1988, 792-814.

Lakshamanam M, Schaffer A, Robbins J, et al, "A Simplified Low Iodine Diet in I-131 Scanning and Therapy of Thyroid Cancer," *Clin Nucl Med*, 1988, 13:866-8.

Schlumberger M, Archangioli O, Piekarski JD, et al, "Detection and Treatment of Lung Metastases of Differentiated Thyroid Carcinoma in Patients With Normal Chest X-rays," *J Nucl Med*, 1988, 29(11):1790-4.

Thyroid Scan

CPT 78006 (single with uptake); 78007 (multiple with uptake); 78010 (thyroid imaging only); 78011 (with vascular flow)

Related Information

Thyroid Metastatic Survey, Iodine-131 *on previous page*

Synonyms Iodine Thyroid Scan; Technetium Thyroid Scan; Thyroid Scintigraphy

Applies to Thyroid Uptake and Thyroid Scanning

Abstract PROCEDURE COMMONLY INCLUDES: The patient receives an intravenous injection of technetium-99m (^{99m}Tc) pertechnetate which is trapped like iodide in the thyroid gland. Images of the thyroid are acquired beginning 20-40 minutes after injection. If radioactive iodine is employed, the dose of either iodine-131 or iodine-123 is given orally and images are acquired at 24 hours. Either ^{99m}Tc or iodine scans are often combined with radioiodine uptake measurements. INDICATIONS: Thyroid imaging is useful in evaluating the location, approximate size, anatomy, and functional status of the thyroid gland. This is especially helpful for thyroid nodules, multinodular goiter, thyroiditis, and possible ectopic thyroid tissue, eg, lingual or mediastinal.

Patient Care/Scheduling PATIENT PREPARATION: Patient should have all RIA blood work performed, or at least drawn, prior to injection of any radioactive material. Patients should be fasting for at least 2 hours before receiving oral radioiodine. There are no special preparations for ^{99m}Tc scans. Any recently ingested iodine or radiographic procedures using iodinated contrast may suppress radioiodine or ^{99m}Tc localization in the thyroid gland. Refer to Limitations. SPECIAL INSTRUCTIONS: Requisition must state the current patient diagnosis in order to select the most appropriate radiopharmaceutical and/or imaging technique. DURATION OF PROCEDURE: 30 minutes to 1 hour RADIOPHARMACEUTICAL: ^{99m}Tc pertechnetate, iodine-131 or iodine-123 sodium iodide.

Specimen CAUSES FOR REJECTION: Other recent Nuclear Medicine procedure may interfere. If uncertain, call the Nuclear Medicine Department. Recent radiographic procedure using iodinated contrast. TURNAROUND TIME: A written report will be sent to the patient's chart and/or to the referring physician.

Interpretation NORMAL FINDINGS: Homogeneous and symmetric distribution of activity throughout the thyroid gland LIMITATIONS: Iodine-containing compounds and foods interfere with any tests using radioactive iodine. The following exogenous iodine sources may suppress uptake measurements or scans for the time indicated:

- iodine compounds (Lugol's, tincture, potassium iodide, kelp): 1-2 weeks.
- seafood, Ovaltine®, vitamin pills, Ornade®, Combid® cough syrups: 3-5 days
- Diodrast, Hypaque®, Renografin®, (ie, intravenous pyelograms, CT with contrast and arteriograms): 4-6 weeks
- lipiodol (ie, bronchograms), Oragrafin® (ie, gallbladder exams), Pantopaque® (ie, myelograms): at least 6 months

- antithyroid drugs (ie, propylthiouracil, Tapazole®): 7 days
- thyroid hormone (ie, desiccated thyroid, thyroxine): 4 weeks
- tri-iodothyronine (Cytomel®): 10-12 days

Call the Nuclear Medicine Department for further information.

ADDITIONAL INFORMATION: A variation of thyroid scanning is performed for detection of metastases from primary thyroid carcinoma. See Thyroid Metastatic Survey, ^{131}Iodine.

References

Chen JJ, LaFrance ND, Allo MO, et al, "Single Photon Emission Computed Tomography of the Thyroid," *J Clin Endocrinol Metab*, 1988, 66(6):1240-6.

Park HM, Tarver RD, Siddiqui AR, et al, "Efficacy of Thyroid Scintigraphy in the Diagnosis of Intrathoracic Goiter," *Am J Roentgenol*, 1987, 148:527-9.

Sandler MP and Patton JA, "Multimodality Imaging of the Thyroid and Parathyroid Glands," *J Nucl Med*, 1987, 28:122-9.

Schneider AB, "Thyroid Nodules Following Childhood Irradiation: A 1989 Update," *Thyroid Today*, 1989, 12:1-7.

Thyroid Scintigraphy *see* Thyroid Scan *on previous page*

Thyroid Suppression Test *see* Thyroid Uptake *on this page*

Thyroid TSH Stimulation Test *see* Thyroid Uptake *on this page*

Thyroid Uptake

CPT 78000 (single); 78001 (multiple)

Synonyms Radioactive Iodine Uptake; Radioiodine Thyroid Uptake and/or Scan; RAI Uptake and/or Scan; Thyroid Uptake and Scan; Uptake and Scan, 6- and/or 24-Hour

Applies to Perchlorate Discharge Test; Thyroid Suppression Test; Thyroid TSH Stimulation Test; Thyroid Uptake and Thyroid Scanning

Abstract **PROCEDURE COMMONLY INCLUDES:** A small oral dose of radioiodine is administered to the patient. A calculation of uptake by the thyroid gland is made at 4-6 hours and usually again at 24 hours by measuring the radioactivity present in the anterior neck over the gland. **INDICATIONS:** The thyroid uptake directly measures the ability of the thyroid gland to trap and organify circulating iodide. Uptake measurements accurately detect and quantify the effects of thyroid disease. Uptake values are used in conjunction with measurement of circulating thyroid hormone levels to differentiate primary and secondary causes of these conditions. They are also used to plan therapy for thyroid disorders, especially therapy involving larger doses of radioiodine. Serial uptake measurements are helpful in long-term management and follow-up of patients.

Patient Care/Scheduling **PATIENT PREPARATION:** Patient should have all RIA blood work performed, or at least drawn, prior to injection of any radioactive material. Patients should be fasting for at least 2 hours before receiving the oral radioiodine dose. They may resume their normal diet 1 hour after the dose is given. Any recently ingested iodine or radiographic procedures using iodinated contrast may suppress uptake measurements. Refer to Limitations. Thyroid suppression, thyroid stimulation, and perchlorate discharge tests involve measurement of baseline thyroid uptake, then pharmacologic intervention, then repeat uptake measurement. Call the Nuclear Medicine Department for consultation when ordering these tests. **SPECIAL INSTRUCTIONS:** Requisition must state the current patient diagnosis in order to select the most appropriate radiopharmaceutical and/or imaging technique. **DURATION OF PROCEDURE:** 24 hours **RADIOPHARMACEUTICAL:** Iodine-131 or iodine-123 sodium iodide.

Specimen **CAUSES FOR REJECTION:** Other recent Nuclear Medicine procedure may interfere. If uncertain, call the Nuclear Medicine Department. **TURNAROUND TIME:** A written report will be sent to the patient's chart and/or to the referring physician at the completion of the procedure.

Interpretation **NORMAL FINDINGS:** Normal values cover a wide range and are somewhat dependent on local variations in dietary iodine consumption by the population and technical differences between laboratories. An approximate normal range is 5% to 15% at 4-6 hours and 10% to 30% at 24 hours. Normal ranges have gradually decreased in the last 50 years due to progressive increases in dietary iodine sources. **LIMITATIONS:** Iodine-containing compounds and foods interfere with any tests using radioactive iodine. The following ex-

(Continued)

Thyroid Uptake *(Continued)*

ogenous iodine sources may suppress uptake measurements or scans for the time indicated:

- iodine compounds (Lugol's, tincture, potassium iodide, kelp): 1-2 weeks
- seafood, Ovaltine®, vitamin pills, Ornade®, Combid® cough syrups: 3-5 days
- Diodrast, Hypaque®, Renografin®, (ie, intravenous pyelograms, CT with contrast and arteriograms): 4-6 weeks
- lipiodol (ie, bronchograms), Oragrafin® (ie, gallbladder exams), Pantopaque® (ie, myelograms): at least 6 months
- antithyroid drugs (ie, propylthiouracil, Tapazole®): 7 days
- thyroid hormone (ie, desiccated thyroid, thyroxine): 4 weeks
- tri-iodothyronine (Cytomel®): 10-12 days

Call the Nuclear Medicine Department for further information.

ADDITIONAL INFORMATION: If iodine-131 treatment of hyperthyroidism is anticipated at a future date, notify the Nuclear Medicine Department when making appointment for uptake and scan. See table.

Special Tests of Thyroid Function

Test	Intervention	Use
Thyroid suppression	24–hour uptake; tri–iodothyronine (T_3) 24 μg/day orally for 8 days; uptake repeated	Assess borderline hyperthyroidism, autonomy of functioning nodules or diffuse enlargement
Thyroid stimulation	24–hour uptake; thyroid stimulating hormone (TSH) 10 IU/day for 3 days; uptake repeated	Differentiate between primary vs secondary hypothyroidism; identify thyroid tissue (by scanning) suppressed by autonomously functioning nodules
Perchlorate discharge	2–hour uptake; potassium perchlorate 1 g orally; uptake repeated hourly for 2 hours	Measures dissociation between trapping and organification of iodide: congenital or acquired defects

These interventions are approximate and may vary in individual departments.

References

Carpenter WR, Gilliland PF, Piziak VR, et al, "Radioiodine Uptake Following Iodine I-131 Therapy for Graves' Disease: An Early Indicator of Need for Retreatment," *Clin Nucl Med*, 1989, 14:15.

Kitchner MI and Chapman IM, "Subacute Thyroiditis: A Review of 105 Cases," *Clin Nucl Med*, 1989, 14:439.

Okamura K, Sato K, Ikenoue H, et al, "Re-evaluation of the Thyroidal Radioactive Iodine Uptake Test With Special Reference to Reversible Primary Hypothyroidism With Elevated Thyroid Radioiodine Uptake," *J Clin Endocrinol Metab*, 1988, 67(4):720-6.

Sarkar SD, "*In Vivo* Thyroid Studies," *Diagnostic Nuclear Medicine*, Gottschalk A, Hoffer PB, and Potchen EJ, eds, Baltimore, MD: Williams & Wilkins, 1988, 756-68.

Thyroid Uptake and Scan *see* Thyroid Uptake *on previous page*

Thyroid Uptake and Thyroid Scanning *see* Thyroid Uptake *on previous page*

Thyroid Uptake and Thyroid Scanning *see* Thyroid Scan *on page 386*

Total Blood Volume *see* Blood Volume *on page 359*

Triple Phase Renal Scan (Renogram, Renal Flow and Scan) *see* Renal Scan *on page 381*

Uptake and Scan, 6- and/or 24-Hour *see* Thyroid Uptake *on previous page*

V/2 Scan *see* Lung Scan, Perfusion *on page 372*

Vascular Dynamic Study *see* Angiogram, Radionuclide *on page 358*

Vascular Flow Study *see* Angiogram, Radionuclide *on page 358*

VCU *see* Voiding Cystourethrogram, Radionuclide *on this page*

VCUG *see* Voiding Cystourethrogram, Radionuclide *on this page*

Venogram, Radionuclide

CPT 78457 (unilateral); 78458 (bilateral)

Related Information

Cardiac Blood Pool Scan, ECG-Gated *on page 363*

Synonyms Isotope Venogram; Lower Extremity Venogram, Radionuclide; Phlebothrombogram, Radionuclide; Radioactive Venogram; Thrombophlebogram, Radionuclide

Abstract PROCEDURE COMMONLY INCLUDES: The patient receives an intravenous injection by one of the following techniques:

- via a vein in the dorsum of each foot with rapid sequence image acquisition of the venous structures of the lower extremities during and immediately following injection; the radiopharmaceutical is usually technetium-99m (^{99m}Tc) MAA and the procedure is usually performed as part of a perfusion lung scan.
- via an arm vein with static images of the lower extremities acquired at equilibrium; the radiopharmaceutical is usually ^{99m}Tc pertechnetate to radiolabel circulating RBC (See Cardiac Blood Pool Scan, ECG-Gated).

INDICATIONS: Radionuclide venography is used as a screening test for detecting deep vein thrombosis of the lower extremities. It can be performed in patients who are allergic to iodinated radiographic contrast media.

Patient Care/Scheduling PATIENT PREPARATION: The patient does not need to be fasting or NPO for this procedure. Patient should have all RIA blood work performed, or at least drawn, prior to the injection of any radioactive material. SPECIAL INSTRUCTIONS: Requisition must state the current patient diagnosis in order to select the most appropriate radiopharmaceutical and/or imaging technique. DURATION OF PROCEDURE: 1 hour RADIOPHARMACEUTICAL: ^{99m}Tc labeled RBC or ^{99m}Tc MAA.

Specimen CAUSES FOR REJECTION: Other recent Nuclear Medicine procedure may interfere. If uncertain, call the Nuclear Medicine Department. TURNAROUND TIME: A written report will be sent to the patient's chart and/or to the referring physician.

Interpretation NORMAL FINDINGS: Symmetric visualization of deep and superficial large venous structures in the lower extremities LIMITATIONS: Radionuclide venograms have less specificity and less sensitivity than radiographic contrast venograms. It can be difficult to differentiate acute thrombosis from patients with chronic changes due to previous thrombotic disease.

References

LeClerc JR, Wolfson C, Arzoumanian A, et al, "Technetium-99m Red Blood Cell Venography in Patients With Clinically Suspected Deep Vein Thrombosis: A Prospective Study," *J Nucl Med*, 1988, 29(9):1498-506.

Lisbona R, "Radionuclide Venography in the Diagnosis of Deep Vein Thrombosis of the Leg," *Current Concepts Diagn Nucl Med*, 1987, 1:4-8.

Rudavsky AZ, "Radionuclide Angiography in the Evaluation of Arterial and Venous Grafts," *Semin Nucl Med*, 1988, 18(3):261-8.

Ventilation Lung Scan *see* Lung Scan, Ventilation *on page 373*

Ventilation-Perfusion Lung Scan *see* Lung Scan, Perfusion *on page 372*

Ventilation-Perfusion Lung Scan *see* Lung Scan, Ventilation *on page 373*

Vitamin B_{12} Absorption Test *see* Schilling Test *on page 383*

Voiding Cystourethrogram, Radionuclide

CPT 78740

Synonyms Bladder Reflux Study; VCU; VCUG

Abstract PROCEDURE COMMONLY INCLUDES: The patient must have an indwelling urinary bladder catheter in place. A dose of technetium-99m (^{99m}Tc) pertechnetate is instilled into the bladder along with a maximally tolerated volume of sterile normal saline solution via the catheter. Sequential static images of the bladder and ureters are acquired during the fill-

(Continued)

Voiding Cystourethrogram, Radionuclide *(Continued)*

ing, postfilling, voiding, and postvoiding phases to detect retrograde vesicoureteral reflux from the bladder and/or abnormally high postvoid residual volume. **INDICATIONS:** The radionuclide VCUG is a useful procedure for the detection and follow-up of pediatric patients with bladder reflux causing recurrent urinary tract infections. The radionuclide study is more sensitive than a radiographic contrast VCUG and imparts only approximately 10% of the radiation dose. However, a contrast VCUG is often recommended at the time of diagnosis of reflux to better delineate any anatomic abnormalities. The radionuclide procedure is then used as the primary follow-up technique for these patients, many of whom will outgrow their reflux and not require surgical intervention.

Patient Care/Scheduling **PATIENT PREPARATION:** The patient does not need to be fasting or NPO for this procedure. Patient should have all RIA blood work performed, or at least drawn, prior to the injection of any radioactive material. **SPECIAL INSTRUCTIONS:** Requisition must state the current patient diagnosis in order to select the most appropriate radiopharmaceutical and/or imaging technique. **DURATION OF PROCEDURE:** 30 minutes **RADIOPHARMACEUTICAL:** ^{99m}Tc pertechnetate.

Specimen **CAUSES FOR REJECTION:** Other recent Nuclear Medicine procedure may interfere. If uncertain, call the Nuclear Medicine Department. **TURNAROUND TIME:** A written report will be sent to the patient's chart and/or to the referring physician.

Interpretation **NORMAL FINDINGS:** Normal bladder activity which clears upon voiding with no reflux into ureters or significant bladder residual volume **LIMITATIONS:** The radionuclide VCUG had less anatomic resolution than the radiographic contrast technique but is more sensitive and has a lower radiation exposure.

References

Strife JL, Bissett GS, Kirks DR, et al, "Nuclear Cystography and Renal Sonography: Findings in Girls With Urinary Tract Infections," *Am J Roentgenol*, 1989, 153:115-9.

Sty JR and Wells RG, "Radionuclide Cystography," *Nucl Med Ann*, 1990, 223-38.

Summerville DA and Treves ST, "Radionuclide Detection of Vesicoureteral Reflux," *Current Concepts Diagn Nucl Med*, 1986, 3:4-9.

Wall Motion Study *see* Cardiac Blood Pool Scan, ECG-Gated *on page 363*

WBC Scan *see* Indium Leukocyte Scan *on page 370*

White Blood Cell Scan *see* Indium Leukocyte Scan *on page 370*

Whole Body Bone Scan *see* Bone Scan *on page 361*

Xenon Lung Scan *see* Lung Scan, Ventilation *on page 373*

ULTRASOUND

Robert K. Desai, MD

The past decade has seen the rapid and ongoing development of diagnostic ultrasound as a diagnostic tool. B-mode scanning provides superb imaging of many anatomic regions and provides increasingly valuable pathologic information. In addition to standard ultrasound imaging, standard Doppler evaluation and more recently color Doppler studies provide an excellent noninvasive means of evaluating vascular disease and vascular abnormalities.

It is important for the clinician to know and realize that the quality of ultrasound examinations is particularly dependent on the expertise of the operator and interpreter. Additionally, differences between older and newer equipment may be profound and often will impact on the reliability of the study results.

Today, well performed ultrasound examinations and procedures provide answers to questions which heretofore required other more complicated or expensive radiologic procedures. In future years, this trend is expected to continue.

Ultrasound, Abdomen

CPT 76700

Synonyms Abdomen Ultrasound

Applies to Follow-up Ultrasound Abdomen; Follow-up Ultrasound Retroperitoneal; Ultrasound Retroperitoneal

Abstract PROCEDURE COMMONLY INCLUDES: Liver, spleen, gallbladder, pancreas, and biliary tree INDICATIONS: Presence of neoplasms, cystic lesions, enlarged lymph nodes, bile ducts, abdominal abscesses, pancreatic mass or pseudocysts, gallbladder calculi, or any malignancies CONTRAINDICATIONS: Open wound or incision overlying examination area, recent barium study.

Patient Care/Scheduling PATIENT PREPARATION: The patient should not have had a barium study within the 3 days prior to study. The examinations may be up to 1 hour each. An emergency exam or an unpredictably long preceding exam may result in additional delay. **Note**: Ultrasound exam is to be scheduled before endoscopy, endoscopic retrograde cholangiopancreatography, colonoscopy, or a barium study. If barium study was done, bowel preparation is needed before doing ultrasound examination. **No** barium studies should have been done for **at least** 2 days preceding exam. NPO after midnight before day of examination. SPECIAL INSTRUCTIONS: All outpatient examinations are by appointment only. All inpatients are placed on the daily schedule as time permits and are performed as scheduled. Nonemergent examinations are given secondary priority and therefore may not be able to be performed the same day scheduled. Patients will generally be asked to stay after the examination until films are reviewed by the radiologist. Instruct the patient that ultrasound uses sound waves to image the different organs. There is **no** radiation involved, therefore, it is not harmful to the patient.

Method EQUIPMENT: Standard B-mode real time ultrasonic imager with 2-5 MHz transducer TECHNIQUE: A gel is applied to the skin and a handheld transducer is swept across the abdomen to image the appropriate organs. Sound waves are used for the imaging and no radiation exposure is present. Images are recorded on x-ray film. DATA ACQUIRED: Transverse, sagittal, and oblique images of upper abdominal organs.

(Continued)

Ultrasound, Abdomen *(Continued)*

Specimen **CAUSES FOR REJECTION:** Bowel gas, barium, eating or drinking, unresponsive or poorly responsive patient, open wound(s) overlying area of study **TURNAROUND TIME:** A typed report will generally be issued within 36 hours. A preliminary verbal report generally can be given to the referring physician on request.

Interpretation **NORMAL FINDINGS:** Absence of abnormal masses, fluid collections, enlarged structures, or calcifications **ADDITIONAL INFORMATION:** Request for this study will result in imaging of liver, gallbladder, pancreas, and spleen. Individual study of any of these organs can be ordered as a specific examination (eg, gallbladder, ultrasound). Solid and cystic abnormalities of each of these organs may be detected as well as adenopathy or retroperitoneal masses. It is not uncommon to be unable to visualize the pancreas and/or retroperitoneum in its entirety due to overlying bowel gas. Common abnormalities detected by this modality include cholelithiasis, biliary tree dilatation, primary carcinomas of liver, gallbladder, and pancreas as well as metastatic disease to any organ studied. Ascites is also readily detected as well as inflammatory masses or collections.

References

Bernardino ME, "The Liver: Anatomy and Examination Techniques," *Radiology*, Taveras JT and Ferrucci JT, eds, Philadelphia, PA: JB Lippincott, 1988.

Cooperberg PL and Rowley VA, "Abdominal Sonographic Examination Technique," *Radiology*, Taveras JT and Ferrucci JT, eds, Philadelphia, PA: JB Lippincott, 1988.

Goldberg BB, *Abdominal Ultrasonography*, New York, NY: John Wiley and Sons Inc, 1984.

Ultrasound, Abscess Drainage, Guided

CPT 75989

Synonyms Aspiration, Ultrasound Guided; Drainage, Ultrasound Guided

Abstract **PROCEDURE COMMONLY INCLUDES:** The location of abnormal fluid collections and insertion of needle and/or drain into the collection. **INDICATIONS:** Diagnostic aspiration of fluid, therapeutic drainage of fluid **CONTRAINDICATIONS:** Inadequate access by ultrasound, bleeding diathesis.

Patient Care/Scheduling **PATIENT PREPARATION:** NPO for 2 hours prior to examination. Referring physician may desire pretreatment with prophylactic I.V. antibiotics. **AFTERCARE:** Check physician order sheet. Monitor vital signs in department for 1-hour postprocedure. **SPECIAL INSTRUCTIONS:** Inpatients only. All procedures are scheduled after consultation with a radiologist. All inpatients are placed on an "on call" schedule. After hours, approval is given by radiologist "on call". Recent (less than 2 weeks) PT and PTT results should be available at the time of the procedure. **COMPLICATIONS:** Hemorrhage, sepsis.

Method **EQUIPMENT:** Standard B-mode real time ultrasonic imager with 2-5 MHz transducer and biopsy guides if desired. Appropriate aspiration needle (18- to 22-gauge) and drain (5-11 F). **TECHNIQUE:** A gel is applied to the skin and a handheld transducer is swept across the area of interest to image the appropriate organs. Sound waves are used for the imaging and no radiation exposure is present. An appropriate access route is chosen and a needle is placed into the abnormal collection. Local anesthesia as well as I.V. analgesia may be given. Images are recorded on x-ray film.

Specimen Fluid aspirated from abnormal collection **CONTAINER:** Aerobic and anaerobic culture containers **STORAGE INSTRUCTIONS:** Culture containers should be sent immediately to the Bacteriology Laboratory. **CAUSES FOR REJECTION:** Contamination of cutaneous entry site, needle traversing bowel, patient unable to remain motionless during the procedure **TURNAROUND TIME:** A typed report will generally be issued within 36 hours. A preliminary verbal report generally can be given to the referring physician on request.

Interpretation **LIMITATIONS:** Fluid unable to be obtained due to inadequate access or increased viscosity **ADDITIONAL INFORMATION:** If therapeutic, this procedure may preclude the need for surgery.

References

Mueller PR and Van Sonnenberg EV, "Abscesses and Fluid Collections: Detection and Drainage," *Radiology*, Taveras JT and Ferrucci JT, eds, Philadelphia, PA: JB Lippincott, 1988.

Rifkin MD and Goldberg BB, "Aspiration and Biopsy Techniques," *Abdominal Ultrasonography*, Goldberg BB, ed, New York, NY: John Wiley and Sons Inc, 1984.

Ultrasound, Amniocentesis

CPT 76947

Synonyms Amniocentesis Ultrasound

Abstract PROCEDURE COMMONLY INCLUDES: Locating appropriate puncture site for amniocentesis and subsequent performance of amniocentesis under direct visualization. INDICATIONS: Used in the last two trimesters of pregnancy to determine postmaturation, deformities, Rh incompatibility, amniotic fluid bilirubin level, amniotic fluid L/S ratio, amniotic fluid α-fetoprotein level, and genetic malformations CONTRAINDICATIONS: Inadequate amount of fluid, anterior placenta, presence of fetal vertex or trunk in needle path.

Patient Care/Scheduling PATIENT PREPARATION: The examination may be long, up to 1 hour including waiting time. An emergency examination or an unpredictably long preceding examination may result in additional delay. **Note**: Each Rh-negative unsensitized woman whose husband is not known to be Rh-negative should receive Rh immune globulin. SPECIAL INSTRUCTIONS: Patient is brought to Radiology and the procedure is performed by a radiologist or obstetrician with the aid of ultrasound. Patient is required to stay in the hospital for a few hours for precautionary measures. COMPLICATIONS: Pain, amnionitis (infection), abortion, hemorrhage, trauma to fetus, rupture of membranes, placental or subchorionic hematoma, Rh sensitization, premature labor, abruptio placenta, maternal death.

Method EQUIPMENT: Standard B-mode real time ultrasonic imager with 2-5 MHz transducer. Biopsy guide if desired; 20- or 22-gauge spinal needle. TECHNIQUE: Under ultrasound guidance, an appropriate location is found to insert a small needle into the amniotic fluid. The skin is marked appropriately and prepared for placement of the needle using sterile technique. Needle is placed and amniotic fluid aspirated. DATA ACQUIRED: Images of area to be sampled.

Specimen Amniotic fluid CAUSES FOR REJECTION: Patient not able to tolerate exam TURNAROUND TIME: A typed report will generally be issued within 36 hours. A preliminary verbal report generally can be given to the referring physician on request.

Interpretation NORMAL FINDINGS: Successful aspiration of adequate amount of amniotic fluid LIMITATIONS: Amniotic fluid not obtainable due to placenta location or lack of suitable puncture site, little or no amniotic fluid available for amniocentesis.

References

Platt LO, Hill LM, DeVore GR, et al, "Amniocentesis: Current Concepts and Techniques," *The Principles and Practice of Ultrasonography in Obstetrics Gynecology*, Sanders and James. eds, Norwalk, CT: Appleton-Century-Crofts, 1985.

Ultrasound, Aorta

CPT 76926

Synonyms Aorta Ultrasound

Abstract PROCEDURE COMMONLY INCLUDES: Abdominal aorta and proximal iliac arteries INDICATIONS: Determine the presence and size of aortic aneurysms CONTRAINDICATIONS: Recent barium study.

Patient Care/Scheduling PATIENT PREPARATION: Patient is held NPO at midnight. Please inform all patients that the examinations may be up to 1 hour including waiting time. An emergency exam or an unpredictably long preceding exam may result in additional delay. **Note**: Ultrasound exam is to be scheduled before endoscopy, endoscopic retrograde cholangiopancreatography, colonoscopy, or a barium study. If a barium study was done, bowel preparation is needed before doing ultrasound examination. **No** barium studies should have been done for **at least** 2 days preceding exam. SPECIAL INSTRUCTIONS: All outpatient exams are by appointment only. All inpatients are placed on a daily schedule and called for exam in order of priority. After hours, approval is given by radiologist "on call". Instruct the patient that ultrasound uses sound waves to image the different organs. There is **no** radiation involved, therefore, it is not harmful to the patient. Patient may be asked to wait until the films are checked to make sure more are not necessary.

Method EQUIPMENT: Standard B-mode real time ultrasonic imager with 2-5 MHz transducer TECHNIQUE: A gel is applied to the skin and a handheld transducer is swept across the aorta to image the appropriate organs. Sound waves are used for the imaging and no radiation exposure is present. Images are recorded on x-ray film. DATA ACQUIRED: Transverse and longitudinal images of abdominal aorta and bifurcation.

(Continued)

Ultrasound, Aorta *(Continued)*

Specimen CAUSES FOR REJECTION: Bowel gas, barium, eating or drinking TURNAROUND TIME: A typed report will be generated within 36 hours. A preliminary verbal report will be given to the referring physician upon request.

Interpretation NORMAL FINDINGS: ≤3 cm maximal transverse diameter CRITICAL VALUES: Maximal transverse diameter >3 cm ADDITIONAL INFORMATION: Ultrasound is a useful modality to evaluate for presence of an abdominal aortic aneurysm, particularly involving the distal aorta. Evaluation of the proximal abdominal aorta may be problematic due to overlying bowel gas.

References

Gooding GA, "B-Mode and Duplex Examination of the Aorta, Iliac Arteries and Portal Vein," *Introduction to Vascular Ultrasonography*, Zweibel WJ, ed, New York, NY: Grune and Stratton Inc, 1986.

Ultrasound Aspiration *see* Ultrasound, Biopsy Localization *on this page*

Ultrasound, Biopsy Localization

CPT 76943

Synonyms Biopsy Localization Ultrasound; Ultrasound Aspiration; Ultrasound Localization

Abstract PROCEDURE COMMONLY INCLUDES: Localization of abnormal mass followed by biopsy under direct visualization. INDICATIONS: Cyst localization, organ or lesion biopsy or aspiration CONTRAINDICATIONS: Bleeding diathesis.

Patient Care/Scheduling PATIENT PREPARATION: NPO for 2 hours prior to examination. The procedure may take up to several hours depending on the complexity of any given individual case. PT and PTT are performed within 48 hours prior to procedure. AFTERCARE: Check physician order sheet. Monitor vital signs in department for 3 hours if patient is an outpatient, 1 hour is patient is an inpatient. SPECIAL INSTRUCTIONS: All outpatient exams are by appointment only. All procedures are scheduled after consultation with radiologist. All inpatients are placed on a daily schedule and called for in order of priority. After hours, approval is given by radiologist "on call". Recent PT and PTT results should be available at time of procedure. COMPLICATIONS: Bleeding, infection.

Method EQUIPMENT: Standard B-mode real time ultrasonic imager with biopsy guide, 2-5 MHz transducer, aspiration or cutting type biopsy needle (18- to 22-gauge). TECHNIQUE: A gel is applied to the skin and a handheld transducer is swept across the area of interest to image the appropriate organs. Sound waves are used for the imaging and no radiation exposure is present. An appropriate access route is chosen and a needle is placed into the abnormal collection. Local anesthesia as well as I.V. analgesia may be given. Images are recorded on x-ray film. DATA ACQUIRED: Tissue and/or fluid samples, images of area and/or organ biopsied.

Specimen Fluid and/or tissue CONTAINER: Sterile saline, sterile slides for cytology, fixative for core tissue samples, culture tubes, tubes for chemistry evaluation SAMPLING TIME: Immediate STORAGE INSTRUCTIONS: Samples should immediately be sent to the appropriate laboratory (ie, cytology, pathology, bacteriology). CAUSES FOR REJECTION: Contamination by nonsterile object TURNAROUND TIME: A typed report will generally be issued within 36 hours. A preliminary verbal report generally can be given to the referring physician on request.

Interpretation LIMITATIONS: Insufficient material for analysis, patient unable to remain still, lesion unable to be visualized secondary to overlying bowel gas ADDITIONAL INFORMATION: Many abnormal masses in the abdomen are approachable by the percutaneous route. Exploratory laparotomy may be avoided and this procedure can be performed on an outpatient basis.

References

Rifkin MD and Goldberg BB, "Aspiration and Biopsy Techniques," *Abdominal Ultrasonography*, Goldberg BB, ed, New York, NY: John Wiley and Sons Inc, 1984.

Ultrasound, Breast

CPT 76645

Synonyms Breast Ultrasound

Abstract PROCEDURE COMMONLY INCLUDES: Specific area of breast which contains a mammographic abnormality. INDICATIONS: To differentiate solid from cystic lesions in the breast.

Patient Care/Scheduling PATIENT PREPARATION: The examination may be long, up to 1 hour including waiting time. An emergency examination or an unpredictably long preceding examination may result in additional delay. SPECIAL INSTRUCTIONS: A recent mammogram **must** accompany the patient or be available at examination time. All outpatient examinations are by appointment only. All inpatients are placed on the daily schedule as time permits and are performed as scheduled. Nonemergent examinations are given secondary priority and therefore may not be able to be performed the same day scheduled. Patients will generally be asked to stay after the examination until films are reviewed by the radiologist. All outpatients are by appointment only.

Method EQUIPMENT: Standard B-mode ultrasonic imager with 5-10 MHz transducer TECHNIQUE: A gel is applied to the skin and a handheld transducer is swept across the breast(s) showing breast tissue. Sound waves are used for the imaging and no radiation exposure is present. Images are recorded on x-ray film. DATA ACQUIRED: Sagittal, transverse, and oblique images of portions of the breast(s).

Specimen TURNAROUND TIME: A typed report will generally be issued within 36 hours. A preliminary verbal report generally can be given to the referring physician on request.

Interpretation NORMAL FINDINGS: Solid breast tissue without focal mass or cyst LIMITATIONS: Patient unable to remain sitting quietly or obese patient ADDITIONAL INFORMATION: This study is most useful in the determination of whether a mammographic abnormality is a simple cyst or a solid mass. If found not to be a simple cyst, malignancy cannot be excluded.

References

Kopans DB, "Other Breast Imaging Modalities," *Radiology*, Taveras JT and Ferrucci JT, eds, Philadelphia, PA: JB Lippincott, 1988.

Ultrasound, Chest Wall

CPT 76604

Synonyms Chest Wall Ultrasound

Abstract PROCEDURE COMMONLY INCLUDES: Specific portion of the chest wall. INDICATIONS: Measurement of distance between anterior surface to chest wall prior to radiation therapy, check for pleural effusions CONTRAINDICATIONS: Open wound or incision overlying examination area.

Patient Care/Scheduling PATIENT PREPARATION: The examination may be long, up to 1 hour including waiting time. An emergency examination or an unpredictably long preceding examination may result in additional delay. SPECIAL INSTRUCTIONS: All outpatient examinations are by appointment only. All inpatients are placed on the daily schedule as time permits and are performed as scheduled. Nonemergent examinations are given secondary priority and therefore may not be able to be performed the same day scheduled. Patients will generally be asked to stay after the examination until films are reviewed by the radiologist.

Method EQUIPMENT: Standard ultrasonic imager with high frequency transducer (5-10 MHz) TECHNIQUE: A gel is applied to the skin and a handheld transducer is swept across the area of interest to image the appropriate organs. Sound waves are used for the imaging and no radiation exposure is present. Images are recorded on x-ray film. DATA ACQUIRED: Transverse, longitudinal, and oblique images of the chest wall with measurements of chest wall thickness.

Specimen TURNAROUND TIME: A typed report will generally be issued within 36 hours. A preliminary verbal report generally can be given to the referring physician on request.

Interpretation ADDITIONAL INFORMATION: Study is generally performed prior to radiation therapy and to identify loculated pleural effusions.

Ultrasound, Colorflow Carotid Doppler

CPT 76926

Synonyms Carotid Ultrasound, Colorflow; Color Encoded Doppler Ultrasound

Applies to Colorflow Miscellaneous Doppler Ultrasound

Abstract PROCEDURE COMMONLY INCLUDES: The carotid arteries to look for plaque, stenosis, or occlusion in the common, internal, or external carotid arteries INDICATIONS: Checking

(Continued)

Ultrasound, Colorflow Carotid Doppler *(Continued)*

the carotid arteries for plaque formation, stenosis, or occlusion; asymptomatic bruit, TIA, stroke, confirm the presence of subclavian steal. **CONTRAINDICATIONS:** Presence of indwelling catheter of any kind, presence of a fresh incision site.

Patient Care/Scheduling **PATIENT PREPARATION:** The examination may be long, up to 1 hour including waiting time. An emergency examination or an unpredictably long preceding examination may result in additional delay.

Method **EQUIPMENT:** Standard B-mode real time ultrasonic imager with Doppler and Colorflow capability. High frequency transducer (7-10 MHz). **TECHNIQUE:** A gel is applied to the skin and a handheld transducer is swept across the area of the carotid arteries. Sound waves are used for the imaging and no radiation exposure is present. Images are recorded on x-ray film. **DATA ACQUIRED:** Transverse and longitudinal images of common carotid, internal, and external carotid arteries. Quantitative Doppler flow parameters throughout visualized vessels.

Specimen **CAUSES FOR REJECTION:** If carotid bifurcation is located past the angle of the jaw, visualization may be not possible **TURNAROUND TIME:** A typed report will be generated within 36 hours. A preliminary verbal report will be given to the referring physician upon request.

Interpretation **NORMAL FINDINGS:** Absence of atherosclerotic plaque, stenosis, or occlusion of common carotid artery or branches **CRITICAL VALUES:** Fifty percent or greater stenosis of studied vessel is considered hemodynamically significant **LIMITATIONS:** Inability of patient to hold head still, high bifurcation of carotid artery **ADDITIONAL INFORMATION:** In addition to all the information obtained in a standard duplex carotid artery ultrasound examination, this examination provides Doppler flow data from the entire visualized lumen of the examined vessel. This is displayed as a spectrum of colors on the screen, with different colors representing velocity and direction. This allows for an easier evaluation of disease present and is inherently more complete. However, the color evaluation provides subjective data and **must** be interpreted together with objective data obtained from standard Doppler flow sampling.

References

Zweibel WJ, "Color-Encoded Blood Flow Imaging," *Seminars in Ultrasound, CT and MR*, 1988, 9(4):320-5.

Ultrasound, Colorflow Extremity Doppler

CPT 76925

Abstract **PROCEDURE COMMONLY INCLUDES:** Peripheral masses **INDICATIONS:** Evaluation of vascular lesions of any extremity or vascularity of a lesion.

Patient Care/Scheduling **PATIENT PREPARATION:** Examinations may be long, lasting up to 1 hour including waiting time. An emergency examination or an unpredictably long preceding examination may result in additional delay. **SPECIAL INSTRUCTIONS:** All outpatient examinations are by appointment only. All inpatients are placed on the daily schedule as time permits and are performed as scheduled. Nonemergent examinations are given secondary priority and therefore may not be able to be performed the same day scheduled. Patients will generally be asked to stay after the examination until films are reviewed by the radiologist.

Method **EQUIPMENT:** Standard B-mode real time ultrasonic imager with 5-10 MHz, Doppler and colorflow capability **TECHNIQUE:** A gel is applied to the skin and a handheld transducer is swept across the area of interest to image the appropriate organs. Sound waves are used for the imaging and no radiation exposure is present. Images are recorded on x-ray film. **DATA ACQUIRED:** Longitudinal and transverse images of vessels studied with Doppler flow parameters.

Specimen **TURNAROUND TIME:** A typed report will generally be issued within 36 hours. A preliminary verbal report generally can be given to the referring physician on request.

Interpretation **ADDITIONAL INFORMATION:** Study may be useful in evaluating the vascularity of a mass lesion. Useful in evaluating for hemangioma, AVM, pseudoaneurysm.

Ultrasound, Colorflow Hepatic Doppler

CPT 76926

Synonyms Color Doppler Ultrasound

Applies to Colorflow, Liver; Duplex Colorflow Ultrasound Liver

Abstract PROCEDURE COMMONLY INCLUDES: Hepatic, portal, and IVC blood flow INDICATIONS: Evaluation of hepatic blood vessels, abnormal hepatic vessels, intrahepatic masses.

Patient Care/Scheduling PATIENT PREPARATION: The examination may be long, up to 1 hour including waiting time. An emergency examination or an unpredictably long preceding examination may result in additional delay. SPECIAL INSTRUCTIONS: All outpatient examinations are by appointment only. All inpatients are placed on the daily schedule as time permits and are performed as scheduled. Nonemergent examinations are given secondary priority and therefore may not be able to be performed the same day scheduled. Patients will generally be asked to stay after the examination until films are reviewed by the radiologist.

Method EQUIPMENT: Standard B-mode real time ultrasonic imager with colorflow Doppler capabilities and a 3-5 MHz transducer. TECHNIQUE: A gel is applied to the skin and a hand-held transducer is swept across the area of interest to image the appropriate organs. Sound waves are used for the imaging and no radiation exposure is present. Images are recorded on x-ray film. DATA ACQUIRED: Longitudinal, transverse, and oblique images with Doppler flow parameters.

Specimen TURNAROUND TIME: A typed report will generally be issued within 36 hours. A preliminary verbal report generally can be given to the referring physician on request.

Interpretation ADDITIONAL INFORMATION: Examination is valuable in evaluating portal and hepatic venous flow. Hepatic arterial flow and flow within the IVC are also studied. The procedure is often performed to evaluate porto-systemic venous shunts and for presence of Budd-Chiari syndrome, cavernous transformation of the IVC, tumor thrombus in the IVC.

Ultrasound, Duplex Carotid

CPT 76926

Synonyms Carotid Ultrasound

Abstract PROCEDURE COMMONLY INCLUDES: The carotid arteries to look for plaque, stenosis, or occlusion in the common, internal, or external carotid arteries INDICATIONS: Checking the carotid arteries for plaque formation, stenosis, or occlusion; asymptomatic bruit, TIA, stroke, confirm the presence of subclavian steal CONTRAINDICATIONS: Presence of indwelling catheter of any kind, presence of a fresh incision site.

Patient Care/Scheduling PATIENT PREPARATION: The examination may be long, up to 1 hour including waiting time. An emergency examination or an unpredictably long preceding examination may result in additional delay.

Method EQUIPMENT: Standard B-mode real time ultrasonic images with Doppler capabilities, 7-10 MHz transducer TECHNIQUE: A gel is applied to the sides of the neck and a hand-held transducer is swept over the area of the carotid arteries. Sound waves are used for the imaging and no radiation exposure is present. Images are recorded on x-ray film. DATA ACQUIRED: Transverse and longitudinal images of common carotid, internal, and external carotid arteries; quantitative Doppler flow parameters throughout visualized vessels.

Specimen CAUSES FOR REJECTION: Inability of patient to hold head still, high bifurcation of carotid artery. If carotid bifurcation is located past the angle of the jaw, visualization may not be possible. TURNAROUND TIME: A typed report will generally be issued within 36 hours. A preliminary verbal report generally can be given to the referring physician on request.

Interpretation NORMAL FINDINGS: Absence of stenosis or occlusion of common carotid artery or branches CRITICAL VALUES: Fifty percent or greater stenosis of studied vessel is considered hemodynamically significant ADDITIONAL INFORMATION: Duplex carotid ultrasound is a very useful means of noninvasively screening for atherosclerotic disease of the carotid arteries. Both the severity of plaque formation as well as an estimate of the degree of stenosis is reliably obtained. When significant disease is detected, angiography should be performed to fully evaluate the extent of disease. This examination is useful in the serial evaluation of patients to rule out progressive disease.

References

Zweibel WJ, "Duplex Carotid Sonography," *Introduction to Vascular Ultrasonography*, Zweibel WJ, ed, New York, NY: Grune and Stratton, Inc, 1986.

Ultrasound, Extremity

CPT 76880

Synonyms Extremity Ultrasound

Abstract PROCEDURE COMMONLY INCLUDES: Specific area of an extremity INDICATIONS: Diagnosis of popliteal aneurysms, Baker's cyst, hematoma CONTRAINDICATIONS: Open wound or incision overlying examination area.

Patient Care/Scheduling PATIENT PREPARATION: No patient preparation is necessary. Examinations may be long, 30 minutes to 1 hour each. An emergency exam or an unpredictably long preceding exam may necessitate waiting on the part of the next patient. SPECIAL INSTRUCTIONS: All outpatient examinations are by appointment only. All inpatients are placed on the daily schedule as time permits and are performed as scheduled. Nonemergent examinations are given secondary priority and therefore may not be able to be performed the same day scheduled. Patients will generally be asked to stay after the examination until films are reviewed by the radiologist. Instruct the patient that ultrasound uses sound waves to image the different organs. There is **no** radiation involved, therefore, it is not harmful to the patient.

Method EQUIPMENT: Standard B-mode ultrasonic imager with 5-10 MHz transducer TECHNIQUE: A gel is applied to the skin and a handheld transducer is swept across the area of interest to image the appropriate organs. Sound waves are used for the imaging and no radiation exposure is present. Images are recorded on x-ray film. DATA ACQUIRED: Longitudinal, transverse and oblique images of the area of interest are obtained.

Specimen TURNAROUND TIME: A typed report will generally be issued within 36 hours. A preliminary verbal report generally can be given to the referring physician on request.

Interpretation ADDITIONAL INFORMATION: This examination is most valuable to evaluate for the presence of abnormal fluid collections. If present, it can determine if the fluid collection is simple or complex in nature.

Ultrasound, Gallbladder

CPT 76705

Synonyms Gallbladder Ultrasound

Abstract PROCEDURE COMMONLY INCLUDES: Gallbladder and biliary tree INDICATIONS: Cholelithiasis, cholecystitis, neoplasms, lesions, polyps, or ductal obstruction CONTRAINDICATIONS: Open wound or incision overlying examination area, recent barium study.

Patient Care/Scheduling PATIENT PREPARATION: Patient should be on a low fat diet the night before the examination with NPO for 10 hours prior to the examination. No laxatives are given the day of the examination. No barium studies should have been performed on the patient for **at least** 2 days preceding the examination. Endoscopy, ERCP, colonoscopy, and abdominal CT should be performed after this examination. Nuclear Medicine studies may be ordered prior to the examination. The examination may be long, up to 1 hour including waiting time. An emergency examination or an unpredictably long preceding examination may result in additional delay. **Note**: Ultrasound exam to be scheduled before a barium study. If barium study was done, bowel preparation is needed before doing ultrasound examination. SPECIAL INSTRUCTIONS: All outpatient examinations are by appointment only. All inpatients are placed on the daily schedule as time permits and are performed as scheduled. Nonemergent examinations are given secondary priority and therefore may not be able to be performed the same day scheduled. Patients will generally be asked to stay after the examination until films are reviewed by the radiologist.

Method EQUIPMENT: Standard B-mode real time ultrasonic imager with 2-5 MHz transducer. TECHNIQUE: A gel is applied to the skin and a handheld transducer is swept across the area of interest to image the appropriate organs. Sound waves are used for the imaging and no radiation exposure is present. Images are recorded on x-ray film. DATA ACQUIRED: Longitudinal, transverse, and oblique views of the gallbladder; longitudinal image of common bile duct.

Specimen CAUSES FOR REJECTION: Gas, barium, oral ingestion of food or fluids, obesity TURNAROUND TIME: A typed report will generally be issued within 36 hours. A preliminary verbal report generally can be given to the referring physician on request.

Interpretation NORMAL FINDINGS: Absence of cholelithiasis CRITICAL VALUES: Common bile duct ≤6 mm prior to cholecystectomy, ≤11 mm after cholecystectomy ADDITIONAL INFOR-

MATION: This is a very sensitive examination for evaluation of the presence of gallstones as well as biliary tree dilatation. Additionally, soft tissue masses, and abnormal collections can be detected.

References

Bernardino ME, "The Liver: Anatomy and Examination Techniques," *Radiology*, Taveras JT and Ferrucci JT, eds, Philadelphia, PA: JB Lippincott, 1988.

Cooperberg PL and Rowley VA, "Abdominal Sonographic Examination Technique," *Radiology*, Taveras JT and Ferrucci JT, eds, Philadelphia, PA: JB Lippincott, 1988.

Goldberg BB, *Abdominal Ultrasonography*, New York, NY: John Wiley and Sons Inc, 1984.

Ultrasound, Hepatic

CPT 76705

Synonyms Hepatic Ultrasound; Liver Ultrasound; RUQ

Abstract PROCEDURE COMMONLY INCLUDES: Liver, biliary tract, gallbladder, right kidney (limited) INDICATIONS: To evaluate for the presence of hepatitis, malignancies, cysts, biliary obstruction.

Patient Care/Scheduling PATIENT PREPARATION: Ultrasound examination should be performed before endoscopy, ERCP, colonoscopy, barium studies, and abdominal CT. Nuclear Medicine studies may be performed first. NPO after midnight. The examination may be long, up to 1 hour including waiting time. An emergency examination or an unpredictably long preceding examination may result in additional delay. SPECIAL INSTRUCTIONS: All outpatient examinations are by appointment only. All inpatients are placed on the daily schedule as time permits and are performed as scheduled. Nonemergent examinations are given secondary priority and therefore may not be able to be performed the same day scheduled. Patients will generally be asked to stay after the examination until films are reviewed by the radiologist.

Method EQUIPMENT: Standard B-mode ultrasonic imager 2-5 MHz transducer TECHNIQUE: A gel is applied to the skin and a handheld transducer is swept across the area of interest to image the appropriate organs. Sound waves are used for the imaging and no radiation exposure is present. Images are recorded on x-ray film. DATA ACQUIRED: Longitudinal, transverse, and oblique images of the liver; limited images of the gallbladder and right kidney.

Specimen CAUSES FOR REJECTION: Gas, barium, oral ingestion of food TURNAROUND TIME: A typed report will generally be issued within 36 hours. A preliminary verbal report generally can be given to the referring physician on request.

Interpretation ADDITIONAL INFORMATION: This examination is useful to evaluate for the presence of hepatic mass lesions, cysts or other collections, calcifications or biliary tree dilatations. Diffuse hepatic parenchymal disease may be detected as well.

References

Cooperberg PL and Rowley VA, "Abdominal Sonographic Examination Technique," *Radiology*, Taveras JT and Ferrucci JT, eds, Philadelphia, PA: JB Lippincott, 1988.

Goldberg BB, *Abdominal Ultrasonography*, New York, NY: John Wiley and Sons Inc, 1984.

Ultrasound, Intraoperative Real Time Scanning

CPT 76986

Synonyms Intraoperative Real Time Scanning Ultrasound

Abstract PROCEDURE COMMONLY INCLUDES: Scanning of organs (eg, brain, spinal cord, kidney, liver, gallbladder, pancreas) with the transducer during surgery and obtaining real time images INDICATIONS: Localization of tumors, cystic mass aspiration, during surgery.

Patient Care/Scheduling SPECIAL INSTRUCTIONS: Study scheduled after consultation with radiologist.

Method EQUIPMENT: Standard B-mode real time ultrasonic imager with 5-10 MHz transducer. TECHNIQUE: A handheld transducer is swept across the area of interest to image the appropriate organs. Sound waves are used for the imaging and no radiation exposure is present. Images are recorded on x-ray film.

Specimen TURNAROUND TIME: A typed report will generally be issued within 36 hours. A preliminary verbal report generally can be given to the referring physician on request.

(Continued)

Ultrasound, Intraoperative Real Time Scanning *(Continued)*

References

Knake JE, Bowerman RA, Silver TM, et al, "Neurosurgical Applications of Intraoperative Ultrasound," *Radiol Clin North Am*, 1985, 23(1):73-90.

Bowerman RA, McCracken S, Silver TM, et al, "Abdominal and Miscellaneous Applications of Intraoperative Ultrasound," *Radiol Clin North Am*, 1985, 23(1):107-19.

Ultrasound, Kidney Biopsy

CPT 76943

Related Information

Kidney Biopsy *on page 145*

Synonyms Kidney Biopsy Ultrasound; Renal Biopsy Ultrasound

Abstract PROCEDURE COMMONLY INCLUDES: Use of real time ultrasound imaging to direct biopsy of renal mass INDICATIONS: Provide tissue sample or fluid sample for diagnostic purposes CONTRAINDICATIONS: Coagulopathy.

Patient Care/Scheduling PATIENT PREPARATION: The examination may be long, up to 1 hour including waiting time. An emergency examination or an unpredictably long preceding examination may result in additional delay. AFTERCARE: Check physician order sheet. Monitor vital signs in department for 1 hour postprocedure. SPECIAL INSTRUCTIONS: All outpatient examinations are by appointment only. All inpatients are placed on the daily schedule as time permits and are performed as scheduled. Nonemergent examinations are given secondary priority and therefore may not be able to be performed the same day scheduled. Patients will generally be asked to stay after the examination until films are reviewed by the radiologist. COMPLICATIONS: Hemorrhage, infection.

Method EQUIPMENT: Standard B-mode real time ultrasonic imager with 2-5 MHz transducer. TECHNIQUE: A gel is applied to the skin and a handheld transducer is swept across the area of interest to image the appropriate organs. Sound waves are used for the imaging and no radiation exposure is present. Images are recorded on x-ray film.

Specimen Fluid and/or tissue CONTAINER: Sterile saline, sterile slides for cytology, fixative for core tissue samples, culture tubes, tubes for chemistry evaluation SAMPLING TIME: Immediate STORAGE INSTRUCTIONS: Samples should immediately be sent to the appropriate laboratory (ie, cytology, pathology, bacteriology). CAUSES FOR REJECTION: Obesity, inability to suspend respiration or lie motionless, inability to locate good access to site TURNAROUND TIME: A typed report will generally be issued within 36 hours. A preliminary verbal report generally can be given to the referring physician on request.

References

Rifkin MD and Goldberg BB, "Aspiration and Biopsy Techniques," *Abdominal Ultrasonography*, Goldberg BB, ed, New York, NY: John Wiley and Sons Inc, 1984.

Ultrasound, Kidney Cyst Puncture

CPT 76938

Synonyms Kidney Cyst Puncture Ultrasound; Renal Cyst Puncture Ultrasound

Abstract PROCEDURE COMMONLY INCLUDES: Use of real time ultrasound imaging to direct aspiration of renal cyst INDICATIONS: Provide fluid or tissue sample for diagnostic purposes CONTRAINDICATIONS: Inadequate access by ultrasound, bleeding diathesis.

Patient Care/Scheduling PATIENT PREPARATION: The examination may be long, up to 1 hour including waiting time. An emergency examination or an unpredictably long preceding examination may result in additional delay. AFTERCARE: Follow physician's orders SPECIAL INSTRUCTIONS: All outpatient examinations are by appointment only. All inpatients are placed on the daily schedule as time permits and are performed as scheduled. Nonemergent examinations are given secondary priority and therefore may not be able to be performed the same day scheduled. Patients will generally be asked to stay after the examination until films are reviewed by the radiologist. COMPLICATIONS: Hemorrhage, infection.

Method EQUIPMENT: Standard B-mode real time ultrasonic imager with 2-5 MHz transducer. TECHNIQUE: A gel is applied to the skin and a handheld transducer is swept across the area of interest to image the appropriate organs. Sound waves are used for the imaging and no radiation exposure is present. Images are recorded on x-ray film. Following sterile preparation of the skin, and use of local anesthesia, a small (20- to 22-gauge) needle is introduced into the suspected cyst under real time ultrasonic visualization. **DATA ACQUIRED:** A sample of fluid and/or tissue is obtained for analysis.

Specimen Fluid and/or tissue **CONTAINER:** Sterile saline, sterile slides for cytology, fixative for core tissue samples, culture tubes, tubes for chemistry evaluation **SAMPLING TIME:** Immediate **STORAGE INSTRUCTIONS:** Samples should immediately be sent to the appropriate laboratory (ie, cytology, pathology, bacteriology). **CAUSES FOR REJECTION:** Obesity, inability to suspend respiration or lie motionless, inability to locate good access to site **TURNAROUND TIME:** A typed report will generally be issued within 36 hours. A preliminary verbal report generally can be given to the referring physician on request.

References

Rifkin MD and Goldberg BB, "Aspiration and Biopsy Techniques," *Abdominal Ultrasonography*, Goldberg BB, ed, New York, NY: John Wiley and Sons Inc, 1984.

Ultrasound, Kidneys

CPT 76700

Synonyms Kidneys Ultrasound; Renal Ultrasound

Abstract **PROCEDURE COMMONLY INCLUDES:** Kidneys **INDICATIONS:** Evaluation of cysts and neoplasms, calcifications, abscess, and hydronephrosis and hydroureter.

Patient Care/Scheduling **PATIENT PREPARATION:** The examination may be long, up to 1 hour including waiting time. An emergency examination or an unpredictably long preceding examination may result in additional delay. **Note**: Ultrasound exam to be scheduled before a barium study. If barium study was done, bowel preparation is needed before doing ultrasound examination. **SPECIAL INSTRUCTIONS:** All outpatient examinations are by appointment only. All inpatients are placed on the daily schedule as time permits and are performed as scheduled. Nonemergent examinations are given secondary priority and therefore may not be able to be performed the same day scheduled. Patients will generally be asked to stay after the examination until films are reviewed by the radiologist.

Method **EQUIPMENT:** Standard B-mode real time ultrasonic imager with 2-5 MHz transducer. **TECHNIQUE:** A gel is applied to the skin and a handheld transducer is swept across the area of interest to image the appropriate organs. Sound waves are used for the imaging and no radiation exposure is present. Images are recorded on x-ray film. **DATA ACQUIRED:** Longitudinal and transverse images of each kidney.

Specimen **CAUSES FOR REJECTION:** Patient unable to cooperate with positioning and respiratory maneuvers; bowel gas, barium, obesity **TURNAROUND TIME:** A typed report will generally be issued within 36 hours. A preliminary verbal report generally can be given to the referring physician on request.

Interpretation **ADDITIONAL INFORMATION:** Rapid, sensitive evaluation for the presence of hydronephrosis. Useful in confirming the cystic nature of lesions. Detection of hydroureter is often problematic.

References

Goldberg BB, *Abdominal Ultrasonography*, New York, NY: John Wiley and Sons Inc, 1984.

Grant DC, "Ultrasound of the Genitourinary Tract," *Radiology*, Taveras JT and Ferrucci JT, eds, Philadelphia, PA: JB Lippincott, 1988.

Ultrasound Localization *see* Ultrasound, Biopsy Localization *on page 396*

Ultrasound, Neonatal Intracranial Real Time

CPT 76506

Synonyms Neonatal Intracranial Ultrasound

Abstract **PROCEDURE COMMONLY INCLUDES:** Examination of calvarial contents through anterior fontanelle **INDICATIONS:** Detection of intracranial hemorrhage, intraventricular hemorrhage, hydrocephalus, porencephaly, Dandy Walker cyst.

Patient Care/Scheduling **PATIENT PREPARATION:** I.V.s that cover the anterior fontanelle should be avoided. If an I.V. butterfly needle is covering the anterior fontanelle it will have to be removed prior to the ultrasound. The examination may be long, up to 1 hour including waiting time. An emergency examination or an unpredictably long preceding examination

(Continued)

Ultrasound, Neonatal Intracranial Real Time *(Continued)*

may result in additional delay. **SPECIAL INSTRUCTIONS:** All outpatient examinations are by appointment only. All inpatients are placed on the daily schedule as time permits and are performed as scheduled. Nonemergent examinations are given secondary priority and therefore may not be able to be performed the same day scheduled. Patients will generally be asked to stay after the examination until films are reviewed by the radiologist.

Method **EQUIPMENT:** Standard B-mode real time ultrasonic imager with 2-5 MHz transducer. **TECHNIQUE:** A gel is applied to the skin and a handheld transducer is swept across the area of interest to image the appropriate organs. Sound waves are used for the imaging and no radiation exposure is present. Images are recorded on x-ray film. **DATA ACQUIRED:** Parasagittal and transverse images.

Specimen **TURNAROUND TIME:** A typed report will generally be issued within 36 hours. A preliminary verbal report generally can be given to the referring physician on request.

Interpretation **NORMAL FINDINGS:** Absence of hydrocephalus, abnormal collections, hemorrhage **LIMITATIONS:** Child's fontanelle size **ADDITIONAL INFORMATION:** Useful in evaluating premature infants in the postpartum period for presence and degree of intracranial hemorrhage and complications. Also useful in the evaluation of structural abnormalities.

Ultrasound, Nephrostomy, Guided

CPT 76999

Applies to Nephrostomy; Percutaneous Nephrostomy

Abstract **PROCEDURE COMMONLY INCLUDES:** Use of real time ultrasound imaging to direct placement of a nephrostomy tube into the dilated renal collecting system **INDICATIONS:** Hydronephrosis **CONTRAINDICATIONS:** Inadequate access by ultrasound, bleeding diathesis.

Patient Care/Scheduling **PATIENT PREPARATION:** The procedure may be long, up to several hours including waiting time. An emergency examination or an unpredictably long preceding examination may result in additional delay. **SPECIAL INSTRUCTIONS:** All procedures performed after consultation with radiologist. All inpatients are placed on the daily schedule as time permits and performed as scheduled. Nonemergent examinations are given secondary priority and therefore may not be able to be performed the same day scheduled. **COMPLICATIONS:** Hemorrhage, sepsis.

Method **EQUIPMENT:** Standard B-mode real time ultrasonic imager with 2-5 MHz transducer and biopsy guide if desired. Appropriate percutaneous nephrostomy kit. **TECHNIQUE:** A gel is applied to the skin and a handheld transducer is swept across the area of interest to image the appropriate organs. Sound waves are used for the imaging and no radiation exposure is present. An appropriate access route is chosen and a needle is placed into the renal collecting system under sterile conditions. Local anesthesia and I.V. analgesia are given. The needle is exchanged for nephrostomy catheter. Images are recorded on x-ray film.

Specimen Urine, infected urine **CONTAINER:** Aerobic and anaerobic culture containers **STORAGE INSTRUCTIONS:** Culture containers should be sent immediately to the Bacteriology Laboratory. **CAUSES FOR REJECTION:** Patient unable to remain motionless during study **TURNAROUND TIME:** A typed report will generally be issued within 36 hours. A preliminary verbal report generally can be given to the referring physician on request.

Interpretation **ADDITIONAL INFORMATION:** Procedure allows decompression of obstructed kidney without surgery.

References

Rifkin MD and Goldberg BB, "Aspiration and Biopsy Techniques," *Abdominal Ultrasonography*, Goldberg BB, ed, New York, NY: John Wiley and Sons Inc, 1984.

Ultrasound, OB, Complete

CPT 76805

Abstract **PROCEDURE COMMONLY INCLUDES:** Examination of the fetus for viability, placenta localization, measurements of the fetus to determine fetal age and weight, and examination of the maternal pelvis to rule out masses. This study also includes the evaluation of the fetal cerebral ventricles, urinary bladder, kidneys, stomach, spine and umbilical cord. **INDICATIONS:** Evaluate for total age and viability, IVGR, placenta position, amount of amniotic fluid and presence of certain anomalies.

Patient Care/Scheduling PATIENT PREPARATION: The examination may be long, up to 1 hour including waiting time. An emergency examination or an unpredictably long preceding examination may result in additional delay. The patient must have a full urinary bladder at the time of study. Patient should drink 32 oz of water 1 1/2 to 1 hour prior to the study. SPECIAL INSTRUCTIONS: All outpatient examinations are by appointment only. All inpatients are placed on the daily schedule as time permits and are performed as scheduled. Nonemergent examinations are given secondary priority and therefore may not be able to be performed the same day scheduled. Patients will generally be asked to stay after the examination until films are reviewed by the radiologist.

Method EQUIPMENT: Standard B-mode real time ultrasonic imager with 2-5 MHz transducer. TECHNIQUE: A gel is applied to the skin and a handheld transducer is swept across the uterus to image the appropriate organs. Sound waves are used for the imaging and no radiation exposure is present. Images are recorded on x-ray film. DATA ACQUIRED: Transverse, longitudinal, and oblique images of the uterus, placenta, and fetus(es). Biparietal diameter (BPD), abdominal circumference (AC), and femur length (FL) are reported in the second through the third trimesters with estimated gestational age (GA) and fetal weight reported. First trimester, gestational sac size, and/or crown to rump length are reported. Survey of cerebral ventricles, urinary bladder, stomach, kidneys, spine, and umbilical cord insertion site into fetus is performed. Fetal age and viability, position of the placenta, and the amount of amniotic fluid are determined.

Specimen TURNAROUND TIME: A typed report will generally be issued within 36 hours. A preliminary verbal report generally can be given to the referring physician on request.

Interpretation ADDITIONAL INFORMATION: When evaluating for intrauterine growth retardation, patient should have two ultrasound exams approximately 4-6 weeks apart. Growth retardation cannot be diagnosed on the basis of one exam. This examination is valuable in evaluating for the presence of fetal structural abnormalities, detection of intrauterine growth retardation, and fetal gestational age. Placenta previa detected and abruptio placenta may be detected.

References

Fleischer AC and James AE, "Obstetric Sonography: Normal Pregnancy and Anatomical Variants," *Radiology*, Taveras JT and Ferrucci JT, eds, Philadelphia, PA: JB Lippincott, 1988.

Platt LO, Hill LM, DeVore GR, et al, "Amniocentesis: Current Concepts and Techniques," *The Principles and Practice of Ultrasonography in Obstetrics Gynecology*, Sanders and James, eds, Norwalk, CT: Appleton-Century-Crofts, 1985.

Ultrasound, OB, Limited

CPT 76815

Synonyms Fetal Age; Gestational Age; Pregnancy, Complete Sonogram; Pregnancy, Echo

Abstract PROCEDURE COMMONLY INCLUDES: Examination of the fetus for viability and well being, placenta localization, measurements of the fetus to determine fetal age, and examination of the maternal pelvis to rule out masses INDICATIONS: Diagnosis of pregnancy, fetal age, placenta localization, multiple pregnancies, fetal position, amniotic fluid, fetal anomalies, fetal viability, growth retardation.

Patient Care/Scheduling PATIENT PREPARATION: The examination may be long, up to 1 hour including waiting time. An emergency examination or an unpredictably long preceding examination may result in additional delay. The patient must have a full urinary bladder at the time of study. Patient should drink 32 oz of water 1 1/2 to 1 hour prior to the study. SPECIAL INSTRUCTIONS: All outpatient examinations are by appointment only. All inpatients are placed on the daily schedule as time permits and are performed as scheduled. Nonemergent examinations are given secondary priority and therefore may not be able to be performed the same day scheduled. Patients will generally be asked to stay after the examination until films are reviewed by the radiologist.

Method EQUIPMENT: Standard B-mode real time ultrasonic imager with 2-5 MHz transducer. TECHNIQUE: A gel is applied to the skin and a handheld transducer is swept across the area of interest to image the appropriate organs. Sound waves are used for the imaging and no radiation exposure is present. Images are recorded on x-ray film. DATA ACQUIRED: Transverse, longitudinal, and oblique images of the uterus, placenta, and fetus(es). Biparietal di-

(Continued)

Ultrasound, OB, Limited *(Continued)*

ameter (BPD), abdominal circumference (AC), and femur length (FL) are reported in the second through the third trimesters with estimated gestational age (GA) reported. First trimester, gestational sac size, and/or crown to rump length are reported. Survey of cerebral ventricles, urinary bladder, stomach, kidneys, spine, and umbilical cord insertion site into fetus is **not** performed. Fetal age and viability, position of the placenta, and the amount of amniotic fluid are determined.

Specimen **TURNAROUND TIME:** A typed report will generally be issued within 36 hours. A preliminary verbal report generally can be given to the referring physician on request.

Interpretation **LIMITATIONS:** The patient not having a full bladder **ADDITIONAL INFORMATION:** When evaluating for intrauterine growth retardation, patient should have two ultrasound exams approximately 4-6 weeks apart. Growth retardation cannot be diagnosed on basis of one exam.

References

Fleischer AC and James AE, "Obstetric Sonography: Normal Pregnancy and Anatomical Variants," *Radiology*, Taveras JT and Ferrucci JT, eds, Philadelphia, PA: JB Lippincott, 1988.

Platt LO, Hill LM, DeVore GR, et al, "Amniocentesis: Current Concepts and Techniques," *The Principles and Practice of Ultrasonography in Obstetrics Gynecology*, Sanders and James, eds, Norwalk, CT: Appleton-Century-Crofts, 1985.

Ultrasound, Pancreas

CPT 76705

Synonyms Pancreas Ultrasound

Abstract **PROCEDURE COMMONLY INCLUDES:** Pancreas, biliary tree, and gallbladder **INDICATIONS:** Evaluate pancreatic size and shape, presence of neoplasm, cystic lesions, pseudocyst, pancreatitis **CONTRAINDICATIONS:** Open wound or incision overlying examination area, (routine study) recent barium study.

Patient Care/Scheduling **PATIENT PREPARATION:** The patient should not have had a barium study within the 3 days prior to study. The examinations may be up to 1 hour each. An emergency exam or an unpredictably long preceding exam may result in additional delay. NPO after midnight before day of examination. **SPECIAL INSTRUCTIONS:** All outpatient examinations are by appointment only. All inpatients are placed on the daily schedule as time permits and are performed as scheduled. Nonemergent examinations are given secondary priority and therefore may not be able to be performed the same day scheduled. Patients will generally be asked to stay after the examination until films are reviewed by the radiologist.

Method **EQUIPMENT:** Standard B-mode real time ultrasonic imager with 2-5 MHz transducer. **TECHNIQUE:** A gel is applied to the skin and a handheld transducer is swept across the area of interest to image the appropriate organs. Sound waves are used for the imaging and no radiation exposure is present. Images are recorded on x-ray film.

Specimen **CAUSES FOR REJECTION:** Gas, barium, oral ingestion of food, body habitus, rib artifacts **TURNAROUND TIME:** A typed report will generally be issued within 36 hours. A preliminary verbal report generally can be given to the referring physician on request.

Interpretation **ADDITIONAL INFORMATION:** Request for this study results in study of the pancreas with limited evaluation of other nearby organs.

References

Cooperberg PL and Rowley VA, "Abdominal Sonographic Examination Technique," *Radiology*, Taveras JT and Ferrucci JT, eds, Philadelphia, PA: JB Lippincott, 1988.

Goldberg BB, *Abdominal Ultrasonography*, New York, NY: John Wiley and Sons Inc, 1984.

Ultrasound, Parathyroids

CPT 76536

Synonyms Parathyroids Ultrasound

Abstract **PROCEDURE COMMONLY INCLUDES:** Parathyroid glands **INDICATIONS:** Evaluation of parathyroid size as well as abnormal masses.

Patient Care/Scheduling **PATIENT PREPARATION:** The examination may be long, up to 1 hour including waiting time. An emergency examination or an unpredictably long preceding examination may result in additional delay. **SPECIAL INSTRUCTIONS:** All outpatient examinations are by appointment only. All inpatients are placed on the daily schedule as time permits and are performed as scheduled. Nonemergent examinations are given secondary priority and therefore may not be able to be performed the same day scheduled. Patients will generally be asked to stay after the examination until films are reviewed by the radiologist.

Method **EQUIPMENT:** Standard B-mode real time ultrasonic imager with 7.5-10 MHz transducer. **TECHNIQUE:** A gel is applied to the skin and a handheld transducer is swept across the area of interest to image the appropriate organs. Sound waves are used for the imaging and no radiation exposure is present. Images are recorded on x-ray film. **DATA ACQUIRED:** Longitudinal, sagittal, and oblique images of parathyroid glands.

Specimen **CAUSES FOR REJECTION:** Overlying thyroid pathology **TURNAROUND TIME:** A typed report will generally be issued within 36 hours. A preliminary verbal report generally can be given to the referring physician on request.

Interpretation **ADDITIONAL INFORMATION:** Patients referred for this examination should have a proven diagnosis of hyperparathyroidism. This test is used to define the anatomy of the parathyroids and not to assess function. It most often is performed in the preoperative evaluation of a patient with hyperparathyroidism.

References

Butch RJ, Simeone JF, and Mueller PR, "Thyroid and Parathyroid Ultrasonography," *Radiol Clin North Am*, 1985, 23(1):57-71.

Simeone JF, "Ultrasound Examination of the Thyroid and Parathyroid," *Radiology*, Taveras JT, and Ferrucci JT, eds, Philadelphia, PA: JB Lippincott, 1988.

Ultrasound, Pelvis

CPT 76856

Synonyms Lower Abdomen Ultrasound; Pelvis Ultrasound

Abstract **PROCEDURE COMMONLY INCLUDES:** Uterus, fallopian tubes, ovaries, bilateral adnexa, appendix region **INDICATIONS:** Pelvic masses and abscess, uterus size, IUD localization, and pregnancy diagnosis. Ectopic pregnancy, dermoid cyst, pelvic inflammatory disease, ovarian cyst, fibroid tumor, and bladder tumor.

Patient Care/Scheduling **PATIENT PREPARATION:** Instruct patient to drink four 8 oz glasses of water 45 minutes prior to exam and not to empty bladder. The examination may be long, up to 1 hour including waiting time. An emergency examination or an unpredictably long preceding examination may result in additional delay. No barium studies should have been performed on the patient for **at least** 2 days preceding exam. **Note:** Ultrasound exam is to be scheduled before a barium study. If barium study was done, bowel preparation is needed before doing ultrasound examination. **SPECIAL INSTRUCTIONS:** All outpatient examinations are by appointment only. All inpatients are placed on the daily schedule as time permits and are performed as scheduled. Nonemergent examinations are given secondary priority and therefore may not be able to be performed the same day scheduled. Patients will generally be asked to stay after the examination until films are reviewed by the radiologist.

Method **EQUIPMENT:** Standard B-mode real time ultrasonic imager with 2-5 MHz transducer. **TECHNIQUE:** A gel is applied to the skin and a handheld transducer is swept across the area of interest to image the appropriate organs. Sound waves are used for the imaging and no radiation exposure is present. Images are recorded on x-ray film. **DATA ACQUIRED:** Longitudinal, transverse, and oblique images.

Specimen **CAUSES FOR REJECTION:** Bowel gas, barium, patient not having full bladder, patient scheduled for barium studies and/or IVP **TURNAROUND TIME:** A typed report will generally be issued within 36 hours. A preliminary verbal report generally can be given to the referring physician on request.

Interpretation **ADDITIONAL INFORMATION:** This study is valuable for the detection of ovarian cysts and neoplasms, uterine abnormalities, presence of abnormal collections such as abscess and endometrioma. May aid in the diagnosis of ectopic pregnancy.

References

Hall DA and Hann LE, "Gynecologic Radiology: Benign Disorders," *Radiology*, Taveras JT and Ferrucci JT, eds, Philadelphia, PA: JB Lippincott, 1988.

(Continued)

Ultrasound, Pelvis *(Continued)*

Lang FC, "Ectopic Pregnancy," *Radiology*, Taveras JT and Ferrucci JT, eds, Philadelphia, PA: JB Lippincott, 1988.
Zornoza J, "Gynecologic Radiology: Malignant," *Radiology*, Taveras JT and Ferrucci JT, eds, Philadelphia, PA: JB Lippincott, 1988.
Zornoza J, "The Pelvis: Anatomy and Examination Techniques," *Radiology*, Taveras JT and Ferrucci JT, eds, Philadelphia, PA: JB Lippincott, 1988.

Ultrasound, Penile

CPT 76999

Related Information

Penile Blood Flow *on page 152*

Synonyms Penile Ultrasound

Abstract **PROCEDURE COMMONLY INCLUDES:** Penis **INDICATIONS:** Primary impotence, vasculogenic impotence.

Patient Care/Scheduling **PATIENT PREPARATION:** The examination may be long, up to 1 hour including waiting time. An emergency examination or an unpredictably long preceding examination may result in additional delay. **SPECIAL INSTRUCTIONS:** Examinations scheduled after consultation with radiologist. All outpatient examinations are by appointment only. All inpatients are placed on the daily schedule as time permits and are performed as scheduled. Nonemergent examinations are given secondary priority and therefore may not be able to be performed the same day scheduled. Patients will generally be asked to stay after the examination until films are reviewed by the radiologist.

Method **EQUIPMENT:** Standard B-mode real time ultrasonic imager with Doppler capability with 7.5-10 MHz transducer. **TECHNIQUE:** A gel is applied to the skin and a handheld transducer is swept across the area of interest to image the appropriate organs. Sound waves are used for the imaging and no radiation exposure is present. Images are recorded on x-ray film. **DATA ACQUIRED:** Doppler flow data of major penile vessels.

Specimen **TURNAROUND TIME:** A typed report will generally be issued within 36 hours. A preliminary verbal report generally can be given to the referring physician on request.

Interpretation **ADDITIONAL INFORMATION:** Examination may be valuable in the evaluation of impotence of vascular origin.

Ultrasound, Peripheral Arteries and Veins

CPT 76925

Synonyms Iliac Arteries Ultrasound; Peripheral Arteries and Veins Ultrasound; Popliteal Ultrasound

Abstract **PROCEDURE COMMONLY INCLUDES:** Peripheral arteries and/or veins **INDICATIONS:** Determine aneurysm, cysts, pseudoaneurysm, deep vein thrombosis (DVT), arterial insufficiency.

Patient Care/Scheduling **PATIENT PREPARATION:** The examination may be long, up to 1 hour including waiting time. An emergency examination or an unpredictably long preceding examination may result in additional delay. **SPECIAL INSTRUCTIONS:** Specific vessels of interest to be studied as well as location must be specified. All outpatient examinations are by appointment only. All inpatients are placed on the daily schedule as time permits and are performed as scheduled. Nonemergent examinations are given secondary priority and therefore may not be able to be performed the same day scheduled. Patients will generally be asked to stay after the examination until films are reviewed by the radiologist.

Method **EQUIPMENT:** Standard B-mode real time ultrasonic imager with Doppler capability with 5-10 MHz transducer. **TECHNIQUE:** A gel is applied to the skin and a handheld transducer is swept across the area of interest to image the appropriate organs. Sound waves are used for the imaging and no radiation exposure is present. Images are recorded on x-ray film.

Specimen **TURNAROUND TIME:** A typed report will generally be issued within 36 hours. A preliminary verbal report generally can be given to the referring physician on request.

Interpretation **NORMAL FINDINGS:** Presence of appropriate flow, compressibility of venous structures **ADDITIONAL INFORMATION:** Examination is valuable in the detection of pseudoaneurysms, aneurysms, arterial insufficiency, and deep venous thrombosis (DVT).

Ultrasound, Pleural Effusion

CPT 76604

Synonyms Pleural Effusion Ultrasound

Abstract PROCEDURE COMMONLY INCLUDES: Chest INDICATIONS: Determine presence of pleural fluid and/or abscess.

Patient Care/Scheduling PATIENT PREPARATION: The examination may be long, up to 1 hour including waiting time. An emergency examination or an unpredictably long preceding examination may result in additional delay. SPECIAL INSTRUCTIONS: All outpatient examinations are by appointment only. All inpatients are placed on the daily schedule as time permits and are performed as scheduled. Nonemergent examinations are given secondary priority and therefore may not be able to be performed the same day scheduled. Patients will generally be asked to stay after the examination until films are reviewed by the radiologist.

Method EQUIPMENT: Standard B-mode real time ultrasonic imager with 5-10 MHz transducer. TECHNIQUE: A gel is applied to the skin and a handheld transducer is swept across the area of interest to image the appropriate organs. Sound waves are used for the imaging and no radiation exposure is present. Images are recorded on x-ray film.

Specimen CAUSES FOR REJECTION: Size of patient, rib artifacts TURNAROUND TIME: A typed report will generally be issued within 36 hours. A preliminary verbal report generally can be given to the referring physician on request.

Interpretation ADDITIONAL INFORMATION: This examination is useful in localizing loculated pleural collections as well as confirming the presence of pleural effusions.

References

Neff CC and Van Sonnenberg E, "Percutaneous Drainage of Pleural Collections," *Radiology*, Taveras JT and Ferrucci JT, eds, Philadelphia, PA: JB Lippincott, 1988.

Ultrasound, Prostate

CPT 76872

Synonyms Prostate Ultrasound

Abstract PROCEDURE COMMONLY INCLUDES: Prostate, seminal vesicles INDICATIONS: Evaluate for the presence of a prostatic lesion CONTRAINDICATIONS: Recent rectosigmoid surgery.

Patient Care/Scheduling PATIENT PREPARATION: Patient should not void 1 hour prior to examination. A cleansing enema should be given to patient 2 hours prior to examination. Patient must not have had recent rectosigmoid surgery. SPECIAL INSTRUCTIONS: All outpatient examinations are by appointment only. All inpatients are placed on the daily schedule as time permits and are performed as scheduled. Nonemergent examinations are given secondary priority and therefore may not be able to be performed the same day scheduled. Patients will generally be asked to stay after the examination until films are reviewed by the radiologist.

Method EQUIPMENT: Standard B-mode real time ultrasonic imager with 2-5 MHz transrectal transducer. TECHNIQUE: A cylindrical transrectal ultrasound transducer is inserted into the rectum. The transducer is then gently rocked back and forth to obtain needed images. DATA ACQUIRED: Sagittal and transverse images of prostate and seminal vesicles.

Specimen TURNAROUND TIME: A typed report will generally be issued within 36 hours. A preliminary verbal report generally can be given to the referring physician on request.

Interpretation ADDITIONAL INFORMATION: This examination may be useful in the detection of prostatic carcinoma.

References

Lee F, Gray JM, McLeary RD, et al, "Prostatic Evaluation by Transrectal Sonography: Criteria for Diagnosis of Early Carcinoma," *Radiology*, 1986, 158:91-5.

Ultrasound, Radiotherapy Plan

CPT 76950

Synonyms Radiotherapy Plan Ultrasound

Abstract PROCEDURE COMMONLY INCLUDES: Specific anatomic area per request INDICATIONS: Measurement of distance between anterior surface to chest wall, mark boundaries of tumor for radiotherapist, measure distance to tumor and dimensions of therapy site.

(Continued)

Ultrasound, Radiotherapy Plan *(Continued)*

Method EQUIPMENT: Standard B-mode real time ultrasonic imager with 5-7 MHz transducer. TECHNIQUE: A gel is applied to the skin and a handheld transducer is swept across the area of interest to image the appropriate organs. Sound waves are used for the imaging and no radiation exposure is present. Images are recorded on x-ray film.

Specimen CAUSES FOR REJECTION: Bowel gas, barium, body habitus on patients with abdominal tumors TURNAROUND TIME: A typed report will generally be issued within 36 hours. A preliminary verbal report generally can be given to the referring physician on request.

Interpretation ADDITIONAL INFORMATION: Examination is limited to demarcating appropriate field used in radiotherapy.

Ultrasound, Renal Transplant

CPT 76778

Synonyms Renal Transplant Ultrasound

Abstract PROCEDURE COMMONLY INCLUDES: Renal transplant.

Patient Care/Scheduling PATIENT PREPARATION: The examination may be long, up to 1 hour including waiting time. An emergency examination or an unpredictably long preceding examination may result in additional delay. SPECIAL INSTRUCTIONS: All outpatient examinations are by appointment only. All inpatients are placed on the daily schedule as time permits and are performed as scheduled. Nonemergent examinations are given secondary priority and therefore may not be able to be performed the same day scheduled. Patients will generally be asked to stay after the examination until films are reviewed by the radiologist.

Method EQUIPMENT: Standard B-mode real time ultrasonic imager with Doppler capability with 2-5 MHz transducer. TECHNIQUE: A gel is applied to the skin and a handheld transducer is swept across the area of interest to image the appropriate organs. Sound waves are used for the imaging and no radiation exposure is present. Images are recorded on x-ray film.

Specimen TURNAROUND TIME: A typed report will generally be issued within 36 hours. A preliminary verbal report generally can be given to the referring physician on request.

Interpretation ADDITIONAL INFORMATION: Detection of perirenal fluid collections such as abscess urinoma or lymphocele. Doppler parameters are obtained to evaluate perfusion.

References

Rifkin MD, Needleman L, Pasto ME, et al, "Evaluation of Renal Transplant Rejection by Duplex Doppler Examination: Value of the Resistive Index," *AJR*, 1987, 148:759-62.

Ultrasound Retroperitoneal *see* Ultrasound, Abdomen *on page 393*

Ultrasound, Soft Tissue Mass

CPT 76999

Synonyms Superficial Soft Tissue Mass Ultrasound

Abstract PROCEDURE COMMONLY INCLUDES: Soft tissue mass INDICATIONS: Evaluate for the presence of mass, determine if a mass is solid or cystic, determine size of a mass.

Patient Care/Scheduling PATIENT PREPARATION: The examination may be long, up to 1 hour including waiting time. An emergency examination or an unpredictably long preceding examination may result in additional delay. SPECIAL INSTRUCTIONS: All outpatient examinations are by appointment only. All inpatients are placed on the daily schedule as time permits and are performed as scheduled. Nonemergent examinations are given secondary priority and therefore may not be able to be performed the same day scheduled. Patients will generally be asked to stay after the examination until films are reviewed by the radiologist.

Method EQUIPMENT: Standard B-mode real time ultrasonic imager with 2-7 MHz transducer. TECHNIQUE: A gel is applied to the skin and a handheld transducer is swept across the area of interest to image the appropriate organs. Sound waves are used for the imaging and no radiation exposure is present. Images are recorded on x-ray film.

Specimen TURNAROUND TIME: A typed report will generally be issued within 36 hours. A preliminary verbal report generally can be given to the referring physician on request.

Interpretation ADDITIONAL INFORMATION: This examination is useful in determining the size of peripheral masses. The examination will determine if the mass is solid, cystic, or complex.

Ultrasound, Spleen

CPT 76705

Synonyms Spleen Ultrasound

Abstract PROCEDURE COMMONLY INCLUDES: Spleen, left kidney (limited) INDICATIONS: Determines size, presence of calcifications, infarction, trauma, mass, cysts.

Patient Care/Scheduling PATIENT PREPARATION: All patients should be NPO for 12 hours prior to the exam. Examination should be performed prior to endoscopy, ERCP, barium studies, colonoscopy. The examination may be long, up to 1 hour including waiting time. An emergency examination or an unpredictably long preceding examination may result in additional delay. SPECIAL INSTRUCTIONS: All outpatient examinations are by appointment only. All inpatients are placed on the daily schedule as time permits and are performed as scheduled. Nonemergent examinations are given secondary priority and therefore may not be able to be performed the same day scheduled. Patients will generally be asked to stay after the examination until films are reviewed by the radiologist.

Method EQUIPMENT: Standard B-mode real time ultrasonic imager with 2-5 MHz transducer. TECHNIQUE: A gel is applied to the skin and a handheld transducer is swept across the area of interest to image the appropriate organs. Sound waves are used for the imaging and no radiation exposure is present. Images are recorded on x-ray film.

Specimen CAUSES FOR REJECTION: Gas, barium, oral ingestion of food, body habitus, rib artifacts TURNAROUND TIME: A typed report will generally be issued within 36 hours. A preliminary verbal report generally can be given to the referring physician on request.

Interpretation ADDITIONAL INFORMATION: This examination is most useful in evaluating for the presence of abnormal splenic collections or masses. Approximate size can also be determined.

References

Goldberg BB, *Abdominal Ultrasonography*, New York, NY: John Wiley and Sons Inc, 1984.

Ultrasound, Testicular

CPT 76870

Synonyms Testicular Ultrasound

Abstract PROCEDURE COMMONLY INCLUDES: Evaluation of scrotal contents INDICATIONS: Lesions, enlargement, epididymitis, torsion.

Patient Care/Scheduling PATIENT PREPARATION: The examination may be long, up to 1 hour including waiting time. An emergency examination or an unpredictably long preceding examination may result in additional delay. SPECIAL INSTRUCTIONS: All outpatient examinations are by appointment only. All inpatients are placed on the daily schedule as time permits and are performed as scheduled. Nonemergent examinations are given secondary priority and therefore may not be able to be performed the same day scheduled. Patients will generally be asked to stay after the examination until films are reviewed by the radiologist.

Method EQUIPMENT: Standard B-mode real time ultrasonic imager with 7-10 MHz transducer. TECHNIQUE: A gel is applied to the skin and a handheld transducer is swept across the testicles to image the appropriate organs. Sound waves are used for the imaging and no radiation exposure is present. Images are recorded on x-ray film.

Specimen CAUSES FOR REJECTION: Lack of patient cooperation, unable to hold still for exam TURNAROUND TIME: A typed report will generally be issued within 36 hours. A preliminary verbal report generally can be given to the referring physician on request.

Interpretation ADDITIONAL INFORMATION: Very useful examination for detecting occult malignancies of the testicle. Other lesions seen include spermatocele, varicocele, hydrocele, hematocele, infarct, orchitis and epididymitis.

References

Krone KD and Carroll BA, "Scrotal Ultrasound," *Radiol Clin North Am*, 1985, 23:121-39.

Ultrasound, Thoracentesis

CPT 76935

Related Information

Thoracentesis *on page 267*

Synonyms Thoracentesis Ultrasound

Abstract PROCEDURE COMMONLY INCLUDES: Use of real time ultrasound to find suitable puncture site for thoracentesis and perform thoracentesis INDICATIONS: Provide a suitable site for thoracentesis.

Patient Care/Scheduling PATIENT PREPARATION: The examination may be long, up to 1 hour including waiting time. An emergency examination or an unpredictably long preceding examination may result in additional delay. AFTERCARE: Check physician order sheet. Chest x-rays on inspiration and expiration are routine to rule out a pneumothorax. SPECIAL INSTRUCTIONS: All outpatient examinations are by appointment only. All inpatients are placed on the daily schedule as time permits and are performed as scheduled. Nonemergent examinations are given secondary priority and therefore may not be able to be performed the same day scheduled. Patients will generally be asked to stay after the examination until films are reviewed by the radiologist.

Method EQUIPMENT: Standard B-mode real time ultrasonic imager with 7-10 MHz transducer. TECHNIQUE: A gel is applied to the skin and a handheld transducer is swept across the area of interest to image the appropriate organs. Sound waves are used for the imaging and no radiation exposure is present. Images are recorded on x-ray film.

Specimen CAUSES FOR REJECTION: Lack of suitable puncture site TURNAROUND TIME: A typed report will generally be issued within 36 hours. A preliminary verbal report generally can be given to the referring physician on request.

References

Neff CC and Van Sonnenberg E, "Percutaneous Drainage of Pleural Collections," *Radiology*, Taveras JT and Ferrucci JT, eds, Philadelphia, PA: JB Lippincott, 1988.

Ultrasound, Thyroid

CPT 76536

Synonyms Thyroid Ultrasound

Abstract PROCEDURE COMMONLY INCLUDES: Thyroid gland INDICATIONS: Prove whether a palpable mass is a simple cyst; enlarged thyroid CONTRAINDICATIONS: Patient unable to lay supine with head hyperextended.

Patient Care/Scheduling PATIENT PREPARATION: The examination may be long, up to 1 hour including waiting time. An emergency examination or an unpredictably long preceding examination may result in additional delay. **Note**: Ultrasound exam to be scheduled before a barium study. If barium study was done, bowel preparation is needed before doing ultrasound examination. SPECIAL INSTRUCTIONS: All outpatient examinations are by appointment only. All inpatients are placed on the daily schedule as time permits and are performed as scheduled. Nonemergent examinations are given secondary priority and therefore may not be able to be performed the same day scheduled. Patients will generally be asked to stay after the examination until films are reviewed by the radiologist.

Method EQUIPMENT: Standard B-mode real time ultrasonic imager with 5-10 MHz transducer. TECHNIQUE: A gel is applied to the skin and a handheld transducer is swept across the area of interest to image the appropriate organs. Sound waves are used for the imaging and no radiation exposure is present. Images are recorded on x-ray film.

Specimen TURNAROUND TIME: A typed report will generally be issued within 36 hours. A preliminary verbal report generally can be given to the referring physician on request.

Interpretation LIMITATIONS: Patient has to have palpable mass and have a cold spot on the Nuclear Medicine thyroid scan. Thyroid exams will not be done without a previous Nuclear Medicine scan unless the referring physician has consulted a radiologist. ADDITIONAL INFORMATION: If patient is pregnant, then Nuclear Medicine thyroid scan is not a prerequisite. Physician should consult a radiologist before ordering exam if patient is pregnant.

References

Butch RJ, Simeone JF, and Mueller PR, "Thyroid and Parathyroid Ultrasonography," *Radiol Clin North Am*, 1985, 23(1)57-71.

Simeone JF, "Ultrasound Examination of the Thyroid and Parathyroid," *Radiology*, Taveras JT and Ferrucci JT, eds, Philadelphia, PA: JB Lippincott, 1988.

Ultrasound, Transcranial Doppler Vascular Examination

CPT 76926

Abstract PROCEDURE COMMONLY INCLUDES: Intracranial common carotid arteries, anterior cerebral, posterior cerebral, middle cerebral, anterior and posterior communicating arteries, vertebral and basilar arteries INDICATIONS: Evaluate velocity of (blood flow) in intracranial arteries, evaluation of presence of vasospasm intracranial arterial stenosis.

Patient Care/Scheduling PATIENT PREPARATION: The examination may be long, up to 1 hour including waiting time. An emergency examination or an unpredictably long preceding examination may result in additional delay. SPECIAL INSTRUCTIONS: All outpatient examinations are by appointment only. All inpatients are placed on the daily schedule as time permits and are performed as scheduled. Nonemergent examinations are given secondary priority and therefore may not be able to be performed the same day scheduled. Patients will generally be asked to stay after the examination until films are reviewed by the radiologist.

Method EQUIPMENT: Pulsed Doppler transcranial ultrasound unit with 2 MHz transducer. TECHNIQUE: A gel is applied to the skin and a handheld transducer is swept across the area of interest to obtain flow velocity data. Sound waves are used for the imaging and no radiation exposure is present.

Specimen TURNAROUND TIME: A typed report will generally be issued within 36 hours. A preliminary verbal report generally can be given to the referring physician on request.

Interpretation ADDITIONAL INFORMATION: Relatively new device to evaluate the intracranial circulation. May be of value to detect stenosis, occlusion, spasm, vascular steals.

References

Arnolds BJ and von Reutern GM, "Transcranial Doppler Sonography. Examination Technique and Normal Reference Values," *Ultrasound Med Biol*, 1986, 12:115-23.

Hennerici M, Rautenberg W, Sitzer G, et al, "Transcranial Doppler Ultrasound for the Assessment of Intracranial Arterial Flow Velocity. Part I. Examination Technique and Normal Values," *Surg Neurol*, 1987, 27:439-48.

Ultrasound, Transvaginal

CPT 76830

Synonyms Transvaginal Ultrasound

Abstract PROCEDURE COMMONLY INCLUDES: Uterus, ovaries, adnexa INDICATIONS: Pelvic masses and abscess, uterus size, IUD localization and pregnancy diagnosis; ectopic pregnancy, dermoid cyst, pelvic inflammatory disease, ovarian cyst, fibroid tumor, and bladder tumor.

Patient Care/Scheduling PATIENT PREPARATION: The examination may be long, up to 1 hour including waiting time. An emergency examination or an unpredictably long preceding examination may result in additional delay. SPECIAL INSTRUCTIONS: All outpatient examinations are by appointment only. All inpatients are placed on the daily schedule as time permits and are performed as scheduled. Nonemergent examinations are given secondary priority and therefore may not be able to be performed the same day scheduled. Patients will generally be asked to stay after the examination until films are reviewed by the radiologist.

Method EQUIPMENT: Standard B-mode real time ultrasonic imager with 3-5 MHz transvaginal transducer. TECHNIQUE: A gel is applied to the skin and a handheld transducer is placed into the vagina to image the pelvis. Sound waves are used for the imaging and no radiation exposure is present. Images are recorded on x-ray film. DATA ACQUIRED: Coronal, sagittal images of uterus and adnexa.

Specimen TURNAROUND TIME: A typed report will generally be issued within 36 hours. A preliminary verbal report generally can be given to the referring physician on request.

Ultrasound, Urinary Bladder

CPT 76856

Synonyms Urinary Bladder Ultrasound

Abstract PROCEDURE COMMONLY INCLUDES: Urinary bladder, prostate (limited) INDICATIONS: Bladder neoplasm, bladder calculi, foreign bodies, prostate hypertrophy, bladder carcinoma.

(Continued)

Ultrasound, Urinary Bladder *(Continued)*

Patient Care/Scheduling **PATIENT PREPARATION:** Outpatient: Instruct patient to drink 16 oz of fluid 1 hour prior to exam and not to empty bladder. Inpatient: Ultrasound will notify the floor when to instruct the patient to drink 16 oz of fluid. The examination may be long, up to 1 hour including waiting time. An emergency examination or an unpredictably long preceding examination may result in additional delay. **SPECIAL INSTRUCTIONS:** All outpatient examinations are by appointment only. All inpatients are placed on the daily schedule as time permits and are performed as scheduled. Nonemergent examinations are given secondary priority and therefore may not be able to be performed the same day scheduled. Patients will generally be asked to stay after the examination until films are reviewed by the radiologist.

Method **EQUIPMENT:** Standard B-mode real time ultrasonic imager with 2-5 MHz transducer. **TECHNIQUE:** A gel is applied to the skin and a handheld transducer is swept across the area of interest to image the appropriate organs. Sound waves are used for the imaging and no radiation exposure is present. Images are recorded on x-ray film.

Specimen **TURNAROUND TIME:** A typed report will generally be issued within 36 hours. A preliminary verbal report generally can be given to the referring physician on request.

Urinary Bladder Ultrasound *see* Ultrasound, Urinary Bladder *on previous page*

ACRONYMS AND ABBREVIATIONS GLOSSARY

This glossary provides a useful listing of many acronyms and abbreviations commonly associated with laboratory medicine. We offer this glossary not as an exhaustive authoritative list, but more as a guide to assist in interpreting frequently used terminology.

ACRONYMS AND ABBREVIATIONS GLOSSARY

A ... apical; artery
A1AT ... alpha$_1$ antitrypsin
A_2 ... aortic second sound
aa ... of each (ana)
AABB ... American Association of Blood Banks
AAC ... antibiotic associated colitis
AACC ... American Association of Clinical Chemistry
AaG ... alveolar arterial gradient
AAL ... anterior axillary line
AAP ... American Academy of Pediatrics
AAPCC ... American Association of Poison Control Centers
AAS ... acute abdominal series
AAT ... alpha antitrypsin
Ab ... antibody
AB ... abort; antibiotic
ABC ... avidin-biotin complex
ABE ... acute bacterial endocarditis
ABG ... arterial blood gas
ABL ... abetalipoprotein
ABLB ... alternate binaural loudness balance
ABO ... ABO blood group
ABPA ... allergic bronchopulmonary aspergillosis
ABR ... auditory brainstem response
ABS ... alkylbenzene sulfonate
ac ... before meals (ante cibum)
Ac ... actinium
AC ... air conduction; alternating current
ACA ... anticardiolipin antibody; Du Pont chemistry analyzer
ACC ... amylase creatinine clearance
ACD ... acid-citrate-dextrose
ACE ... angiotensin converting enzyme
AChR ... acetylcholine receptor antibody
ACLS ... advanced cardiac life support
ACOG ... American College of Obstetrics and Gynecology
AcP ... acid phosphatase
ACT ... activated clotting time
ACTH ... adrenocorticotropic hormone
ad ... right ear; up to (ad)
ADCC ... antibody-dependent cell-mediated cytotoxicity
ADH ... alcohol dehydrogenase; antidiuretic hormone
ADL ... active daily living
ad lib ... as desired (ad libitum)
ADM ... admission
ADNase ... anti-DNAse
ADP ... adenosine 5-diphosphate
ADT ... adenosine triphosphate; alternate-day treatment
AED ... anticonvulsant drugs
AEP ... average evoked potential
AF ... acid-fast; amniotic fluid; artrial fibrillation
AFB ... acid-fast bacillus
AFP ... alphafetoprotein
Ag ... antigen; silver
A/G ... albumin/globulin ratio
AGA ... accelerated growth area
AGL ... acute glomerular nephritis
$AgNO_3$ ... silver nitrate
AGS ... adrenogenital syndrome
AH ... antihyaluronidase
A-H ... atrial-HIS
AHA ... acquired hemolytic anemia; autoimmune hemolytic anemia
AHBC ... hepatitis B core antibody
AHF ... antihemophilic factor

AHG .... antihemophilic globulin
AHT .... antihyaluronidase titer
AI .... allergy index; aortic insufficiency
AICC .... anti-inhibitor coagulant complex
AIDS .... acquired immune deficiency syndrome
AIHA .... autoimmune hemolytic anemia
AIP .... acute intermittent porphyria; average intravascular pressure
AJ .... ankle jerk
AK .... adenylate kinase; above the knee
Al .... aluminum
ALA .... aminolevulinic acid
alb .... albumin
alk .... alkaline
AlkP .... alkaline phosphatase
ALL .... acute lymphoblastic leukemia; acute lymphocytic leukemia
$Al(OH)_3$ .... aluminum hydroxide
ALP .... alkaline phosphatase
ALPI .... alkaline phosphatase isoenzymes
ALS .... advanced life support; amyotrophic lateral sclerosis; antilymphocyte serum
ALT .... alanine aminotransferase
Am .... americium
AM .... morning
AMA .... against medical advice; American Medical Association; antimitrochondrial antibody
AMI .... acute myocardial infarction
AML .... acute myeloblastic leukemia
AMP .... adenosine monophosphate
AMPS .... acid mucopolysaccharide
ANA .... antinuclear antibody
ANF .... antinuclear factor
ANLL .... acute nonlymphocytic leukemia
A & O .... alert and oriented
AODM .... adult onset diabetes mellitus
AOS .... acridine orange staining
AP .... antepartum; anteroposterior
A & P .... anterior and posterior; assessment and plans
APCA .... antiparetial cell antibody
APhA .... American Pharmaceutical Association
APP .... alum-precipitating pyridine
APTT .... activated partial thromboplastin time
APUD .... amine precursor uptake and decarboxylation
aq .... water (aqua)
Ar .... argon
ARA .... antireticulin antibody
ARD .... antimicrobial removal device; acute respiratory distress
ARDS .... adult respiratory distress syndrome
ARF .... acute renal failure
Ars .... arylsulfatase
ART .... arterial line
as .... left ear
As .... arsenic
AS .... anal sphincter; ankylosing spondylitis; aortic stenosis
ASA .... acetylsalicylic acid
AsA .... arylsulfatase A
ASAP .... as soon as possible
AsB .... arylsulfatase B
ASCP .... American Society of Clinical Pathologists
ASCVD .... arteriosclerotic cardiovascular disease
ASD .... atrial septal defect
ASHD .... arteriosclerotic heart disease

ASHP ....American Society of Hospital Pharmacists
ASK ....antistreptokinase
ASKA ....antiskeletal antibody
ASLO ....antistreptolysin O
ASMA ....antismooth muscle antibody
ASO ....antistreptolysin O; arterioselerosis obliterans
AST............aspartate aminotransferase
ASVD ....arteriosclerotic vascular disease
At ....astatine
AT III ....antithrombin III
ATN ....acute tubular necrosis
ATP............adenosine triphosphate
ATPase.........adenosine triphosphatase
ATS............American Thoracic Society
au ....each ear (auris utro)
Au ....gold
^{198}Au ....radioisotope of gold
A-V ....arteriovenous; atrioventricular; audiovisual
AVA ....availability
AVM ....arteriovenous malformation
A & W ....alive and well
Ax ....axillary

B ....boron
Ba ....barium
BAC ....blood alcohol concentration
BAE ....barium enema
BAEP ....brainstem auditory evoked potential
BAER ....brainstem auditory evoked response
BAL............bronchial alveolar lavage
BAO ....basal acid output
BBB ....blood brain barrier; bundle branch block
BBPRL ....big big prolactin
BBT ....basal body temperature
BC ....bone conduction
BCG ....bacillus Calmette-Guérin
BCP ....birth control pills; blood cell profile
bcr ....breakpoint cluster region
BD ....bronchodilators
Be ....beryllium
BE.............bacterial endocarditis; barium enema
BEP ....brainstem evoked potential
BERA ....brainstem evoked response auditory
BF ....black female
BFT............bentonite flocculation test
BHB ....beta-hydroxybutyrate
BHI ....brain heart infusion
Bi ....bismuth
bid ....twice a day (bis in die)
B-J ....Bence Jones
BJ ....biceps jerk; bone and joint
Bk ....berkelium
BK.............below knee
Bl Obs ....bladder observation
BLS............basic life support
BM ....black male; bone marrow; bowel movement; breast milk
BMR ....basal metabolic rate
BNO ....bladder neck obstruction
BP.............blood pressure
BPD ....biparietal diameter
BPH ....benign prostatic hypertrophy

Br .... bromine; bromide
BR............ bathroom; bedrest
BrdU 5-bromodeoxyuridine
BRP .... bathroom privileges
BRU .... bromide urine
BS............ blood sugar; bowel sounds; breath sounds
bsa .... body surface area
BSEP .... brainstem evoked potential
BSO .... bilateral salpingo-oophorectomy
BSP .... bromsulfophthalein
BTG .... beta thromboglobulin
BTL........... bilateral tubal ligation
BUN .... blood urea nitrogen
BVL........... bilateral vas ligation
BW .... birth weight; body weight
Bx .... biopsy

c .... with (cum)
C............. carbon
C_2 .... second cervical vertebra
Ca............ calcium
CA .... cancer antigen; cardiac arrest; chronological age
CAB .... coronary artery bypass
CABG .... coronary artery bypass graft
CAC .... circulating anticoagulant
CaCl .... calcium chloride
$CaCO_3$ .... calcium carbonate
CAD .... coronary artery disease
CaEDTA .... calcium disodium edetate
CAH .... chronic active hepatitis
CALLA .... common acute lymphoblastic leukemia antigen
cAMP .... cyclic AMP
CAPD .... chronic ambulatory peritoneal dialysis
CAT .... computed axial tomography
CBAT .... Coulter battery
CBC .... complete blood count
CBD .... common bile duct
CBF .... cerebral blood flow
CBG .... capillary blood gases
CBIL .... conjugated bilirubin
CBS .... chronic brain syndrome
CBT .... computerized body tomography
CC .... chief complaint; closing capacity
CCI .... corrected count increment
CCK .... cholecystokinin
CCK-OP .... cholecystokinin-octapeptide
CCU .... cardiac care unit; coronary care unit
Cd............ cadmium
CDA .... congenital dyserythropoietic anemia
CDC .... Center for Disease Control
CDP .... continuous distending pressure; cytidine diphosphate
CDU .... cumulative dose unit
Ce............ cerium
CEA .... carcinoembryonic antigen
Cf .... californium
CF............ cardiac failure; caucasian female; complement fixation; cystic fibrosis
CFU .... colony forming units
CGL .... chronic granulocytic leukemia
CH .... congenital hypothyroidism
CHBHA........ congenital Heinz body hemolytic anemia
CHD .... congenital heart disease

CHF ....congestive heart failure
CI ....cardiac index; color index; confidence intervals
CIC ....circulating immune complexes
CIE ....counterimmunoelectrophoresis
CIF ....clone-inhibiting factor
CIN ....cervical intraepithelial neoplasia
CIP ....cellular immunocompetence profile
CIPD ....chronic inflammatory demyelinating polyradiculoneuropathy
CJD ....Creutzfeldt-Jakob disease
CK ....creatine kinase
Cl ....chlorine
CLL...........chronic lymphocytic leukemia
cm ....centimeter
cm^2 ....square centimeter
Cm ....curium
CM ....caucasian male; contrast media; culture media
CMG ....cystometrogram
CML ....cell mediated lysis; chronic myelogenous leukemia
cmm ....square centimeter cm^2
CMP ....cardiomyopathy; cervical mucus penetration
CMPT ....cervical mucous penetration test
CMV ....cytomegalovirus
CMVS ....culture midvoid specimen
CN ....cyanogen
CNS ....central nervous system
CNSHA ....congenital nonspherocytic hemolytic anemia
Co ....cobalt
^{57}Co ....radioisotope of cobalt
^{60}Co ....radioisotope of cobalt
CO ....carbon monoxide; cardiac output
C/O ....complaint of
CO_3...........carbonate
coag ....coagulation
COHb ....carboxyhemoglobin
COLD ....chronic obstructive lung disease
COP ....chronic obstructive pulmonary
COPD ....chronic obstructive pulmonary disease
C & P ....cystoscopy and pyelogram
CPA ....carotid phonoangiography
CPAP ....continuous positive airway pressure
CPB ....cardiopulmonary bypass
CPD ....cyst disease protein; citrate phosphate dextrose
CPDA ....citrate phosphate dextrose adenine
CPE ....cytopathogenic effects
CPI ....coronary prognostic index
CPK ....creatine phosphokinase
cpm ....counts per minute
CPP ....cerebral perfusion pressure
CPPB ....continuous positive pressure breathing
CPPD ....calcium pyrophosphate dihydrate
CPR ....cardiopulmonary resuscitation
cps ....cycles per second
CPS ....Compendium of Pharmaceuticals and Specialties
CPT ....chest physiotherapy
Cr ....chromium
^{51}Cr...........radioisotope of chromium
CRA ....central retinal artery
Cre ....creatinine
creat ....creatinine
CRF ....chronic renal failure; corticotropin releasing factor
CRM ....cross reacting material
CRP ....C-reactive protein

CRS . . . . catheter related sepsis
CRST . . . . calcinosis, Raynaud's phenomenon, sclerodactylia, telangiectasis
CRT . . . . cathode ray tube
Cs . . . . cesium
CS . . . . cesarean section; coronary sclerosis
C & S . . . . culture and sensitivity
CS & CC . . . . . . culture, sensitivity and colony count
CSF . . . . cerebrospinal fluid
CSP . . . . chemistry screening profile
CSR . . . . corrected sedimentation rate
CT . . . . circulation time; clotting time; computerized tomography
CTA . . . . Committee on Thrombolytic Agents
CTAB . . . . cetyltrimethylammonium bromide
CTD . . . . carpal tunnel decompression; congenital thymic dysplasia
CTM . . . . *Chlamydia* transport media
CTT . . . . computerized transaxial tomography
Cu . . . . copper
CUC . . . . chronic ulcerative colitis
CV . . . . cardiovascular; coefficient of variation; conjugata vera
CVA . . . . cerebrovascular accident
CVE . . . . cerebrovascular evaluation
CVI . . . . cerebral vascular insufficiency; continuous venous infusion
CVP . . . . central venous pressure
CVS . . . . cardiovascular system; clean voided specimen
Cx . . . . cervical; cervix
CXR . . . . chest x-ray

D_5W . . . . 5% dextrose in water solution
DALA . . . . delta aminolevulinic acid
DAT . . . . direct antiglobulin test
db . . . . decibel
DB . . . . deep breath
DBI . . . . development at birth index
DBP . . . . diastolic blood pressure
DC . . . . direct current
D & C . . . . dilatation and curettage
DCG . . . . dynamic electrocardiogram
DCH . . . . delayed and cutaneous hypersensitivity
DD . . . . differential diagnosis
DDD . . . . degenerative disc disease
DDT . . . . dichloro-diphenyltrichloroethane
DDX . . . . differential diagnosis
DEA . . . . Drug Enforcement Agency
DEAE . . . . diethylaminoethyl
DER . . . . dermatone evoked response
DFA . . . . direct fluorescent antibody
dg . . . . decigram
DH . . . . dermatitis herpetiformis
DHA . . . . dehydroepiandrosterone
DHEA . . . . dehydroepiandrosterone
DHEA-S . . . . dehydroepiandrosterone sulfate
DHL . . . . diffuse histiocytic lymphoma
DHS . . . . duration of hospital stay
DHT . . . . dihydrotestosterone
DI . . . . diabetes insipidus
DIC . . . . disseminated intravascular coagulation
diff . . . . differential
DIP . . . . dichlorophenolindophenol
DISIDA . . . . diisopropyl-iminodiacetic acid
DJD . . . . degenerative joint disease
DKA . . . . diabetic ketoacidosis

dL . . . . deciliter
D-L . . . . Donath-Landsteiner
DLCO . . . . diffusing capacity of the lung for carbon monoxide
DLE . . . . discoid lupus erythematosus
DLF . . . . digoxin-like factors
dm . . . . decimeter
DM . . . . diabetes mellitus; diastolic murmur
DMO . . . . dimethyloxazolidinedione
DMSO . . . . dimethylsulfoxide
DNA . . . . deoxyribonucleic acid
DNase . . . . deoxyribonuclease
DNBT . . . . dinitroblue
DNPH . . . . dinitrophenylhydrazine
DOA . . . . date of admission; dead on arrival
DOB . . . . date of birth
DOC . . . . deoxycorticosterone
DOE . . . . dyspnea on exertion
DOI . . . . date of injury
dos . . . . dose (dosis)
DP . . . . diastolic pressure
DPG . . . . diphosphoglycerate
DPH . . . . diphenylhydantoin
DPT . . . . diphtheria toxoid, pertussis vaccine, tetanus toxoid
DQ . . . . developmental quotient
Dr . . . . doctor
DR . . . . donor related
DRG . . . . diagnostic related group(s)
DSA . . . . digital subtraction angiography
DSD . . . . discharge summary dictated; dry sterile dressing
ds-DNA . . . . double stranded DNA
DSF . . . . disulfiram
DST . . . . dexamethasone suppression test
DT . . . . delirium tremons; duration tetany; dye test
dtd . . . . let such doses be given (dentur tales doses)
DTM . . . . dermatophyte test medium
DTR . . . . deep tendon reflex
dU . . . . deoxyuridine
DVT . . . . deep vein thrombosis
Dx . . . . diagnosis
Dy . . . . dysprosium

EA . . . . early antigen
EAC . . . . external auditory canal
EACA . . . . epsilon-aminocaproic acid
EB . . . . Epstein-Barr
EBEA . . . . Epstein-Barr early antigen
EBNA . . . . Epstein-Barr nuclear antigen
EBV . . . . Epstein-Barr virus
EB-VCA . . . . Epstein-Barr viral capsid antigen
EBVEA . . . . Epstein-Barr virus, early antigen
EBVNA . . . . Epstein-Barr virus, nuclear antigen
EC . . . . *Escherichia coli*; extracellular
ECA . . . . external carotid artery
ECG . . . . electrocardiogram
ECT . . . . emission computed tomography
EDTA . . . . ethylenediaminetetraacetic acid
EDX . . . . electrodiagnosis
EEG . . . . electroencephalography
EENT . . . . eyes, ears, nose, throat
EF . . . . ejection fraction; extended-field
EFA . . . . essential fatty acids

EFM .... external fetal monitoring
eg .... example
EGA .... estimated gestational age
EGD .... esophagogastroduodenoscopy
EH .... enlarged heart; essential hypertension
EHEC .... enterohemorrhagic *E. coli*
EIA .... enzyme immunoassay
EID .... electroimmunodiffusion
EIEC .... enteroinvasive *E. coli*
EKG .... electrocardiogram
ELISA .... enzyme-linked immunosorbent assay
ELT .... euoglobulin lysis time
EM .... electron microscopy
EMA .... endomysial antibody
EMG .... electromyogram
EMS .... eosinophil myalgia syndrome
ENA .... extractable nuclear antigen
ENG .... electronystagmography
ENT .... ear, nose and throat
EOG .... electro-oculogram
eos .... eosinophil
EPA .... Environmental Protection Agency
EPBI .... exercise penile-brachial index
EPEC .... enteropathogenic *E. coli*
EPIS .... episiotomy
EPS .... electrophysiologic studies
Eq .... equivalent
Er .... erbium
ER .... emergency room; estrogen receptors
ERA .... estrogen receptor assay; evoked response audiometry
ERCP .... endoscopic retrograde cholangiopancreatography
ERG .... electroretinogram
ERPF .... effective renal plasma flow
ERV .... expiratory reserve volume
Es .... Einsteinium
ES .... electrical stimulation
ESP .... extrasensory perception
ESR .... erythrocyte sedimentation rate
ESRD .... end-stage renal disease
EST .... electroshock therapy
et .... and (et)
ETEC .... enterotoxigenic *E. coli*
EtOH .... ethyl alcohol
ETT .... extrathyroidal thyroxine
EU .... Ehrlich unit
EVI .... endocardial, vascular, and interstitial

F .... fluorine
FA .... fatty acid; filterable agent; fluorescent antibody
FAB .... French-American-British
FACP .... Fellow of the American College of Physicians
FAD .... flavin adenine dinucleotide
FAMA .... fluorescent antibody to membrane antigen
FANA .... fluorescent antinuclear antibody
FAS .... fetal alcohol syndrome
FB .... finger breadths; foreign bodies
FBC .... functional bactericidal concentration
FBP .... fibrin breakdown product
FBS .... fasting blood sugar
Fc .... portion of antibody molecule bound by membrane receptors
FDA .... Federal Drug Administration

FDP . . . . fibrin degradation product; fructose diphosphate
Fe . . . . iron
$FeCl_3$ . . . . ferric chloride
FEF . . . . forced expiratory flow
FEP . . . . free erythrocyte protoporphyrin
FES . . . . functional electrical stimulation
FETI . . . . fluorescent energy transfer immunoassay
FEV . . . . forced expiratory volume
FF . . . . filtration fraction; force fluids
FFA . . . . free fatty acids
FFP . . . . fresh frozen plasma
fg . . . . femtogram
FH . . . . family history
FHH . . . . familial hypocalciuric hypercalcemia
FHR . . . . fetal heart rate
FHS . . . . fetal heart sounds
FIC . . . . functional inhibitory concentration
FIF . . . . forced inspiratory flow
FITC . . . . fluorescein isothiocyanate
FIVC . . . . forced inspiratory vital capacity
fL . . . . femtoliter; fluid
Fm . . . . fermium
fmol . . . . femtomole
FMULC . . . . free monoclonal urinary light chains
FNA . . . . fine needle aspiration
FOB . . . . fiberoptic bronchoscopy
FOS . . . . fiberoptic sigmoidoscopy
FP . . . . false-positive
Fr . . . . francium
FRA . . . . fluorescent rabies antibody
FRC . . . . functional residual capacity
FS . . . . frozen section
FSH . . . . follicle stimulating hormone
FSI . . . . foam stability index
FSP . . . . fibrin split products
ft . . . . make (fiat, fiant)
FTA . . . . fluorescent treponemal antibody
FTA-ABS . . . . . . fluorescent treponemal antibody absorption
FTI . . . . free thyroxine index
FTND . . . . full-term normal delivery
FUO . . . . fever of undetermined origin
FVC . . . . forced vital capacity
Fx . . . . fracture
FX . . . . factor X

g . . . . gram
G-6-PD . . . . glucose 6-phosphate dehydrogenase
Ga . . . . gallium
GABA . . . . gamma-aminobutyric acid
GAL . . . . galactosemia
GAW . . . . airway conductance
GAZT . . . . glucuronide derivative of azidothymidine
GB . . . . gallbladder
GBM . . . . glomerular basement membrane
GC . . . . geriatric chair; gonorrhea culture; gas chromatography
GC-MS . . . . gas chromatography - mass spectrometry
Gd . . . . gadolinium
g/dL . . . . gram percent
Ge . . . . germanium
GE . . . . gastroesophageal
GFR . . . . glomerular filtration rate

GGCT . . . . ground glass clotting time
GGT . . . . gamma-glutamyltransferase
GH . . . . growth hormone
GHB . . . . glycohemoglobin
GI . . . . gastrointestinal
GIH . . . . gastric inhibitory hormone
GIP . . . . gastric inhibitory polypeptide
GIS . . . . gastrointestinal series
GK . . . . galactokinase
GLC . . . . gas-liquid chromatography
GM . . . . geometric mean
GMS . . . . Grocott-Gomori methenamine-silver
GnRH . . . . gonadotropin releasing hormone
GOT . . . . glutamic-oxaloacetic transaminase
GP . . . . glycoprotein
GPK . . . . guinea pig kidney
GPT . . . . glutamic-pyruvic transaminase
GPUT . . . . glactose phosphate uridyl transferase
GR . . . . glutathione reductase
GSD . . . . glycogen storage disease
GSH . . . . glutathione; growth stimulating hormone
GSR . . . . galvanic skin response; generalized Schwartzman reaction
GSSR . . . . generalized Sandarelli-Shwartzman reaction
GT . . . . gait training; gamma-glutamyltransferase
GTP . . . . glutamyl transpeptidase
GTT . . . . glucose tolerance test
gtt(s) . . . . drop(s) (gutta)
GU . . . . genitourinary; gastric ulcer; gonococcal urethritis
GVHD . . . . graft versus host disease
GXT . . . . graded exercise test
gyn . . . . gynecological

h . . . . hour (hora)
H . . . . hydrogen
Ha . . . . hahnium
HA . . . . headache
HABA . . . . hydroxybenzeneazobenzoic acid
HAI . . . . hemagglutination inhibition
HANE . . . . hereditary angioneurotic edema
HAV . . . . hepatitis A virus
HAVAB . . . . hepatitis A virus antibody
Hb . . . . hemoglobin
HBAB . . . . hepatitis B antibody
HB_c . . . . hepatitis B core
HBD . . . . hydroxybutric dehydrogenase
HBDH . . . . hydroxybutyrate dehydrogenase
HB_eAg . . . . hepatitis B e antigen
HBP . . . . high blood pressure
HB_sAg . . . . hepatitis B surface antigen
HBV . . . . hepatitis B virus
HC . . . . homocystinuria
HCFA . . . . Health Care Financing Administration
hCG . . . . human chorionic gonadotropin
HCl . . . . hydrochloric acid
HCO_3 . . . . bicarbonate
HCS . . . . human chorionic somatomammotropin
Hct . . . . hematocrit
HD . . . . Hodgkin's disease
HDL . . . . high density lipoprotein
HDLC . . . . high density lipoprotein cholesterol

HDN . . . . hemolytic disease of the newborn
HDP . . . . hydroxydimethylpyrimidine
He . . . . helium
HEMPAS . . . . . . here. erythroblastic multinuclearity with positive acidified serum
HEp . . . . human epithelial cells
HES . . . . acute hypereosinophilic syndrome
Hf . . . . hafnium
HFI . . . . hereditary fructose intolerance
Hg . . . . mercury
^{197}Hg . . . . radioisotope of mercury
^{203}Hg . . . . radioisotope of mercury
HG . . . . herpes gestationis
HGA . . . . homogentisic acid
Hgb . . . . hemoglobin
HGG . . . . human gamma globulin
HGH . . . . human growth hormone
HGPRT . . . . hypoxanthine guanine phosphoribosyl transferase
HHC . . . . home health care
HHD . . . . hypertensive heart disease
HHH . . . . hyperornithinemia, hyperammonemia-homocitrullinuria
HHM . . . . humoral hypercalcemia of malignancy
HHT . . . . head holter traction
HI . . . . hydriodic acid
HIAA . . . . hydroxyindoleacetic acid
HIB . . . . *Haemophilus influenzae* B
HIDA . . . . acetanilidoiminodiacetic acid
HIP . . . . humoral immunocompetence profile
HIV . . . . human immunodeficiency virus
HK . . . . hexokinase
HL . . . . hearing level
HLA . . . . human leukocyte antigen
HMO . . . . Health Maintenance Organization
HMS . . . . hexose monophosphate shunt
HMW . . . . high molecular weight
HMWK . . . . high molecular weight kininogen
HN . . . . head nurse
Ho . . . . holmium
HO . . . . house officer
H/O . . . . history of
HOB . . . . head of bed
HP . . . . hot packs
H & P . . . . history and physical
hpf . . . . high power field
HPFH . . . . hereditary persistence of fetal hemoglobin
HPI . . . . history of present illness
HPL . . . . human placental lactogen
HPLC . . . . high-performance liquid chromatography; high-pressure liquid chromatography
HPN . . . . home parenteral nutrition
HPP . . . . human pancreatic polypeptide
HPPH . . . . hydroxyphenyl-phenylhydantoin
HPT . . . . hyperparathyroidism
HPV . . . . human papilloma virus
HR . . . . heart rate; hospital record
HRANA . . . . histone reactive ANA
HRLM . . . . high resolution light microscopy
hs . . . . at bedtime (hora somni)
HS . . . . herpes simplex; hereditary spherocytosis
HSV . . . . herpes simplex virus
HT . . . . hypertension; hypodermic tablet
HTLV . . . . human T-lymphotropic virus
HTN . . . . hypertension

HTP . . . . hydroxytrytophan
HTVD . . . . hypertensive vascular disease
HUS . . . . hemolytic-uremic syndrome; hyaluronidase unit for semen
H-V . . . . HIS-ventricular
HVA . . . . homovanillic acid
Hx . . . . history
Hz . . . . hertz

I . . . . iodine
^{125}I . . . . radioisotope of iodide
^{131}I . . . . radioisotope of iodide
Ia . . . . antigen
IAA . . . . indole acetic acid
I-3-AA . . . . indole-3-acetic acid
IABP . . . . intra-aortic balloon pump
IADH . . . . inappropriate antidiuretic hormone
IAT . . . . indirect antiglobulin test
Ib . . . . a glycoprotein
IBC . . . . iron binding capacity
IC . . . . immune complexes; inspiratory capacity
ICA . . . . internal carotid artery
ICD . . . . isocitrate dehydrogenase
ICDH . . . . isocitrate dehydrogenase
ICG . . . . indocyanine green
ICN . . . . intensive care neonatal
ICS . . . . intercostal space
ICSH . . . . interstitial cell stimulating hormone
ICT . . . . indirect Coombs' test
ICU . . . . intensive care unit
ID . . . . identification; immunodiffusion; infectious disease; intradermal(ly)
IDA . . . . iron deficiency anemia; image display and analysis
IDAT . . . . indirect antiglobulin test
IDDM . . . . insulin dependent diabetes mellitus
IDL . . . . intermediate-density lipoprotein
IEF . . . . isoelectric focusing
IEM . . . . inborn errors of metabolism
IEP . . . . immunoelectrophoresis
IF . . . . immunofluorescence; inspiratory force; interstitial fluid; intrinsic factor
IFA . . . . indirect fluorescent antibody
IFIX . . . . immunofixation
Ig . . . . immunoglobulin
IGT . . . . impaired glucose tolerance
IHA . . . . indirect hemagglutination
IIb-IIIa . . . . glycoproteins found on platelet membranes
IIF . . . . indirect immunofluorescence
I.M. . . . . intramuscular
IMD . . . . inherited metabolic disorders
IMP . . . . impression
IMV . . . . intermittent mandatory ventilation
In . . . . indium
INH . . . . isonicotinic acid hydrazide; isoniazid
IOFNA . . . . intraoperative fine needle aspiration
IOL . . . . intraocular lens
IOP . . . . intraocular pressure
IOT . . . . intraocular tension
IP . . . . intraperitoneal(ly)
I-PAO . . . . insulin induced peak acid output
IPF . . . . idiopathic pulmonary fibrosis
IPG . . . . impedence phlebograph
IPPB . . . . intermittent positive pressure breathing
Ir . . . . iridium

IR . . . . infrared
IRDS . . . . infant respiratory distress syndrome
IRG . . . . immunoreactive glucose
IRGH . . . . immunoreactive growth hormone
IRI . . . . immunoreactive insulin
IRMA . . . . immunoradiometric assay
IRT . . . . immunoreactive trypsinogen
ISD . . . . isosorbide dinitrate
ISE . . . . ion-selective electrode
IT . . . . inhalation therapy; intrathecal(ly)
ITP . . . . idiopathic thrombocytopenic purpura
ITT . . . . insulin tolerance test
IU . . . . International unit
IUD . . . . intrauterine device
IUGR . . . . intrauterine growth retardation
IUP . . . . intrauterine pregnancy
I.V. . . . . intravenous
IVAC . . . . I.V. infusion control device
IVC . . . . inferior vena cava; intravenous cholangiography
IVP . . . . intravenous push; intravenous pyelogram
IVPB . . . . intravenous piggyback
IVSD . . . . intraventricular septal defect

JVD . . . . jugular-venous distenion
JVP . . . . jugular venous pressure; jugular venous pulse

K . . . . potassium
K-B . . . . Kleihauer-Betke
kcal . . . . kilocalorie
KCl . . . . potassium chloride
KCN . . . . potassium cyanide
kg . . . . kilogram
KGS . . . . ketogenic steroids
kL . . . . kiloliter
km . . . . kilometer
KO . . . . keep open
KOH . . . . potassium hydroxide
Kr . . . . krypton
KS . . . . ketosteroids; Kaposi's sarcoma
KU . . . . Karmen units
KUB . . . . kidney and urinary bladder
KVO . . . . keep vein open
KW . . . . Keith-Wagener

L . . . . left; liter; lumbar
L_2 . . . . second lumbar vertebra
La . . . . lanthanum
LA . . . . left artrium; local anesthetic
LAD . . . . left anterior descending (artery)
LAI . . . . labioincisal
LAO . . . . left anterior oblique
Lap . . . . laparotomy
LAP . . . . leucine aminopeptidase; leukocyte alkaline phosphatase
LATS . . . . long acting thyroid stimulating hormone
LBBB . . . . left bundle branch block
LBM . . . . lean body mass
LBW . . . . low birth weight
LC . . . . lethal concentration

LCI .... lung clearance index
LCIS .... lobular carcinoma *in situ*
LCM .... lymphocytic choriomeningitis
LCS .... Leydig cell stimulation
LD .... lactate dehydrogenase; lethal dose; light difference
LD_1 .... lactate dehydrogenase fraction 1
LDH .... lactate dehydrogenase
LDHI .... LDH isoenzymes
LDL .... low density lipoprotein
LDLC .... low density lipoprotein cholesterol
LDV .... lactate dehydrogenase virus
LE .... lower extremity; lupus erythematosus
LEA .... lower extremity arterial
LES .... lower esophageal sphincter
LEV .... lower extremity venous
LFT .... liver function test
LGV .... lymphogranuloma venereum
LH .... luteinizing hormone
LHRF .... luteinizing hormone releasing factor
LHRH .... luteinizing hormone releasing hormone
LHV .... left ventricular hypertrophy
Li .... lithium
LISS .... low ionic strength saline
L-J .... Löwenstein-Jensen
LKM .... liver/kidney microsomes
LKS .... liver, kidneys, spleen
LLA .... lupus like anticoagulant
LLDH .... liver lactate dehydrogenase
LLL .... left lower lobe
LLQ .... left lower quadrant
LM .... light microscopy
LMN .... lower motor neuron
LMP .... last menstrual period
LMWH .... low molecular weight heparin
LOA .... left occipital anterior
LOM .... limitation of motion
LOS .... length of stay
LP .... light perception; lumbar puncture
LPC .... leukocyte-poor cells
lpf .... low power field
LPO .... left posterior oblique
LPRBC .... leukocyte-poor red blood cells
LRC .... Lipid Research Clinic
L/S .... lecithin/sphingomyelin ratio
LSD .... lysergic acid diethylamide
LSG .... labial salivary gland
LTC .... long term care
LTCPs .... L-tryptophan-containing products
LTT .... lymphocyte transformation test
Lu .... lutetium
LUL .... left upper lobe
LUQ .... left upper quadrant
LV .... lung volume
LVET .... left ventricular ejection time
LVH .... left ventricular hypertrophy
LVOT .... left ventricular outflow tract
LVW .... lateral vaginal wall
Lw .... lawrencium
L & W .... living and well
Lytes .... electrolytes

m . . . . meter
m^2 . . . . square meter
m^3 . . . . cubic meter
M . . . . mix (misce)
mA . . . . milliampere
MA-1 . . . . a type of respirator
MAA . . . . microaggregatedalbumin
MAI . . . . *Mycobacterium avium-intracellulare*
MAO . . . . monoamine oxidase
MAR . . . . mixed antiglobulin reaction
MB . . . . a fraction of creatine kinase
MBC . . . . minimum bactericidal concentration; maximum breathing capacity
MBD . . . . maximum bactericidal dilution
MBP . . . . myelin basic protein
mc . . . . millicurie
MC-Ab . . . . monoclonal antibody
mcg . . . . microgram
MCH . . . . mean corpuscular hemoglobin
MCHC . . . . mean cell hemoglobin concentration
mCi . . . . millicurie
MCL . . . . midclavicular line; midcostal line
MCT . . . . medium chain triglycerides
MCTD . . . . mixed connective tissue disease
MCV . . . . mean corpuscular volume
Md . . . . mendelevium
MD . . . . medical doctor
MDM . . . . minor determinant mixture
MDP . . . . mentodextra posterior
MDR . . . . minimum daily requirement
MDV . . . . multiple dose vial
MEA . . . . mercaptoethylamine; multiple endocrine adenomatosis
MED . . . . minimal erythemal dose
MEET . . . . multistage exercise electrocardiographics test
MEN . . . . multiple endocrine neoplasia
mEq . . . . milliequivalent
METS . . . . metastases
MF . . . . mycosis fungoides
MFC . . . . minimum fungicidal concentration
mg . . . . milligram
Mg . . . . magnesium
$MgCl_2$ . . . . magnesium chloride
$MgCO_3$ . . . . magnesium carbonate
MGP . . . . methyl green pyronine
$MgSO_4$ . . . . magnesium sulfate
MH . . . . malignant hyperthermia; marital history; menstrual history; mental health
MHA . . . . microhemagglutination
MHA-TP . . . . microhemagglutination *Treponema pallidum*
MHPG . . . . methoxyhydroxyphenylglycol
MHz . . . . megahertz
MI . . . . myocardial infarction; maturation index
MIC . . . . minimum inhibitory concentration
μ . . . . micron
μg . . . . microgram
μL . . . . microliter
μm . . . . micrometer
μm^3 . . . . cubic micrometer
μmol . . . . micromole
μmol/L . . . . micromolar
μOsm . . . . micro-osmolar
μU . . . . microunit
MID . . . . maximum bactericidal dilution

MIF . . . . merthiolate-iodine-formalin; migration inhibitory factor
MIT . . . . migration inhibition test
mIU . . . . milli International unit
mL . . . . milliliter
MLC . . . . mixed leukocyte culture; mixed lymphocyte culture
MLD . . . . metachromatic leukodystrophy; minimum lethal dose
MLR . . . . mixed lymphocyte reaction
MLV . . . . monitored live voice
mm . . . . millimeter
mm^2 . . . . square millimeter
mm^3 . . . . cubic millimeter
MMA . . . . methylmalonic acid
MMC . . . . minimal medullary concentration
MMEF . . . . mean midexpiratory flow
MMF . . . . maximal midexpiratory flow rate
mm Hg . . . . millimeters of mercury
mmol . . . . millimole
mmol/L . . . . millimolar
MMPI . . . . Minnesota multiple personality inventory
MMT . . . . manual muscle test
Mn . . . . manganese
MNS . . . . MNS blood group
Mo . . . . molybdenum
MO . . . . mesio-occlusal
mol . . . . mole
mol/L . . . . molar
mOsm . . . . milliosmole
mph . . . . miles per hour
MPHD . . . . methoxyhydroxphenolglycerol
MPS . . . . mucopolysaccharidosis
MPV . . . . mean plasma volume
MR . . . . moderately resistant
mrad . . . . millirad
MRI . . . . magnetic resonance imaging
MRSA . . . . methicillin-resistant *S. aureus*
MS . . . . mental status; mitral stenosis; multiple sclerosis
MSD . . . . metabolic screening disorders
msec . . . . millisecond
MSL . . . . midsternal line
MSLT . . . . multiple sleep latency test
MSUD . . . . maple syrup urine disease
mt . . . . send of such (mitte talis)
MT . . . . medical technologist
MTB . . . . mycobacterium tuberculosis
^{99m}Tc . . . . radioisotope of technetium Tc 99m
MTRX . . . . methotrexate
MTX . . . . methotrexate
mU . . . . milliunit
MUGA . . . . multiple gated scan
MUP . . . . monitor unit potential
MV . . . . minute volume
MVP . . . . mitral valve prolapse
MVV . . . . maximum voluntary ventilation
MW . . . . molecular weight
MZ . . . . monozygotic

N . . . . nitrogen; normal
Na . . . . sodium
NA . . . . not applicable
NACI . . . . National Advisory Committee on Immunization
NaCl . . . . sodium chloride

Na_2CO_3 . . . . sodium carbonate
NAD . . . . nicotinamide adenine dinucleotide; no acute distress; no apparent distress
NADH . . . . reduced form of NAD
NADP . . . . nicotinamide adenine dinucleotide phosphate
NADPH . . . . reduced form of NADP
NaF . . . . sodium fluoride
NaOH . . . . sodium hydroxide
NAPA . . . . n-acetylprocainamide
NAS . . . . no added salt
NATP . . . . neonatal autoimmune thrombocytopenic purpura
Nb . . . . niobium
NBIL . . . . neonatal bilirubin
NBT . . . . nitro blue tetrazolium
NC . . . . nerve conduction
NCA . . . . nonspecific cross reacting antigen
NCEP . . . . National Cholesterol Education Program
NCI . . . . National Cancer Institute
NCS . . . . nerve conduction study
NCV . . . . nerve conduction velocity
Nd . . . . neodymium
Ne . . . . neon
ng . . . . nanogram
NGU . . . . nongonococcal urethritis
NH_4Cl . . . . ammonium chloride
NH_4OH . . . . ammonium hydroxide
Ni . . . . nickel
NICU . . . . neonatal intensive care unit
NIH . . . . National Institute of Health
NK . . . . natural killer
NKA . . . . no known allergies
nL . . . . nanoliter
NL . . . . normal
nm . . . . nanometer
NMJ . . . . neuromuscular junction disease
nmol . . . . nanomole
nmol/L . . . . millimicromolar
NMR . . . . nuclear magnetic resonance
No . . . . nobelium
noc . . . . in the night (nocturnal)
non rep . . . . do not repeat; no refills
Np . . . . neptunium
NP . . . . nasopharynx
NPO . . . . nothing by mouth
NPT . . . . nocturnal penile tumescence
NPTM . . . . nocturnal penile tumescence monitoring
nr . . . . do not repeat (non repetatur)
NRBCs . . . . nucleated red blood cells
NRC . . . . National Research Council; Nuclear Regulatory Commission
NS . . . . normal saline; not seen; not significant
NSA . . . . no salt albumin
NSE . . . . neuron specific enolase
NSR . . . . normal sinus rhythm
NST . . . . nonstress test
NSU . . . . nonspecific urethritis
NSVD . . . . normal spontaneous vaginal delivery
NT . . . . nasotracheal
N & T . . . . nose and throat
NTI . . . . nonthyroidal illness; nonthyroidal index
N & V . . . . nausea and vomiting
NVD . . . . nausea, vomiting, diarrhea

NYD . . . . not yet diagnosed

O . . . . oxygen
OB . . . . obstetrics; occult blood
OBS . . . . organic brain syndrome
OC . . . . on call; oral contraceptive
OCG . . . . oral cholecystogram
OCT . . . . ornithine carbamyl transferase
od . . . . right eye (oculus dexter)
OD . . . . overdose
ODC . . . . oxygen dissociation curve
ODE . . . . O-desmethylencainide
ODm . . . . ophthalmodynamometry
O/E . . . . on examination
OGTT . . . . oral glucose tolerance test
OH . . . . hydroxide; hydroxyl
OHCS . . . . hydroxycorticosteroid
OIF . . . . oil immersion field
OKT . . . . a group of monoclonal antibodies for typing lymphocytes
OM . . . . otitis media
OOB . . . . out of bed
OPG . . . . ocular plethysmography
OPV . . . . out patient visit; oral polio vaccine
O.R. . . . . operating room
os . . . . left eye (oculus sinister)
Os . . . . osmium
OT . . . . old tuberculin
OTC . . . . ornithine transcarbamylase
ou . . . . each eye (oculus uterque)
ov . . . . ovarian

P . . . . phosphorus; pulse
^{32}P . . . . radioisotope of phosphorus
p^{50} . . . . half saturation (oxygen)
Pa . . . . protactinium
PA . . . . phenylalinine; platelet associated; pernicious anemia; physician's assistant
P & A . . . . percussion and auscultation
PABA . . . . para-aminobenzoic acid
PAC . . . . premature atrial contraction
PAH . . . . phenylalanine hydroxylase
PAI . . . . plasminogen activator inhibitor
PAO . . . . peak acid output
Pap . . . . Papanicolaou's stain
PAP . . . . peroxidase antiperoxidase; pri. atypical pneum.; prostate acid phosphatase
PAR . . . . pulmonary arteriolar resistance
PAS . . . . para-aminosalicylic acid; periodic acid Schiff stain
PAT . . . . paroxysmal atrial tachycardia; preadmission testing
Pb . . . . lead
PBC . . . . primary biliary cirrhosis
PBG . . . . porphobilinogen
PBI . . . . protein-bound iodine
PBL . . . . peripheral blood lymphocytes
PBS . . . . peripheral blood smear
pc . . . . after meals (post cibum)
PC . . . . porto-caval; present complaint
pc1 . . . . platelet count pretransfusion
pc2 . . . . platelet count post-transfusion
PCA . . . . parietal cell antibody; percutaneous coronary angioplasty

PCE . . . . pseudocholinesterase
PCG . . . . pneumocardiogram
PCH . . . . paroxysmal cold hemoglobinuria
PCHE . . . . pseudocholinesterase
PCI . . . . prothrombin consumption index
PCP . . . . phencyclidine
PCR . . . . polymerase chain reaction
PCT . . . . prothrombin consumption test
PCV . . . . packed cell volume
Pd . . . . palladium
PD. . . . . postural drainage
PDR . . . . *Physician's Desk Reference*
PDW . . . . platelet distribution width
PE . . . . physical examination; pleural effusion; pulmonary embolism
PEEP . . . . positive end-expiratory pressure
PEF . . . . peak expiratory flow
PEFR . . . . peak expiratory flow rate
PEFT. . . . . peak expiratory flow time
PEG . . . . polyethylene glycol
PEP. . . . . phosphoenolpyruvate
PERLA . . . . pupils equal, reactive to light and accommodation
PET . . . . positron emission tomography; pre-eclamptic toxemia
PF . . . . platelet factor; preservative free
PFK. . . . . phosphofructoaldolase
PFS. . . . . penile flow study; prefilled syringe
PFT . . . . pulmonary function test
pg . . . . picogram
PG . . . . phosphatidyl glycine
PGD . . . . phosphogluconate dehydrogenase
PGI . . . . phosphoglucose isomerase
PGK . . . . phosphoglycerokinase
PgR. . . . . progesterone receptor
pH . . . . measurement of acidity or alkalinity
pHa. . . . . arterial blood pH
PHA . . . . phytohemagglutinin activation
PhD. . . . . Doctor of Philosophy
PHI . . . . phosphohexoseisomerase
PHP . . . . persistent hyperphenylalaninemia
PHT . . . . peroxide hemolysis test
pi. . . . . platelet count increment
PI . . . . phosphatidylinositol; protamine insulin; pulmonary infarction
PID . . . . pelvic inflammatory disease
PK. . . . . pyruvate kinase
PKU . . . . phenylketonuria
Pm . . . . promethium
PM . . . . afternoon
PMD . . . . primary myocardial disease; progressive muscular dystrophy
PMH . . . . past medical history
PM-I . . . . platelet membrane antigen
PMN . . . . polymorphonuclear neutrophil
pmol . . . . picomole
PMP . . . . previous menstrual period
PM & R . . . . physical medicine and rehabilition
PMS . . . . premenstrual syndrome
PNH . . . . paroxysmal nocturnal hemoglobinuria
PNP . . . . nonprotein nitrogen
pNPP . . . . paranitrophenylphosphate
Pnx . . . . pneumothorax
po . . . . by mouth (per os)
Po . . . . polonium
POMR . . . . problem oriented medical record
POR . . . . problem oriented record

PP .... postprandial
PPBS .... postprandial blood sugar
PPD .... purified protein derivative
PPF .... plasma protein fraction
PPG .... photoplethysmography
PPLO .... pleuropneumonia-like organisms
ppm .... parts per million
ppt .... precipitate
Pr .... praseodymium; presbyopia
PR .... per rectum
PRA .... plasma renin activity; progesterone receptor assay
PRBCs .... packed red blood cells
PRG .... phleborheography
PRL .... prolactin
prn .... as needed (pro re nata)
PROM .... premature rupture of membranes; prolonged rupture of membranes
PRP .... polyribophosphate
PRSM .... peripheral smear
PSA .... prostate specific antigen
PSG .... polysomnography
PSIS .... posterior/superior iliac spine
PSP .... phenolsulfonphthalein
PSRO .... Professional Standards Review Organization
PSS .... progressive systemic sclerosis
PS-VER .... pattern shift – visual evoked response
Pt .... platinum
PT .... physical therapy; prothrombin time
P & T .... Pharmacy & Therapeutics
PTA .... platelet thromboplastin antecedent; prothrombin activity
PTAH .... phosphotungstic acid hematoxylin
PTC .... phenylthiocarbamide; plasma thromboplastin component
PTH .... parathyroid hormone
PTP .... prothrombin-proconvertin
PTT .... partial thromboplastin time
Pu .... plutonium
PU .... peptic ulcer
PUD .... peptic ulcer disease
pulv .... a powder (pulvis)
PV .... plasma volume
PVA .... polyvinyl alcohol
PVC .... premature ventricular contraction
PVD .... peripheral vascular disease
PVR .... pulse volume recording
PVT .... paroxysmal ventricular tachycardia
PWM .... pokeweed mitogen
PYP .... pyrophosphate

q .... every (quaque)
QBCA .... quantitative buffy coat analysis
qd .... every day (quaque die)
qh .... every hour (quaque hora)
qhr .... every hour (quaque hora)
qid .... four times a day (quarter in die)
QNS .... quantity not sufficient
qod .... every other day
qs .... sufficient quantity (quantum sufficiat)
qs ad .... sufficient quantity to make (quantum sufficiat ad)
QTC .... quantitative tip culture
qv .... as much as you will (quam volveris)

R . . . . respiration; right
Ra . . . . radium
RA. . . . . rheumatoid arthritis; right atrium
RAD . . . . radiation absorbed dose
RAF . . . . rheumatoid arthritis factor
RAI . . . . radioactive iodine
RAO . . . . right anterior oblique
RAP . . . . rheumatoid arthritis precipitins
RAW . . . . airway resistance
Rb . . . . rubidium
RBC . . . . red blood cell
RC . . . . red cell; retrograde cystogram
RCM . . . . radiographic contrast media; right costal margin
RCMI. . . . . red cell morphology index
rd . . . . rutherford
RDS . . . . respiratory distress syndrome
RDW . . . . red cell distribution width
Re . . . . rhenium
REM . . . . rapid eye movement
repet . . . . to be repeated (repetatur)
Rf . . . . rutherfordium
RF . . . . renal failure; rheumatoid factor
Rh . . . . rhodium; rhesus
RhIG . . . . Rh_o(D) immune globulin
RI . . . . reticulocyte index
RIA . . . . radioimmunoassay
RID . . . . radial immunodiffusion
RIPA . . . . radioimmunoprecipitation
RISA . . . . radioiodinated serum albumin
RK. . . . . radial keratotomy
RLL . . . . right lower lobe
RLQ . . . . right lower quadrant
RMSF . . . . Rocky Mountain spotted fever
Rn . . . . radon
RN . . . . registered nurse
RNA . . . . ribonucleic acid
RNP . . . . ribonucleoprotein
RO . . . . routine order
R/O . . . . rule out
RODAC . . . . replicate organism detection and counting
ROM . . . . range of motion
ROS . . . . review of symptoms; review of systems
RPBI . . . . resting penile-brachial index
RPF. . . . . renal plasma flow
RPGN . . . . rapidly progressive glomerulonephritis
RPI . . . . reticulocyte production index
rpm . . . . revolutions per minute
RPO . . . . right posterior oblique
RPR . . . . rapid plasma reagin
RPT. . . . . right occipital transverse
RQ . . . . respiratory quotient
RR. . . . . recovery room; respiratory rate
RRA . . . . right renal artery
RSV . . . . respiratory syncytial virus
RTA . . . . renal tubular acidosis
Ru . . . . ruthenium
RUG . . . . right upper quadrant
RUL . . . . right upper lobe
RUQ . . . . right upper quadrant
RV. . . . . reserve volume
RVH . . . . right ventricular hypertrophy
RVVT . . . . Russell viper venom test

Rx . . . . a recipe

s . . . . without (sine)
S . . . . sulfur
S_1 . . . . first heart sound
S_2 . . . . second heart sound
SA . . . . surface area; sinoatrial
SACE . . . . serum angiotensin converting enzyme
SAH . . . . subarachnoid hemorrhage
SAL . . . . suction assisted lipectomy
Sb . . . . antimony
SBB . . . . small bowel biopsy
SBE . . . . subacute bacterial endocarditis
SBL . . . . serum bactericidal level
SBP . . . . systemic blood pressure; systolic blood pressure
Sc . . . . scandium
SC . . . . sickle cell; subclavian; subcutaneous
SCAT . . . . sheep cell agglutination test
SCE . . . . sister chromatid exchange
SCID . . . . severe combined immunodeficiency
Scl . . . . scleroderma; scleroderma antibody
SD . . . . senile dementia; spontaneous delivery; standard deviation
S-D . . . . strength duration
SDFP . . . . single donor frozen plasma
SDS . . . . same day surgery
Se . . . . selenium
SEM . . . . scanning electron microscopy; standard error of the mean
SEP . . . . serum electrophoresis; somatosensory evoked potential
SER . . . . somatosensory evoked response
SF-EMG . . . . single fiber electromyography
SG . . . . specific gravity
SGPT . . . . serum glutamic pyruvic transaminase
SH . . . . serum hepatitis
SHBG . . . . sex hormone binding globulin
Si . . . . silicon
SI . . . . Système International (SI) units
SIADH . . . . syndrome of inappropriate antidiuretic hormone
SIDS . . . . sudden infant death syndrome
Sig . . . . mark, write (signa)
SISI . . . . short increment sensitivity index
SK . . . . streptokinase
SKAB . . . . skeletal antibody
SKSD . . . . streptokinase-streptodornase
SL . . . . sublingual(ly)
SLCG . . . . sulfolithoecholylglycine
SLE . . . . systemic lupus erthyematosus
Sm . . . . samarium; Smith antigen
SMA . . . . sequential/serial multiple analysis; smooth muscle antibody
Sn . . . . tin
SNF . . . . skilled nursing facility
SOAP . . . . subjective, objective, assessment and plans
SOB . . . . short of breath
SOD . . . . superoxide dismutase
sos . . . . if there is need (si opus sit)
SPC . . . . standard plate count
SPCA . . . . serum prothrombin conversion accelerator
SPECT . . . . single-photon emission tomography
SPEP . . . . serum protein electrophoresis
SPI . . . . selective protein index
SPL . . . . sound pressure level
SPS . . . . sodium polyanetholsulfonate; sulfite polymyxin sulfadiazine

SQ . . . . subcutaneous(ly)
Sr . . . . strontium
SR . . . . sedimentation rate; sustained release; systems review
SRAW . . . . specific airway resistance
SRIF . . . . somatotropin releasing inhibiting factor
SRT . . . . speech reception threshold
ss . . . . one-half (semis)
SS . . . . *Salmonella-Shigella*; saturated solution; subaortic stenosis
SS-A . . . . Sjögren's syndrome A antibody
SS-B . . . . Sjögren's syndrome B antibody
SS-DNA . . . . single stranded DNA
SSEP . . . . somatosensory evoked potential
SSKI . . . . saturated solution of potassium iodide
SSPE . . . . subacute sclerosing panencephalitis
stat . . . . st once (statim)
STD . . . . skin test dose; sexually transmitted disease
STH . . . . somatotropic hormone
STI . . . . systolic time intervals
STIC . . . . serum trypsin inhibitory capacity
STP . . . . standard temperature and pressure
STS . . . . serologic test for syphillis
supp . . . . suppository (suppositorium)
SVC . . . . slow vital capacity
SVR . . . . systemic vascular resistance
SW . . . . short wave
Sx . . . . signs; symptom(s)
syr . . . . syrup (syrupus)

T . . . . temperature
Ta . . . . tantalum
TA . . . . thyroglobulin autoprecipitins
T & A . . . . tonsillectomy and adenoidectomy
TAb . . . . therapeutic abortion
tab . . . . tablet (tabella)
TAD . . . . tricyclic antidepressant drug
TAH . . . . total abdominal hysterectomy
tal . . . . such
tal dos . . . . such doses
TAT . . . . thematic apperception test; toxin-antitoxin
Tb . . . . terbium
TB . . . . tuberculosis
TBA . . . . to be administered; to be admitted
TBG . . . . thyroxine binding globulin
TBGI . . . . thyroid binding globulin index
TBI . . . . thyroid binding index; thyroxine binding index
TBM . . . . tuberculous meningitis
TBPA . . . . thyroxine binding prealbumin
TBW . . . . total body water
Tc . . . . technetium
TC . . . . throat culture; total cholesterol
T & C . . . . type and crossmatch
TCA . . . . trichloracetic acid
TCBS . . . . thiosulfate citrate bile salts sucrose
TCM . . . . tissue culture medium
TCT . . . . thrombin clotting time
TDM . . . . therapeutic drug monitoring
TdT . . . . terminal deoxynucleotidyl transferase
Te . . . . tellurium
TEAC . . . . tetraethylammonium chloride
TeBG . . . . testosterone-estradiol-binding globulin
TEE . . . . transesophageal echocardiography

TENS .... transcutaneous electrical nerve stimulation
TET .... treadmill exercise test
TG .... triglyceride
TGT .... thromboplastin generation test
TGV .... thoracic gas volume
th .... thoracic
Th .... thorium
THA .... transient hemispheric attack
THb .... total hemoglobin
THC .... tetrahydrocannabinol
Ti .... titanium
TI .... total iron
TIA .... transient ischemic attack
TIBC .... total iron binding capacity
tid .... three times a day (ter in die)
TIUV .... total intrauterine volume
TK .... transketolase
TKO .... to keep open
Tl .... thallium
TL .... tubal ligation
TLA .... translumbar aortogram
TLC .... thin layer chromatography; total lung capacity
Tm .... thulium
TMB .... transient monocular blindness
TMJ .... temporomandibular joint
TMP .... trimethoprim
TMP-SMX ...... trimethoprim-sulfomethoxazole
TNS .... transcutaneous nerve stimulation
TOS .... thoracic outlet syndrome
TP .... total protein
TPA .... *Treponema pallidum* agglutination
TPC .... telescoping plugged catheter
TPI .... *Treponema* immobilization test; triose phosphate isomerase
TPN .... total parenteral nutrition
TPP .... thiamine pyrophosphate
TPR .... temperature, pulse, respiration
TRAP .... tartrate resistance leukocyte acid phosphatase
TRH .... thyroid releasing hormone
TRIC .... trachoma inclusion conjunctivitis
trig .... triglycerides
TRIS .... tris(hydroxymethyl)aminomethane
trit .... triturate (tritura)
TRP .... tubular reabsorption of phosphorus
TS .... total solids
TSB .... trypticase soy broth
TSH .... thyroid stimulating hormone
TSI .... thyroid stimulating immunoglobulin
tsp .... teaspoon
TT .... thrombin time
TTP .... thrombotic thrombocytopenic purpura
TU .... thiouracil; Todd unit; toxic unit; tuberculin unit
TUR .... transurethral resection
TURP .... transurethral resection of prostate
TV .... total volume
TVC .... triple voiding cystogram
Tx .... therapy; treatment

U .... uranium
UA .... uric acid; urinalysis
UAO .... upper airway obstructions
UB12BC .... unsaturated B_{12} binding capacity

UBBC . . . . unsaturated vitamin B_{12} binding capacity
UBC . . . . unsaturated binding capacity
UCG . . . . urinary chorionic gonadotropin
ud . . . . as directed (ut dictum)
UDP . . . . uridine diphosphate
UDPG . . . . uridinediphosphoglucose
UEA . . . . upper extremity arterial
UES . . . . upper esophageal sphincter
UFC . . . . urinary free cortisol
UGI . . . . upper GI
UIBC . . . . unbound iron binding capacity
U-I-S . . . . uroporphyrinogen-I-synthetase
UK . . . . urokinase
UMN . . . . upper motor neuron
ung . . . . ointment (unguentum)
URI . . . . upper respiratory infection
US . . . . ultrasound
U.S. . . . . United States
USAN . . . . United States Adopted Names
USP . . . . United States Pharmacopeia
ut dict . . . . as directed (ut dictum)
UTI . . . . urinary tract infection
UUN . . . . urine urea nitrogen
UV . . . . ultraviolet

V . . . . vanadium
VA . . . . visual activity
VBG . . . . venous blood gases
VC . . . . vena cava; vital capacity
VCA . . . . viral capsid antigen
VCA-EB . . . . viral capsid antigen, Epstein-Barr
VCG . . . . vectorcardiogram
VCT . . . . venous clotting time
VCU . . . . voiding cystourethrogram
VCUG . . . . voiding cystourethrogram
VD . . . . venereal disease
VDRL . . . . Venereal Disease Research Laboratory; test for syphilis
VE . . . . visual efficiency
VEP . . . . visual evoked potential
VER . . . . visual evoked response
VF . . . . ventricular fibrillation; vision field
VIP . . . . vasoactive intestinal polypeptide
VLDL . . . . very low density lipoprotein
VLM . . . . visceral larva migrans
VMA . . . . vanillylmandelic acid
vo . . . . verbal order
VP . . . . venous pressure
VS . . . . vital signs
VSD . . . . ventricular septal defect
VSS . . . . vital signs stable
VSV . . . . vesicular stimatitis virus
VT . . . . ventricular tachycardia
VTM . . . . virus transport media
VU . . . . voltage unit
vW . . . . von Willebrand
vWD . . . . von Willebrand's disease
vWF . . . . von Willebrand factor
V-Z . . . . varicella-zoster
VZIG . . . . varicella-zoster immune globulin

VZV . . . . varicella-zoster virus

W . . . . tungsten
wa . . . . while awake
WB . . . . weight bearing; whole blood
WBC . . . . white blood cell
WD . . . . well developed
WDHA . . . . watery diarrhea-hypokalemia-achlorhydria
WDHH . . . . watery diarrhea-hypokalemia-hypochlorhydria
WF . . . . white female
W-F . . . . Weil-Felix
WM . . . . white male
WN . . . . well nourished
WNL . . . . within normal limits
WP . . . . whirlpool
WPW . . . . Wolff-Parkinson-White syndrome
WSR . . . . Westergren sedimentation rate

Xe . . . . xenon
XO . . . . gonadal dysgenesis of Turner type

y . . . . year
Y . . . . yttrium
YAG . . . . yttrium-argon-garnet - a type of laser
Yb . . . . ytterbium

Z-E . . . . Zollinger-Ellison
ZIG . . . . zoster immune globulin
ZIP . . . . zoster immune plasma
Zn . . . . zinc
ZPP . . . . zinc protophorhyrin
Zr . . . . zirconium
ZSR . . . . zeta sedimentation rate

KEY WORD INDEX

The Key Word Index provides a reference to the test name based on a diagnostic property, disease entity, organ system, or syndrome in which the test might be useful. This reference focuses the physician's attention on specific tests available to support his clinical diagnosis or rule out other diagnostic possibilities.

Each laboratory test relevant to the indexed diagnosis is listed and weighted. Two symbols (••) indicate that the test is diagnostic, that is, it documents the diagnosis if the expected result is found. A single symbol (•) indicates a test frequently used in the diagnosis or management of the particular disease. The other listed tests are useful on a selective basis with consideration of clinical factors and specific aspects of the case.

Diagnoses with *International Classification of Disease—Ninth Revision—Clinical Modification* (ICD-9-CM) codes are indicated within the [ ] symbol.

(Continued)

(Continued)

(Continued)

(Continued)

(Continued)

(Continued)

(Continued)

(Continued)

(Continued)

(Continued)

(Continued)

CURRENT PROCEDURAL TERMINOLOGY (CPT-4) INDEX

Current Procedural Terminology (CPT-4) codes are provided with each test for reference, as a basis for documentation of diagnostic procedures performed and to facilitate financial and patient record keeping. The codes are current. Applications of codes may vary by region of the country and in some instances the application of a specific code to a given procedure is a matter of individual interpretation.[1]

[1] Coy JA, Ely EA, Kirschner CG, et al, eds, *Physicians' Current Procedural Terminology (CPT 1990)*, 4th ed, Chicago, IL: American Medical Association, 1989.

ALPHABETICAL INDEX

The Alphabetical Index provides all test names and synonyms listed in this book by page number for quick and easy reference.

NOTES

NOTES